1997
YEAR BOOK OF
PEDIATRICS®

Statement of Purpose

The YEAR BOOK Service

The YEAR BOOK series was devised in 1901 by practicing health professionals who observed that the literature of medicine and related disciplines had become so voluminous that no one individual could read and place in perspective every potential advance in a major specialty. In the final decade of the 20th century, this recognition is more acutely true than it was in 1901.

More than merely a series of books, YEAR BOOK volumes are the tangible results of a unique service designed to accomplish the following:

- to *survey* a wide range of journals of proven value
- to *select* from those journals papers representing significant advances and statements of important clinical principles
- to provide *abstracts* of those articles that are readable, convenient summaries of their key points
- to provide *commentary* about those articles to place them in perspective

These publications grow out of a unique process that calls on the talents of outstanding authorities in clinical and fundamental disciplines, trained literature specialists, and professional writers, all supported by the resources of Mosby, the world's preeminent publisher for the health professions.

The Literature Base

Mosby and its Editors survey more than 1,000 journals published worldwide, covering the full range of the health professions. On an annual basis, the publisher examines usage patterns and polls its expert authorities to add new journals to the literature base and to delete journals that are no longer useful as potential YEAR BOOK sources.

The Literature Survey

The publisher's team of literature specialists, all of whom are trained and experienced health professionals, examines every original, peer-reviewed article in each journal issue. More than 250,000 articles per year are scanned systematically, including title, text, illustrations, tables, and references. Each scan is compared, article by article, to the search strategies that the publisher has developed in consultation with the 270 outside experts who form the pool of YEAR BOOK editors. A given article may be reviewed by any number of editors, from one to a dozen or more, regardless of the discipline for which the paper was originally published. In turn, each editor who receives the article reviews it to determine whether or not the article should be included in the YEAR BOOK. This decision is based on the article's inherent quality, its probable usefulness to readers of that YEAR BOOK, and the editor's goal to represent a balanced picture of a given field in each volume of the YEAR BOOK. In addition, the editor indicates when to include figures and tables from the article to help the YEAR BOOK reader better understand the information.

Of the quarter million articles scanned each year, only 5% are selected for detailed analysis within the YEAR BOOK series, thereby assuring readers of the high value of every selection.

The Abstract

The publisher's abstracting staff is headed by a seasoned medical professional and includes individuals with training in the life sciences, medicine, and other areas, plus extensive experience in writing for the health professions and related industries. Each selected article is assigned to a specific writer on this abstracting staff. The abstracter, guided in many cases by notations supplied by the expert editor, writes a structured, condensed summary designed so that the reader can rapidly acquire the essential information contained in the article.

The Commentary

The YEAR BOOK editorial boards, sometimes assisted by guest commentators, write comments that place each article in perspective for the reader. This provides the reader with the equivalent of a personal consultation with a leading international authority—an opportunity to better understand the value of the article and to benefit from the authority's thought processes in assessing the article.

Additional Editorial Features

The editorial boards of each YEAR BOOK organize the abstracts and comments to provide a logical and satisfying sequence of information. To enhance the organization, editors also provide introductions to sections or individual chapters, comments linking a number of abstracts, citations to additional literature, and other features.

The published YEAR BOOK contains enhanced bibliographic citations for each selected article, including extended listings of multiple authors and identification of author affiliations. Each YEAR BOOK contains a Table of Contents specific to that year's volume. From year to year, the Table of Contents for a given YEAR BOOK will vary depending on developments within the field.

Every YEAR BOOK contains a list of the journals from which papers have been selected. This list represents a subset of the more than 1,000 journals surveyed by the publisher and occasionally reflects a particularly pertinent article from a journal that is not surveyed on a routine basis.

Finally, each volume contains a comprehensive subject index and an index to authors of each selected paper.

The 1997 Year Book Series

Year Book of Allergy, Asthma, and Clinical Immunology: Drs. Rosenwasser, Borish, Gelfand, Leung, Nelson, and Szefler

Year Book of Anesthesiology and Pain Management®: Drs. Tinker, Abram, Chestnut, Roizen, Rothenberg, and Wood

Year Book of Cardiology®: Drs. Schlant, Collins, Gersh, Graham, Kaplan, and Waldo

Year Book of Chiropractic®: Dr. Lawrence

Year Book of Critical Care Medicine®: Drs. Parrillo, Balk, Calvin, Franklin, and Shapiro

Year Book of Dentistry®: Drs. Meskin, Berry, Kennedy, Leinfelder, Roser, Summitt, and Zakariasen

Year Book of Dermatologic Surgery®: Drs. Greenway, Papadopoulos, and Whitaker

Year Book of Dermatology®: Drs. Sober and Fitzpatrick

Year Book of Diagnostic Radiology®: Drs. Federle, Clark, Gross, Dalinka, Maynard, Rebner, Smirniotopolous, and Young

Year Book of Digestive Diseases®: Drs. Greenberger and Moody

Year Book of Drug Therapy®: Drs. Lasagna and Weintraub

Year Book of Emergency Medicine®: Drs. Wagner, Dronen, Davidson, King, Niemann, and Roberts

Year Book of Endocrinology®: Drs. Bagdade, Braverman, Haas, Horton, Kannan, Landsberg, Molitch, Morley, Nathan, Odell, Poehlman, Rogol, and Ryan

Year Book of Family Practice®: Drs. Berg, Bowman, Davidson, Dexter, and Scherger

Year Book of Geriatrics and Gerontology®: Drs. Beck, Burton, Ostwald, Rabins, Reuben, Roth, Shapiro, and Whitehouse

Year Book of Hand Surgery®: Drs. Amadio and Hentz

Year Book of Hematology®: Drs. Spivak, Bell, Ness, Quesenberry, Wiernik, and Blume

Year Book of Infectious Diseases®: Drs. Keusch, Barza, Bennish, Poutsiaka, Skolnik, and Snydman

Year Book of Medicine®: Drs. Klahr, Cline, Petty, Frishman, Greenberger, Malawista, Mandell, and O'Rourke

Year Book of Neonatal and Perinatal Medicine®: Drs. Fanaroff and Klaus

Year Book of Nephrology, Hypertension, and Mineral Metabolism:

Year Book of Neurology and Neurosurgery®: Drs. Bradley and Wilkins

Year Book of Nuclear Medicine®: Drs. Gottschalk, Blaufox, Neumann, Strauss, and Zubal

Year Book of Obstetrics, Gynecology, and Women's Health: Drs. Mishell, Herbst, and Kirschbaum

Year Book of Occupational and Environmental Medicine®: Drs. Emmett, Frank, Gochfeld, and Hessl

Year Book of Oncology®: Drs. Ozols, Cohen, Glatstein, Loehrer, Tallman, and Wiersma

Year Book of Ophthalmology®: Drs. Wilson, Augsburger, Cohen, Eagle, Flanagan, Grossman, Laibson, Maguire, Nelson, Rapuano, Sergott, Spaeth, Tipperman, and Ms. Salmon

Year Book of Orthopedics®: Drs. Sledge, Poss, Cofield, Dobyns, Griffin, Springfield, Swiontkowski, Wiesel, and Wilson

Year Book of Otolaryngology–Head and Neck Surgery®: Drs. Paparella and Holt

Year Book of Pain®: Drs. Gebhart, Haddox, Jacox, Janjan, Marcus, Rudy, and Shapiro

Year Book of Pathology and Laboratory Medicine: Drs. Mills, Bruns, Gaffey, and Stoler

Year Book of Pediatrics®: Dr. Stockman

Year Book of Plastic, Reconstructive, and Aesthetic Surgery®: Drs. Miller, Cohen, McKinney, Robson, Ruberg, Smith, and Whitaker

Year Book of Podiatric Medicine and Surgery®: Dr. Kominsky

Year Book of Psychiatry and Applied Mental Health®: Drs. Talbott, Ballenger, Breier, Frances, Meltzer, Schowalter, and Tasman

Year Book of Pulmonary Disease®: Dr. Petty

Year Book of Rheumatology®: Drs. Sergent, LeRoy, Meenan, Panush, and Reichlin

Year Book of Sports Medicine®: Drs. Shephard, Drinkwater, Eichner, Torg, Anderson, and Mr. George

Year Book of Surgery®: Drs. Copeland, Bland, Deitch, Eberlein, Howard, Luce, Seeger, Souba, and Sugarbaker

Year Book of Thoracic and Cardiovascular Surgery®: Drs. Ginsberg, Wechsler, and Williams

Year Book of Urology®: Drs. Andriole and Coplin

Year Book of Vascular Surgery®: Dr. Porter

1997

The Year Book of PEDIATRICS®

Editor

James A. Stockman, III, M.D.

President, The American Board of Pediatrics; Clinical Professor of Pediatrics, University of North Carolina at Chapel Hill; Consultant Professor, Duke University Medical Center, Durham, North Carolina

Contributing Editors

Daniel P. Krowchuk, M.D.

Associate Professor of Pediatrics and Dermatology; Director of Adolescent Medicine, Bowman Gray School of Medicine of Wake Forest University, Winston-Salem, North Carolina

Walter W. Tunnessen, Jr., M.D.

Senior Vice-President, The American Board of Pediatrics, Chapel Hill, North Carolina

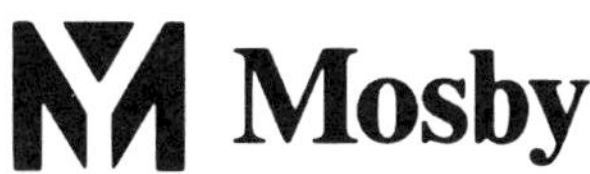 Mosby

St. Louis   Baltimore   Boston   Carlsbad   Chicago   Naples   New York   Philadelphia   Portland
London   Madrid   Mexico City   Singapore   Sydney   Tokyo   Toronto   Wiesbaden

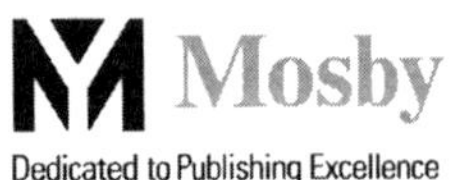 Mosby

Dedicated to Publishing Excellence

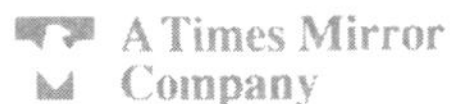 A Times Mirror
Company

Vice President and Publisher, Continuity Publishing: Kenneth H. Killion
Director, Editorial Development: Gretchen C. Murphy
Developmental Editor, Continuity: Kelly J. Poirier
Acquisitions Editor: Linda M. Sheehan
Illustrations and Permissions Coordinator: Lois M. Ruebensam
Director, Continuity–EDP: Maria Nevinger
Project Supervisor, Editing: Rebecca Nordbrock
Assistant Project Supervisor: Sandra Rogers
Freelance Staff Supervisor: Barbara M. Kelly
Director, Editorial Services: Edith M. Podrazik, B.S.N., R.N.
Information Specialist: Kathleen Moss, R.N.
Circulation Manager: Lynn D. Stevenson

1997 EDITION
Copyright © January 1997 by Mosby–Year Book, Inc.

Printed in the United States of America
Composition by Reed Technology and Information Services, Inc.
Printing/binding by Maple-Vail

Mosby–Year Book, Inc.
11830 Westline Industrial Drive
St. Louis, MO 63146

Editorial Office:
Mosby–Year Book, Inc.
161 North Clark Street
Chicago, IL 60601

International Standard Serial Number: 0084–3954
International Standard Book Number: 0–8151–9724–1

Table of Contents

Journals Represented

Mosby and its Editors survey more than 1,000 journals for its abstract and commentary publications. From these journals, the Editors select the articles to be abstracted. Journals represented in this YEAR BOOK are listed below.

Acta Paediatrica
American Journal of Emergency Medicine
American Journal of Human Genetics
American Journal of Hypertension
American Journal of Perinatology
American Journal of Preventive Medicine
American Journal of Psychiatry
American Journal on Mental Retardation
American Surgeon
Annals of Emergency Medicine
Annals of Internal Medicine
Annals of Surgery
Archives of Disease in Childhood
Archives of Otolaryngology–Head and Neck Surgery
Archives of Pediatrics and Adolescent Medicine
Australian and New Zealand Journal of Psychiatry
Biological Psychiatry
Blood
British Journal of Obstetrics and Gynaecology
British Journal of Urology
British Medical Journal
Canadian Journal of Psychiatry
Cancer
Child Development
Cleft Palate-Craniofacial Journal
Clinical Endocrinology (Oxford)
Clinical Infectious Diseases
Clinical Orthopaedics and Related Research
Clinical Pediatrics
Contraception
European Journal of Cancer
European Journal of Oral Sciences
International Journal of Cancer
International Journal of Eating Disorders
International Journal of Pediatric Otorhinolaryngology
Journal of Acquired Immune Deficiency Syndromes and Human Retrovirology
Journal of Adolescent Health
Journal of Bone and Joint Surgery (American Volume)
Journal of Burn Care and Rehabilitation
Journal of Clinical Anesthesia
Journal of Clinical Microbiology
Journal of Clinical Oncology
Journal of Dentistry for Children
Journal of Family Practice
Journal of General Internal Medicine
Journal of Heart and Lung Transplantation
Journal of Pediatric Gastroenterology and Nutrition

Journal of Pediatric Ophthalmology and Strabismus
Journal of Pediatric Orthopedics
Journal of Pediatric Surgery
Journal of Pediatrics
Journal of Perinatology
Journal of Thoracic and Cardiovascular Surgery
Journal of Urology
Journal of the American Academy of Child and Adolescent Psychiatry
Journal of the American Board of Family Practice
Journal of the American College of Cardiology
Journal of the American Medical Association
Lancet
Laryngoscope
Medical Journal of Australia
New England Journal of Medicine
Paraplegia
Pediatric Dentistry
Pediatric Emergency Care
Pediatric Infectious Disease Journal
Pediatric Nephrology
Pediatric Neurology
Pediatric Pulmonology
Pediatric Research
Pediatrics
Plastic and Reconstructive Surgery
Prenatal Diagnosis
Public Health Reports

STANDARD ABBREVIATIONS

The following terms are abbreviated in this edition: acquired immunodeficiency syndrome (AIDS), cardiopulmonary resuscitation (CPR), central nervous system (CNS), cerebrospinal fluid (CSF), computed tomography (CT), deoxyribonucleic acid (DNA), electrocardiography (ECG), health maintenance organization (HMO), human immunodeficiency virus (HIV), intensive care unit (ICU), intramuscular (IM), intravenous (IV), magnetic resonance (MR) imaging (MRI), and ribonucleic acid (RNA).

NOTE

The YEAR BOOK OF PEDIATRICS is a literature survey service providing abstracts of articles published in the professional literature. Every effort is made to ensure the accuracy of the information presented in these pages. Neither the editors nor the publisher of the YEAR BOOK OF PEDIATRICS can be responsible for errors in the original materials. The editors' comments are their own opinions. Mention of specific products within this publication does not constitute endorsement.

To facilitate the use of the YEAR BOOK OF PEDIATRICS as a reference tool, all illustrations and tables included in this publication are now identified as they appear in the original article. This change is meant to help the reader recognize that any illustration or table appearing in the YEAR BOOK OF PEDIATRICS may be only one of many in the original article. For this reason, figure and table numbers will often appear to be out of sequence within the YEAR BOOK OF PEDIATRICS.

Introduction

"Give me ambiguity, or give me something else"
The diversity of articles selected for inclusion in this year's YEAR BOOK OF PEDIATRICS again demonstrates how complex the practice of pediatrics has become. It has become more complex at a time when our discipline is facing many challenges. The health care system providing care for today's children has undergone a dramatic transformation, a transformation similar to what is occurring in other areas of medicine. The failure of major health care reform legislation did not slow changes that were previously under way, changes catalyzed by the increasing emergence of managed care systems.

The implications of such events for those who practice general pediatrics or one of its subspecialties are not minor, especially given the enormity of the unknowns regarding the future of our discipline. What will be the role of the pediatric generalist in the future? What will be that role in relation to others who provide care to children, including family physicians and nurse practitioners? How will changes in these types of relationships affect workforce requirements in pediatrics? Will general pediatrics remain rooted as a broadly generalist discipline, or will pediatricians increasingly be expected to assume responsibility for subspecialty management problems? What are the likely changes that will occur in the relationship between the generalist pediatrician and the pediatric subspecialist? Is it conceivable that pediatrics might evolve into the British model, where the generalist pediatrician principally functions as a consultant to the general practitioner? Will there be a need for fewer of us, both generalists and subspecialists?

Pediatrics, fortunately, has not created for itself the type of problem currently facing practitioners within internal medicine. Clearly the latter discipline has become oversubspecialized. In recent years, more than two thirds of internal medicine residents have gone on to fellowship training, producing significant surpluses of adult subspecialists in several areas of the country. In pediatrics, only 16% of pediatricians are subspecialists. Even so, we don't know for sure whether we have too many or too few subspecialists, or generalists, for that matter. There are several "wild cards" that will affect our workforce requirements. Managed care could increase the need for generalist physicians, including pediatricians, although this isn't clear at the present time. If managed care requires generalist pediatricians to assume greater roles in the diagnosis and management of patients previously referred for consultation and treatment, fewer subspecialists may be needed.

There are factors, however, that could increase our requirements for both generalists and subspecialists in pediatrics. Currently, with the failure of governmental resources to adequately provide support for the care of children, there continue to be some 12 million youngsters under the age of 18 who do not receive codified care either by a generalist or subspecialist. Should adequate health care funding exist for them, the need for physician resources could increase. Also, it's likely that we will see a continuation of a slow trend toward a decrease in the number of hours worked each week by health care providers, a phenomenon that does affect workforce requirements in an upward manner.

Workforce requirements represent a balance of supply and demand. Pediatrics as a generalist discipline remains highly interesting as a career pathway for medical students. The number of filled residency positions has increased by more than one third in the past decade alone. It seems likely that interest in general pediatrics will remain extremely strong, given the primary care imperative in this country. Fortunately for pediatricians, we have not intended to oversupply our subspecialty fields and there is still time to prospectively adjust the number of specialists we train to meet current and projected future requirements. That's the good news. The less-than-good news is that there is still much work to be done in fine-tuning the direction in which our discipline is moving.

To date, much of the change that has occurred has happened without a clear national policy for addressing both the needs of children and the workforce required to meet those needs. Our pediatric community has relied on a 1978 American Academy of Pediatrics report, "The Future of Pediatric Education," for overall guidance on the specific needs of the pediatric population and the training required by pediatrician providers to meet those needs. This document has served us well for the better part of two decades, but nothing lasts forever. A new 3-year project, "The Task Force on the Future of Pediatric Education II," has just been initiated. This task force will examine all the issues noted above and will update the findings and conclusions of the earlier report. We cannot teach the pediatricians of the future without having a clear understanding of all the issues that face our discipline, including who will be doing what and under what circumstances. The Task Force includes working groups on the future role of the pediatric generalist and subspecialist, the financing of graduate medical education, the implications of the new roles of the generalist and subspecialist, and what we need to teach in this regard. Lastly, and as importantly, the Task Force will attempt to make definitive statements about our workforce requirements. Funding for this extensive project has been provided by a major grant from the Center for the Future of Children of the David and Lucille Packard Foundation, with additional support from the American Academy of Pediatrics, the American Board of Pediatrics Foundation, and the Association of Medical School Pediatric Department Chairmen.

Not all aspects of the Task Force's work will require 3 years to complete. The working group dealing with the requirements for generalists and subspecialists in pediatrics hopes to report its conclusions soon. Those interested in following the progress of this extraordinary and critically important effort can do so by communicating with the Task Force at the e-mail address: futpededII@aap.org, established by the American Academy of Pediatrics as a means of providing information and receiving input about this project.

At this point, the reader may wonder why this introduction to the YEAR BOOK has dealt with a topic that seems at arm's length from the 300 or so abstracts and commentaries contained herein. Au contrairé. None of us can be ambiguous about what we think the future holds. The YEAR BOOK must adapt its content to reflect where pediatrics is headed. We who work on the YEAR BOOK OF PEDIATRICS will be following the work of the Task Force closely to be certain that what we present to you does reflect what is current and important within our discipline, even as that discipline changes over time.

James A. Stockman, III, ·M.D.

1   The Newborn

Timing of Sexual Intercourse in Relation to Ovulation: Effects on the Probability of Conception, Survival of the Pregnancy, and Sex of the Baby
Wilcox AJ, Weinberg CR, Baird DD (Natl Inst of Environmental Health Sciences, Research Triangle Park, NC)
N Engl J Med 333:1517–1521, 1995   1–1

Objective.—It is agreed that conception must take place near the time of ovulation, but the precise timing and duration of fertility remain uncertain. The timing of intercourse was monitored in 221 healthy women who were planning to conceive.

Methods.—Daily first-morning urine specimens were collected from the time the participants stopped using birth control and were analyzed for estrogen and progesterone metabolites. Specimens were collected up to week 8 of clinical pregnancy or for up to 6 months. A total of 625 ovulatory cycles in 217 women were available for analysis.

Findings.—Without exception, conception was associated with at least 1 episode of intercourse in the 6-day period ending on the day of ovulation. None of 31 cycles lacking intercourse during this time resulted in conception. When intercourse took place only once during the 6-day period, it most commonly was on the day of ovulation. The chance of conception decreased substantially with intercourse less often than every other day during the 6-day period. Only 6% of conceptions were definitively related to fertilization by sperm that were 3 or more days old. No particular pattern of intercourse could be related to infant sex.

Implications.—The fertile period of the cycle lasts approximately 6 days and ends on the day of ovulation. The present findings do not support limiting the frequency of intercourse to achieve pregnancy. Deliberately timing intercourse for the day of ovulation will not aid gender selection.

▶ Imagine that you live in a rural community and are covering for the town's only obstetrician who has had to leave because of an emergency. The first call you receive is from a young married couple that has had difficulties conceiving. They fire off a number of questions and refuse to wait for a response until the obstetrician returns to town. Their questions include the following: How many days in a menstrual cycle is a woman fertile? When is this? Will sperm that have aged in the female reproductive tract before

1

ovulation result in a less viable fetus? Can the couple influence the sex of their infant by timing their intercourse in relation to ovulation?

The article abstracted is your best source for these answers. For example, the fertile period during a menstrual cycle is now accepted to be 6 days. The fertile period ends on the day of ovulation. Historically, couples who have been advised to maximize their chance of pregnancy by timing their intercourse to coincide with ovulation (for example, using kits to detect the surge of luteinizing hormone) were ill-advised. Because the probability of conception is now understood to decrease quickly after ovulation, couples who abstain from intercourse until they have evidence of ovulation may miss their best shot for conception, which is in the several days before ovulation. This also means that there no longer is support for a recommendation that normal couples seeking pregnancy should limit the frequency of sexual intercourse (not true if the man has a marginal sperm count). Also, aging sperm do not decrease the viability of a resulting conceptus.

Lastly, we've all seen a number of theories about when to have intercourse to rig the odds for having a baby boy or a baby girl. The most recent data, however, show no association between the sex of an infant and the timing of intercourse in relation to ovulation. The deliberate timing of intercourse around the day of ovulation adds no practical value in sex selection.

All of these data can be summarized in a brief sentence or two. For normal couples who wish to conceive, the best time to have sex is on every conceivable occasion, literally and figuratively. The chance that a baby will be born a boy or a girl is 100%.

While on the topic of fertility, are you aware of what group has the highest fertility rate recorded in the world? The clearest evidence in response to this query has been reported in the Hutterites, a sect of Anabaptist refugees from Europe who settled in North America over a century ago. Although their fertility has fallen in recent years, this community has the highest age-specific fertility rates anywhere. This is because the sect forbids any fertility control. Nonetheless, the group enjoys extraordinarily high standards of living and health care. In the 1950s, women in this sect were giving birth to an average of 11 infants each, with a peak fertility age of about 30 years. Interestingly, half of Hutterite women deliver their last child by age 40, when only 1% would be expected to be postmenopausal. Thus, even Hutterites get their childbearing done relatively early.

The Analgesic Effect of Sucrose in Full Term Infants: A Randomised Controlled Trial
Haouari N, Wood C, Griffiths G, et al (Leeds Gen Infirmary, England)
BMJ 310:1498–1500, 1995   1–2

Background.—All newborns have at least 1 heel-prick procedure done in the hospital, and some have several of these procedures. The value of sucrose in reducing pain in neonates undergoing routine blood sampling by heel prick was studied.

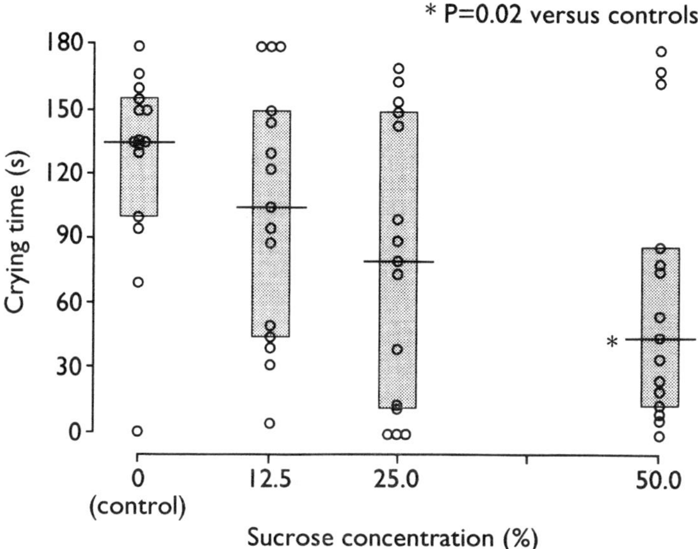

FIGURE 1.—Total time crying in first 3 minutes after heel prick in 60 infants given sterile water (controls) or 12.5%, 25%, or 50% sucrose. *Points* are individual values. *Horizontal lines* are median values. *Shaded areas* are interquartile ranges. (Test for trend across groups: $P = 0.007$.) (Courtesy of Haouari N, Wood, C, Griffiths G, et al: The analgesic effect of sucrose in full term infants: A randomised controlled trial. *BMJ* 310:1498–1500, 1995.)

Methods.—Sixty healthy infants, born at 37– 42 weeks' gestation, were included. Postnatal ages ranged from 1 to 6 days. The infants were assigned randomly to receive 2 mL of 1 of 4 solutions on the tongue 2 minutes before heel-prick sampling for serum bilirubin concentrations. Placebo or sucrose, 12.5%, 25%, or 50%, was given.

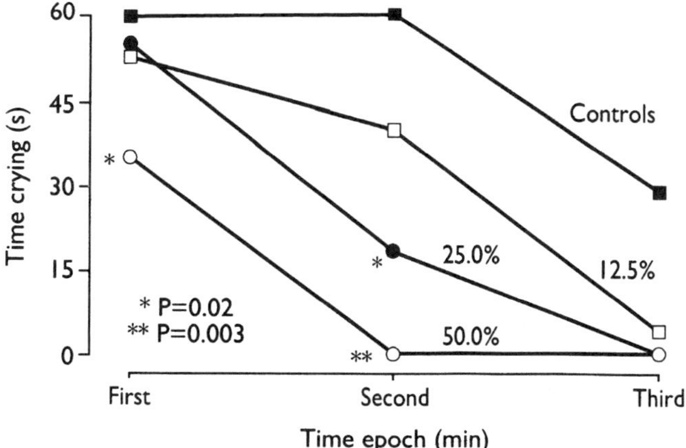

FIGURE 2.—Time crying during each 1-minute epoch after heel prick in infants given sterile water (*controls*) or 12.5%, 25%, or 50% oral sucrose. *Points* are median values for each group. (Courtesy of Haouari N, Wood C, Griffiths G, et al: The analgesic effect of sucrose in full term infants: A randomised controlled trial. *BMJ* 310:1498–1500, 1995.)

Findings.—The infants receiving 50% sucrose had a significant decrease in overall crying time and heart rate after 3 minutes compared with those given placebo. The reduction was greatest 1 minute after heel prick. In newborns given 25% sucrose, the decrease in overall crying time and heart rate was statistically significant 2 minutes after heel prick. There was a significant trend for crying time reduction with increasing concentrations of sucrose during the first 3 minutes (Figs 1 and 2).

Conclusions.—In healthy normal newborns, concentrated sucrose solution appears to reduce crying and the autonomic effects of a painful procedure. Sucrose may be a useful, safe analgesic for minor painful procedures in infants.

▶ A newborn must wonder what kind of world he or she is born into when, in the first few hours of life, various assaults occur. These include invasions of the nose and other parts of the airway and at least 2 or 3 painful procedures: a heel stick for neonatal screening purposes, an IM injection with vitamin K, and for boys, at least, a circumcision. In the hospital from which this report originated, every infant had at least 1 heel-prick procedure, 15% of infants had 2–5 blood samples taken, and 2% had 5 or more such procedures. Is a spoonful of sugar (sucrose) the answer to the discomfort associated with such procedures, as this report suggests? The answer appears to be an unequivocal yes, not just from this report, but from several others that have appeared in recent years.[1-3]

What's important about this study is that it tells us exactly how much sucrose should be used and when the painful procedure should be performed after the administration of the sugar water. Specifically, use a 50% sucrose solution. Place 2 mL of it in the mouth. Wait 1 minute and perform the needed procedure. Sucrose not only reduces the duration of crying, if any crying occurs at all, but also reduces the tachycardia induced by painful procedures. Most fascinating is the observation of Blass et al.,[4] who have demonstrated that sucrose does what it does by some sort of opiate effect, because any benefit of sucrose is ablated by naloxone.

If you're going to use sugar water, use the real stuff. Artificial sweeteners such as saccharine, and presumably aspartame, don't juice up your endogenous opiate pathways.[5]

References

1. Miller A, et al: *Pain* 56:175, 1994.
2. Schoen EJ, et al: *Clin Pediatr* 30:429, 1991.
3. Blass EM, et al: *Pediatrics* 87:215, 1991.
4. Blass E, et al: *Pharmacol Biochem Behav* 26:483, 1987.
5. Lieblich I, et al: *Science* 97:871, 1983.

Increased Maternal Age and the Risk of Fetal Death

Fretts RC, Schmittdiel J, McLean FH, et al (Harvard Med School, Boston; Harvard School of Public Health, Boston; McGill Univ, Montreal)
N Engl J Med 333:953–957, 1995   1–3

Introduction.—In recent decades, the number of women older than 40 years having their first pregnancy has increased. The current risk of fetal death associated with older maternal age and nulliparity is not clear. Therefore, the rate of fetal death was studied in a large obstetric population during a 30-year period, and the significance of older maternal age and nulliparity as risk factors for fetal death was analyzed after controlling for potential confounding factors.

Methods.—Data on infants born alive or stillborn between 1961 and 1993 were extracted from the database at a tertiary care teaching hospital. The rate of fetal deaths per 1,000 births was calculated for each decade and for 2 periods: 1961–1974 and 1978–1993. The risk of fetal death in older and nulliparous women was compared with that in women younger than 30 years of age and having their second or third child. A logistic regression model was used to control for potentially confounding obstetric and patient factors.

Results.—The perinatal mortality rate per 1,000 births was 25.2 during the 1960s and decreased to 6.6 in 1990 through 1993 (Table 1). From 1978 through 1993, the fetal death rate for women of all ages was about half that in the earlier period (Fig 1). Compared with younger women, the odds ratio for fetal death among women older than 35 years was 1.5 in the 1960s and 2.2 in 1990 through 1993. Compared with women having their second or third child, the risk of fetal death was associated with both nulliparity and high parity in the earlier part of the study and with only high parity in the later period. Women older than 35 years of age also had a higher prevalence of multiple gestation, hypertension, diabetes mellitus, placenta previa, placental abruption, previous abortion, and previous fetal

TABLE 1.—Total Births and Fetal, Neonatal, and Perinatal Mortality From the 1960s Through the 1990s*

Variable	1960s	1970s	1980s	1990–1993
Total births	28,844	17,499	35,338	12,665
Fetal deaths				
Total no.	331	142	174	41
No./1,000 total births	11.5	8.1	4.9	3.2
Neonatal deaths				
Total no.	396	159	198	43
No./1,000 live births	13.9	9.2	5.6	3.4
Perinatal mortality	25.2	17.2	10.5	6.6
(per 1,000 total births)				

*Total births include both live births and stillbirths. Data collection for the 1960s began in 1961. Information on births from 1975 through 1977 was not available and was therefore not included. Excluded are 2 births for which the date of delivery was not entered into the database.

(Reprinted by permission of *The New England Journal of Medicine* from Fretts RC, Schmittdiel J, McLean FH, et al: Increased maternal age and the risk of fetal death. *N Engl J Med* 333:953–957, Copyright 1995, Massachusetts Medical Society.)

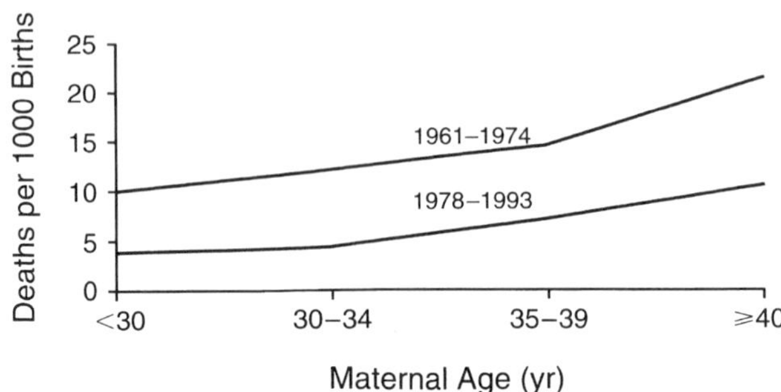

FIGURE 1.—Fetal deaths per 1,000 total births, according to maternal age and study population. (Reprinted by permission of *The New England Journal of Medicine* from Fretts RC, Schmittdiel J, McLean FH, et al: Increased maternal age and the risk of fetal death. *N Engl J Med* 333:953–957, Copyright 1995, Massachusetts Medical Society.)

death. After controlling for these factors, age older than 40 years, nulliparity, and high parity were all associated with an increased risk of fetal death during the early period, whereas age older than 35 years and high parity, but not nulliparity, were associated with an increased risk of fetal death during the later period.

Conclusions.—The fetal death rate decreased by more than 70% during the 3 decades of the study, probably because of changes in the obstetric population and in obstetric practice. However, older age is still a predictor of an increased risk of fetal death, even after controlling for age-related medical confounders and complications of pregnancy.

▶ When this editor was in medical school, there was a socially indelicate term commonly applied to those who were 35 years or older when they had their first baby: "elderly primigravida." We don't hear that term, first adopted in 1959 by the International Federation of Obstetricians and Gynecologists, used very much anymore. The reason is that there now are more than 500,000 pregnancies in women between the ages of 35 and 39 years and more than 100,000 in women 40 years and older. This reflects the observation that as older and often well-educated women make up for previous delays in childbearing, they elect to become pregnant. The number of women in their thirties who remain childless has increased sharply during the past 2 decades. At the start of this decade, 20% of women 35 years of age had not yet had children, compared with only 9% of those who were 35 years old just 20 years ago. According to a survey performed by the Bureau of the Census, half of the married, childless women who reach 35 years of age are expected to have at least 1 child.[1] Put these statistics together with the fact that there are a disproportionately large number of women of childbearing age right now—a product of the baby boom that followed World War II—and you now have more older women having babies than at any other time in history.

As we see from this report, maternal age can be a problem for the infant as well as for the mother. Potential complications resulting from maternal diabetes, hypertension, and premature separation of the placenta increase the hazards to the infant by as much as 2½ -fold, and to the mother by more than 4-fold. These risks technically have not decreased during the past 35 years. One reason is that in the 1960s, a 40-year-old pregnant woman was having her last child, not her first. Today, women older than 40 years are more likely to be unmarried than their counterparts in the 1960s and 1970s and to have had 1 or more induced abortions. Also, as the result of assisted-reproduction technique, older women are having triplet and higher-order multiple gestations. In vitro fertilization, in particular, carries with it significant increases in maternal and neonatal morbidity. A report by Tallo et al. shows that mothers who have undergone in vitro fertilization have a 21% prevalence of pregnancy-induced hypertension, a 44% chance of premature labor, and a 37% chance of preterm delivery.[2] Their infants have about a 42% chance of having 1 of the following complications: being of low birth weight, having a longer hospital stay, or having respiratory distress syndrome, patent ductus arteriosus, or sepsis. The rate of stillbirth is twice as high among older women, with or without in vitro fertilization.

So, is the cup half empty or half full for "elderly primigravida?" As much as these data suggest a "negative" overview, the overview is hardly negative at all. Think of it this way: pregnant women older than 35 years who have undergone early screening for fetal anomalies have a live birth rate of 994 per 1,000 (compared with 997 per 1,000 for their younger counterparts). This relatively small, although statistically significant, difference is a tiny price to pay for women who wish to be mothers for the first time.

References

1. Report. Bureau of the Census. Series p-20. No. 436. Washington, DC: Government Printing Office, June 1989.
2. Tallo CP, et al: *J Pediatr* 127:794, 1995.

Apparent Life-threatening Events in Presumed Healthy Neonates During the First Three Days of Life
Grylack LJ, Williams AD (Columbia Hosp for Women, Washington, DC)
Pediatrics 97:349–351, 1996   1–4

Background.—Little is known about sudden infant death syndrome (SIDS) and apparent life-threatening events (ALTEs) in mature infants in the first few days of life. The historical, clinical, and pneumographic correlates of ALTEs were studied in a term newborn nursery population during the first 3 days of life in a maternity hospital.

Methods and Findings.—During a 3-year period, 20 of about 15,000 newborns had ALTEs. The most common initial symptom was apnea, usually accompanied by cyanosis. Treatment most often consisted of tactile stimulation and oxygen. Airway clearance, intermittent positive pressure ventilation, and cardiac massage were performed less commonly. The causes were potentially identifiable in 40% of the events. These included CNS abnormality, airway obstruction, and persistent fetal cardiovascular shunt. Analysis of the multichannel recordings done after the ALTEs

TABLE 1.—Apparent Life-Threatening Events: Clinical Characteristics of Initial Events

Event	Primary Symptoms, n	Secondary Symptoms, n
Apnea	15	
Cyanosis	5	12
Bradycardia		6
Pallor		3
Hypotonia		2

(Courtesy of Grylack LJ, Williams AD: Apparent life-threatening events in presumed healthy neonates during the first three days of life. *Pediatrics* 97:349–351. Reproduced by permission of *Pediatrics*, Copyright 1996.)

showed desaturation of less than 85% in 11 infants, apneic pauses of more than 15 seconds in 10, and bradycardia of less than 80 beats/min in 4 infants. Eighteen infants were discharged with home monitors. Medication was prescribed for 4 infants. Four infants had recurrent ALTEs before discharge and 1 infant after discharge. None of the infants died (Table 1).

Conclusions.—Apparent life-threatening events can occur in low-risk, term neonates in the first 3 days of life. In most infants, the causes of these events are not discovered. Multichannel recordings may show abnormalities. The likelihood of an ALTE recurring is higher in the first week than in the following 2 months.

▶ No larger survey exists on the subject of ALTEs in the first few days of life than the report abstracted here. The term ALTE, of course, has replaced the terms "near-miss SIDS," "aborted SIDS," and "aborted crib death," largely because of a lack of consensus regarding the relationship between ALTEs and SIDS. We tend not to think of ALTEs as occurring in the newborn period, but the data from this study clearly indicate that about 1 in 750 otherwise absolutely well newborns will have an ALTE. It is quite obvious from this series that the causes of such events remain unknown in the majority of cases, although multichannel recordings do show abnormalities in some of these infants. All are deserving of follow-up because recurrent episodes do occur.

One infant in 750 otherwise normal infants having an ALTE is a chilling statistic for a care provider. It goes to show that when it comes to the well-baby nursery, wellness is a relative term at best.

Parous Patients' Estimate of Birth Weight in Postterm Pregnancy

Chauhan SP, Sullivan CA, Lutton TC, et al (Univ of Mississippi, Jackson)
J Perinatol 15:192–194, 1995
1–5

Introduction.—Delivery of a macrosomic fetus (birth weight ≥ 4,000 g) may be difficult to predict by sonographic means. A simple and reliable method to estimate birth weight would be valuable in the management of

TABLE 2.—Comparison of Clinical vs. Maternal Estimate of Birth Weight Among 40 Post-Term Parous Patients

Method of Estimating Fetal Weight	Mean Absolute Error (g) ± SD	Mean Standardized Error (g/kg) ± SD	Percent of Estimates Within ± 10% of Actual Birth Weight
Clinical	378 ± 232	75 ± 71	65.0
Maternal	349 ± 331	92 ± 81	67.5
Significance	*P* = NS	*P* = NS	*P* = NS

Abbreviation: NS, not significant.
(Courtesy of Chauhan SP, Sullivan CA, Lutton TC, et al: Parous patients' estimate of birth weight in postterm pregnancy. *J Perinatol* 15:192–194, 1995.)

these high-risk pregnancies. Several studies report that parous women in labor are able to provide an estimate of birth weight as accurate as those obtained by clinical examination or sonography. Seventy postterm parous women were asked for their estimates during early labor, and these estimates were compared with those of obstetric providers.

Methods.—Women eligible to participate in the study were postterm, parous, in early active labor with a singleton gestation, had a vertex presentation, and had no evidence of fetal distress. Each patient was asked to estimate, on the basis of past experience, the birth weight of her newborn. For the last 40 women in the study group, an obstetrician or midwife also offered an estimate.

Results.—Birth weight was ≥ 4,000 g in 18 (25.7%) of the 70 neonates. The mean of the mothers' estimate of birth weight was 3,545 g, and 71.4% of mothers made an estimate that was within ± 10% of the actual birth weight. Maternal estimates for birth weight ≥ 4,000 g had a specificity of 94% and a positive predictive value of 77%. Among the 40 deliveries with a concurrent clinical and maternal estimate of birth weight, the mean standardized error was comparable for clinical (75 g/kg) and maternal (92 g/kg) predictions. Approximately two thirds of clinical and maternal estimates were within ± 10% of actual birth weight (Table 2). For the 11 macrosomic newborns who underwent both methods of birth weight estimation, the mean standardized error between estimates was not significantly different.

Conclusion.—Postterm parous women were at risk for delivery of a macrosomic fetus and were able to predict with good accuracy the birth weight of their newborns. The maternal estimates were comparable to those derived clinically and may prove to be as accurate as those obtained sonographically.

▶ The report abstracted was the topic of some dinner-table discussion in our home. I asked the question: "Who is better able to more accurately predict a baby's birth weight—an obstetrician with 4 years of medical school and 5 years of residency training or the mother carrying that baby?" Meredith, our 17-year-old daughter, a high school senior, gave a candid response. She said, "Most of the doctors were probably men. They don't have a clue. How can a man know what it's like to carry a 9-pound baby?"

In fact, as this report shows, obstetricians are no better than mothers who have had babies when asked to provide such estimates.

The conclusion: Don't ask the delivery person. Mother knows best.

Maternal and Fetal Responses to Low-impact Aerobic Dance
McMurray RG, Katz VL, Poe MP, et al (Univ of North Carolina, Chapel Hill)
Am J Perinatol 12:282–285, 1995   1–6

Introduction.—Aerobic dance, compared with aerobic walking, has been shown to produce a higher heart rate without a proportional increase in oxygenation and higher blood pressures. The effects of these changes on pregnant women and their fetuses have not been established. Therefore, the effects on pregnant women and their fetuses of low-impact aerobic dance or of treadmill walking at a similar intensity were compared.

Methods.—Ten women with singleton pregnancies at 21–28 weeks' gestation all completed both a 40-minute aerobic dance program and a 40-minute treadmill walk, which produced the same maternal heart rate responses. Each trial consisted of 10 minutes of warm-up and increasing intensity, 20 minutes of moderate to high intensity, and 10 minutes of decreasing intensity and cool-down. Maternal oxygen uptake ($\dot{V}O_2$) and fetal heart rate (with ultrasound evaluation) were measured at 10-minute intervals, and maternal heart rate was measured at 5-minute intervals throughout the exercise period. During the 20 minutes of recovery after the trials, maternal heart rate and fetal heart rate and movement were assessed at 5-minute intervals.

Results.—The average maternal heart rate was similar in the 2 trials. However, the average $\dot{V}O_2$ values were 4 mL/kg/min lower during aerobic dance than during walking. Fetal heart rates averaged 172 beats/min during aerobic dance and 149 beats/min during walking. The significant differences in fetal heart rates were gradually reduced during the recovery period. There were no instances of fetal bradycardia or uterine contractions during any trial.

Conclusions.—Pregnant women can perform 40 minutes of either aerobic dance or walking with fairly high intensity. However, a walking program will produce a higher maternal metabolic rate and induce less of the transient fetal heart rate responses than will aerobic dance. The clinical significance of the fetal response requires further study.

▶ Talking about learning to exercise early! This report shows how a fetus is no innocent bystander when a mother decides that her need for physical fitness is important, pregnancy or no pregnancy. What a pregnant woman does, in regard to strenuous activity, affects the cardiovascular status of her unborn infant, and the effect is very much dependent on the nature of that strenuous activity. Maternal walking is theoretically "safer" than aerobic dancing, even if the latter is low impact. Why this is so is what this article is all about. Apparently, at comparable maternal heart rates during exercise, a woman is able to increase her oxygen uptake much better during simple walking than during aerobic dancing. If that is true, the consequence to the fetus is a potential decrease in oxygenation, with a consequent compensatory increase in heart rate during maternal aerobic dancing. This study showed the latter. Aerobic dancing caused greater fetal heart rates than walking, differences as high as 25 beats/min.

The only real issue with this topic is whether exercising on the part of a pregnant woman actually harms her unborn infant. This important query has no answer as of now. Until the answer is known, it seems sensible that although women should not lose fitness during pregnancy, they should not go overboard with an activity that might create more challenge for their unborn infants than perhaps for themselves.

Severe Retinopathy of Prematurity in Extremely Low Birth Weight Infants After Short-term Dexamethasone Therapy

Ramanathan R, Siassi B, deLemos RA (Univ of Southern California, Los Angeles)
J Perinatol 15:178–182, 1995   1–7

Background.—With the significant increase in survival rates for extremely low birth weight (ELBW) infants, a concomitant increase in the incidence and severity of retinopathy of prematurity (ROP) has occurred. Dexamethasone therapy for chronic lung disease (CLD) may now be added to the factors identified as contributors to ROP. Despite the widespread use of dexamethasone in ELBW infants with CLD, its potential short-term and long-term complications are not clear. The association between short-term dexamethasone therapy and severe ROP in ELBW infants was retrospectively studied.

TABLE 1.—Clinical Characteristics of the Study Population ($n = 90$)

	Dexamethasone ($n = 38$)	No Dexamethasone ($n = 52$)	Significance
Birth weight (gm)	820 ± 138	828 ± 115	$p = 0.78$
Gestational age (wk)	26.5 ± 1.6	26.9 ± 1.6	$p = 0.21$
Apgar score ≤5 at 1 min	20/38	19/52	$p = 0.13$
Apgar score ≤5 at 5 min	2/38	3/82	$p = 0.9$
Male sex	18/28	24/52	$p = 0.9$
Inborn	11/38	14/52	$p = 0.83$
Sepsis	13/38	21/52	$p = 0.55$
PDA	28/38	18/52	$p < 0.0003$
Ductal ligation	12/38	7/52	$p < 0.03$
Mechanical ventilation (days)	44 ± 23	26 ± 15	$p < 0.001$
Oxygen therapy (days)	57 ± 28	29 ± 23	$p < 0.001$
Surfactant therapy	17/38	11/52	$p < 0.017$

Note: Continuous data are expressed as mean ± SD, and categoric data are expressed as number.
Abbreviation: PDA, patent ductus arteriosus.
(Courtesy of Ramanathan R, Siassi B, deLemos RA: Severe retinopathy of prematurity in extremely low birth weight infants after short-term dexamethasone therapy. *J Perinatol* 15:178–182, 1995.)

TABLE 2.—Clinical Characteristics of Infants With Severe Retinopathy of Prematurity ($n = 16$)

	Dexamethasone ($n = 12$)	No Dexamethasone ($n = 4$)	Significance
Birth weight (gm)	780 ± 128	727 ± 54	$p = 0.45$
Gestational age (wk)	264 ± 1.8	262 ± 1	$p = 0.87$
Cryotherapy	9/12	4/4	$p = 0.94$
Mechanical ventilation (days)	51 ± 23	41 ± 23	$p = 0.48$
Oxygen therapy (days)	68 ± 26	45 ± 24	$p = 0.12$

Note: Continuous data are expressed as mean ± SD, and categoric data are expressed as number.

(Courtesy of Ramanathan R, Siassi B, deLemos RA: Severe retinopathy of prematurity in extremely low birth weight infants after short-term dexamethasone therapy. *J Perinatol* 15:178–182, 1995.)

Methods.—Dexamethasone use was monitored for all ELBW infants admitted to a newborn ICU between October 1989 and December 1992. Data examined included gestational age, surfactant use, the presence of patent ductus arteriosus (PDA), and use of supplemental oxygen. Ophthalmologic examinations were performed at 6–7 weeks after delivery, with follow-up weekly or biweekly. Dexamethasone, given at the discretion of the individual neonatologist, was generally started at 0.5 mg/kg/ day and gradually tapered over a 2-week period. Indications were respiratory failure necessitating high ventilatory pressures and supplemental oxygen, lack of clinical improvement, and development of the exudative phase of CLD.

Results.—Of the 115 infants who weighed less than 1 kg and were admitted to the neonatal ICU, 90 survived until hospital discharge. Thirty-eight of these 90 infants were treated with dexamethasone, starting at a mean postnatal age of 21 days and continuing for a mean of 12 days. Infants treated and not treated with dexamethasone did not differ significantly in mean birth weight or gestational age. Treated infants, however, had a significantly higher incidence of PDA, required surgical ligation more often, had a significantly longer duration of positive-pressure ventilation and supplemental oxygen, and were more likely to have received surfactant therapy (Table 1). Stage III ROP developed in 16 infants, 12 of whom had been treated with dexamethasone (Table 2). Of the 13 infants requiring cryotherapy, 9 had received dexamethasone.

Conclusion.—Retinopathy of prematurity has been attributed to a number of clinical variables, all related to severity of illness. The findings indicate an association between dexamethasone therapy for CLD in ELBW infants and ROP. Other studies suggest that the occurrence of ROP may be affected by the dosage, duration, and time of initiation for dexamethasone.

▶ Steroids are increasingly used for the prevention and treatment of CLD in ELBW infants. This is not the first report to raise concerns about the effects of steroids on the immature retina of preterm infants. It is one of the few studies that have attempted to apply some rigor to the issues involved, but unfortunately without a convincing degree of success.

The use of supplemental oxygen, the duration of oxygen treatment, hypoxia, hyperoxia, hypercarbia, the presence of sepsis, intraventricular hemorrhage, light exposure, and blood transfusions have all been proved or suspected to play a role in causing ROP. It would be literally impossible to tease out the effects of an additional factor, such as the use of dexamethasone as an isolated variable. The only way to do so would be by a randomized, controlled trial. However, in a recent report, 78% of surveyed neonatologists in the United States and Canada would not participate in a study that attempted to isolate the effects of steroids.[1] Therefore, it remains impossible to answer the question of safety of steroid use for CLD.

What does all this mean? Because there is little likelihood of there being decent prospective studies to tell us how to use steroids to prevent CLD, at least in terms of the risk of certain kinds of complications, we're just going to have to use something unique to tell us what to do. Try common sense. Common sense would dictate that steroids are valuable, in moderation. Nonetheless, in view of their putative potential for increasing the prevalence of severe retinopathy, don't be blind to this potential complication.

Reference

1. Solimano A, et al: *Pediatr Res* 33:237A, 1993.

Children Whose Mothers Had Second Trimester Amniocentesis: Follow Up at School Age
Finegan J-AK, Sitarenios G, Bolan PL, et al (Hosp for Sick Children, Toronto)
Br J Obstet Gynaecol 103:214–218, 1996   1–8

Introduction.—The decision to undergo amniocentesis for prenatal diagnosis is not an easy one for potential parents. A previous report on amniocentesis performed in the second trimester of pregnancy showed that up to 20% of children exposed to amniocentesis had minimal brain damage. Design problems leave questions about the accuracy of this report. The long-term psychological and physical effects of amniocentesis were compared in 86 children exposed to second-trimester amniocentesis and 44 children whose mothers declined the procedure.

Methods.—This same cohort of children underwent evaluation at age 4, at which time the only between-group difference was a higher incidence of middle ear infections in the amniocentesis group. The mean patient age at the follow-up reported here was 7.1 years. The mean fetal age at amniocentesis was 16.5 weeks. Between-group maternal background characteristics did not differ significantly. Children in both groups underwent evaluation of level of intelligence, reading abilities, mathematical skills, speech articulation, visual-motor-perceptual abilities, fine motor coordination, behavioral problems, hyperactivity, social competence, temperament, height, weight, occipital-frontal head circumference, and health history (including frequency of ear infections).

TABLE 1.—Outcome Measures

	Amniocentesis (n = 86)	Comparison (n = 44)	P values
Intelligence			
IQ score*	119·90 (22·70)	119·67 (14·09)	0·93 NS
Academic achievement			
Reading (grade levels)			
Word identification	2·32 (1·07)	2·31 (1·01)	0·93 NS
Passage comprehension	2·02 (0·84)	2·06 (0·89)	0·81 NS
Total reading	2·23 (0·99)	2·23 (0·97)	0·98 NS
Mathematics (raw scores)			
Numeration	13·60 (1·71)	13·93 (1·85)	0·31 NS
Addition	7·00 (1·27)	7·50 (1·17)	0·03 NS
Subtraction	5·42 (1·23)	5·50 (1·07)	0·73 NS
Numerical reasoning	6·60 (1·98)	6·57 (2·13)	0·93 NS
Word problems	6·05 (1·77)	6·09 (1·95)	0·90 NS
Visual-motor-perceptual ability			
Raw score	13·97 (2·40)	13·82 (2·13)	0·73 NS
Age equivalence	7·56 (1·50)	7·36 (1·32)	0·45 NS
Fine motor coordination			
Raw score	18·41 (3·15)	18·14 (2·96)	0·64 NS
Age equivalence	9·98 (3·21)	9·68 (2·86)	0·59 NS
Speech			
Articulation errors†	3·10 (3·30)	3·36 (3·99)	0·74 NS
Centile (SE)	62·26 (28·41)	60·14 (26·97)	0·68 NS

Note: Values are shown as mean (standard deviation), except where indicated. Because a large number of statistical tests were conducted, a conservative α level was used for determining significant findings. Using Bonferroni's procedure, $P <$ 0.003 (0.05/15 variables) was considered statistically significant.

* Normative mean = 100, SD = 15.

† Comparisons were made on log transformations of the data because of skewed distributions.

Abbreviation: NS, not significant.

(Courtesy of Finegan J-AK, Sitarenios G, Bolan PL, et al: Children whose mothers had second trimester amniocentesis: Follow up at school age. *Br J Obstet Gynaecol* 103:214–218, 1996, Blackwell Science Ltd.)

Results.—There were no significant between-group differences for measures of intelligence, academic achievement, visual-motor-perceptual abilities, fine motor coordination, or speech articulation (Table 1). Parent-reported measures of child behavior did not differ between groups. There

TABLE 2.—Physical Growth and Health

	Amniocentesis (n = 86)	Comparison (n = 44)	P values
Height (cm)	125·08 (4·78)	125·07 (4·00)	0·99 NS
Weight (kg)	25·65 (4·06)	26·18 (3·89)	0·47 NS
Head circumference (cm)	53·07 (1·68)	53·15 (1·27)	0·78 NS
Ear infections in past year	0·84 (1·25)	0·70 (1·17)	0·54 NS
General health	1·46 (0·74)	1·47 (0·77)	0·92 NS

Note: Values are shown as mean (standard deviation). Because several statistical tests were conducted, a conservative α level was used for determining significant findings. Using Bonferroni's procedure, $P < 0.01$ (0.05/5) was considered statistically significant.

Abbreviation: NS, not significant.

(Courtesy of Finegan J-AK, Sitarenios G, Bolan PL, et al: Children whose mothers had second trimester amniocentesis: Follow up at school age. *Br J Obstet Gynaecol* 103:214–218, 1996, Blackwell Science Ltd.)

were no between-group differences in measures of height, weight, head circumference, number of ear infections in the past year, or general health (Table 2).

Conclusion.—Parents considering prenatal diagnosis have concerns about the long-term implications of amniocentesis for the child. Findings indicate that children exposed to second-trimester amniocentesis do not differ from those whose mothers declined the test in a number of psychological, behavioral, and physical evaluations, using reliable and standardized measures.

▶ Why, pray tell, would anyone think that merely because a child is a product of a pregnancy that had undergone an amniocentesis, that child would be at any greater risk for developmental problems? Unfortunately, however, this is what has been reported in prior studies. For example, 62 Swedish children, 5–7 years of age, whose mothers had amniocentesis were compared with 60 controls in the following areas: gross and fine motor skills, visual perception, speech/language, and attention. Of the children exposed to amniocentesis, 30% were reported to have a marked dysfunction in at least one area.[1] Of these, 20% received a diagnosis of minimal brain dysfunction. Since this type of information has crept into the literature, the discussion that parents undergo regarding decisions related to amniocentesis has become more complicated. Thus, the report abstracted here comes none too soon. This investigation appears to be the only one in which children exposed to amniocentesis have been studied prospectively from birth all the way to school age in a carefully controlled manner.

The findings of this study are comforting. Children exposed to second-trimester amniocentesis are not different in physical growth or health at age 7. Physical growth was looked at because it is known that 5% to 6% of fetuses undergoing amniocentesis actually have puncture wounds as a result of the procedure. The number of children with orthopedic problems does not differ. Although children in the group exposed to amniocentesis showed more ear problems than those in the control group in the preschool phase of this study, by 7 years there are no higher rates of infections. The findings of this report also do not support those of the Swedish investigators, who found high rates of minimal brain dysfunction. This study from Canada is better controlled in the sense that the comparison group, who did not undergo amniocentesis, were the offspring of mothers who had the same indications for amniocentesis but who declined the procedure.

What this report means to us pediatricians is pretty straightforward. For most couples, the decision to undergo prenatal diagnosis is a difficult one at best. One commonly raised question is the long-term implications of the procedure for the child. Assuming that these data hold up, children exposed to second-trimester amniocentesis do not differ from their peers when tested with a broad range of psychological and physical examinations. Parents no longer need to worry that they are putting their healthy offspring at unusual risk by undergoing amniocentesis for genetic diagnostic purposes.

Reference

1. Gillberg C, et al: *Clin Genet* 21:69, 1982.

Limb Defects and Chorionic Villus Sampling: Results From an International Registry, 1992–94
Froster UG, Jackson L (Universitätsspital Zürich, Switzerland; Jefferson Med College, Philadelphia)
Lancet 347:489–494, 1996

1–9

Background.—The safety of chorionic villus sampling (CVS) during pregnancy has been questioned. Several reports have described limb defects in infants exposed to this procedure. The World Health Organization (WHO) began an international registration of post-CVS limb defects in 1992 to address these concerns.

Methods.—Seventy-seven of 138,996 infants or fetuses reported to the WHO CVS registry between May 1992 and May 1994 had limb defects. Affected infants and fetuses were evaluated by the standard methods—by excluding syndromes, inherited disorders, and defects occurring in previable fetuses. Pattern analysis was performed on the limb deficiencies reported.

Findings.—In 64.4% of the affected infants and fetuses, defects occurred in the upper limbs (Table 2). Lower limbs were affected in 12.5% (Table 3). Both upper and lower limbs were affected in 20.8%. These values are consistent with limb defect distribution figures in several large population-based studies (Fig 1). Limb defects were transverse in 40.8% and longitudinal in 59.2%, compared with 42.7% and 57.3%, respectively, in a population not exposed to prenatal CVS.

Conclusion.—These findings do not suggest that the risk of limb defects is increased by CVS. The overall frequency and pattern distribution of limb deficiencies in the cohort studies did not differ significantly from the background population. Also, gestational age at CVS was uncorrelated with the severity of defects.

▶ Another report dealing with potential complications of prenatal testing. Although a number of infants have been reported with transverse limb deficiencies after their mothers had undergone CVS, it has been unclear whether the procedure actually caused these defects. From a biological point of view, a connection between placental disruption caused by an invasive procedure and a subsequent limb deficiency is an attractive proposition. It is also plausible that the earlier in pregnancy this disruption occurs, the more likely it is that a fetal defect will result.

What exactly is the story behind the putative relationship between CVS and limb deficiencies? In 1991, a group in Oxford, England, reported 5 limb deficiencies among 289 infants after CVS had been done before 69 days of gestation.[1] A second cluster of 4 limb deficiency defects among 394 infants

TABLE 2.—Deficiencies of Upper Limb in 42 Liveborns

Gestational age at sampling (days)	Limb deficiencies	Remarks
53	Amelia lower, i.e. Tt, radius/ulna, r/le	45, XX, t(13;14) pat; micrognathia; hypoglossia (case 2, ref 20)
63	Tl, ulna, le	
76	Tt, radius/ulna, le	Mother HBsAg pos; acyclovir in first trimester
73	Tt, radius/ulna, r	
72	Tt, radius/ulna, le	
73	Tt, radius/ulna, r	45, XXX, t(13;14) mat;
59	Tt, hand, r/le Tt, foot, le	micrognathia (case 1, ref 6)
88	Tt, hand, le	
62	Tt, hand, r/le	
75	Tt, hand, unilat	
79	Tt, hand, le Tl, digits, r Tt, foot, r/le	
64	Tt, hand, le	
76	Tt, hand, le; Tl, digits II-V, r Tl, foot, r/le	Scalp hemangioma
73	Tt, hand le	
68	Tt, hand, r; Tl, fingers, le Tt, foot, r	
66	Tt, hand, le	Micrognathia; hypoplastic maxilla
73	Tt, hand, le	
63	Tt, hand, le	
67	Tt, hand, r/le Tt, foot, r	Cleft lip (case 7, ref 20)
58	Tt, hand r Tl, digits I/V, le toes II/IV/V	Telecanthus; micrognathia; camptodactyly; paralysis VIIth nerve; strabismus
70	Tt, hand, le Tl, digits IV-V, r Tt, foot, r, le	Sickle cell carrier
101	Tl, digits III/IV, le	
87	Tl, digits I-IV, r/le	
47	Tl, digits II, V, r/le Tl, toes V, r/le	
77	Tl, digits II-V, le	
63	Tl, digits II-IV, le	
68	Tl, digits II-IV, unilat	
73	Tl, digits II-III, r Tl, digits I-III, le Tl, toe II, le Tl, toes, R	Umbilical hernia; talipes equinovarus
70	Tl, digits I-III, r	Placental cyst
70	Tl, digits III-V, le	
63	Tl, digits III-V, r	Syndactyly left hand, left foot
70	Tl, digits II-IV, le	
69	Tl, digits II-III, le	
64	Tl, digits II, unilat	
73	Tl, digit V, le	
73	Tl, digit II, r Tl, toes II, le	Neck hemangioma
63	Tl, digits II-IV, le	
65	Tl, digits II/III, le	
69	Tl, digits III, le	Dysmorphic face
73	Tl, digits II-IV, r/le	Syndactyly
73	Tt, digits, unilat	Tepicanthus; broad nasal bridge
73	Tl, digit II, le	

Abbreviations: T, terminal; *t*, transverse; *l*, longitudinal; *r*, right; *le*, left.
(Courtesy of Froster UG, Jackson L: Limb defects and chorionic villus sampling: Results from an international registry, 1992–94. *Lancet* 347:489–494, copyright by The Lancet Ltd. 1996.)

TABLE 3.—Deficiencies of Lower Limbs Only in 6 Liveborns

Gestational age at sampling (days)	Limb deficiency	Remarks
70	Tl, toe, l, le II/III, le	Syndactyly toes
76	Tl, femur, fibula, r Tl, tibia, le	Radiohumeral synostosis; FFU
75	Tl, toes II-V, le	
78	Tt, toes, le Tl, toes II/III, r	
80	Tl, toes I-III, le Tl, toes II-IV, r	
79	Tl, toes II-V, le	t(13;14)mat

Abbreviations: T, terminal; *t,* transverse; *l,* longitudinal; *r,* right; *le,* left.
(Courtesy of Froster UG, Jackson L: Limb defects and chorionic villus sampling: Results from an international registry, 1992–94. *Lancet* 347:489–494, copyright by The Lancet Ltd. 1996.)

exposed to CVS was then reported by Burton.[2] These earlier reports clearly presented a dilemma for women desiring an early prenatal test and for those providing care to these patients. In response to these initial reports, the Food and Drug Administration responded by advising that CVS should not be undertaken before 70 days' gestation. On the other hand, the WHO experts questioned whether there was any association between CVS and limb deficiencies. It is on this WHO CVS Registry that the report abstracted bases its data. This latest analysis does not reveal significant differences in the number or nature of limb defects.

Where exactly do these results leave a woman who desires an early prenatal diagnosis? For an overview of this topic, see the excellent commentary by Evans and Hamerton.[3] In an editorial, these individuals suggest that the study abstracted, although the largest report of limb deficiencies in infants exposed to CVS, is flawed. The flaw lies in the noncomparability of sources of the data that were entered into the registry. Of equal concern is

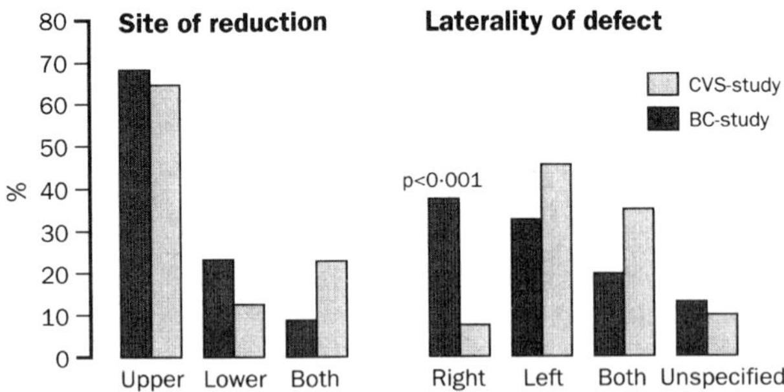

FIGURE 1.—Site of limb defect and laterality. *CVS* designates chorionic villus sampling; *BC* designates British Columbia, site of a population-based study. (Courtesy of Froster UG, Jackson L: Limb defects and chorionic villus sampling: Results from an international registry, 1992–94. *Lancet* 347:489–494, copyright by The Lancet Ltd. 1996.

the fact that the registry cases come from a single voluntary source of ascertainment, whereas the population-based data are derived from multiple sources including records from a universal health plan. Thus, the CVS registry cases are likely to be incomplete and not representative of limb deficiencies in the overall CVS-exposed group. Add to these concerns a recent report from the National Center for Environmental Health of the Centers for Disease Control and Prevention, which shows a 1.7-fold increased risk of limb deficiency after CVS, and, more specifically, a 6.4-fold increased risk of transverse digital deficiency.[4] The latter risk clearly increased with earlier gestational exposure.

These data leave us in limbo. Limbo is a lonely place for a pregnant woman concerned about the risk to her baby of a prenatal diagnostic procedure. Because an ideal study (e.g., a large, national, randomized trial with vaginal ultrasonic determination of gestational age and detailed evaluation of all fetuses and infants) is unlikely to be attempted, we are left with studies that are replete with methodologic limitations and contradictory results.

The decision as to whether to undergo CVS must remain with the woman herself; the decision as to whether to inform her of the potential, yet unproven, increased risk of limb defects must remain with the conscience of the care provider. The only consolation to be offered is that the potential incremental risk, if any at all, must be quite small.

References

1. Firth HV, et al: *Lancet* 337:762, 1991.
2. Burton BK: *Obstet Gynecol* 79:726, 1992.
3. Evans JA, et al: *Lancet* 347:44, 1996.
4. Olney RS, et al: *Teratology* 51:20, 1995.

The Natural History of Meconium Peritonitis Diagnosed In Utero

Dirkes K, Crombleholme TM, Craigo SD, et al (Tufts Univ, Boston)
J Pediatr Surg 30:979–982, 1995   1–10

Objective.—Although obstetric ultrasound has made it easier to diagnose meconium peritonitis (MP) in utero, there is little information about the natural history of prenatally diagnosed MP. Cases of prenatally diagnosed MP were reviewed.

Methods.—Sonographic criteria for diagnosing MP prenatally included the detection of intra-abdominal calcifications with acoustic shadowing. Nine cases of MP were diagnosed sonographically in fetuses between 18 and 37 weeks of gestation. Cases were divided into 2 groups; those with simple meconium peritonitis (SMP) had no associated bowel abnormalities, whereas those with complex meconium peritonitis (CMP) had associated bowel abnormalities (Fig 1). Patients were followed for 3–24 months.

Results.—Five fetuses had SMP diagnosed at 18, 23, 30, 34, and 37 weeks of gestation, and 4 had CMP diagnosed at 26, 26, 31, and 37 weeks

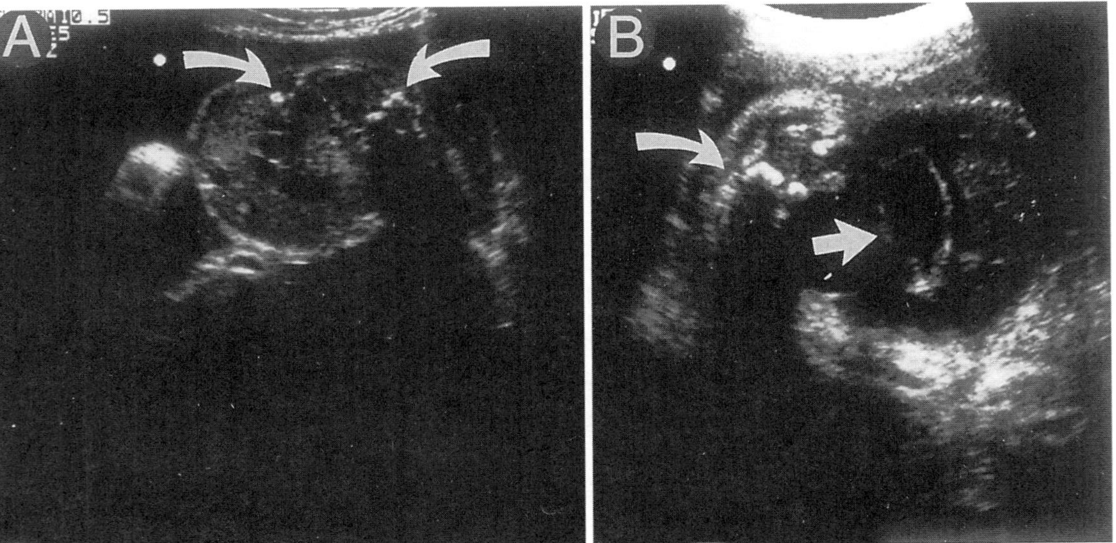

FIGURE 1.—**A,** sonogram obtained at 26 weeks of gestation showing simple meconium peritonitis with acoustic shadowing, intra-abdominal calcification (*arrows*), but no evidence of bowel dilatation, pseudocyst, or ascites. **B,** sonogram obtained at 30 weeks' gestation in a fetus with complex meconium peritonitis, which in addition to intra-abdominal calcifications (*curved arrow*) shows a meconium pseudocyst and dilated loops of bowel (*straight arrow*). (Courtesy of Dirkes K, Crombleholme TM, Craigo SD, et al: The natural history of meconium peritonitis diagnosed in utero. *J Pediatr Surg* 30:979–982, 1995.)

of gestation. All patients with SMP were delivered normally at term. Three had normal bowel gas patterns, and 2 had intra-abdominal calcifications. All were fed uneventfully, and all were healthy at a mean age of 15 months. All 4 fetuses with CMP had bowel dilatation; 2 had meconium cysts, 1 associated with polyhydramnios and the other with ascites. After birth, the 2 infants with meconium cysts required resection of the ileum and ileostomy for ileal perforation and atresia, respectively. One of these infants later died of complications after a liver transplant, and the other is doing well at 24 months of age. The other 2 patients had normal bowel gas patterns and were fed uneventfully. At 24 months of age, they were healthy.

Conclusion.—Fetal age was not correlated with outcome or severity of disease. Fetuses with CMP are at higher risk of bowel complications at birth, including perforation and obstruction.

▶ As much as we know about MP diagnosed postnatally, we know practically nothing about the natural history of MP diagnosed before birth. That is the relevance of this report because it shows us that the natural history of MP diagnosed in utero is markedly different from that of MP diagnosed in the newborn nursery. As many as half of infants with MP diagnosed after birth die. Death is an unusual occurrence when MP occurs in utero. Furthermore, the overall prognosis is otherwise better, and prenatal MP has a much lower incidence of an associated cystic fibrosis.

The ability of ultrasound to pick up calcifications is the principal reason we can now diagnose MP in utero. Calcifications detected by prenatal ultrasound do not automatically mean perforated bowel, however. There are biliary, vascular, intraluminal, solid organ, and tumor calcifications that can mimic the calcifications seen with MP. Associated findings such as dilated loops of bowel, pseudocyst, ascites, or polyhydramnios characterize CMP. When these findings are present, there is about a 50% chance that surgical intervention will be required in a newborn. Such infants should be delivered in a tertiary care setting with a surgeon on hand. Once an infant with CMP is born, an abdominal examination should be done immediately, and a plain radiograph of the abdomen and an ultrasound examination should be performed. An upper gastrointestinal study and small-bowel follow-through using water-soluble contrast may be necessary to confirm or exclude perforation, stenosis, atresia, or a meconium pseudocyst.

When MP is diagnosed before birth, there is a temptation to undertake parental DNA testing to define the fetal risk for cystic fibrosis. Because what will be will be, it would seem that this is not likely to be cost-effective, certainly in cases of SMP. On the other hand, for all cases of MP, it seems reasonable to recommend to parents that a simple, inexpensive sweat test be obtained post partum on the infant to exclude the chance of cystic fibrosis.

Early Meconium Evacuation: Effect on Neonatal Hyperbilirubinemia

Chen J-Y, Ling U-P, Chen J-H (Chung Shan Med and Dental College, Taichung, Taiwan)
Am J Perinatol 12:232–234, 1995

1–11

Introduction.—Neonatal jaundice, a common problem in newborns, is caused by the overproduction, impaired hepatic clearance, and increased enterohepatic circulation of bilirubin. Enterohepatic circulation of bilirubin can be increased in infants with delayed meconium passage, increasing the risk of neonatal jaundice. The effect of early meconium evacuation using glycerin enema on the incidence of neonatal hyperbilirubinemia was studied prospectively.

Methods.—During a 1-year period, 265 healthy newborns were randomly assigned to either the experimental or the control group. The experimental group (130 neonates) was given a glycerin enema within 30 minutes after birth and again 12 hours after birth. The control group (135 neonates) was given no glycerin enemas. All the infants were given infant formula, beginning within 6 hours after birth. The times at the passage of the first meconium stool and of the first transitional stool, the number and weight of stools during the first 24 hours after birth, and the cumulative weight of the stools until the passage of the first transitional stool were compared in the 2 groups. Total serum bilirubin levels were measured daily for 7 days.

Results.—All infants in the experimental group passed the first meconium stool within 30 minutes after birth, whereas 5 infants in the control group passed the first meconium stool more than 24 hours after birth. There was a significantly greater number and weight of stools during the first 24 hours in the experimental than in the control group, and neonates passed the first transitional stool significantly earlier in the experimental group than in the control group (Table 2). However, there were no significant differences between the 2 groups in either peak serum bilirubin levels or daily serum bilirubin levels (Table 3). Phototherapy was given to

TABLE 2.—Number and Weight of Stools During the First Day After Birth and Age at Passage of First Transitional Stool

	Group 1 (Glycerin Enema) (*n* = 130)	Group 2 (Control) (*n* = 135)
No. stools during the first day	51 ± 1.5	2.5 ± 0.8*
Weight of stools during the first day (g)	117 ± 20	50 ± 25*
Age at passage of first transitional stool (h)	230 ± 5.3	49.2 ± 8.5*
Cumulative weight of stools until passage of first transitional stool (g)	135 ± 29	138 ± 41

Values are mean ± SD.

*P < 0.001.

(Reprinted with permission from *American Journal of Perinatology* 12:232–234, 1995, Thieme Medical Publishers, Inc.)

TABLE 3.—Serum Bilirubin Concentration in Neonates Treated With and Without Glycerin Enema

Postnatal age	Serum Bilirubin Concentration (mg/dL)		P Value*
	Glycerin Enema Group (*n* = 130)	Control Group (*n* = 135)	
24 hours	4.6 ± 1.3	4.4 ± 1.3	NS
2 days	8.1 ± 2.4	7.7 ± 2.4	NS
3 days	10.6 ± 3.0	10.5 ± 3.2	NS
4 days	11.3 ± 3.3	11.2 ± 2.8	NS
5 days	11.0 ± 3.2	10.2 ± 3.2	NS
6 days	10.2 ± 3.2	9.1 ± 3.2	NS
7 days	9.0 ± 3.0	8.1 ± 3.3	NS

*Values are mean ± SD.
Abbreviation: NS, not significant.
(Reprinted with permission from *American Journal of Perinatology* 12:232–234, 1995, Thieme Medical Publishers, Inc.)

20 neonates in the experimental group and 18 neonates in the control group who had serum bilirubin levels of at least 15 mg/dL.

Conclusions.—Early meconium evacuation induced by glycerin enema does not affect serum bilirubin levels during the first week of life.

▶ This study from Taiwan is not as silly as it might seem at first. East Asian, including Chinese, newborn infants have mean maximal serum bilirubin concentrations higher than those of white populations. Most studies show that the average bilirubin concentration in such infants is approximately double those of white and black populations. Add to this situation a higher prevalence of significant variants of glucose-6-phosphate dehydrogenase deficiency and you have a group of infants who might have a higher risk of getting into trouble with neonatal jaundice. How early meconium evacuation might help is fairly straightforward. Newborn infants have fewer bacteria in the small and large bowel and greater enzyme activity that deconjugates bilirubin. A large portion of conjugated bilirubin is hydrolyzed to unconjugated bilirubin, which is then reabsorbed and constitutes a significant factor contributing to neonatal jaundice.

This is not the first report to study the effects of early meconium passage on peak bilirubin levels. Oral administration of nonabsorbable substances such as activated charcoal or agar, which bind bilirubin, have been observed to lower serum bilirubin levels, although differences in the latter were so marginal that there has been no stampede to incorporate their use in routine newborn care. Simply taking a rectal temperature stimulates meconium passage, fostering bilirubin clearance, but again the effects are marginal. In the study abstracted, glycerin enemas within half an hour of birth and again at 12 hours later do facilitate meconium passage, but the same percentage of treated infants achieve bilirubin levels of 15 mg/dL as those who never receive enemas.

Enemas are an unnatural thing. They should be reserved for those who are plugged up. Nature never meant enemas to facilitate what nature was going to do in her own good time. This applies to adults as well as to newborns.

Drug Screening in Newborns and Mothers Using Meconium Samples, Paired Urine Samples, and Interviews

Bibb KW, Stewart DL, Walker JR, et al (Univ of Louisville, Ky)
J Perinatol 15:199–202, 1995   1–12

Introduction.—The infants of women who use cocaine while pregnant are at increased risk of premature birth and complications of delivery. What is known about the extent of peripartum drug use comes mainly from maternal self-report and sporadic toxicologic tests. The prevalence of illicit substance abuse was assessed by testing of meconium and paired urine samples and by maternal interview.

Methods.—The blinded, prospective study took place at an urban hospital that served a mainly indigent population. A total of 580 mother-infant pairs were studied. Urine samples collected from the mothers and infants, and meconium samples collected from the infants, were tested for illicit substances. The mothers were unaware of the reasons for the specimen collections. On admission, the mothers were asked about their use of alcohol, tobacco, and street drugs, and those with a positive history of illegal substance use were evaluated by Child Protective Services. However, identification of drug users by the screening studies remained blinded.

Results.—Cocaine was detected in 3.4% of maternal urine specimens and tetrahydrocannabinol in 2.5%. Women who used cocaine were more likely not to have received prenatal care. Infants of mothers who used cocaine were more likely to be premature and to have a lower birth weight, a shorter length, and a smaller head circumference. For mother-infant pairs with positive drug screening results for cocaine, the interview, maternal urine sample, and meconium sample were equally sensitive. The newborn urine sample showed poor correlation (Table 2).

Conclusions.—Drug screening in newborns could be made more reliable by obtaining a urine sample from the mother and a meconium sample from

TABLE 2.—Results of Positive Tests When All 3 Specimens With a Common Number Were Present for Analysis (*n* = 29)

	Meconium	Newborn urine	Maternal urine
Cocaine	13 (4.5%)	8 (2.7%)	14 (4.8%)
THC	4 (1.4%)	0 (0%)	11 (3.8%)

Note: Cocaine includes cocaine metabolites. Cocaine was positive if the value was greater than 300 mg/mL urine and 150 ng/g meconium. Tetrahydrocannabinol (*THC*) was positive with values greater than 100 ng/mL urine and greater than 50 ng/g meconium.

(Courtesy of Bibb KW, Stewart DL, Walker JR, et al: Drug screening in newborns and mothers using meconium samples, paired urine samples, and interviews. *J Perinatol* 15:199–202, 1995.)

the newborn, in addition to asking the mother about drug use. The newborn urine sample is not as helpful. This screening approach could be especially valuable for mothers with complications associated with illicit substance abuse or infants with symptoms of drug abstinence syndrome. Lack of perinatal care may be a useful marker of substance abuse.

▶ The problems that infants who are born to cocaine-abusing mothers have include prematurity, greater complications of labor and delivery, a higher frequency of stillbirth, and increased rates of spontaneous abortion and abruptio placentae. These infants are at risk of being small for gestational age in both weight and head circumference. They have an increased incidence of congenital anomalies, including genitourinary malformations and heart defects, as well as CNS abnormalities, including cystic changes, atrophy, and infarction. Later they may show evidence of an increased probability of death from sudden infant death syndrome, presumably as a result of an abnormal ventilatory response to carbon dioxide. Other problems they encounter include necrotizing enterocolitis and a better-than-even chance of having attention-deficit hyperactivity disorder and difficulties in concentration, abnormal play patterns, and a flat affect. For reasons not easily explained, cocaine-exposed infants have a 2½-fold increased incidence of urinary tract infections early in life (14% vs. 4% of controls).[1]

This complication list is astounding both in its number and breadth. Because many of the complications of cocaine exposure in utero could be at least partially ameliorated if it was known which infant had such an exposure, it would seem reasonable to think about screening all mothers and/or their infants at the time of delivery to determine whether there is any risk for the development of such problems. This report shows that a combination of a maternal interview, a maternal urine sample, and an infant's meconium tested for cocaine will have a high degree of sensitivity and specificity. A newborn urine sample need not be included because it doesn't correlate well, largely because it may be falsely negative.

The trick with all of this is pretty obvious. How do you, legally and otherwise, identify infants at risk without infringing on personal freedoms of the mother? The analogy with perinatal HIV testing is obvious. All women should have access to prenatal care, as well as comprehensive drug treatment and other supportive services. The same is true of infants born to such mothers. The current climate of prosecution and criminalization of substance abuse may contribute to adverse perinatal outcomes by deterring women from seeking prenatal care and chemical-dependency treatment during their pregnancies. Opponents of universal drug screening are concerned about the involvement of government, the cost of testing, and the overloading of social agencies with cases. Universal screening is costly. The cost of a urine test ranges from $20 to $100 in individual hospitals. The most cost-effective assay, of course, would be meconium testing because it eliminates many false negatives. Meconium can be used to detect cocaine, marijuana, opiates, and a score of other drugs. More importantly, these drugs stay in meconium even if they were not used by a mother within the last 20 weeks before delivery of a term infant.[2]

Unbiased samples in the United States show that about 5% of all pregnant women deliver an infant who has been exposed to cocaine. In selected populations, this figure rises to 65%. There are probably not enough social agencies in our nation to deal with the total breadth of the problem. That means being selective. Who will do the selecting?

References

1. Gottbrath-Flaherty EK, et al: *J Perinatol* 15:203, 1995.
2. MecStat (brochure). Chicago, US Drug Testing Laboratory, 1993.

Prophylactic Indomethacin Therapy in the First Twenty-four Hours of Life for the Prevention of Patent Ductus Arteriosus in Preterm Infants Treated Prophylactically With Surfactant in the Delivery Room
Couser RJ, Ferrara TB, Wright GB, et al (Children's Health Care, Minneapolis; Children's Heart Clinic, Minneapolis)
J Pediatr 128:631–637, 1996   1–13

Objective.—For infants with hyaline membrane disease, treatment with surfactant may lead to a more rapid decrease in pulmonary vascular resistance and, thus, greater susceptibility to the development of hemodynamically significant patent ductus arteriosus (PDA). Previous studies have suggested that prophylactic indomethacin treatment can reduce problems with PDA. Infants receiving prophylactic surfactant therapy were studied to see whether low-dose indomethacin treatment can decrease the incidence of PDA.

Methods.—The prospective, randomized, placebo-controlled trial included 90 infants with birth weights of 600 to 1,250 g who received prophylactic surfactant therapy in the delivery room. They were assigned to receive either indomethacin, 0.1 mg/kg, or placebo once within 24 hours and again every 24 hours for 6 doses. The patients underwent echocardiography on the first day of life, before the start of treatment, and again on day 7, 24 hours after treatment. Additional, out-of-study echocardiograms were obtained to evaluate suspected PDA. For patients who did not respond to the study treatment, standard indomethacin therapy or ligation was performed.

Results.—Forty-three infants received indomethacin and 47 received placebo. Echocardiography showed a PDA in 86% of infants on the first day of life, before the start of treatment. The PDAs were classified as moderate-sized or large in 84% of indomethacin-treated patients vs. 93% of placebo-treated patients. Twenty-one percent of infants treated with indomethacin failed to respond to the study dose, whereas 47% of placebo-treated infants were nonresponders. The number of infants undergoing surgical ligation in the indomethacin group was half that in the placebo group. Long-term outcomes were similar between groups, including intraventricular hemorrhage, duration of oxygen therapy, endotracheal intuba-

TABLE 3.—Outcome

Variable	Birth weight 600 to 1250 gm		Birth weight <1000 gm	
	Indomethacin (*n* = 43)	Placebo (*n* = 47)	Indomethacin (*n* = 25)	Placebo (*n* = 32)
Survived	42 (98%)	46 (98%)	24 (96%)	32 (100%)
Duration (days)				
Endotracheal intubation	23.3 ± 21	21.4 ± 14	31.2 ± 22	26.7 ± 14
Oxygen therapy	44.5 ± 46	34.0 ± 28	60.4 ± 52	44.6 ± 27
Length of stay at level 3	42.7 ± 25	39.7 ± 19	53.8 ± 23	46.8 ± 15
Total length of stay	86.3 ± 42	79.2 ± 23	101 ± 46	88 ± 20
Regain birth weight	16.3 ± 7	16.4 ± 7	16.4 ± 7	15.8 ± 7
Reach full calories	27.9 ± 11	25.2 ± 8	32.0 ± 11	27.8 ± 8
Bronchopulmonary dysplasia	28 (65%)	23 (49%)	23 (92%)	20 (63%)
Retinopathy of prematurity (≥stage 3)	6 (14%)	4 (9%)	5 (21%)	4 (13%)
Inotrope dose (mg/kg)	48.9 ± 41	64.5 ± 43	55.0 ± 45	63.5 ± 41
Duration of inotrope therapy (days)	5.2 ± 4	6.0 ± 4	5.6 ± 4	6.3 ± 4

Note: Values are expressed as occurrence, percentage, or mean value ± standard deviation. The *P* values were not significant for all comparisons.

(Courtesy of Couser RJ, Ferrara TB, Wright GB, et al: Prophylactic indomethacin therapy in the first twenty-four hours of life for the prevention of patent ductus arteriosus in preterm infants treated prophylactically with surfactant in the delivery room. *J Pediatr* 128:631–637, 1996.)

tion, length of stay in the neonatal ICU, time to regain birth weight or achieve full caloric intake, incidence of bronchopulmonary dysplasia, and survival (Table 3). Neither were there any significant differences in the occurrence of adverse events, i.e., oliguria, elevated plasma creatinine concentration, thrombocytopenia, pulmonary hemorrhage, or necrotizing enterocolitis (Table 4).

Conclusion.—Low-dose indomethacin therapy, given within 24 hours after birth, can decrease the incidence of hemodynamically significant PDA in low–birth weight infants who receive prophylactic surfactant. This treatment reduces the need for surgical ligation, although it does not produce any differences in other outcome variables. Early low-dose indomethacin treatment may become a useful part of the overall manage-

TABLE 4.—Analysis of Adverse Events

Variable	Indomethacin (n = 43)	Placebo (n = 47)
Necrotizing enterocolitis	1	2
Pulmonary hemorrhage		
Mild	4	4
Severe	1	3
Urine output		
< 0.5 ml/kg/hr	2	1
< 1.0 ml/kg/hr	8	5
Creatinine >1.8 mg/dl	5	4
Platelets <50,000	0	0

Note: Values are expressed as occurrence. The *P* values were not significant for all comparisons.

(Courtesy of Couser RJ, Ferrara TB, Wright GB, et al: Prophylactic indomethacin therapy in the first twenty-four hours of life for the prevention of patent ductus arteriosus in preterm infants treated prophylactically with surfactant in the delivery room. *J Pediatr* 128:631–637, 1996.)

ment of very low birth weight infants who receive prophylactic surfactant therapy.

▶ The incidence of PDA continues to vary inversely with postconceptional age, affecting more than 40% of very low birth weight infants. The current use of surfactant has caused symptomatic PDA to present earlier than it did during the presurfactant era. The presence of a large, symptomatic PDA that persists throughout the first week of life increases the likelihood of a variety of problems. These problems include intraventricular cerebral hemorrhage, necrotizing enterocolitis, bronchopulmonary dysplasia, and death. Although it is well known that surgical closure of the PDA can decrease these various morbidities and mortalities related to PDA, the trick is to avoid surgery if possible.

Currently, indomethacin is the only nonsteroidal anti-inflammatory drug commonly used for the treatment and prophylaxis of the newborn and is quite effective in closing the PDA once opened. As this study shows, the prophylactic use of low doses of indomethacin—when initiated in the first 24 hours of life in low–birth weight infants who have received prophylactic surfactant in the delivery room—does decrease the incidence of left-to-right shunting at the level of the PDA. However, in other series, indomethacin has been noted to have several potential adverse side effects in newborns including transient or permanent alterations in renal function, necrotizing enterocolitis, gastrointestinal hemorrhage, and impairment in cerebral blood flow.

If indomethacin is not your cup of tea, you may wish to consider another nonsteroidal anti-inflammatory drug: ibuprofen. The administration of 3 doses of ibuprofen within 3 hours after birth in preterm infants also reduces the incidence of PDA without causing notable early adverse drug reactions.[1] A number of studies have shown that ibuprofen does not affect cerebral blood flow, cerebral metabolic rates, or intestinal or renal hemodynamics. In fact, ibuprofen may enhance cerebral autoregulation and can protect neurologic function after oxidative stress.

Reference

1. Varvarigou A, et al: *JAMA* 275:539, 1996.

Case-control Study of Antenatal and Intrapartum Risk Factors for Cerebral Palsy in Very Preterm Singleton Babies
Murphy DJ, Sellers S, MacKenzie IZ, et al (Radcliffe Infirmary, Oxford, England; John Radcliffe NHS Trust, Oxford, England)
Lancet 346:1449–1454, 1995   1–14

Background.—Advances in neonatal intensive care in the 1980s led to an increase in the survival rate of very preterm infants. Unfortunately, a sharp increase in the rate of cerebral palsy among infants with birth weights of less than 1,500 g accompanied this increased survival. The relationship between antenatal and intrapartum variables and the occur-

TABLE 2.—Antenatal Variables Among Cases of Cerebral Palsy and Controls

Factor	Number of:		Odds ratio
	Cases (n=59)	Controls (n=234)	(95% CI) for cerebral palsy
Antenatal complications			
Prolonged rupture of membranes	25 (42%)	64 (27%)	2.3 (1.2–4.2)
Chorioamnionitis	10 (17%)	8 (3%)	4.2 (1.4–12.0)
Maternal infection	22 (37%)	40 (17%)	2.3 (1.2–4.5)
Antepartum haemorrhage	23 (40%)	72 (31%)	1.0 (0.5–1.8)
Abruptio placentae*	16 (27%)	35 (15%)	1.5 (0.7–3.0)
Pre-eclampsia	6 (10%)	56 (24%)	0.4 (0.2–0.9)
Antenatal treatment			
Antihypertensives	6 (10%)	51 (22%)	0.4 (0.2–1.0)
Steroids	2 (3%)†	15 (6%)	0.5 (0.1–2.3)
Antibiotics	10 (17%)	35 (15%)	1.2 (0.5–2.5)
Tocolytics	5 (8%)†	20 (9%)	1.0 (0.4–2.8)

*Severe (≥200 mL) hemorrhage after 20 weeks' gestation with at least 2 of the following: pain plus tense uterus, retroplacental clot at delivery, histologic evidence of abruption.

† Small numbers.

Abbreviation: CI, confidence interval.

(Courtesy of Murphy DJ, Sellers S, MacKenzie IZ, et al: Case-control study of antenatal and intrapartum risk factors for cerebral palsy in very preterm singleton babies. *Lancet* 346:1449–1454, Copyright by The Lancet Ltd., 1995.)

rence of cerebral palsy in this infant population has not been established. Adverse and protective antenatal and intrapartum factors were identified in a case-control study.

Methods.—The case patients were 59 infants born at less than 32 gestational weeks in whom cerebral palsy developed. The control group consisted of 234 infants of comparable gestational age who survived to hospital discharge and did not have cerebral palsy. Multiple births were excluded from the study. Fifty-two antenatal factors were investigated.

Findings.—As gestational age and birth weight increased among these infants, the frequency of cerebral palsy decreased. Seventy-three percent of the women had antenatal complications. After adjustment for gestational age, factors that were correlated with an increased risk of cerebral palsy included chorioamnionitis, with an odds ratio of 4.2; prolonged rupture of the membranes, with an odds ratio of 2.3; and maternal infection, with an odds ratio of 2.3. Pre-eclampsia and delivery without labor were correlated with a decreased risk of cerebral palsy (odds ratios 0.4 and 0.3, respectively). The risk of cerebral palsy was not increased in infants with intrauterine growth retardation (Table 2).

Conclusions.—These findings suggest several etiologic hypotheses about the development of cerebral palsy in very preterm infants, as well as possible preventive strategies. For example, rigorous management of common adverse antenatal factors may help reduce the frequency of cerebral palsy in the infant population. Well-designed, randomized, controlled trials should be done to test this hypothesis.

▶ Read this report in detail. There is more to it than meets the eye. My first reading left me cold. I found it difficult to believe that anyone was still reporting that the sharp rate of increase in number of cases of infants affected with cerebral palsy correlates with the proportion of very preterm infants who survive. No news there. A second reading of this report, however, showed that the story wasn't as simple. It seems that it isn't prematurity alone that is the problem. The specific disease entities causing preterm labor are the source of the problem. Of 52 antenatal factors associated with preterm births, prolonged rupture of membranes, maternal infection, and chorioamnionitis were significantly associated with an increased risk of cerebral palsy, after adjustment for the confounding effect of gestational age. A number of earlier studies have found that chorioamnionitis is present in preterm delivery in up to 50% of very low birth weight infants. Because cerebral palsy represents the end effect of infants who have sustained an in utero ischemic insult or an insult that occurred shortly after birth, it would seem imperative to see what the link might be with intrauterine infection. Current data also suggest that bacterial vaginosis is a major risk factor for prematurity itself.[1]

This report is important to all of us because it raises several possibilities that could be investigated to diminish the likelihood of cerebral palsy in association with preterm labor and delivery. It has been suggested that some pregnant women mount an excessive response to infection while they are pregnant by producing tumor necrosis factor (TNF), which results in disturbances to the fetal cerebral vasculature and causes fetal strokes, infarcts, and bleeds. It is known that TNF stimulates prostaglandin production, and it is possible that a combination of factors, including prostaglandins, contribute to disturbances in the cerebral vasculature of the developing brain. Increased prostaglandin E_2 concentration in fetal membranes has been found in association with very early preterm labor when chorioamnionitis is present. There are pharmacologic agents that affect, in a beneficial way, all of these mechanisms.

Thus, this report turns out to be quite important. Not only does it raise several hypotheses as to the cause of cerebral palsy, but it points to several possible preventive strategies. It's tempting to speculate that rigorous management of common antenatal factors, such as infection and the by-products of infection, could lead to a reduction in the frequency of cerebral palsy in preterm infants.

Reference

1. Hillier SL, et al: *N Engl J Med* 333:1737, 1995.

Predictors of Neonatal Encephalopathy in Full Term Infants

Adamson SJ, Alessandri LM, Badawi N, et al (Inst for Child Health Research, West Perth, Western Australia; Princess Margaret Hosp for Children, Subiacco, Western Australia)
BMJ 311:598–602, 1995

1–15

Background.—Few studies of the development of neonatal encephalopathy in unselected populations have considered the contribution of

TABLE 3.—Cases of Neonatal Encephalopathy With Possible Intrapartum Asphyxia

Case No.	Antepartum factors	Intrapartum factors	Others
		Cases with important contribution from antepartum events	
1	Pregnancy-induced hypertension	Spontaneous labor Severe shoulder dystocia 13 minutes to deliver baby Fresh meconium No cardiotocograph Apgar scores 0, 0, 0*	Adrenal hemorrhage Hematuria Large for gestational age (4,980 g) Neonatal death
2	Mother smoked 5–10 cigarettes a day Pregnancy-induced hypertension at 33 weeks Placental infarctions	Spontaneous labor No meconium Fetal bradycardia 45 minutes before delivery Apgar scores 1, 5, 6* Cord pH 6.7	
3	Pregnancy-induced hypertension at term	Induced because of pregnancy-induced hypertension Face presentation Pronounced dips and severe decelerations with no beat-to-beat variation; bradycardia 40 beats/min No meconium Apgar scores 0, 3, –*	
4	Mother smoked 20–30 cigarettes a day Chorioamnionitis	Occipitoposterior, spontaneous labor Wrigley's forceps Fresh meconium No cardiotocograph Apgar scores 0, 0, 2*	Neonatal death
5	Antepartum hemorrhage at 22 weeks	Spontaneous labor, failed vacuum, forceps delivery Bradycardia to 40 beats/min lasting 40 mins with decelerations Fresh meconium Apgar scores 1, 1, –*	Hematuria Oliguria Neonatal death

(Continued)

TABLE 3 (cont.)

Case No.	Antepartum factors	Intrapartum factors	Others
6	Mother smoked 10–15 cigarettes a day Mother intellectual disability Sibling intellectual disability *Trichomonas vaginalis* infection Decreased fetal movements Abnormal Cardiotocograms Presented on numerous occasions for decreased fetal movements Abdominal trauma Suspicion of substance abuse Calcified placenta	Induced at 40 weeks Meconium Baseline bradycardia Apgar scores 1, 3, ⁻* Cord pH 7.37 BE +2	Neonatal death
7	Breech Failed external cephalic version 2 weeks before birth	Spontaneous labor Bradycardia in second stage No meconium Apgar scores 1, 4, 7*	
8	Hereditary bleeding disorder Crohn's disease Hospitalized for threatened preterm labor at 32 weeks Mild hypertension Calcified placenta Iris coloboma in baby	Induced for postterm and mild hypertension Vacuum delivery for maternal distress and failure to progress Meconium No cardiotocograph Apgar scores 2, 3, 10*	

Cases with important contribution from intrapartum events

Case No.	Antepartum factors	Intrapartum factors	Others
9	Two urinary tract infections	Spontaneous labor Meconium Bradycardia for 18 minutes Vacuum extraction after nonelective cesarean section refused Apgar scores 1, 2, 3*	Renal failure Coagulopathy Subgaleal bleed Syndrome of inappropriate antidiuretic hormone secretion

Case No.	Antepartum factors	Intrapartum factors	Others
10	Urinary tract infection at 28 weeks	Induced at 40 weeks Profound prolonged maternal hypotension, baby delivered with high forceps Bradycardia No meconium Apgar scores 1, 2, 3*	Depressed fracture left frontal bone Left facial palsy
11	No abnormality detected	Spontaneous labor Cord tight around the neck Meconium No cardiotocograph Apgar scores 0, 4, 6*	Placenta showed pronounced vascular congestion probably caused by an acute intrapartum event
12	No abnormality detected	Induced for post dates Forceps delivery for cord prolapse Large decelerations for bradycardia for 16 minutes Meconium Apgar scores 1, 2, 4* Cord pH 7.28	Acute renal failure Neonatal death
13	Decreased fetal movements day before delivery with nonreactive nonstress test†	Induced due to decreased fetal movements Meconium staining at artificial rupture of membranes Low-lying placenta Vasa praevia Intrapartum hemorrhage of 400 ml 30 minutes before delivery by nonelective cesarean section Bradycardia 70 beats/min after the antepartum hemorrhage Apgar scores 1, 2, 4* Cord pH 6.778 BE–15 · 8	Transient acute renal failure

*Apgar scores measured at 1, 5, and 10 minutes.
†Despite presence of antepartum factors in this case, it is included in this group because the vasa praevia with intrapartum hemorrhage could account for the encephalopathy in its own right.
(Courtesy of Adamson SJ, Alessandri LM, Badawi N, et al: Predictors of neonatal encephalopathy in full term infants. *BMJ* 311:598–602, 1995.)

causes other than intrapartum hypoxia. The contribution of factors in family and maternal history, pregnancy, and birth to encephalopathic features was investigated in full-term newborn infants.

Methods.—All 89 full-term singleton neonates born in an 8-month period in 1992 fulfilling 1 or more of 6 criteria during the first week of life were studied. These criteria were seizures, abnormal conscious state, persistent hypertonia or hypotonia, and feeding or respiratory difficulties of central origin. Each case infant was matched to 1 control infant by sex, hospital of delivery, time of day and day of the week of birth, and maternal health insurance status.

Findings.—In the first week of life, the estimated incidence of moderate or severe encephalopathy was 3.75 per 1,000 full-term live births. Thirteen infants with encephalopathy and none of those without it showed evidence of important intrapartum hypoxia (Table 3). The neurologic condition at birth was attributed to events during the intrapartum period in only 5 of these infants. In a univariate conditional logistic regression analysis, there were significant between-group differences in maternal vaginal bleeding during pregnancy, maternal thyroxine treatment, congenital abnormalities, labor induction, interval between membrane rupture and delivery, maternal pyrexia in labor, augmentation of labor, abnormal intrapartum cardiotocograms, and meconium in labor. A family history of convulsions approached statistical significance between groups.

Conclusions.—Intrapartum hypoxia is apparently not the cause of neonatal encephalopathy in most patients in this population. Many of the causes of neonatal encephalopathy seem to originate in the antepartum period.

▶ There has only recently been a challenge to the concept of what causes neonatal encephalopathy. The assumption that most neonatal encephalopathy is caused by "intrapartum asphyxia" has served to maintain the impetus for the high level of obstetric intervention in labor. These interventions may have little or no influence on encephalopathy because of factors other than hypoxia, but they are associated with an appreciable degree of maternal and infant morbidity. The assumption that hypoxia is the singular significant cause of neonatal encephalopathy is the prime ingredient in most obstetric litigation these days. If the results of this study hold up, we will probably have to change our thinking because the preliminary findings suggest that intrapartum hypoxia, according to currently used criteria, is not the cause of most neonatal encephalopathy. The recipe of causes has so many ingredients that it really is not possible to tease out any single one as the bad actor when it comes to neonatal brain difficulties.

In the order of causes of neonatal encephalopathy, hypoxia is potentially well down on the list (a contributor in only 6% of cases). Maternal vaginal bleeding, fever during labor, and a longer interval between membrane rupture and delivery are associated with neonatal encephalopathy. Fetal sepsis is as well.

The results of this study have implications for pediatricians, obstetricians, and legal practitioners. With hypoxia on the sidelines, it becomes incumbent on all of us to look for other causes of neonatal encephalopathy, hopefully preventable or treatable ones. One clue to whether intracranial hemorrhage has occurred has recently been defined. Blood lactate levels are almost twice as high in such patients.[1]

Reference

1. Grayck EN, et al: *Pediatrics* 96:914, 1995.

Antimicrobial Therapy in Expectant Management of Preterm Premature Rupture of the Membranes

Mercer BM, Arheart KL (Univ of Tennessee, Memphis)
Lancet 346:1271–1279, 1995   1–16

Background.—Isolated case reports suggest that antimicrobial treatment may be effective in preterm premature rupture of the membranes (pPROM) before 37 weeks' gestation. A number of clinical trials have also been done to assess the efficacy of this treatment. The available prospective clinical trials were reviewed to determine the impact of antimicrobial therapy and fetal outcome during expectant management of pPROM.

Methods.—Three databases were searched: MEDLINE, from 1966 to 1994; Excerpta Medica, from 1972 to 1994; and the Cochrane database of systemic reviews. Unpublished data from a randomized, placebo-controlled clinical trial of ceftizoxime were also reviewed. Studies selected for review were randomized controlled trials of systemic antimicrobial treatment for prolongation of gestation in nonlaboring women after pPROM.

Data Synthesis.—Antimicrobial treatment after pPROM was associated with a decrease in the number of women delivering within 1 week and in the diagnosis of maternal morbidity, including chorioamnionitis and postpartum infection. In addition, fetal diagnoses of confirmed sepsis, pneumonia, and intraventricular hemorrhage were less common. In a separate analysis of the 6 placebo-controlled trials, the odds of pregnancy prolongation, chorioamnionitis, neonatal sepsis, postpartum infection, positive infant blood cultures, and pneumonia were similar or improved.

Conclusions.—Antimicrobial treatment in the expectant management of pPROM prolongs pregnancy and reduces the diagnosis of maternal and infant morbidity. Additional research should focus on determining optimal antimicrobial therapy, increasing pregnancy prolongation, and enhancing corticosteroid therapy for the induction of pulmonary maturity after pPROM.

▶ One more report showing that infection may precede premature rupture of membranes and therefore is a major cause of preterm delivery before 37 weeks' gestation. Although previous isolated case reports have suggested that antibiotic therapy might be useful in treating intrauterine infection related to premature rupture of membranes, this is the only study that summarizes a 30-year body of literature of all available prospective clinical trials demonstrating the impact of antibiotic therapy on fetal outcome as related to the management of premature rupture of membranes. There is a beneficial effect from antibiotics that allows some pregnancies to continue. What this study does not show is whether antibiotic therapy reduces the severity of complications among infants who do have perinatal morbidity. It doesn't indicate the optimal route and duration of antibiotic therapy in the management of women seen with premature rupture of membranes. It doesn't point out which subpopulation of women with this problem is more likely to benefit from antibiotic treatment. Lastly, it doesn't give a clue as to whether tocolytic therapy can be used to prolong pregnancy, allowing time for antibiotics to work.

Despite all of these unanswered questions, antibiotics are a promising adjunctive therapy for the expectant management of premature rupture of membranes. They allow nature to keep some infants where they should be for a few more days or weeks.

Remember the Gallo vineyards motto: "no wine before its time"; the same applies to newborns.

Uncertain Value of Electronic Fetal Monitoring in Predicting Cerebral Palsy
Nelson KB, Dambrosia JM, Ting TY, et al (Natl Inst of Neurological Disorders and Stroke, Bethesda, Md; Howard Hughes Med Inst, Bethesda, Md; Univ of Pennsylvania, Philadelphia; et al)
N Engl J Med 334:613–618, 1996   1–17

Introduction.—Electronic fetal monitoring was introduced in the hope of preventing birth injuries caused by hypoxia or asphyxia and thus reducing the frequency of cerebral palsy and mental retardation. The widespread use of fetal monitoring has probably contributed to the rising rate of cesarean section; however, there has been no accompanying decrease in the incidence of cerebral palsy. There are few reliable data on whether specific fetal heart rate patterns detectd by electronic monitoring are useful in predicting long-term neurologic outcomes. The value of fetal monitoring in predicting the diagnosis of cerebral palsy was evaluated in a population-based study.

Methods.—The subjects were drawn from a population of nearly 156,000 children born in 4 California counties in a 2-year period. Ninety-five children with moderate to severe cerebral palsy who survived to 3 years of age and had birth weights of no less than 2,500 g were identified. They were compared with 378 randomly selected controls; 78 of the children with cerebral palsy and 300 of the control children had intrapartum fetal monitoring. The results of fetal monitoring were analyzed in terms of the interpretations made at the time by the attending physicians. Known risk factors for cerebral palsy, including vaginal bleeding during pregnancy, breech presentation, meconium in the amniotic fluid, gestational age less than 37 weeks, and maternal infection, were evaluated for univariate association with cerebral palsy and with electronic fetal monitoring abnormalities.

Results.—Certain fetal monitoring characteristics were associated with an elevated risk of cerebral palsy. These were multiple late decelerations in the heart rate, i.e., heart rate slowing well after the start of uterine contractions, odds ratio (OR) 3.9; and decreased beat-to-beat variability, OR 2.7. Cerebral palsy was unrelated to the highest or lowest recorded fetal heart rate. After adjustment for other risk factors, fetal monitoring abnormalities were still associated with an elevated risk of cerebral palsy, OR 2.7. The previously identified risk factors were significantly associated with cerebral palsy.

However, the fetal monitoring abnormalities identified were not present in all children with cerebral palsy and were present in many children without cerebral palsy. Although 21 children with cerebral palsy had multiple late decelerations or decreased heart rate variability, they accounted for only 0.19% of all infants in the study population with these findings. The associated false negative rate was therefore 99.8%.

Conclusions.—Although certain fetal heart rate abnormalities are associated with an increased risk of cerebral palsy, the vast majority of infants with these findings will not go on to have cerebral palsy. If these abnormalities were used as indications for cesarean section, many such deliveries would be performed with no benefit but with significant risk to the mother. The emphasis on the rare outcome of cerebral palsy may be distracting attention from other important factors that could lead to injury or maldevelopment of the infant brain.

▶ Any obstetrician who has lost a malpractice suit on the basis of a pregnancy and delivery that resulted in a child with evidence of cerebral palsy, a child who was the product of a pregnancy associated with multiple late decelerations or decreased variability in heart rate, should ask for his or her money back. This impressive report from the National Institute of Neurologic Disorders and Stroke shows how statistics should be used to put this problem into perspective. Yes, specific abnormalities on electronic monitoring of the fetal heart are associated with an increased risk of cerebral palsy. No, one cannot use these in any effective way to make decisions about cesarean section largely because the false positive rate is so high. (This editor has never seen a report where a false positive rate was higher.) Only 0.19% of infants exhibiting these types of findings are subsequently shown to have evidence of cerebral palsy. To perform a cesarean section on 100% of such babies means that 998 out of 1,000 were not benefited by the procedure. Is this good and effective medical care?

This is a very complex topic to say the least. Readers of the YEAR BOOK OF PEDIATRICS are encouraged to read the commentary on this *New England Journal of Medicine* article, a commentary by Dermot MacDonald. Dr. MacDonald closes his commentary with the following words, "Despite intensive care obstetrics of the last 25 years, with increasing attention directed to prenatal care, reduction of birth trauma, and greater use of cesarean section for high-risk deliveries, the frequency of cerebral palsy remains unchanged at about two cases per 1,000 term infants. There is a pressing need to inform the public, as well as the medical and legal professions, that cerebral palsy is not often caused by the events during labor and that the cause in most cases remains unknown."[1] Dr. MacDonald says it all.

Reference

1. MacDonald D: *N Engl J Med* 334:659, 1996.

Prolonged Episodes of Hypoxemia in Preterm Infants Undetectable by Cardiorespiratory Monitors
Poets CF, Stebbens VA, Richard D, et al (Children's Hosp, Hannover, Germany; Univ of Keele, Stoke-on-Trent, England; Transvaal Provincial Hosps, Johannesburg, South Africa)
Pediatrics 95:860–863, 1995   1–18

Background.—Although continuous monitoring of oxygenation is typically performed only in preterm infants receiving additional inspired oxygen and/or intermittent positive pressure ventilation, apnea, bradycardia, and hypoxemia commonly develop in preterm infants breathing room air, for whom monitoring is usually limited to surveillance of breathing movements and/or heart rates. However, few studies have investigated whether cardiorespiratory monitors reliably detect episodic hypoxemia in preterm infants. Whether episodes of prolonged hypoxemia occur in the absence of prolonged apneic pauses and bradycardia in preterm infants who appear well was determined.

Methods.—Ninety-six infants born at 28–36 weeks' gestation, with a median of 34 weeks, were assessed. Long-term recordings of arterial oxygen saturation were measured by pulse oximetry, photoplethysmographic waveforms from the oximeter, and breathing movements. Recordings were begun at a median age of 4 days.

Findings.—During a median recording duration of 25 hours, 15 infants had 88 episodes in which pulse oximetry dropped to 80% or less, remaining there for 20 seconds or longer. The median duration of these desaturations was 27 seconds. In 73 episodes, or 83%, pulse oximetry continued to decline to 60% or less. Twenty-three desaturations were associated with prolonged apneic pauses, and 54 were associated with bradycardia. Nineteen of these were related to both apnea and bradycardia. Thirty-four percent of the desaturations occurred without bradycardia or prolonged apnea.

Conclusions.—Some apparently well preterm infants have episodes of severe, prolonged hypoxemia unassociated with prolonged apneic pauses or bradycardia. Episodes such as these would be difficult to detect by the monitoring of only breathing movements and heart rate. Thus, indications for oxygenation monitoring in preterm infants need to be reconsidered.

▶ It's pretty unusual for a nursery in the United States to do anything other than use monitoring of breathing movement and heart rate in infants breathing room air. Continuous monitoring of oxygenation generally is done only in preterm infants who are receiving additional inspired oxygen and/or intermittent positive pressure ventilation. This study challenges the concept that apnea monitors and heart rate monitors can detect all episodes of significant hypoxemia. The findings are dramatic. Ten percent of apparently well preterm infants had prolonged episodes of hypoxemia (oxygen saturations of less than 80%) lasting as long as 81 seconds and saturations less than 60% for periods of up to 36 seconds. These episodes were not accompanied by apnea or bradycardia.

If you are an aficionado of the medical literature, you will quickly recognize that the findings of this report are not new. Peabody et al.,[1] some 17 years ago, noted the failure of conventional monitoring to detect apnea resulting in hypoxemia. Unfortunately, this message of the late 1970s has been lost somewhere. Clearly, hypoxemia of the severity and duration observed in the present study, particularly if occurring repetitively, can be harmful. Repeated episodes of hypoxemia have been identified as risk factors for several diseases to which preterm infants are particularly liable, such as retinopathy of prematurity, necrotizing enterocolitis, and periventricular leukomalacia. Recurrent hypoxemia, when reflecting airway hypoxia, also may increase the resistance of pulmonary blood vessels and airways and thus may lead to further impairments in gas exchange in patients who are already vulnerable.

For all these reasons, the early detection of episodic hypoxemia in preterm infants seems to be of clinical importance. The results of this, and earlier studies, suggest that such detection cannot be reliably achieved by means of cardiorespiratory monitoring alone. As important as this message is, it produces a real dilemma for many nurseries because this report seems to recommend the monitoring of oxygenation in all hospitalized preterm infants. There are not enough monitors in most nurseries to do this. If resources are limited, as is frequently the case, the authors suggest that oxygenation should be monitored in at least those infants who are known to have recurrent apnea and/or are born at less than 32 weeks' gestation and have a postconceptional age of less than 36 weeks.

Preterm infants are crazy little creatures. There is probably not another mammal on earth that can look so terribly good with an oxygen saturation of less than 60%. It just goes to show that appearances can be deceiving.

Reference

1. Peabody JL, et al: *Birth Defects* 15:276, 1979.

Association Between Duration of Neonatal Hospital Stay and Readmission Rate

Lee K-S, Perlman M, Ballantyne M, et al (Hosp for Sick Children, Toronto; Women's College Hosp, Toronto; Univ of Toronto; et al)
J Pediatr 127:758–766, 1995   1–19

Objective.—Recently the duration of neonatal hospital stays in Ontario, Canada, declined; at the same time, the number of infants admitted from home to the hospital within 2 weeks after birth increased. Hospital discharge data for Ontario were reviewed during a 7-year period to determine whether these observations reflect a regional trend.

Study Population.—Both population-based and single hospital–based reviews were conducted, comprising 920,554 healthy infants born in Ontario during 1987–1994 whose birth weight was at least 2,500 g. Infants born during the same time who were readmitted to the Hospital for Sick Children before age 15 days for jaundice or dehydration were specifically reviewed.

Findings.—The mean length of stay for healthy newborn infants in Ontario decreased from 4.5 to 2.7 days during the 7-year period under review. The rate of readmission in the first 2 weeks of life increased from 12.9 to 20.7 per 1,000. Readmissions for jaundice in the first week of life increased as the neonatal length of stay declined (Fig). Jaundice accounted for approximately one third of all 2-week readmissions in 1987–1988, and for half in 1993–1994 (Table 2). Infants readmitted for jaundice had increasingly higher serum bilirubin levels during the years under review,

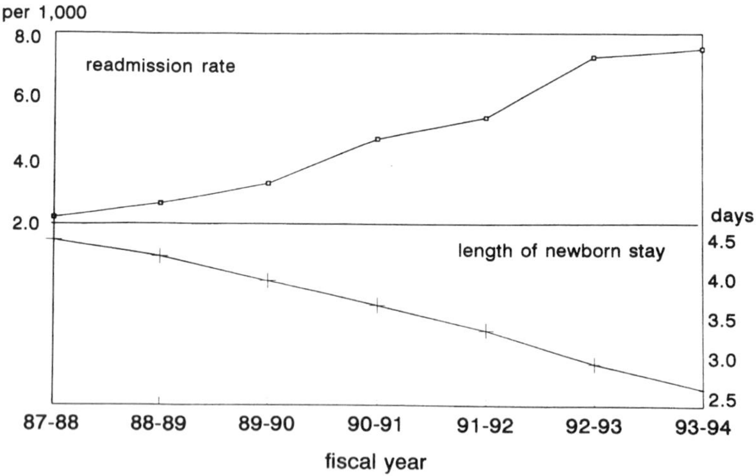

FIGURE.—Association between duration of newborn stay and first-week readmission rate for jaundice. (Courtesy of Lee K-S, Perlman M, Ballantyne M, et al: Association between duration of neonatal hospital stay and readmission rate. *J Pediatr* 127:758–766, 1995.)

TABLE 2.—Readmission Rates at Age 14 Days or Younger for Specific Diagnostic Groups (per 1,000 Healthy Newborn Infants)

	1987–1988	1988–1989	1989–1990	1990–1991	1991–1992	1992–1993	1993–1994	P*	OR (95% CI)†
Jaundice	3.3	3.6	4.7	6.5	6.9	9.0	9.3	0.000‡	2.80 (2.50, 3.14)
Dehydration	0.07	0.09	0.17	0.15	0.27	0.35	0.58	0.000‡	7.84 (3.81, 16.73)
Lower bowel obstruction	0.11	0.06	0.08	0.08	0.11	0.12	0.14	0.057	1.37 (0.63, 3.02)
Defect, left side of heart	0.10	0.08	0.15	0.13	0.10	0.20	0.14	0.079	1.37 (0.63, 3.02)
Defect, right side of heart	0.12	0.07	0.07	0.06	0.10	0.17	0.12	0.081	1.05 (0.48, 2.26)
Remaining diagnoses	9.2	8.8	8.8	9.4	9.8	10.4	10.7	0.000‡	1.16 (1.07, 1.26)
All diagnoses	12.9	12.8	13.9	16.3	17.2	20.2	20.7	0.000‡	1.61 (1.52, 1.72)

* Chi-square test for linear trend in binomial proportions.
† Rate in 1987–1988 used as the reference, the odds ratio for the rate in 1993–1994.
‡ Statistically significant.
(Courtesy of Lee K-S, Perlman M, Ballantyne M, et al: Association between duration of neonatal hospital stay and readmission rate. *J Pediatr* 127:758–766, 1995.)

and those readmitted for dehydration had higher serum sodium levels. Two infants died of hypernatremic dehydration during 1992–1994.

Conclusion.—In Ontario, shorter neonatal hospital stays have been associated with more early readmissions for jaundice or dehydration. Discharge decisions should rest on careful assessment of the individual infant.

▶ This is another report in the debate about the ideal duration of neonatal hospital stay. Very few seem to be without opinion in this regard. Take, for example, the commentary by Downs and Loda that accompanied this article.[1] They comment: "The interest of legislators in setting health policy may disturb physicians, but it may be a needed counterbalance at this time to the zeal of those who view cost reduction as the highest priority. At the same time, health care providers need to use this opportunity to identify the best approaches to reducing neonatal risk at the lowest cost consistent with patient safety."

These commentators also note that no "magic" time of discharge will ever be identified that will relieve the physician of the responsibility of weighing all the variables that determine the risk of sending an infant home. Some of these variables include discharge of infants who will, if breast-fed, not do well and become dehydrated. There is a risk of jaundice being missed. There is a risk that neonatal screening may be performed in a less-than-adequate way. For example, only 48% of institutions that discharge the majority of their infants by 24 hours of age have mandatory rescreening of these infants. Without rescreening, detecting phenylketonuria will be a problem. A similar dilemma exists for newborn screening for congenital hypothyroidism. When the blood test is performed within the first day, the surge of maternal thyroid hormone obscures the accuracy of the newborn test. Many suspect that there will be more children with subclinical hypothyroidism and possibly significantly lower intelligence quotients as a result of misdiagnosis in a genetic screening that is performed too early.

To read more on the topic of early discharge, see the overviews by Charles and Prystowsky and the recommendations of the American Academy of Pediatrics Committee on Fetus and Newborn.[2,3]

When the pendulum finally stops swinging regarding the most appropriate time for neonatal hospital discharge, there probably will be a reemergence of the debate about midwives and infants being birthed at home, a dialogue that should not happen. Infants are put at too serious a risk. Remember, home delivery is for pizza.

References

1. Downs SM, Loda F: *J Pediatr* 127:736, 1995.
2. Charles S, Prystowsky B: *Pediatrics* 96:746, 1995.
3. Committee on Fetus and Newborn: *Pediatrics* 96:788, 1995.

2 Infectious Disease and Immunology

Trends in Infectious Diseases Mortality in the United States
Pinner RW, Teutsch SM, Simonsen L, et al (Natl Ctr for Infectious Diseases, Ctrs for Disease Control and Prevention, Atlanta, Ga)
JAMA 275:189–193, 1996   2–1

Background.—The occurrence of infectious diseases has not waned in the United States, as was once predicted. Numerous reports of the emergence and reemergence of such diseases have appeared. Trends in deaths from infectious diseases between 1980 and 1992 were investigated.

Methods.—A scheme was developed for assessing the burden of infectious diseases in data sources using the *International Classification of Diseases, Ninth Revision* (ICD-9) to classify diseases. Data were obtained on all individuals dying of infectious diseases between 1980 and 1992 in the United States.

Findings.—The number of deaths from infectious diseases increased from 41 to 65 per 100,000 population between 1980 and 1992. This was a 58% increase. Age-adjusted mortality caused by infectious diseases increased by 39% during that time. Death rates increased 25% among patients aged 65 years and older with infectious diseases. Among individuals aged 25–44 years, the increase was 6.3-fold. Death from respiratory tract infections increased by 20%, from 25 to 30 deaths per 100,000 population. In 1992, the incidence of deaths from HIV was 13 per 100,000, compared with none in 1980. The rate of death from septicemia increased from 4.2 to 7.7 per 100,000—an 83% increase (Fig 3).

Conclusions.—The rate of death from infectious disease has risen by more than 50% since 1980. Age-adjusted infectious disease mortality has risen by 39%. In 1992, infectious disease was the third leading cause of death in the United States.

▶ One of the cornerstones of pediatric care is a knowledge of infectious diseases. Despite this, it wasn't that long ago that many predicted that a subspecialty of pediatric infectious diseases would never mature to reality because from every perspective it appeared that infectious diseases would wane in this country and elsewhere. Immunizations, better antibiotics, and

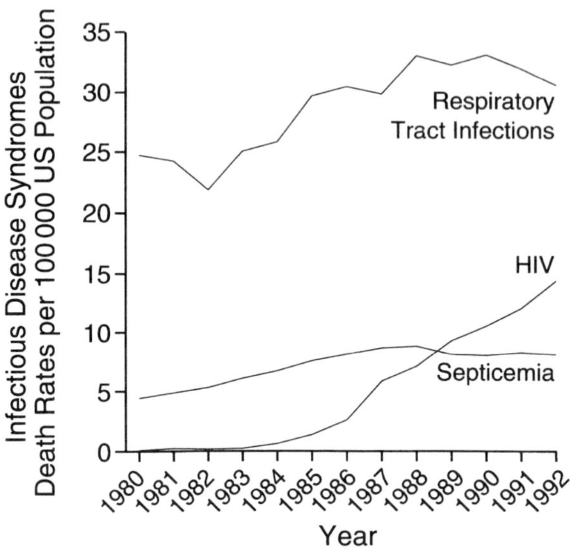

FIGURE 3.—Trends in deaths per 100,000 population caused by leading infectious disease syndromes in the United States between 1980 and 1992. From National Center for Health Statistics underlying cause-of-death data. (Courtesy of Pinner RW, Teutsch SM, Simonsen L, et al: Trends in infectious diseases mortality in the United States. *JAMA* 275:189–193, Copyright 1996, American Medical Association.)

antiviral therapies surely would do the trick. Well, apparently they haven't. Look what's happened in the last 10 years alone. We've seen the continuing emergence of HIV infection. A previously unrecognized hantavirus has caused an outbreak of fatal respiratory illness in the American Southwest. Contamination of a public water supply with *Cryptosporidium* was responsible for an outbreak that caused more than 400,000 cases of diarrhea and resulted in more than 4,000 hospitalizations in Milwaukee. The more recent outbreak of Ebola hemorrhagic fever in Zaire infected hundreds, with an 80% mortality rate. The outbreak of plague in India in 1994 even raised the potential possibility of importation of this disease into the United States. Without even including AIDS, death rates caused by infectious diseases have increased rather than decreased in the last couple of decades, as this report documents.

At the turn of this millennium, most would have hoped that the vast majority of infectious diseases would have been gone but not forgotten. They are neither forgotten nor gone. It is very clear that those factors that influence the emergence of infectious diseases need to be better understood. Factors such as increasing population size and age, decreasing age ("micropremieism"), changes in behaviors, and rapid changes in technology and industry are all creating new niches for microbial pathogens and have contributed to recent increases in infectious diseases mortality in the United States.

Humans, including infectious disease experts, are pretty smart. Bugs are pretty smart, too. Worse yet, they're more adaptable to change than we are.

Predicting the Risk of Bacteremia in Children With Fever and Neutropenia

Rackoff WR, Gonin R, Robinson C, et al (James Whitcomb Riley Hosp for Children, Indianapolis, Ind; Indiana Univ, Indianapolis)

J Clin Oncol 14:919–924, 1996   2–2

Background.—Children with suspected infectious complications of neutropenia are routinely treated with broad-spectrum IV antibiotics as inpatients. Identification of patients at low risk of bacteremia would reduce hospitalization and antibiotic use. Therefore, patients with neutropenic fever were studied prospectively to identify risk factors for bacteremia.

Methods.—All children admitted with fever and neutropenia during a 10-month period were studied. The data available at admission were analyzed in those with or without positive blood cultures with univariate and multiple logistic regression analysis to identify factors significantly associated with bacteremia. Fifty-seven episodes of neutropenic fever were studied retrospectively to validate the resulting predictive model for the risk of bacteremia.

Results.—During the prospective study period, 115 episodes of neutropenic fever were treated in 72 children with cancer. A positive blood culture was initially found in 24 of these 115 episodes. Although the mean admission absolute neutrophil count was not significantly associated with bacteremia, the mean admission absolute monocyte count (AMoC) was significantly higher in patients with than without bacteremia. Multiple logistic regression analysis revealed only 2 significant predictors of bacteremia: admission AMoC and admission temperature. Using a recursive partitioning model, cutpoint values were established for the various risk levels as follows: low risk was defined by an AMoC of at least 100/µL; intermediate risk was defined by an AMoC of less than 100/µL and a temperature at admission of less than 39°C; and high risk was defined by an AMoC of less than 100/µL and a temperature higher than 39°C (Table 4). In the validation group of 57 episodes of neutropenia fever, no bacteremia occurred in the low-risk group as defined by the predictive model, whereas progressively higher rates of bacteremia occurred in the intermediate-risk (4%) and high-risk (43%) groups.

Discussion.—The relative risk of bacteremia may be determined by the patient's monocyte count and temperature at admission. It is possible that patients in the low-risk group and with no other indications for hospitalization could be treated with a single IV dose of a long-acting broad-spectrum antibiotic with outpatient treatment and patients in the intermediate-risk group could be given initial inpatient IV antibiotic treatment with early discharge. Further study is needed to determine the safety and efficacy of these strategies.

▶ Predicting which child with fever and neutropenia is at risk of bacteremia and which is not is a problem that all of us have faced. The pursuit of factors that predict bacteremia has followed a tortuous pathway. For ex-

TABLE 4.—Characteristics of Episodes Grouped by Risk for Bacteremia

Risk Group	Total Episodes		Risk Group With Bacteremia		Risk Group With Other Reason for Hospital Admission*		Median Days From Admission Until ANC $\geq 100/\mu L$
	No.	%	No.	%	No.	%	
Low							
AMoC $\geq 100/\mu L$							
Any temperature	19/115	17	0/19	0	3/19	16	2.0
Intermediate							
AMoC $< 100/\mu L$							
Temperature $< 39°C$	75/115	65	14/75	19	18/75	24	6.0
High							
AMoC $< 100/\mu L$							
Temperature $\geq 39°C$	21/115	18	10/21	48	10/21	48	6.0

* Diagnosis of acute myeloid leukemia, positive finding on chest radiograph, rectal abscess, central venous catheter tunnel tract infection, severe mucositis, septic/ill appearance, cellulitis, or the need for an IV fluid bolus.

Abbreviations: ANC, absolute neutrophil count; *AMoC,* absolute monocyte count.

(Courtesy of Rackoff WR, Gonin R, Robinson C, et al: Predicting the risk of bacteremia in children with fever and neutropenia. *J Clin Oncol* 14:919–924, 1996.)

ample, Pizzo et al.[1] were unable to define any predictor that adequately differentiated the child who was going to get into trouble with fever and neutropenia from the one who was not. Even those who have thought that they had figured this problem out have had the rules change under them. For example, one would think that the use of progressively higher doses of chemotherapy in recent years would result in more frequent and prolonged periods of neutropenia, but with the introduction of granulocyte and granulocyte macrophage colony-stimulating factors (G-CSF and GM-CSF), chemotherapy-induced episodes of neutropenia have become much shorter in duration. For these reasons, it does seem appropriate to take another look at whether one can define risk factors for bacteremia in those who are neutropenic. This is exactly what these authors did.

What the authors found in this study is pretty straightforward. The greatest predictor of being bacteremic is the admission absolute monocyte count, not just the neutrophil count. Recall that the presence of monocytes is a fairly accurate early predictor of bone marrow recovery and that children who have no neutrophils, but who have some monocytes ($\geq 100/\mu L$) are soon to be out of the woods.

If the results of this study are validated, it may be possible to design studies to determine whether outpatient antibiotics can be safely used in those at low risk for bacteremia. Such an approach for this potentially life-threatening complication of cancer chemotherapy would achieve the goals of better quality of life and lower cost of medical care while providing appropriate levels of treatment for those at highest risk of bacteremia.

A closing comment about drawing blood: Do you know what a swaboholic is? A swaboholic is a person who believes in the use of alcohol-soaked swabs. If you are a swaboholic, you may become a member of a vanishing species, because recent data have shown that there is no value whatsoever in routinely swabbing the skin with alcohol before a venipuncture.[2] Similar studies have shown that giving injections without skin preparation does not cause local or systemic infections.[3] Swabs are a potential health hazard because they are frequently used to stem a bleeding point, allowing patients' blood to soak through the wafer-thin pads onto a user's fingers.

It is perplexing to find that most health care professionals continue to use the alcohol swab even though swabbing for a few seconds has no useful function that has ever been documented. Read what Liauw and Archer say about alcohol swabs: "When a procedure has been shown to have no scientific foundation and might be a potential hazard, it should be discontinued. To persist with this archaic ritual is illogical and reflects the difficulty in altering long-standing routine practices. Modern medicine should reflect the appliance of science and, therefore, we recommend the routine use of alcohol swabs be abandoned."[4]

Great recommendation! (But try to explain that to parents as you approach their children with a needle without first cleaning their skin.)

References

1. Pizzo PA, et al: *Medicine* 61:163, 1982.

2. Malathi I, et al: *Arch Dis Child* 69:312, 1993.
3. Dann TC, et al: *Lancet* ii:96, 1969.
4. Liauw J, et al: *Lancet* 345:1648, 1995.

Efficacy of an Observation Scale in Detecting Bacteremia in Febrile Children Three to Thirty-six Months of Age, Treated as Outpatients
Teach SJ, and the Occult Bacteremia Study Group (Children's Hosp of Buffalo, NY; et al)
J Pediatr 126:877–881, 1995   2–3

Background.—The Yale Observation Scale (YOS) is a 6-point clinical assessment system designed for the detection of bacteremia in young, febrile patients (Table 1). It has proven useful in identifying febrile children with the most toxic illness and those with serious illness. Its ability to detect occult bacteremia was evaluated in febrile children with no apparent signs or symptoms of severe infection and with no focal infection.

Methods.—The study included 6,611 children, aged 3–36 months, with a temperature of at least 39.0°C and a nonfocal, nontoxic-appearing illness—or uncomplicated otitis media—who were being treated on an outpatient basis. All underwent both YOS scoring and blood culture as part of a prospective, multicenter, randomized trial of oral and IM antibiotics to prevent complications of occult bacteremia.

Results.—One hundred ninety-two children had bacteremia. The median YOS score was 6 for patients with and without bacteremia. However, the mean rank by Mann-Whitney U test was significantly greater for patients with bacteremia. A YOS score of greater than 10 had a sensitivity of 5.2%, a specificity of 96.7%, a positive predictive value of 4.5%, and a negative predictive value of 97.1% in detecting occult bacteremia (Table 2).

Conclusions.—Febrile children with occult bacteremia have higher YOS scores than those without bacteremia. However, the YOS is not clinically useful in detecting occult bacteremia among febrile pediatric outpatients with nonfocal, apparently nontoxic infection.

▶ Everybody wants to know the score. Everybody. If these data are correct, however, knowing the YOS score isn't going to help you figure out which infant with a high fever, who otherwise looks well, has bacteremia. To be fair about this, realize that the YOS was never intended to be used for this purpose. A little background explanation is in order.

In 1980, McCarthy et al.,[1] in New Haven, developed and applied a 6-point clinical assessment system for febrile children that has come to be known as the YOS (see Table 1). This scale has been validated to demonstrate its ability in identifying those febrile children who have the most toxic illness or who are otherwise seriously ill. The current study is an attempt to extend the principles of objective assessment of McCarthy et al. to a narrower

TABLE 1.—Yale Observation Scales

Observation	Normal (1 point)	Moderate Impairment (3 points)	Severe Impairment (5 points)
Quality of cry	Strong with normal tone *or* content and not crying	Whimpering *or* sobbing	Weak *or* moaning *or* high-pitched
Reaction to parent stimulation	Cries briefly then stops *or* content and not crying	Cries off and on	Continual cry *or* hardly responds
State variation	If awake, stays awake, *or* if asleep and stimulated, wakes up quickly	Eyes close briefly, then awakes *or* awakes with prolonged stimulation	Falls to sleep *or* will not arouse
Color	Pink	Pale extremities *or* acrocyanosis	Pale *or* cyanotic *or* mottled *or* ashen
Hydration	Skin and eyes normal *and* mucous membranes moist	Skin and eyes normal *and* mouth slightly dry	Skin doughy *or* tented *and* dry mucous membranes *and/or* sunken eyes
Response (talk, smile) to social overtures	Smiles *or* alerts (≤2 mo)	Smiles briefly *or* alert briefly (≤2 mo)	No smile, face anxious, dull, expressionless, *or* not alerted (≤2 mo)

(From Teach SJ, and the Occult Bacteremia Study Group: Efficacy of an observation scale in detecting bacteremia in febrile children three to thirty-six months of age, treated as outpatients. *J Pediatr* 126:877–881, 1995. Courtesy of McCarthy PL, Lembo RM, Baron MA, et al: Predictive value of abnormal physical examination findings in ill-appearing and well-appearing febrile children. Reproduced by permission of *Pediatrics*, Vol 76, page 167, Copyright 1985.)

TABLE 2.—Efficacy of an Elevated YOS Score in Detecting Occult Bacteremia in a Cohort of 6,611 Febrile Patients, 3–36 Months of Age

YOS Score	Patients With Bacteremia		Patients Without Bacteremia		Sensitivity (%)	Specificity (%)	PPV (%)	NPV (%)
	No.	%	No.	%				
> 6	55	28.6	1122	17.5	28.6	82.5	4.7	97.4
> 8	32	16.7	522	8.1	16.7	91.9	5.8	97.3
> 10	10	5.2	210	3.3	5.2	96.7	4.5	97.1
> 12	1	0.5	75	1.2	0.5	98.8	1.3	97.1

Abbreviations: YOS, Yale Observation Scale; *PPV,* positive predictive value; *NPV,* negative predictive value.
(Courtesy of Teach SJ, and the Occult Bacteremia Study Group: Efficacy of an observation scale in detecting bacteremia in febrile children three to thirty-six months of age, treated as outpatients. *J Pediatr* 126:877–881, 1995.)

problem—the detection of occult bacteremia in ambulatory, febrile patients from 3 to 36 months of age, who are considered to have neither a toxic nor a serious focal illness. The investigators therefore applied the YOS to a population for whom it was not originally designed. The treatment of such patients is difficult because a finite number have bacteremia and are at risk of focal complications, but such risks are quite low. However, the risk does exist, and therefore the problem being evaluated is of great concern and controversy to all of us.

The authors of this report conclude that YOS is a poor means of detecting occult bacteremia in this specific patient population. When you think, however, of how many patients you see who have temperatures of 39°C or more, and in whom you find nothing on physical examination, particularly when the infant otherwise looks well, you can easily see why a study such as this needed to be done. It's merely a shame that it did not yield useful information. Thus, we are stuck with having to do what we need to do, which is to culture and to treat IF you don't want to miss any patients with bacteremia. This is a big IF because many of these infants and toddlers will do perfectly well without anything being done to them, even if they are bacteremic.

The report abstracted represents a monumental effort on the part of the Occult Bacteremia Study Group, which consists of more than a dozen institutions scattered throughout the United States. Yale was not one of these institutions (Harvard was), but the results are still valid.

Reference

1. McCarthy PL, et al: *Pediatrics* 65:1090, 1980.

Effect of Number of Blood Cultures and Volume of Blood on Detection of Bacteremia in Children
Isaacman DJ, Karasic RB, Reynolds EA, et al (Univ of Pittsburgh, Pa; Children's Hosp of Pittsburgh, Pa)
J Pediatr 128:190–195, 1996   2–4

Background.—In making the diagnosis of bacteremia in children, many clinicians use only a single culture containing as little as 1 mL of blood per sample. This "minimalist" approach is followed despite the lack of data on the optimal number of blood cultures and volume of blood needed to detect bacteremia in children. The effects of each of these issues on the ability to detect bacteremia were examined.

Methods.—The prospective study included 300 children with suspected bacteremia. Two samples from separate sites—a 2-mL sample (sample A) and a 9.5-mL sample (sample B) were obtained from each patient. Sample B was subsequently divided into a 2-mL sample (sample B1), a 6-mL sample (sample B2), and a 1.5-mL sample for quantitative culture (sample ISO). The effects of number of blood cultures and of sample volume on the speed and completeness of bacteremia detection were evaluated.

Results.—In 10% of patients, at least 1 of the blood cultures permitted isolation of a pathogen. The pathogen recovery rate at 24 hours was 72% for the large B2 sample, compared with 37% and 33% for the smaller A and B1 samples, respectively; 47% for the combination of the A and B1 samples; and 21% for the ISO sample. The 7-day pathogen recovery rate was 83% for the B2 sample. This was significantly better than the 60% rate achieved with the B1 sample but similar to the 73% rate observed with the combination of the A and B1 samples.

Conclusion.—Collecting a larger blood sample can help to ensure timely detection of bacteremia in children. This is a practical approach that maximizes pathogen recovery while avoiding the cost and pain of an additional venipuncture. Obtaining a single, small-volume blood culture misses a significant number of cases of bacteremia in children.

▶ This article was selected for inclusion in the YEAR BOOK to annoy those readers who have become pretty much fed up with hearing about how much blood should be taken for bacterial culture. You have a right to be put off by this topic because if the same amount of time were taken to carefully obtain a blood culture as has been spent in writing about it, perhaps we would see a higher and more accurate rate of detection of bacteremia. When will we see an end to such articles?

The only light on the horizon likely to shed new and important insights regarding the detection of bacteremia is the use of techniques to detect bacterial DNA in the blood of those who are septic. This was commented on in the 1996 YEAR BOOK[1] based on the important report by McCabe et al.[2] Hopefully, in the not-too-distant future, we will not even have to culture blood to detect bacteremia; DNA analysis should prove to be a precise tool that allows one to triage for sepsis. It will certainly be a better tool than the complex clinical algorithms that we currently live with and rely on to tell which febrile neonate or toddler is in deep trouble. Because bacterial DNA detection can be accomplished in just a few hours, the molecular biology laboratory will become an extension of the emergency department or office. This technology comes none too soon. When it is finally here, perhaps we will see the end of the publication of articles such as the one abstracted.

References

1. 1996 YEAR BOOK OF PEDIATRICS, p 76.
2. McCabe KM, et al: *Pediatrics* 95:165, 1995.

Detection of *Mycobacterium tuberculosis* in Clinical Specimens From Children Using a Polymerase Chain Reaction

Smith KC, Starke JR, Eisenach K, et al (Univ of Texas, Houston; Baylor College of Medicine, Houston; Univ of Arkansas, Little Rock)
Pediatrics 97:155–160, 1996   2–5

Objective.—Tuberculosis is difficult to diagnose in children because symptoms are atypical and typical laboratory tests are frequently negative. A new polymerase chain reaction (PCR) test has shown good sensitivity and specificity in adults but has not been well studied in children. The usefulness of PCR as a diagnostic test for tuberculosis in children was prospectively examined in a controlled, blinded study.

Methods.—Clinical specimens were collected from 83 children, aged 4 days to 17 years, admitted to 4 Texas hospitals between January 1992 and March 1994 for diagnosis or evaluation of tuberculosis. Polymerase chain reaction was used to detect the IS*6110* loci identifying *Mycobacterium tuberculosis*. After gel electrophoresis, the presence of the 123–base pair fragment was considered a positive test. Southern blot analysis was also performed.

Results.—The active study group consisted of 35 children. Thirty children with no disease or with tuberculosis infection but not active disease were used as controls. Sixteen children were not evaluable. A total of 150 specimens from 65 children were cultured and sent for PCR (Table 3). Cultures and PCR together identified 19 of 35 children with tuberculosis. Fourteen of 35 children with tuberculosis were identified by PCR, for a sensitivity of 40%. Twenty-four of 30 controls without tuberculosis disease were properly identified by PCR, for a specificity of 80%. Polymerase chain reaction gave 6 false positive results. One of these patients had infection but no disease, 4 had nontuberculous mycobacterial disease, and 2 had *Mycobacterium avium* lymphadenitis.

Conclusion.—Although the study was small, PCR showed a sensitivity similar to that of culture for detecting *M. tuberculosis* in children. Because the specificity of PCR is low, it must be used in conjunction with other tests. Improvements in PCR techniques are expected to improve the specificity.

▶ This report comes none too soon. Tuberculosis is particularly difficult to diagnose in children because of the poor yield of standard laboratory tests and the lack of characteristic symptoms in many children. Put these difficulties together with the fact that tuberculosis is increasingly being reported even in the developing world (including this country), and one sees the value of any laboratory technique that aids in diagnosis. Absent PCR, it takes 3–6 weeks for culture results to become positive in most instances. A positive culture is, in fact, a best-case scenario because under ordinary conditions, yields from gastric aspirates in children with tuberculosis are well under 50%. Gastric aspirate acid-fast stains from children are almost never positive.

TABLE 3.—Numbers and Types of Specimens Sent for Culture and Polymerase Chain Reaction (PCR) for All Children, With Percentage of Specimens Positive by Type Among Cases

Specimen Type	No. of Samples for Culture	No. of Samples for PCR	Children With Tuberculosis Disease	
			No. of Specimens Culture +/No. From Cases (%)	No. of Specimens PCR+/No. From Cases (%)
Gastric aspirate	119	106	19/78 (24%)	22/67 (33%)
Cerebrospinal fluid	16	15	1/5 (20%)	2/5 (40%)
Sputum	7	4	2/6 (33%)	1/3 (33%)
Tracheal aspirate	4	3	1/4 (25%)	2/2 (100%)
Pericardial fluid	3	3	0/3 (0%)	1/3 (33%)
Pleural fluid	1	0	0/1 (0%)	0/0 (0%)
Bronchoalveolar lavage	0	1	0/0 (0%)	0/1 (0%)
Total	150	132		

(Courtesy of Smith KC, Starke JR, Eisenach K, et al: Detection of *Mycobacterium tuberculosis* in clinical specimens from children using a polymerase chain reaction. Reproduced by permission of *Pediatrics*, Vol 97, pp 155–160, Copyright 1996.)

The only thing to be careful about with PCR technology is the false positive result that is occasionally seen, which was noted in this report. There are 2 explanations for such false positive PCR results. The most common problem is carry-over of DNA from previous reactions. Another source of false positive results is cross contamination with *M. tuberculosis* DNA isolated from positive clinical samples or positive control samples during the processing procedure. The frequency with which these problems occurs is difficult to determine. In clinical practice, such false positive results could halt a clinical evaluation, obscure the true diagnosis, and obligate a patient to a lengthy and unnecessary treatment. This is particularly true with respect to meningitis, for which PCR detection is increasingly used.

Until advances in PCR technology improve its specificity, PCR alone is insufficient as a single diagnostic test for tuberculosis in children. Epidemiologic and clinical factors remain the most important consideration in the diagnosis of tuberculosis in culture-negative children. However, the benefit of rapid results with PCR (48 hours compared with 3–6 weeks for culture), as well as a sensitivity equal to or better than that of culture, offers an appreciable advantage over traditional techniques.

One last comment on tuberculosis in children. Read the very important Committee on Infectious Diseases statement updating us on tuberculosis skin testing of children.[1] This committee of the American Academy of Pediatrics reminds us that we should focus tuberculin skin testing on children who are at increased risk of acquiring tuberculosis. Routine tuberculin testing (such as school-based programs that include populations at low risk) has a large number of false positive results and represents an inefficient use of limited health resources. Therefore, children without risk factors and who reside in low-prevalence regions do not need routine tuberculosis skin testing. The original recommendation for skin testing at 1 year of age had been based on the theoretical concept that administration of measles vaccine might reactivate dormant *M. tuberculosis*. This concern has not been supported by any data. Routine skin testing at this age is not warranted. Children who have no risk factors but who reside in high-prevalence regions, and children whose histories for risk factors are incomplete or unreliable, should be considered for tuberculin (Mantoux) skin testing at 4–6 and 11–16 years of age. Children with HIV infection should receive annual tuberculin testing (5 tuberculin units, Mantoux).

The guidelines for interpretation of tuberculin tests have changed slightly. You may wish to read about this in more detail. The guidelines are contained in the Committee on Infectious Diseases statement on tuberculosis skin testing.[1]

Quiz: What is the origin of the word scrofula? The term scrofula, referring to tuberculous lymphadenitis of the neck, is a diminutive of the Latin word "scrofa," a breeding cow supposedly prone to the disease, which was recorded by Aristotle. The word corresponds etymologically to the Greek for "pig," but it has been questioned whether it should be taken in the figurative sense meaning a stone, reflecting the scirrhous hardness of the lymph glands when inflamed, as described by Galen. The current term scrofula is first encountered in the medical writings of the school of Salerno, Italy, in the early 16th century.

Reference

1. Committee on Infectious Diseases: *Pediatrics* 97:282, 1996.

School-based Screening for Tuberculous Infection: A Cost-benefit Analysis
Mohle-Boetani JC, Miller B, Halpern M, et al (County of Santa Clara Public Health Dept, San Jose, Calif; Ctrs for Disease Control and Prevention, Atlanta, Ga; Batelle Ctrs for Public Health Research and Evaluation, Arlington, Va)
JAMA 274:613–619, 1995   2–6

Introduction.—In the past 3 decades, public health programs have recommended school-based screening for tuberculous infection either for all children or only for children at high risk for tuberculous infection. Because there are limited public health resources for tuberculosis control activities, a cost-benefit analysis evaluated and compared the relative usefulness of routine screening and targeted screening.

Methods.—All kindergartners at 40 selected schools and all students at 18 selected high schools were tested with the Mantoux test. A high-risk

TABLE 2.—Annual Rate of Development of Active TB and TB Case-Fatality Rate Among Tuberculin Skin-Test Reactors by Age Group

Age Group y,	TB Cases per 100,000 Reactors per y	TB Case-Fatality Rate, %*
5–9	77	0.45
10–14	84	0.45
15–19	95	1.2
20–24	90	1.2
25–29	90	2.9
30–34	64	2.9
30–39	64	3.7
40–44	101	3.7
45–49	101	5.7
50–54	130	5.7
55–59	130	8.8
60–64	95	8.8
65–69	95	16
70–74	174	16
75–79	212	16
80–84	212	16
≥85	212	16

* Calculated as age-specific TB deaths divided by age-specific cases in 1990.
Abbreviation: TB, tuberculosis.
(Courtesy of Mohle-Boetani JC, Miller B, Halpern M, et al: School-based screening for tuberculous infection: A cost-benefit analysis. *JAMA* 274:613–619, Copyright 1995, American Medical Association.)

TABLE 3.—Baseline Estimates of Costs for Screening, TB Treatment, and Contact Tracing

Category	Item	Cost, $	Source
Screening	TST and reading	8.00	SCCTC
	Chest radiograph and one physician visit	58.00	SCCTC
	Six follow-up visits and 6 mo of INH	100.85	SCCTC
	Total per TST reactor	**166.85**	...
Inpatient followed by outpatient treatment for TB	20-d hospitalization	18 588.00	Brown et al
	Physician charges	2318.00	Brown et al
	Outpatient visits and medication after discharge (160 d)	2051.00	Brown et al
	Total	**22 957.00**	...
Outpatient treatment for TB	Outpatient visits and medication (180 d)	2300.00	Brown et al
Treatment cost per TB case (with a 60% hospitalization rate)		14 696.00	Brown et al
Contact tracing	Locate 8.5 contacts per case	144.50	Brown et al, CDC
	Screen 8.5 contacts per case	69.79	Brown et al CDC
	Chest radiograph and initial visit for 1.7 reactors per case	59.50	Brown et al
	INH for reactors	172.70†	SCCTC
	TB treatment of 1% of contacts per case	1249.16‡	Brown et al
Total cost of treatment and contact tracing per TB case		**16 391.66**	

* Costs were estimated from charges or expenditures.
† Calculated as $127 for preventive therapy × 1.7 reactors (20% of 8.5 contacts) × 80% adherence to isoniazid.
‡ Calculated as 0.085 contacts per case (1% of 8.5 contacts) with active TB × $14,696 for treatment of TB.
Abbreviations: TB, tuberculosis; *TST*, tuberculin skin test; *INH*, isoniazid; *SCCTC*, Santa Clara County TB Clinic; *CDC*, Centers for Disease Control and Prevention.
(Courtesy of Mohle-Boetani JC, Miller B, Halpern M, et al: School-based screening for tuberculous infection: A cost-benefit analysis. *JAMA* 274:613–619, Copyright 1995, American Medical Association.)

TABLE 4.—Impact of 2 Programs of Tuberculin Screening of Kindergartners and High School Entrants in Santa Clara County, California, With Baseline Assumptions

Strategy	Group	Program Cost, $	Benefits, $	Cases Prevented (Discounted Cases Prevented)	Net Annual Cost (Net Benefits), $	Incremental Cost per Case Prevented, $*	Benefit-Cost Ratio
Screen all	Kindergartners	183 868	58 201	11.1 (3.9)	125 628	103 758	0.31
	High school entrants	287 452	217 176	37.2 (16.1)	70 276	17 393	0.76
	Both	471 320	275 377	48.3 (20.0)	195 904	34 656	0.58
Targeted screening	Kindergartners	42 218	41 099	7.9 (2.7)	1 119	...	0.97
	High school entrants	155 925	169 136	28.9 (11.3)	(13 211)	...	1.08
	Both	198 143	210 235	36.8 (14.0)	(12 092)	...	1.06

* Compares the screen-all strategy with the targeted screening strategy.

(Courtesy of Mohle-Boetani JC, Miller B, Halpern M, et al: School-based screening for tuberculous infection: A cost-benefit analysis. *JAMA* 274:613–619, Copyright 1995, American Medical Association.)

group was defined as students born in countries with a high prevalence of tuberculosis. Screening effectiveness was determined for routine screening and for targeted screening by calculating the number of cases prevented per 10,000 children, compared with published age-specific prevalence expectations (Table 2). Cost calculations included the direct medical costs of screening, chest radiography, and preventive therapy. Cost benefits included savings from the prevention of tuberculosis treatment and of screening and treatment of patient contacts (Table 3). The benefit-cost ratios were then calculated.

Results.—Screening all students prevented the following number of cases per 10,000 children screened: 6.4 kindergartners, 25 high school students, and 14.9 cases overall. Screening only targeted students prevented the following number of cases per 10,000 children screened: 74.8 kindergartners, 88.9 high school students, and 84.8 cases overall. Benefit-cost analysis revealed that every dollar spent in the screening program saved $0.58 with the routine screening program and $1.06 with the targeted screening program (Table 4). Screening all children would result in savings only if the reactor rate were at least 20%.

Conclusions.—The costs of screening compared with the benefits of prevention are much higher with routine screening than with targeted screening. A high proportion of low-risk students will have false positive reactions, leading to unnecessary radiographic evaluation and preventive therapy. Therefore targeted, rather than universal, screening of children is recommended.

▶ If you want to read more about tuberculosis screening in children, read the superb editorial by Jeffrey Starke that accompanied this *JAMA* report.[1] Dr. Starke reminds us that there are only 2 ways in which a child in the United States can be infected with *Mycobacterium tuberculosis:* the child can be infected in a foreign country and then bring latent tuberculosis infection with him or her during immigration, or the child can be infected here by a contagious adolescent or adult. In theory, if we could conduct perfect contact investigations for tuberculosis and test all foreign-born children at or soon after immigration, we would find virtually all infected children and no additional testing for children would be needed. It is our inability or unwillingness to perform these 2 basic activities that has led to the perceived need to engage in other activities such as universal school-based tuberculin testing. This study by Mohle-Boetani et al. is one of the first (and probably the best) attempts to analyze the usefulness of school-based tuberculosis screening in light of our current tuberculosis epidemic. They find that targeted screening of high-risk children (in this case, foreign-born students) is more efficient and less costly than screening all students.

When you screen large populations at relatively low risk for entities such as tuberculosis, you will pick up a lot of false positive skin reactions. False positive tuberculin skin tests are usually the result of cross reactions with nontuberculous mycobacterial infection or may result from nonspecific reactivity. False positive reactions cannot be distinguished from true positives without fairly detailed and potentially expensive follow-up. This low specificity of the tuberculin skin test and the concentration of tuberculosis infection in pockets of high-risk individuals led the Centers for Disease Control and Prevention (CDC) and the American Academy of Pediatrics to abandon the call for universal tuberculin screening of children and to emphasize targeted testing of high-risk children.

The real challenge is to develop expedient but reliable strategies to identify the truly high-risk child who may have had contact with an adult with contagious tuberculosis. To say this differently, most risk factors for acquiring tuberculosis infection in children are really the risk factors of the adults in their lives.

In a world of finite dollars for health care, a cost-benefit analysis does seem to favor targeted screening. Yes, one can do universal screening, but this study confirms an age-old adage: Something that is not worth doing, is not worth doing well. Pick your targets carefully.

To learn more about the fight against tuberculosis and how it has gotten down to the molecular level, read the excellent commentary by Anthony Fauci, Director of the National Institute of Allergy and Infectious Diseases.[2]

One additional comment concerning tuberculosis. What is the chance you might contract tuberculosis on a commercial airliner? The answer to this question is a complex one but is highlighted by a recent report involving a passenger with infectious multiresistant tuberculosis. This person traveled on commercial airline flights from Honolulu to Chicago and from Chicago to Baltimore and returned one month later retracing his route. As a result of exposure to the infected index patient, a number of people on the airplanes involved had tuberculin skin-test conversions.[3]

From what little information the CDC has, approximately 1 out of every 9 million airline passengers has active tuberculosis. This is probably an underestimate of the risk of exposure to tuberculosis because reporting is likely to be incomplete. From July through December of 1994, the CDC received unsolicited reports of 30 airline passengers with tuberculosis, including 10 whose diagnosis was already known at the time of travel. Assuming 300 passengers per international flight and 150 per domestic flight, it is estimated that as many as 10,000 passengers may have been exposed to *M. tuberculosis* on airliners during that time period, or approximately 1 of every 26,000 passengers who flew in late 1994.

That's the long answer to the question. The short answer is that the risk of getting tuberculosis on a commercial jetliner is pretty small.

References

1. Starke J: *JAMA* 274:652, 1995.
2. Fauci AS: *JAMA* 274:786, 1995.
3. Kenyon TA, et al: *N Engl J Med* 334:933, 1996.

The Family Pet as an Unlikely Source of Group A Beta-hemolytic Streptococcal Infection in Humans
Wilson KS, Maroney SA, Gander RM (Univ of Texas Southwestern Med Center, Dallas)
Pediatr Infect Dis J 14:372–375, 1995   2–7

Introduction.—Several studies have suggested that domestic animals might be a reservoir for group A β-hemolytic streptococcal infections in humans. To determine whether transmission of group A β-hemolytic streptococci (GABS) from family pets to children does occur, oropharyngeal cultures were obtained from various groups of children and pets.

Methods.—Forty-six children with acute pharyngitis were studied. Of the 42 households represented, 26 had a child with culture-proven GABS pharyngitis; children in the remaining 16 households had non-GABS pharyngitis. Within 72 hours of obtaining cultures from the children, throat cultures were collected from 43 dogs and 25 cats in these homes. Also cultured were 10 healthy children without pharyngitis and their 13 pets. Cultures were collected as well from 149 randomly selected dogs and cats seen at a veterinary hospital in the area. Sites collected in these animals included the oropharynx, axilla, and vagina.

Results.—No pet from any households of children with pharyngitis had a positive throat culture for GABS. Three pets, all from households with human culture–proven GABS, had β-hemolytic streptococci, but none of the isolates were group A. One of the 10 healthy children had a throat culture positive for group B streptococci, and a dog in that home had a group G streptococcus. And although 2 asymptomatic children from a single household were colonized with GABS, the family dog had no β-hemolytic streptococci isolated. Finally, no GABS were recovered from the 371 body sites cultured from the veterinary clinic animals.

Conclusion.—The suggestion that household pets serve as a reservoir for GABS and transmit the infection to humans was not supported by this investigation. Although isolated case reports have implicated domestic animals in the transmission of GABS infection to children, negative findings from a total of 230 dogs and cats indicate that the possibility of this source of infection is remote.

▶ Rover has been implicated in causing everything from *Toxocara canis* to GABS infection. In the case of the latter, apparently it just ain't so, or so say Wilson et al. from Dallas. These investigators have looked at enough 4-legged creatures to document that GABS is not a natural inhabitant of the airways of dogs or cats. It isn't found in their axillae or vaginas either. These data do not support the premise of prior reports, which have suggested that household pets may serve as reservoirs for GABS.

The absence of GABS from any animal culture in this study suggests that the transmission of this organism from animal to human is unlikely. This conclusion is also supported by results from another recent survey of the bacterial flora of dogs and cats.[1]

The flip side of this story relates to an interesting report by Roos et al.,[2] who have described an isolated case of a cat harboring a strain of GABS sharing the same serotype as GABS isolates recovered from children of a household. These children were repeatedly contracting streptococcal tonsillitis. This report raises the alternative possibility of transmission from human to animal. In fact, Stallings et al.[3] reported a case of potential transmission of another streptococci, *Streptococcus pneumoniae,* from an infant to the family cat.

What does all this mean? For a long time, we've been teaching our residents that if a child has recurrent streptococcal pharyngitis and you can find no reason to explain the repetitive nature of such an illness, culture the family dog and cat. This teaching is probably wrong. As far as GABS is concerned, our pets probably have more to fear from us than we from them. Also, this report comes none too soon. There isn't a chance in Hades that you're going to get a culture of your dog's throat paid for these days in an era of managed care.

References

1. Devriese LA, et al: *J Appl Bacteriol* 73:421, 1992.
2. Roos K, et al: *Lancet* 2:1072, 1988.
3. Stallings B, et al: *J Am Vet Med Assoc* 191:703, 1987.

Prognostic Factors in Childhood Bacterial Meningitis
Kaaresen PI, Flægstad T (Univ Hosp of Tromsø, Norway)
Acta Paediatr 84:873–878, 1995

2–8

Background.—Despite better antibiotic therapy and intensive care, bacterial meningitis continues to be a major cause of mortality and morbidity among children. The associated mortality is about 5%, and permanent neurologic sequelae occur in 10% to 20% of patients. The findings of previous studies on the association between symptom duration and outcome in patients with bacterial meningitis have been conflicting. The influence of symptom duration and prehospital antibiotic treatment, as well as possible risk factors related to poor prognosis in childhood bacterial meningitis, were investigated.

Methods and Findings.—Ninety-two children aged 1 month to 13.8 years were studied. Four children died (4.3%). Permanent neurologic complications occurred in 14, or 15.2%. The most common sequela was hearing impairment, which was strongly correlated with the length of symptom duration. In a multiple logistic regression analysis, risk factors independently related to subsequent death or sequelae were symptom duration of more than 48 hours, prehospital seizures, peripheral vasoconstriction, fewer than $1,000 \times 10^6$/L leukocytes in CSF, and a temperature of 38°C or greater on admission. Prehospital antibiotic treatment, given orally or parenterally, was unrelated to outcome (Table 2).

TABLE 2.—Association Between Various Risk Factors and Outcome (Death During Hospital Stay or Neurologic Sequelae) as Evaluated at Follow-up Examination

	Sequelae or death ($n = 18$ (%))	Healthy ($n = 74$ (%))	Odds ratio (95% CI)
Pre-admission history			
Duration			
≤24 h	7 (39)	38 (51)	1.5 (0.3–6.3)
25–≤48 h	3 (17)	24 (33)	1.0
>48 h	8 (44)	12 (16)	5.3 (1.3–22.4)
Seizures	6 (32)	4 (5)	8.8 (2.5–30.6)
On admission			
Neck stiffness	10 (56)	59 (80)	0.3 (0.1–0.9)
Peripheral vasoconstriction	8 (42)	13 (17)	3.5 (1.2–10.1)
Hypoventilation	3 (17)	1 (1)	14.6 (2.3–92.8)
Temperature ≥38.0°C	12 (67)	70 (95)	0.1 (0.03–0.4)
< 1000 × 10^6/l leucocytes in CSF	7 (39)	15 (20)	2.5 (0.8–7.4)
Leukocyte count < 5.0 × 10^9/l	5 (26)	7 (9)	3.5 (1.0–12.1)
Serum sodium ≤ 135 mmol/l	12 (67)	33 (45)	2.5 (0.9–7.2)
pH ≤7.35	6 (43)	11 (20)	3.0 (0.9–10.2)
During hospital stay			
Seizures	7 (39)	13 (18)	3.0 (1.0–8.9)
Thrombocyte count < 100 × 10^9/l	7 (39)	8 (11)	5.3 (1.7–16.3)

Abbreviation: CI, confidence interval.
(Courtesy of Kaaresen PI, Flægstad T: Prognostic factors in childhood bacterial meningitis. *Acta Paediatr* 84:873–878, 1995.)

Conclusions.—Until effective prophylaxis against bacterial meningitis is available, early recognition of high-risk patients plus new treatment strategies, such as dexamethasome and anticytokine therapy, may help improve prognosis. The risk factors identified may be useful in determining who is at high risk for death or morbidity. Further research is needed to examine the impact of length of prediagnostic history.

▶ Another report, one of many in the history of pediatrics, that delineates the prognostic factors in childhood meningitis. Children with meningitis who either die or have significant neurologic sequelae are those who have a history of illness untreated for more than 48 hours, have seizures before admission, or at the time of admission have fewer than 1,000 cells × 10^6/L in their CSF. They also have a leukocyte count less than 5,000/mm^3 and a serum sodium level less than 135 mmol/L. They are acidotic and have a platelet count less than 100,000/mm^3. Add to this list of less than pleasant signs and symptoms the presence of pneumococcus as a causative agent, and the prognosis becomes poor. If all of these variables are in place in any given child, there is probably better than a 60% chance of the child dying or having significant morbidity.

There were really no surprises in this report. It was comforting to see that there was no significant association between pretreatment with antibiotics and a negative outcome. Preadmission parenteral antibiotic therapy is recommended in patients with suspected meningitis who will have a long transport to a treatment facility. The data from this report show that there is no reason for abandoning this practice, preferably after obtaining a blood culture.

A closing comment about meningitis and lumbar punctures. If one were to do repeat lumbar punctures at 24–36 hours after the onset of treatment for meningitis, which child is likely to have a lower CSF glucose concentration and a higher protein concentration: the child with *Hemophilus influenzae, Neisseria meningitidis,* or *Streptococcus pneumoniae* meningitis? It would be very difficult to do a study to answer this question in the United States. One was done, however, recently in Santiago, Chile.[1] The findings were very dramatic. Slow recovery of CSF glucose and protein concentrations clearly distinguishes pneumococcal forms of meningitis from *H. influenzae* and *N. meningitidis* as a cause of meningitis in children. Even with proper treatment, the CSF glucose with pneumococcal meningitis averages 23 mg/dL after 24–36 hours, compared with the CSF glucose of patients in other forms of meningitis, which quickly returns to normal. The CSF protein at this same period is still markedly elevated at 177 mg/dL with pneumococcal meningitis.

We need a pneumococcal vaccine that works.

Reference

1. Roine I, et al: *Pediatr Infect Dis J* 14:905, 1995.

No Lumbar Puncture in the Evaluation for Early Neonatal Sepsis: Will Meningitis Be Missed?

Wiswell TE, Baumgart S, Gannon CM, et al (Thomas Jefferson Univ, Philadelphia)
Pediatrics 95:803–806, 1995

2–9

Introduction.—During the first month of life, bacterial meningitis occurs more frequently than at any other time during an individual's life. The only method of confirming the diagnosis of bacterial meningitis is with a lumbar puncture to examine CSF. Recently, it has been proposed by some to eliminate lumbar puncture from the evaluation of sepsis among newborns younger than 1 week. Selective approaches to performing lumbar punctures as part of early neonatal sepsis evaluation were assessed to determine whether they could potentially result in a delayed or missed diagnosis of bacterial meningitis.

Methods.—During a 5-year period, the records of 169,849 infants were retrospectively reviewed to identify those who had culture-positive meningitis during the first 72 hours of life. Collected data included maternal risks for infection, history of administration of antibiotics, and symptoms manifested by the infant (Table).

Results.—In the first 72 hours of life, the incidence of meningitis was 0.25 per 1,000 live births. Organisms were isolated from CSF in 43 infants: 30 had group B streptococcus; 10 had *Escherichia coli;* 1 had

TABLE.—Characteristics of 43 Infants Less Than 72 Hours of Age With CSF Culture-Positive Bacterial Meningitis

Characteristic	Overall ($n = 43$)	GBS* ($n = 30$)	Non-GBS ($n = 13$)
Male gender	20	12	8
Female gender	23	18	5
Mean gestational age in wk (range)	38.8 (29–42)	39.2 (31–42)	37.1 (29–42)
Gestational age $\geq$ 36 wk	7	2	5
Mean birth weight in g (range)	3,160 (1,070–5,100)	3,285 (1,780–4,560)	2,850 (1,070–5,100)
Birth weight < 2,500 g	7	2	5
Maternal risk factors			
Chorioamnionitis	13	10	3
ROM >12 hr	16	11	5
Positive GBS culture from lower vagina	2	2	0
Urinary tract infection	2	2	0
Maternal intrapartum antibiotic therapy	8	7	1
Median age at evaluation (hr)	12	12	12
Mean I:T neutrophil ratio	0.41	0.42	0.38
I:T ratio < 0.20	6	4	2
Baby asymptomatic, LP performed for other reasons	7	5	2
Respiratory distress	17	11	6
Respiratory distress syndrome	6	1	5
Negative blood cultures	12	9	3
Negative blood culture if maternal antibiotics	7	6	1
Seizures during neonatal hospitalization	11	9	2
Abnormal neurologic examination at discharge	5	3	2
Deaths	3	2	1

Abbreviation: GBS, group B streptococcus; *LP*, lumbar puncture.

(Courtesy of Wiswell TE, Baumgart S, Gannon CM, et al: No lumbar puncture in the evaluation for early neonatal sepsis: Will meningitis be missed? Reproduced by permission of *Pediatrics*, Vol 95, pp 803–806, Copyright 1995.)

Listeria monocytogenes; 1 had *Citrobacter diversus*; and 1 had *Streptococcus pneumoniae.* The mean gestational age was 38.8 weeks, the median age at evaluation was 12 hours, and the mean birth weight was 3,163 g. Maternal risk factors were chorioamnionitis in 13 mothers; rupture of membranes greater than 12 hours in 16 mothers; group B streptococcus cultured from the lower vagina in 2 mothers; and intrapartum antibiotic therapy in 8 mothers.

Conclusion.—If advocated selective criteria were used as the basis for not performing lumbar puncture, the diagnosis of bacterial meningitis would have been delayed or missed in 16 (37%) of 43 infants. Of these 16 infants, 8 were born at term with no CNS symptoms and negative blood cultures; 5 were born prematurely with suspected respiratory distress syndrome; and 3 were born at term, asymptomatic but with positive blood cultures.

▶ Are there legitimate reasons not to do a lumbar puncture (LP) in the neonate?

Sure. Lumbar puncture can sometimes cause a clinically important cardio-respiratory compromise in the neonate. Other potential problems of LP include trauma ("bloody tap"), infectious complications, intraventricular hemorrhage, and spinal epidermoid tumor. Some 15% to 40% of infants undergoing an LP will have CSF results that are difficult (or impossible) to interpret because of bloody taps.

The authors try to determine the appropriate balance between the good reasons not to do an LP and the good reasons to perform one. They examine the use of currently advocated selective criteria that are an indication for LP in the evaluation of early neonatal sepsis. Some nurseries limit LPs to those infants who have symptoms. Some limit the use of an LP to those infants who have had a positive blood culture. Some nurseries have used LPs as part of the evaluation of infants born to mothers who have received intra-partum antibiotics for group B streptococcal colonization or for suspected chorioamnionitis.

Is such a conservative approach to performing an LP appropriate? These data from Army neonatologists suggest not. If limited indications for perfor-mance of an LP had been the manner by which Army neonatologists had made decisions, some 37% of infants with meningitis would have been missed. One cannot do much better than a study of 170,000 infants born during a 5-year period to prove the point.

About a quarter of a century ago, it was recognized that studies of outpatient consultations showed that 86% of diagnosis depends entirely on what the patients say, their own story. What physicians found on examina-tion merely added another 6%, and technical investigations such as radiog-raphy and blood tests added another 8%. Because neonates can't talk to you, the role of your physical examination and your ability to perform appro-priate tests, including LPs, makes the need for laboratory assessment even more important in the nursery.[1] In other words, an LP is indicated, except when it is not.

Reference

1. Hampton JR, et al: *BMJ* 2:46, 1975.

Relation Between Passive Tobacco Smoke Exposure and the Development of Bacterial Meningitis in Children
Bredfeldt RC, Cain SR, Schutze GE, et al (Univ of Arkansas, Little Rock)
J Am Board Fam Pract 8:95–98, 1995   2–10

Introduction.—Exposure to household cigarette smoke has been established as a risk factor in numerous childhood illnesses. One previous study reported a possible link between passive tobacco smoke exposure and bacterial meningitis in children. This association was investigated further.

Methods.—The caregivers of 93 children older than 2 months treated between 1989 and 1992 for bacterial meningitis were contacted for a telephone interview to determine the child's exposure to passive tobacco smoke in the home or day-care setting. The caregivers of a control group of children admitted for abdominal surgery and matched for age and sex were also surveyed.

Results.—The response rates were 78.6% in the meningitis group and 79.6% in the control group. Of the 73 children who had meningitis and complete survey information, 45 were exposed to passive cigarette smoke at the time of admission, as compared with 30 of the 74 control children. The meningitis group had increased exposure to passive cigarette smoke even when only household exposure was considered.

Conclusions.—Passive exposure to cigarette smoke increases the risk of bacterial meningitis in children. Further studies are needed to elucidate the mechanisms involved. Possible mechanisms include depressed immune systems or an adverse effect of passive smoking on local defense mechanisms in the nasopharynx, allowing longer exposure to infecting organisms.

▶ How many more reports before Congress finally recognizes that tobacco is a dirty weed? Previous articles in the YEAR BOOK OF PEDIATRICS have mentioned the following risks that result from exposure to smoking (active or passive):

- Asthma
- Otitis media
- Otitis media with effusion
- Chronic respiratory disease
- Sudden infant death syndrome
- Hearing deficits
- Lower intelligence quotients
- Increased risk of inflammatory bowel disease
- Hypertension

- Diminished height in children with cystic fibrosis in households of those who smoke

- Destruction of the rain forest (In many parts of the world, tobacco is flue cured with wood smoke. In Tanzania, 12% of all trees that are felled are used for this purpose.)

Add to this lengthy list, which in fact is only a partial list, the results of this study, which show a relationship between passive tobacco smoke exposure and the development of bacterial meningitis in children. Children in households where they are bathed in smoke have a 2.5-fold increased risk of meningitis. Why this happens is unclear but probably relates to the overall increased risk of upper respiratory tract infections in children who are so exposed.

It seems unlikely that in our lifetime the sale of tobacco will be totally banned. If that realization is accepted, we could get on with more effective ways of diminishing the frequency with which teenagers and adults smoke. Each package of cigarettes should be surtaxed in an amount equivalent to what epidemiologists and health research investigators tell us is an appropriate amount to cover all the added health care costs to society that result from both direct and passive smoking. In a country such as ours, which is predicated on a free market, the likelihood is that the price will be high enough to price cigarettes out of the average household income. It's time for a package of cigarettes to cost more than your average color TV.

A Controlled Trial of Two Acellular Vaccines and One Whole-cell Vaccine Against Pertussis
Greco D, and the Progetto Pertosse Working Group (Istituto Superiore di Sanità, Rome; et al)
N Engl J Med 334:341–348, 1996   2–11

Background.—The use of whole-cell pertussis vaccines has been controversial because of concerns about the frequency and severity of adverse reactions. Acellular vaccines, containing purified proteins, are available. The efficacy and safety of whole-cell and acellular pertussis vaccines were evaluated in a double-blind, randomized clinical trial.

Methods.—Infants seen at 62 public health clinics in Italy during a 1-year period were randomly assigned to receive either a whole-cell pertussis vaccine, 1 of 2 acellular vaccines, or a diphtheria-tetanus (DT) preparation only. The 2 acellular vaccines were either genetically detoxified or detoxified with formalin and glutaraldehyde. Both also contained filamentous hemagglutinin and pertactin. All the vaccines were administered in 3 doses between the ages of 6 and 12 weeks, 13 and 20 weeks, and 21 and 28 weeks. The patients were followed up with monthly surveillance to record coughing episodes for at least 2 years. A coughing illness lasting

TABLE 3.—Confirmed Cases of Pertussis, Vaccine Efficacy, and Relative Risk, According to Vaccine Group and Number of Doses*

Vaccine and No. of Doses	No. of Children	No. of Person-Days at Risk	No. of Cases	Incidence/ 100 Person-Years	Vaccine Efficacy (95% CI) %	Relative Risk (95% CI)†
SmithKline acellular DTP						
3 doses	4481	2,354,321	37	0.56	83.9 (75.8–89.4)	0.25 (0.17–0.36)
≥1 dose	4696	3,099,438	46	0.54	81.5 (73.1–87.4)	0.28 (0.20–0.39)
Biocine acellular DTP						
3 doses	4452	2,342,952	36	0.55	84.2 (76.2–89.7)	0.25 (0.17–0.36)
≥1 dose	4672	3,089,325	41	0.48	83.5 (75.6–88.9)	0.25 (0.17–0.36)
Connaught whole-cell DTP						
3 doses	4348	2,262,810	141	2.2	36.1 (14.2–52.1)	1.0
≥1 dose	4678	3,062,822	162	1.9	34.0 (12.8–49.8)	1.0
Biocine DT						
3 doses	1470	758,646	74	3.5	—	1.6 (1.2–2.1)
≥1 dose	1555	1,010,145	81	2.9	—	1.5 (1.1–2.0)

* Pertussis was defined clinically as 21 days or more of paroxysmal cough beginning 30 days or more after the third vaccine dose or immediately after the first dose.

† Relative risks are expressed in relation to the incidence in the group given the whole-cell DTP vaccine.

Abbreviations: CI, confidence interval; *DTP*, diphtheria-tetanus-pertussis; *DT*, diphtheria-tetanus.

(Reprinted by permission of *The New England Journal of Medicine*, from Greco D, and the Progetto Pertosse Working Group: A controlled trial of two acellular vaccines and one whole-cell vaccine against pertussis. *N Engl J Med* 334:341–348, Copyright 1996, Massachusetts Medical Society.)

more than 7 days prompted sampling and culturing of serum and nasopharyngeal mucus, as well as weekly surveillance of symptoms until resolution. Immunogenicity was assessed with analysis of antibody to pertussis antigens in the serum 1 month after the third dose in 10% of the children. Local and systemic symptoms for the 8 days after each dose were also monitored.

Results.—A total of 14,751 infants completed the study. Withdrawals before the third dose were significantly more common among those receiving the whole-cell vaccine. During follow-up, there were 474 episodes of cough associated with positive cultures for *Bordetella pertussis*. The efficacy of the whole-cell vaccine after 3 doses in preventing pertussis cases was 36%, compared with an efficacy of 84% with both acellular vaccines after 3 doses (Table 3). There was a 94% rate of serologic response to pertussis antigens after acellular diphtheria-tetanus-pertussis (DTP) vaccination, whereas the serologic response was minimal after whole-cell DTP vaccination. Both common and severe adverse events occurred significantly more frequently in patients given the whole-cell DTP vaccine than in those given either acellular vaccine.

Conclusions.—The acellular DTP vaccines demonstrate superior efficacy and safety compared with whole-cell DTP vaccines, and are therefore highly recommended for routine immunization of infants.

▶ There is so much written about acellular and whole-cell pertussis vaccines that it's difficult to keep track of this ever-evolving topic. The article abstracted was accompanied by another one in the same issue of *The New England Journal of Medicine*, which showed that a 5-component acellular pertussis vaccine is recommended for general use because it shows favorable safety profiles and confirmed sustained protection against pertussis, in comparison with a 2-component acellular vaccine. The currently available whole-cell vaccine is much less efficacious.[1]

The search for a more perfect pertussis vaccine has an interesting history. Before vaccines became available in this country, there were 9,000 deaths from each year and 260,000 cases of pertussis. With vaccine in 1976, there were only 7 deaths and about 1,000 cases of pertussis. The vaccine, however, was associated with such devastating events as sudden infant death. Although most studies suggest no causal relation, the current pertussis vaccine remains a source of concern to physicians and to families. In countries such as Britain, Sweden, and Japan, dissatisfaction with the pertussis vaccine has led to a decline in its use, causing a resurgence of pertussis. This resurgence is what stimulated the Japanese to accelerate their efforts to develop a more highly purified (acellular) pertussis vaccine.

To read more about the status of pertussis vaccines, see the excellent commentary by Edwards and Decker.[2] This commentary ends with the following sentence: "They [the acellular vaccines] represent a triumph for all involved in this effort over the past decade—scientists, manufacturers, government agencies, clinicians, and parents of infants and young children." A triumph it is.

A closing query about vaccines. You've just given a DTP injection to a 6-month-old. The injection obviously hurt the infant, who is now screaming and hollering. To console the child, the baby's mother gently massages the site of the injection. Fearing that her actions might somehow disturb the way in which this vaccine becomes effective, you tell her to stop. Are you right in this assumption? You are dead wrong. Local massage after DTP vaccination is associated with enhanced, not lower, immunogenicity. But just to prove that there's no gain without pain, local massage does increase the frequency of local pain (to 66% from 53%) and fever (to 74% from 62%).[3]

Should you routinely massage an immunization site? Chances are you will not become a believer, especially if your patients begin to refer to you as "my doctor, my masseuse."

References

1. Gustaffson L, et al: *N Engl J Med* 334:349, 1996.
2. Edwards KM, et al: *N Engl J Med* 334:391, 1996.
3. Shu C-Y, et al: *Pediatr Infect Dis J* 14:567, 1995.

Comparison of 13 Acellular Pertussis Vaccines: Adverse Reactions
Decker MD, Edwards KM, Steinhoff MC, et al (Vanderbilt Univ, Nashville, Tenn; Johns Hopkins Univ, Baltimore, Md; Univ of Maryland, Baltimore; et al)
Pediatrics 96:S557–S566, 1995   2–12

Background.—Although conventional whole-cell pertussis vaccines have effectively prevented clinical pertussis, they have also been associated with clinically significant and possibly catastrophic adverse events. Acellular vaccines, composed of specific purified pertussis antigens, have been developed and appear to cause fewer adverse events. To identify promising acellular vaccines, the reactogenicity of 13 acellular pertussis vaccines was evaluated and compared with a commercial whole-cell vaccine.

Methods.—A total of 2,342 healthy infants between the ages of 6 and 12 weeks were randomly assigned to receive either 1 of 13 acellular pertussis vaccines plus diphtheria and tetanus toxoids (DTaP) or a conventional whole-cell vaccine (WCL) in combination with diphtheria and tetanus toxoids. The parents were asked to complete reaction assessment forms 3 and 6 hours after immunization, at bedtime for each of the first 7 nights, and on the fourteenth night after each vaccination. The frequency and severity of adverse events were compared. At approximately 1 year after the last vaccination, long-term follow-up was assessed.

Results.—There were significant variations in adverse reactions associated with the 13 DTaP vaccines, but all reactions except vomiting were significantly more prevalent and more severe in association with WCL than with any of the DTaP vaccines. There was no difference in the rate of vomiting between WCL and DTaP recipients. There were similar reaction patterns after each inoculation, with adverse reactions beginning as early as 3 hours after vaccination, peaking on the first or second evening, then diminishing. In addition, both DTaP and WCL recipients had an increased prevalence and severity of fever, redness, and swelling, as well as a decreased prevalence of drowsiness, with successive inoculations; however, no changes in the prevalence of pain, fussiness, anorexia, vomiting, or the use of antipyretics were noted. There were no differences among the vaccination groups in the long-term rates of hospitalization, developmental delay, seizure, other neurologic problems, failure to thrive, prolonged cough, or serious infection. None of these events could be linked to pertussis immunization. Pertussis developed in 1 patient given a DTaP vaccine.

Conclusions.—Although there were significant differences in the frequency and severity of adverse reactions associated with DTaP vaccination, these were all significantly less frequent and less severe than occurred in association with WCL vaccination. Therefore, decisions regarding development or study of DTaP vaccines should be based primarily on findings of immunogenicity and purity rather than on reactogenicity.

▶ The DTP vaccine has been a lifesaver, but it has also been a problem. Since the introduction of DTP in the United States, the annual attack rate of pertussis has declined from 200 cases per 100,000 population to fewer than 2 cases per 100,000 population. Nonetheless, most of us consider DTP the least satisfactory routinely used childhood vaccine because of associated adverse reactions. The common ones, including high fever, persistent crying or screaming, as well as local and systemic reactions, are annoying and certainly disconcerting to parents. Less common, but more worrisome, are the reports (albeit infrequent) of seizure or collapse after receiving the pertussis vaccine. Worse yet is the concern that the pertussis vaccine may be responsible for rare but catastrophic adverse effects. None of these are seen with the new acellular vaccines composed of specific purified pertussis antigens. Although slow to be introduced in the United States, they have been used routinely in Japan since 1981. The report abstracted shows that DTaP vaccine produces fewer reactions in every respect other than vomiting.

The real issue with the acellular pertussis vaccine has to do with the problem of "no pain, no gain." To say this differently, does a vaccine that has fewer side effects produce the same level of immunity? All indications are that the vaccine does what it is supposed to do. A comparison of 13 acellular pertussis vaccines shows this, as does a multicenter acellular pertussis vaccine trial sponsored by the National Institutes of Health.[1, 2] The latter trial was the first multicenter acellular pertussis study to compare numerous acellular products with conventional WCL vaccine among infants using a standardized protocol and centralized laboratory serologic assessment.

There isn't much left to convince most of us that the only way to proceed with pertussis vaccination is with acellular products. To learn more about these, read the supplement to *Pediatrics* that appeared in September 1995. That supplement will tell you more than you ever wanted to know about DTaP vaccines.

A closing comment. We all expect "immunization days" to be successful, but what was the single most effective immunization day in history? Actually, the single most effective immunization day turned out to be 2 days because there was no way to stop the ball once it was rolling. China has conducted national immunization days in each of the past several years. The most successful were 2 consecutive days when more than 80 million children were immunized with the oral polio vaccine.[3] China is a country in which polio had been very rampant, but in 1994 only 5 cases of wild polio virus were confirmed.[4] The World Health Organization estimates that about $100 million will be needed over the next 4 years to eradicate polio from the face of the earth. If one is talking about cost-effective medicine, this $100 million investment should yield global savings of about $10 billion...Not a bad deal!

References

1. Edwards KM, et al: *Pediatrics* 96:548, 1995.
2. Klein DL: *Pediatrics* 96:547, 1995.
3. Bart KJ, et al: *Bull World Health Organ*, In press.
4. Centers for Disease Control and Prevention: *MMWR Morb Mortal Wkly Rep* 44:273, 1995.

A Placebo-controlled Trial of a Pertussis-toxoid Vaccine

Trollfors B, Taranger J, Lagergård T, et al (Göteborg Univ, Sweden; Natl Inst of Child Health and Human Development, Bethesda, Md; Natl Inst of Allergy and Infectious Diseases, Bethesda, Md)
N Engl J Med 333:1045–1050, 1995   2–13

Background.—Reported efficacy rates for inactivated *Bordetella pertussis* vaccines range from 40% to 90%. The protective moieties in whole-cell vaccines have not been identified. In the hope of minimizing side effects, a single-component, pharmacologically inert pertussis toxoid has been evaluated. The acellular vaccine consists of pertussis toxin inactivated by hydrogen peroxide.

Study Design.—A randomized, double-blind, placebo-controlled trial was undertaken in healthy full-term Swedish infants. A total of 1,726 infants received only diphtheria and tetanus toxoids (DT). Another 1,724 infants received pertussis toxoid in addition (DTP). The infants were immunized when 3, 5, and 12 months of age.

Results.—No serious reactions were encountered, but local reactions were slightly more frequent when pertussis vaccine was administered. During an average surveillance period of 17.5 months, the World Health Organization criteria for pertussis were met by 276 infants in the DT group and 92 in the DTP group. No child had to be hospitalized because of *Bordetella* infection. The pertussis toxoid vaccine was 71% effective. Those DTP recipients in whom pertussis developed, coughed for a shorter time than affected recipients of DT, and fewer of them whooped or vomited (Table 5). Two doses of vaccine were 55% effective.

Conclusion.—This pertussis toxoid vaccine is both immunogenic and safe, and it decreases the risk of severe pertussis.

TABLE 5.—Comparison of Clinical Symptoms Among Recipients of DTP Toxoids and of DT Toxoids During the Main Period of Follow-Up, According to the Classification of Pertussis*

| | WHO Definition† | | Göteborg Classification‡ | |
| | DTP-toxoids Group | DT-toxoids Group | DTP-toxoids Group | DT-toxoids Group |
Symptom	(N = 72)	(N = 240)	(N = 125)	(N = 258)
	median no. of days (percentage of children with symptoms)			
Cough	49	59	37	59
Paroxysmal cough	42	51	28	50
Vomiting	0 (46)	20 (78)	0 (35)	20 (76)
Whooping	0 (39)	24 (78)	0 (28)	22 (74)

* $P < 0.001$ for all comparisons between the groups.

† Only patients who had 21 or more days of paroxysmal cough are included because this is 1 of the criteria in WHO definition.

‡ All confirmed and probable cases with 7 or more days of cough are included.

Abbreviations: DT, diphtheria and tetanus toxoids; DTP, diphtheria-tetanus-pertussis toxoids; WHO, World Health Organization.

(Reprinted by permission of *The New England Journal of Medicine,* from Trollfors B, Taranger J, Lagergård T, et al: A placebo-controlled trial of a pertussis-toxoid vaccine. N Engl J Med 333:1045–1050, Copyright 1995, Massachusetts Medical Society.)

▶ This is the third and final article in this year's YEAR BOOK dealing with pertussis vaccines. There has been so much written recently about pertussis vaccines that it has been difficult to select only those articles that provide the most valuable information. This report from Sweden falls into this category.

Any report from Sweden is likely to attract great attention because infant vaccination against pertussis was stopped in Sweden in 1979. About 30 years ago, something happened in the production process that made the Swedish-manufactured whole-cell vaccine ineffective. Beginning in the early 1970s, pertussis became endemic in that country; when the incidence of pertussis increased despite widespread vaccinations, the infant vaccine was withdrawn in 1979. Since then, Sweden has had no licensed pertussis vaccine. In what better population could one experiment with a new vaccine than a country that essentially has had an unimmunized population? Such a population allows a relatively easy assessment of the efficacy of the acellular pertussis-toxoid vaccines. Although these vaccines were proven not to be perfect (the efficacy of the vaccine was 71%), they were nonetheless capable of conferring a reasonably substantial protection with no serious side effects. The pertussis vaccine given along with DT caused no more in the way of temperature elevations. Although DTP toxoids caused slightly more redness and swelling, they had none of the serious neurologic consequences that are seen with the whole-cell vaccine.

Sweden is so enamored with this acellular vaccine that they now consider it essential and sufficient for the vaccination of children and adults. They are pursuing mass vaccination of children with pertussis toxoid to eliminate pertussis from their country, as happened in Sweden and elsewhere in the case of diphtheria, another noninvasive, toxin-mediated respiratory disease. It is well known that diphtheria toxoid also is incapable of causing complete individual protection, yet use of the vaccine has essentially eliminated diphtheria under endemic or epidemic conditions.

It is likely that we will continue to hear more about acellular pertussis vaccines. The literature will move from efficacy and complication reporting to techniques of mass immunization/reimmunization, for the first time including methods to protect quintagenarians.

Clinical Course of Pertussis in Immunized Children

Bortolussi R, Miller B, Ledwith M, et al (Dalhousie Univ, Halifax, Canada)
Pediatr Infect Dis J 14:870–874, 1995   2–14

Background.—Although pertussis is generally effectively prevented with vaccination, infection has been reported in immunized patients. It was hypothesized that immunized children might have different clinical features of pertussis than the classic features described in nonimmunized children. The clinical respiratory features of children with pertussis and their household contacts were studied prospectively in a well-immunized population.

Methods.—Patients with suspected pertussis were tested for the presence of *Bordetella pertussis* in the nasopharyngeal aspirate. When the pathogen was isolated, a nurse performed weekly home visits for 4 weeks to review the clinical features, including the nature and date of onset of all symptoms, in the index case and all family members. Data on immunization history were checked.

Results.—Of the 518 children with documented *B. pertussis* infection, complete clinical data were obtained for 189 patients, of whom 103 were younger than 5 years. All but 4 of these 189 patients were appropriately immunized for their age. In 34% of the patients, congestion preceded the onset of cough by 7 days or less. Paroxysmal coughing developed by the seventh day after the onset of cough in 68%. Among the 62 patients with early diagnosis, 85.5% had a pertussis-specific symptom (paroxysmal cough, vomiting, whoop, cyanosis, or apnea) within 7 days of the onset of cough. Among the patients younger than 2 years, 97% had a pertussis-specific symptom within 7 days of the coughing illness. Overall, 88% had the features specified by the World Health Organization and 93% had the features specified by the Centers for Disease Control and Prevention. Among patients younger than 5 years, coughing lasted 16–91 days (median, 48 days) and 32% had paroxysms for more than 42 days. Treatment with erythromycin reduced the median durations of cough and paroxysms, particularly when given early in the disease course (Fig 4). A total of 48 secondary cases were diagnosed among family members; these patients had a significantly less prolonged and less severe course than did the index cases.

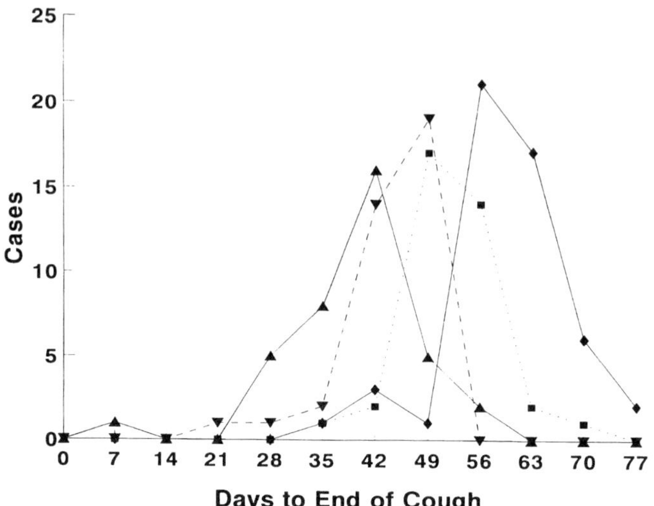

FIGURE 4.—Duration of cough among subjects of any age who were treated with erythromycin in their first (*triangle*, 39 patients), second (*inverted triangle*, 44 patients), and third (*square*, 38 patients) week, or after 21 days (*diamond*, 62 patients) of their coughing illness. (Courtesy of Bortolussi R, Miller B, Ledwith M, et al: Clinical course of pertussis in immunized children. *Pediatr Infect Dis J* 14:870–874, 1995.)

Conclusions.—The course of pertussis is typically less severe and less prolonged in immunized than in unimmunized patients. However, the symptoms are similar to those seen in classic pertussis and should be readily diagnosed.

▶ This report is from Nova Scotia, where immunization rates are extraordinarily high (well in excess of 90% by time of school entry). The province of Nova Scotia has used only diphtheria-pertussis-tetanus–inactivated polio vaccine with whole-cell pertussis for many years now. Despite this widespread vaccination, these Canadian investigators, as well as those in the United States, continue to report cases of whooping cough in an immunized population. It just goes to show you that the whole-cell vaccine is hardly perfect. If the data from this report are to be believed, one can easily diagnose pertussis in a previously immunized child because the presentation is similar to that of natural pertussis infection, albeit milder. The 3 stages of clinical illness are characterized by the classic pattern: catarrhal, paroxysmal, and convalescent. Persistent coughing is the hallmark.

Before accepting the study results as gospel, recognize that these children who were culture positive for pertussis may represent a selected population who were diagnosable only because they had classic symptoms. Are there many more fully immunized children in whom pertussis develops without the typical triad of findings? Probably so. Perhaps their infection, presumably mild, will leave them with a better and lasting immunity in comparison with the immunity acquired from the whole-cell vaccine.

Trends of Diarrheal Disease–associated Mortality in US Children, 1968 Through 1991

Kilgore PE, Holman RC, Clarke MJ, et al (Natl Ctr for Infectious Diseases, Atlanta, Ga)

JAMA 274:1143–1148, 1995

2–15

Objective.—Diarrheal illness not only is a very prominent cause of child deaths worldwide, but it still is a lethal condition in the United States. Patterns of diarrhea-related mortality were examined by reviewing national death certificate data for children 1 month through 4 years of age who died of diarrhea from 1968 through 1991. There were 14,137 such deaths, 78% of which involved infants 1–11 months of age.

Findings.—The cause of diarrhea was not specified in more than 90% of cases. Mortality from diarrhea in infants decreased 79% between 1968 and 1985 (Fig 1). Most of this decrease occurred in the first 6 years of the review period. Diarrheal deaths were most prevalent in whites, males, and those living in the South. The decrease in mortality was shared by all racial, sex, and regional groups. In all years, diarrheal mortality was greatest in young children and declined with advancing age. Geographic trends are shown in Figure 4. The peak in winter deaths associated with rotavirus infection in the earlier years virtually disappeared after 1985.

Conclusions.—Diarrheal deaths in the United States have decreased approximately 75% in recent decades. Many of these deaths still may be prevented by early rehydration, suggesting the need for efforts to better educate health care providers and to teach mothers to start rehydration at an early stage and seek medical help.

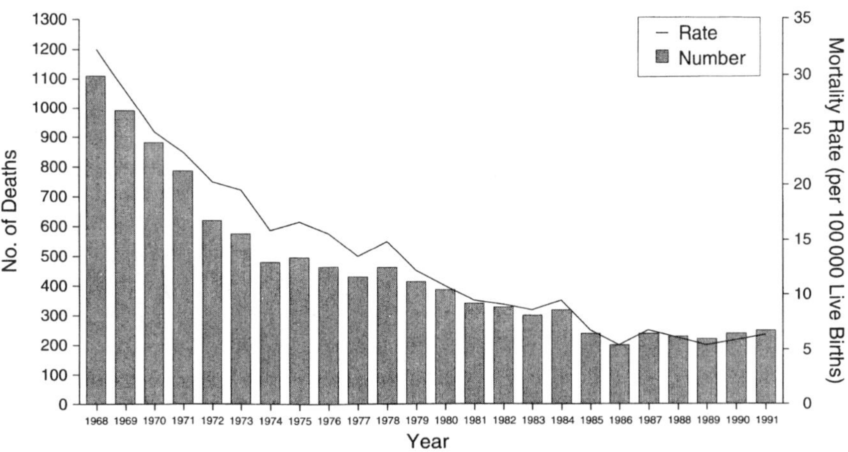

FIGURE 1.—Number of annual diarrheal deaths (*shaded bars*) and mortality rates (*solid line*) among infants in the United States, 1968 through 1991. (Courtesy of Kilgore PE, Holman RC, Clarke MJ, et al: Trends of diarrheal disease-associated mortality in US children, 1968 through 1991. *JAMA* 274:1143–1148, Copyright 1995, American Medical Associations.)

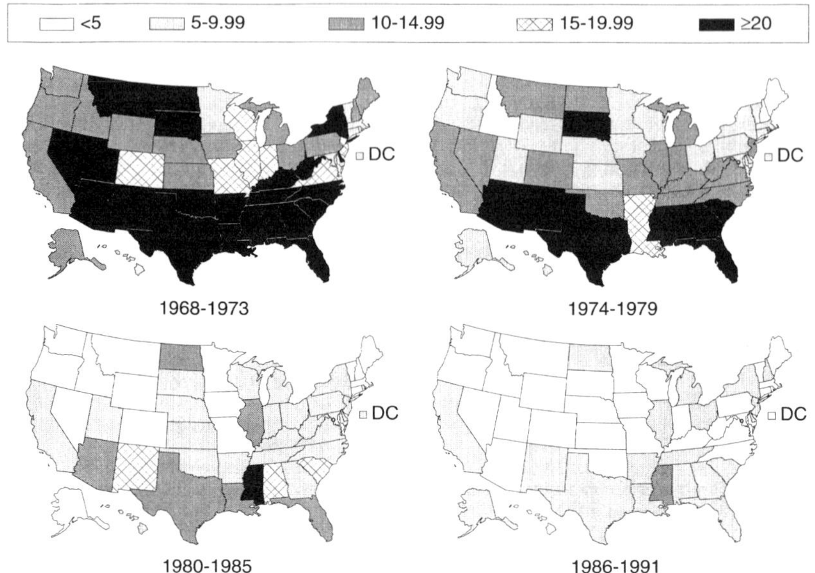

FIGURE 4.—Geographic distribution of diarrheal mortality rates (per 100,000 live births) among infants during 4 periods in the United States from 1968 through 1991. *Abbreviation:* DC, District of Columbia. (Courtesy of Kilgore PE, Holman RC, Clarke MJ, et al: Trends of diarrheal disease-associated mortality in US children, 1968 through 1991. *JAMA* 274:1143-1148, Copyright 1995, American Medical Association.)

▶ There have been many studies of mortality related to diarrhea in this country. In 1989, Ho and colleagues analyzed United States mortality data from 1973 to 1983 and suggested that mortality caused by diarrhea was, to a great extent, preventable.[1] Large racial and geographic differences in mortality were evident: black infants and residents of the southern states had disproportionately higher mortality rates than whites living in the northern or western states. Studies of linked birth and death records in Mississippi identified maternal characteristics—black race, young age, unmarried status, low educational level, and lack of prenatal care—to be associated with increased diarrheal disease–associated mortality in children. Ho and colleagues also identified a distinct seasonal peak of deaths and hospitalizations that began in the Southwest during November and moved progressively across the United States, reaching the Northeast during March, a phenomenon that matched the pattern of laboratory-confirmed rotavirus infections and permitted specific estimates of rotavirus-associated morbidity and mortality in United States children.

The report abstracted is important because in the past 24 years, changes have occurred that might have reduced this mortality and morbidity caused by diarrhea, including the introduction of oral rehydration, mass immunization against measles (decreasing the delayed complication of diarrhea), and improvements in food processing, food handling, and water quality. As this *JAMA* report indicates, diarrheal deaths nationwide have decreased 75% from 1968 to 1985, although there has been further decline since then.

The current analysis suggests that although children continue to die of diarrhea, characteristics of the high-risk children have changed over time. Children at risk are now younger than in the past. Although complications of diarrhea remain the most frequent secondary cause of death, prematurity is now a common secondary diagnosis, suggesting that preterm infants may comprise a group at high risk. Lastly, the pronounced racial and regional differences in rates of diarrheal mortality suggest that social factors continue to play a role in determining infant and child survival.

What will produce the next dramatic phase of decreased mortality caused by diarrhea? Chances are, it will be the introduction and widespread use of rotavirus vaccines. They come none too quickly, because it is not likely that in the short-term we can do much about the underlying social issues in this country that otherwise determine many of these morbidity and mortality factors.

While on the topic of diarrhea, how many individuals did "Typhoid Mary" infect, and whatever became of her, anyway?

In the summer of 1906, before the world had ever heard of a Typhoid Mary, typhoid struck a home in Oyster Bay on Long Island's north shore. Among the 4 family members and 7 servants in the house, 6 contracted the high and extended fever characteristic of typhoid. These individuals were found to be *Salmonella* typhi positive. When Long Island public health officials failed to identify the cause of the Oyster Bay outbreak, the owner of the house hired sanitary engineer George Soper, of New York's Department of Health, to investigate. It turns out that Mary Mallon, the household cook, had only begun working for the affected family 3 weeks before the first member of the household became ill. New York records indicated that typhoid had struck most of the homes where she had previously worked. Soper caught up with Mallon while she was employed at a Park Avenue residence. An ambulance containing 2 interns, 3 policemen, and a physician carried Mary Mallon off to a communicable diseases hospital in New York when she refused to cooperate, including declining giving up being a cook again.

Mary Mallon died in 1938, after 26 years of enforced isolation on the grounds of the Riverside Hospital for Communicable Diseases, located on remote North Brother Island in the East River. All she had to do to get out was to declare she would never be a cook again, but she refused. In the end, Typhoid Mary infected at least 51 people with the disease, 3 of whom died.

Reference

1. Ho M-S, et al: *JAMA* 260:3281, 1988.

A National Outbreak of *Salmonella enteritidis* Infections From Ice Cream

Hennessy TW, and the Investigation Team (Minnesota Dept of Health, Minneapolis)
N Engl J Med 334:1281–1286, 1996   2–16

Introduction.—Eating undercooked eggs that have been contaminated with *Salmonella enteritidis* is a major contributor to the occurrence of *Salmonella* disease in human beings. *Salmonella* infection is often associated with homemade ice cream or unpasteurized commercial ice cream but not generally with ice cream made from pasteurized ingredients. A large *Salmonella* outbreak caused by contamination of a national brand of ice cream was reported.

Methods.—The outbreak began in 1994, when health authorities in Minnesota noted an increasing number of reported *S. enteritidis* infections. One national brand of ice cream was implicated in a case-control study, prompting a product recall and additional epidemiologic and microbiological studies. A national surveillance study was implemented, and consumers who bought the implicated brand of ice cream were surveyed. The manufacturing process was compared for ice cream that was and was not associated with infection, matched for the manufacture date. Bacterial cultures were performed on ice cream samples at the ice cream plant, and in tanker trailers that had brought ice cream premix to the manufacturing plant.

Results.—Estimates suggested that eating the implicated brand of ice cream was associated with 224,000 cases of *S. enteritidis* gastroenteritis in the United States. Diarrhea and other symptoms occurred in about 7% of subjects who ate that brand of ice cream. Investigations suggested that the ice cream became contaminated because of premix transported by tanker trailers that had carried nonpasteurized eggs on their previous trip. Three percent of ice cream culture samples grew *S. enteritidis* compared with none of the samples from the ice cream plant or the tanker trailers.

Conclusion.—The largest United States outbreak of *Salmonella* infection appears to have resulted from contamination of ice cream premix when it was transported in trucks that had previously carried nonpasteurized eggs. Future outbreaks of this type could be avoided by making sure food products that are not destined for repasteurization are transported in dedicated containers. To detect *Salmonella* infection and other food-borne illnesses, the clinician must maintain a high level of suspicion, order appropriate laboratory tests, and report positive culture results to the public health department.

▶ When picking up this article, this editor could not understand why outbreaks of *Salmonella enteritidis* infections were still being reported in *The New England Journal of Medicine,* especially an outbreak related to what some might call a "no name" ice cream company. If you read the abstract, however, you will see why this report has received nationwide attention.

When an estimated quarter of a million cases of diarrhea result from a single common source, that's news. That's big news.

When it comes to finger pointing, the Schwan Ice Cream Company wasn't even at fault. The source of the contamination was an ice cream premix supplier that, between deliveries to the Schwan Ice Cream Company, used its tanker trucks to deliver liquid unpasteurized eggs to another customer. Obviously, their technique of sterilizing a tanker truck must have left a lot to be desired. A huge tanker is able to haul the contents of several million cracked eggs. Currently, in the United States, about 1 in 10,000 eggs is *Salmonella* positive. Sure as shooting, a tanker full of eggs is an 18-wheel biological moving hazard.

To learn more about the hazards of getting sick from eating, read the excellent commentary on lessons to be learned from this outbreak of salmonellosis.[1] Even alfalfa sprouts have been implicated as a source of *Salmonella* infection.[2] Clearly, food is not sterile, and eating anything is not totally risk-free. But watch out for off-brands of ice cream. Stick with well-known names. If you are feeling especially flush, revel in Ben & Jerry's.

P.S: If you are wondering where the Schwan Ice Cream plant is, it is located in Marshall, Minnesota. I can't find it on a state map, however...must be near Lake Wobegone.

This commentary closes with a query. When was the period of the highest number of pet-associated reported cases of *Salmonella* infection in the United States? That was in 1970 and 1971, when an estimated 280,000 cases of turtle-associated salmonellosis occurred in the Unted States. During that period, some 15 million turtles were sold annually here. Infection was so common that a ban on importation and interstate traffic of turtles occurred, and subsequently a 77% reduction in the frequency of salmonellosis caused by serotypes associated with turtles and an 18% reduction in salmonellosis in children ages 1–9 years occurred.[3]

As turtles have exited stage left, coming on stage right have been iguanas. Since 1978, the number of iguanas imported into the United States has increased more than 1500%, and it is estimated that approximately 2.8 million housholds own a pet reptile of this sort. This growing demand for pet iguanas has been met by a large supply of inexpensive juvenile iguanas raised on farms in Colombia and El Salvador. Overcrowding on breeding farms, during shipment, and in pet stores may provide opportunities for infection with *Salmonella*. More than three quarters of captured lizards are *Salmonella* "Marys" in the sense that they are asymptomatic carriers.

Unless you're willing to culture the doo-doo of an iguana, it would be a wise decision to keep these critters out of the home.

References

1. Blaser MJ: *N Engl J Med* 334:1325, 1996.
2. Ponka A: *Lancet* 345:462, 1995.
3. Cohen ML: *JAMA* 243:1247, 1980.

Clinical and Laboratory Characteristics of Human Granulocytic Ehrlichiosis

Bakken JS, Krueth J, Wilson-Nordskog C, et al (Duluth Clinic Ltd, Minn; Univ of Maryland, Baltimore)
JAMA 275:199–205, 1996   2–17

Background.—Human ehrlichiosis was first reported in 1987. The underlying infectious agent is *Ehrlichia chaffeensis,* a previously unknown obligate intracellular *Rickettsia*-like coccobacillus. Patients with human granulocytic ehrlichiosis (HGE) were retrospectively studied to characterize the clinical and laboratory features of this illness and to determine the value of diagnostic tools.

Methods.—Two hundred twenty-eight patients from Minnesota and Wisconsin who were seen for an acute febrile illness between June 1990 and May 1995 were included in the review. Patient ages ranged from 3 to 91 years. Forty-one patients (18%) had confirmed or probable HGE. Seventy-eight percent of these patients were male, aged 6–91 years, and 22% were female, aged 41–75 years.

Findings.—At the initial assessment, all patients with HGE had a temperature of 37.6°C or greater. Most patients also had headaches, myalgias, and chills, as well as various combinations of leukopenia, anemia, and thrombocytopenia. Morulae in the cytoplasm of peripheral blood neutrophils were present in 80% of the patients tested. Of 37 patients assessed by polymerase chain reaction, only 16 were positive for HGE. However, serum immunofluorescent antibody assays of acute or convalescent blood

TABLE 3.—Signs and Symptoms Observed in 41 Patients During the
Acute Phase of Human Granulocyte Ehrlichiosis

Sign or Symptom	No. (%)
Temperature ≥37.6°C	41 (100)
Malaise	40 (98)
Rigors	40 (98)
Myalgias	40 (98)
Sweats	40 (98)
Headache	35 (85)
Nausea	16 (39)
Anorexia	15 (37)
Vomiting	14 (34)
Arthralgias	11 (27)
Cough	12 (29)
Confusion	7 (17)
Prostration/weakness	7 (17)
Diarrhea	4 (10)
Pneumonia	4 (10)
Vertigo	2 (5)
Upper gastrointestinal tract bleeding	2 (5)
Seizure	1 (2)
Rash	1 (2)

(Courtesy of Bakken JS, Krueth J, Wilson-Nordskog C, et al: Clinical and laboratory characteristics of human granulocytic ehrlichiosis. *JAMA* 275:199–205, Copyright 1996, American Medical Association.)

TABLE 5.—Laboratory Findings in Patients With Acute Human Granulocytic Ehrlichiosis

Variable	Reference Range	No. of Patients	Mean Value (SD)	Median Value	Patient Range
White blood cell count, ±10⁹/L					
$\pm10^9$/L	4.0–10.7	36	4.6 (2.8)	3.3	1.1–16.4
Hemoglobin, g/L	130–170	36	135 (22)	134	86–170
Platelet count, $\times10^9$/L	150–450	36	66 (46)	79	13–435
Erythrocyte sedimentation rate, mm/h	0–21	18	29 (22)	27	5–94
C-reactive protein, mg/L	4–8	7	138 (88)	160	59–312
Aspartate aminotransferase, U/L	16–40	22	148 (157)	91	19–750
Lactate dehydrogenase, U/L	80–175	17	774 (1019)	313	183–3230
Creatinine, µmol/L	27–115	21	156 (106)	123	80–506
[mg/dL]	[0.3–1.3]		[1.8 (1.2)]	[1.3]	[0.8–5.7]

(Courtesy of Bakken JS, Krueth J, Wilson-Nordskog C, et al: Clinical and laboratory characteristics of human granulocytic ehrlichiosis. *JAMA* 275:199–205, Copyright 1996, American Medical Association.)

samples revealed antibodies against *Ehrlichia equi* in 38 of 40 patients evaluated. Two patients died. The calculated case death rate was 4.9% (Tables 3 and 5).

Conclusions.—An increasing number of HGE cases are being reported in Wisconsin and Minnesota. The severity of illness is correlated with advanced age, anemia, an increased percentage of neutrophils and a reduced percentage of lymphocytes in the peripheral blood, and the presence of morulae in neutrophils. Human granulocyte ehrlichiosis should be included in the differential diagnosis for patients with influenza-like illness after a tick bite. The fastest, most practical screening method for diagnosing HGE is currently microscopic assessment of the acute-phase blood smear for neutrophilic morulae.

▶ Human granulocytic ehrlichiosis is an acute, sometimes fatal, febrile illness. Unlike Lyme disease, it is usually accompanied by leukopenia, thrombocytopenia, and elevated serum aminotransferase levels. The first human ehrlichial infection to be recognized was Sennetsu fever, a mononucleosis-like illness described in Japan in 1954. The first report of infection in the United States was in 1986: a man acquired the infection from a tick bite while traveling in Arkansas. Human granulocytic ehrlichiosis is increasingly recognized now in northwestern Wisconsin, northeastern Minnesota, and other geographic regions where *Ixodes* species of ticks are found.

Human granulocytic ehrlichiosis should be suspected in previously healthy individuals in whom a febrile influenza-like illness suddenly develops, particularly if this occurs after outdoor activity in the upper Midwest. A history of tick exposure or an actual tick bite during the preceding weeks should further strengthen the suspicion of this disease. Infected patients characteristically complain of headaches, myalgias, and shaking chills. They are febrile. The physical examination is unlikely to reveal any abnormalities, although the younger the patient is, the greater the chance that a rash will be present. A rash, however, is not an intrinsic feature of this illness, which distinguishes it to some extent from the other commonly thought of tick-borne infection, Lyme disease.

The likelihood of being infected with the agent causing HGE varies inversely to the values of the absolute white blood cell count and the platelet count. The diagnosis is usually confirmed by a careful examination of the peripheral blood smear, which shows organisms in the neutrophils. The actual sensitivity of the peripheral blood smear as a diagnostic screening tool is unknown. Certainly a negative blood smear should not rule out the diagnosis of HGE.

To learn more about the agent that causes this fascinating entity, see the article that follows (Abstract 2–18).

Direct Cultivation of the Causative Agent of Human Granulocytic Ehrlichiosis

Goodman JL, Nelson C, Vitale B, et al (Univ of Minnesota, Minneapolis; Grantsburg Clinic, Wis; Univ of California, Davis; et al)
N Engl J Med 334:209–215, 1996   2–18

Objective.—Human granulocytic ehrlichiosis, transmitted by ticks, is a potentially fatal disease usually accompanied by leukopenia, thrombocytopenia, and elevated serum aminotransferase levels. Because symptoms are nonspecific, it is difficult to diagnose. The causative agent has never been cultured. The isolation and culture of this organism from 3 patients were described.

Patients.—A woman, 66 years of age, and 2 men, 61 and 64 years of age, from Wisconsin and Minnesota were admitted to hospitals with a variety of symptoms including unexplained fever, nausea or vomiting, granulocytopenia, and thrombocytopenia. Patients were treated successfully with either doxycycline or chloramphenicol.

Methods.—Blood from patients was incubated with the HL60 leukemia cell line and stained with Giemsa stain. The DNA was amplified by polymerase chain reaction (PCR).

Results.—Despite the fact that only 1 patient had ehrlichial inclusions in neutrophils, blood samples from all 3 patients contained ehrlichial DNA. Blood from patients caused infection in HL60 cells and lysis within 12–14 days after inoculation. Corroboration of the presence of ehrlichia in cultures was provided by immunofluorescence microscopy, DNA sequencing, and PCR analysis. Sequences of 16S ribosomal DNA from all 3 patients were identical but all differed from the animal agents *Ehrlichia equi,* with adenine rather than guanine at nucleotide 84, and *Ehrlichia phagocytophila.*

Conclusion.—The causative agent of human granulocytic ehrlichiosis has been cultured in HL60 cells. Isolation and identification of this agent should facilitate the diagnosis and treatment of infected patients.

▶ It was only recently that Everett et al. described the ability to detect in peripheral blood the agent that may cause human ehrlichiosis.[1] This was done with the use of PCR assay. This particular PCR assay has been continuously improved over the last 2 years and now has excellent sensitivity (86%) and specificity (100%) for the *Ehrlichia chaffeensis* organism. Unfortunately, PCR analysis of blood for confirming acute human granulocytic ehrlichiosis is currently limited to a few research institutions; hence, microscopic examination of acute-phase peripheral blood samples is currently the easiest and quickest method for making a provisional diagnosis in patients infected in high-risk areas of the United States such as the upper Midwest.

Why this report is important is fairly obvious. When you see a patient with myalgias, headache, thrombocytopenia, and elevated serum aminotransferase levels, you should immediately think of human granulocytic ehrlichiosis, but you might have a difficult time diagnosing it because the symptoms are nonspecific and the intraleukocytic inclusions may not be seen in every patient. What can be done, as these authors show, is to inoculate into cell culture the blood of infected patients and then show that the laboratory cultures are PCR positive for the causative agent.

The easiest way to make a diagnosis of ehrlichiosis is to think of it. Patients who have fever, headache, and generalized myalgia within 1 month after exposure to a tick should be considered potentially infected. If, during the course of infection leukopenia and thrombocytopenia occur, particularly if accompanied by evidence of mild hepatitis, think ehrlichiosis and consider treatment. Renal failure, respiratory insufficiency, and CNS involvement may occur. Because the estimated fatality rate is relatively high, about 5%, you probably will want to initiate therapy just on the basis of your suspicions. Therapy should not be delayed until a serologic diagnosis is established, which will take several weeks. Chances are, you will not be able to make a diagnosis by PCR because only a few laboratories have this technology. Even if organisms cannot be seen in peripheral blood white cells, start treatment with tetracycline or doxycycline. These antibiotics may be given orally or intravenously. If tetracyclines are contraindicated, chloramphenicol is the alternative. Therapy should continue for a minimum of 7 days. Unlike Lyme disease, there are no data to support the use of prophylactic treatment with antibiotics, either after a tick bite or before potential exposure to ticks. Such practices should be discouraged. Recommend the use of insect repellent for your patients who like to travel about in the woods.

Webster's dictionary defines a tick as any of a large group of wingless, blood-sucking insects that infest man, cattle, sheep, or other animals. These are degenerate creatures. They pass on all sorts of bad infections. Unless you want to get ticked off, avoid them like the plague.

Reference

1. Everett ED, et al: *Ann Intern Med* 120:730, 1994.

Mosquito-transmitted Malaria in New York City, 1993

Layton M, Parise ME, Campbell CC, et al (New York City Dept of Health; Ctrs for Disease Control and Prevention, Atlanta, Ga; Natl Ctr for Infectious Diseases, Atlanta, Ga; et al)
Lancet 346:729–731, 1995

2–19

Background.—Since the eradication of malaria in the United States in the mid-1950s, almost all malaria cases have been reported in travelers returning from a malarious area. However, some cases in patients with no history of travel or bloodborne exposure still occur. The epidemiologic investigation of 1 outbreak in New York City was presented.

Investigation.—Three cases of *Plasmodium falciparum* malaria in residents of Queens were reported in August 1993. None of the patients had traveled recently or had been exposed through blood, although 1 patient had been to Thailand 2 years before the malaria was diagnosed. The 3 patients lived in separate houses in the same neighborhood and became ill within a day of one another. Patient interviews were conducted, and active attempts were made to find other cases. New York flight and shipping arrivals were reviewed. An entomological survey was also conducted in search of anopheline mosquitoes and breeding sites.

Findings.—Although the area was dry and neither adult nor larval anophelines were found at the time of the investigation, the weather conditions at the probable time of infection were very different. It was determined that malaria was probably transmitted to 2 patients by local anopheline mosquitoes that had bitten infected human hosts. Because there was no evidence of ongoing transmission, mosquito-control measures were not implemented.

Conclusions.—This occurrence of mosquito-transmitted malaria in New York City demonstrates that malaria transmission can be reintroduced into regions that are no longer endemic for the disease. Continued surveillance and prompt investigations are needed when malaria occurs in patients without risk factors.

▶ Another report dealing with malaria within the boundaries of our shores. You will recall from prior YEAR BOOKS OF PEDIATRICS the suggestion that some malaria in the United States is carried by mosquitoes brought to our continent on international airliners (a phenomenon now dubbed "airport malaria").[1, 2] In the past few years, there has been a change in the epidemiology of locally acquired malaria in the United States, with transmission occurring in more densely populated and developed areas. Before 1990, almost all cases were transmitted in rural settings. Since 1990, it has been reported in highly populated parts of California and suburban New Jersey, albeit in just 3 cases. Between 1957 and 1992, the Centers for Disease Control and Prevention has documented 69 cases of locally acquired malaria in our country, the most common species identified being *Plasmodium vivax*. The patients reported in the abstract above are unique in that *P. falciparum* was acquired in an urban setting, and all 3 individuals probably were infected within a close period by mosquitoes that had fed on the blood of immigrants from malaria-endemic countries.

What to do about this problem isn't entirely clear. Nothing was done in Queens. New York City officials believed that there was not an active breeding site of mosquitoes for which they could do anything. They were right, because after these 3 cases appeared, no others occurred.

The occurrence of local transmission of malaria demonstrates the importance of considering this fascinating infectious disorder in the differential diagnosis of any fever of unknown origin, even in the absence of identifiable risk factors. A thick preparation of peripheral blood is cheap and diagnostic.

Nine out of 10 patients who die of malaria are children. A recent article on this topic shows that the main marker of a serious bout of malaria that can lead to death is presentation with respiratory distress associated with acidosis and pulmonary edema.[3]

References

1. Brooke JH, et al: *N Engl J Med* 331:22, 1994.
2. Isaacson M: *Bull World Health Organ* 67:737, 1989.
3. Marsh K, et al: *N Engl J Med* 332:1399, 1995.

Structured Guidelines for the Use of Influenza Vaccine Among Children With Chronic Pulmonary Disorders
Hayden GF, Frayha H, Kattan H, et al (Univ of Virginia, Charlottesville; King Faisal Specialist Hosp and Research Centre, Riyadh, Saudi Arabia)
Pediatr Infect Dis J 14:895–899, 1995   2–20

Background.—Influenza remains a prominent cause of illness and death in children who are predisposed to severe infection. Annual vaccination has been recommended for children at high risk, but many of these patients still are not immunized each year, possibly in part because pediatricians are not always familiar with those high-risk conditions that warrant vaccination. Vaccination has been recommended in particular for children aged 6 months or older who have chronic pulmonary disorders.

Objective.—A pilot study was carried out to develop specific and detailed guidelines for influenza immunization. The guidelines (Table 1) were established after reviewing a number of published sources, including the International Classification of Diseases.

Patient Base.—Hospital records were reviewed for 73 children aged 6 months and older who, in the past month, had visited an allergy clinic or a developmental high-risk neonatology clinic.

Study Plan.—Four reviewers independently examined the charts to determine whether vaccination was warranted based on the child's pulmonary status. Two reviewers, a general pediatrician and a pediatric infectious diseases specialist, used the guidelines in making their decisions. The other 2, a general pediatrician and a specialist in pediatric pulmonary

TABLE 1.—Suggested Indications for Influenza Vaccination of Children Older Than 6 Months With Chronic Pulmonary Disease

Underlying Chronic Pulmonary Disorder	ICD-9 Code
Asthma of moderate to high severity including	493.*
chronic obstructive asthma	493.2
Bronchiectasis	494.
Also congenital bronchiectasis	748.61
Also tuberculous bronchiectasis	011.5
Also Kartagener's syndrome	759.3*
Chronic pulmonary disease arising in the neonatal period, including bronchopulmonary dysplasia, interstitial pulmonary fibrosis of infancy and Wilson-Mikity syndrome	770.7
Cystic fibrosis	277.00–01
Other chronic pulmonary disorder with impaired lung function† including	
Pulmonary alveolar proteinosis	516.0
Idiopathic pulmonary hemosiderosis	516.1
Idiopathic fibrosing alveolitis (includes diffuse pulmonary fibrosis)	516.3
Obstructive chronic bronchitis	491.2
Chronic airway obstruction (includes nonspecific COPD)	496.
Sarcoidosis with lung involvement	135. and 517.8
Systemic lupus erythematosus with lung involvement	710.1 and 517.8
Alpha 1-antitrypsin deficiency	277.6*
Congenital emphysema	770.2
Chronic recurrent aspiration	507.0*
Tracheostomy	31.1–2
Agenesis of lung	748.5
Lobar atelectasis	518.0*
Lipoid pneumonia, exogenous	507.1
Other unspecified	
Neuromuscular or orthopedic disorder affecting the chest and associated with impaired lung function†	
Duchenne muscular dystrophy	359.1*
Myotonic disorders	359.2
Myasthenia gravis	358.0
Quadriplegia	344.0
Werdnig-Hoffman disease (progressive spinal atrophy)	335.0
Asphyxiating thoracic dystrophy	756.4*
Other unspecified	

* ICD-9 code is nonspecific and includes other diseases.

† Impaired lung function defined as follows: for restrictive disease, vital capacity less than 60% to 80% of predicted; for obstructive disease, peak expiratory flow rate less than 60% to 80% of predicted; or hospitalization in previous year because of impaired lung function.

Abbreviations: ICD, International Classification of Diseases; *COPD*, chronic obstructive pulmonary disease.

(Courtesy of Hayden GF, Frayha H, Kattan H, et al: Structured guidelines for the use of influenza vaccine among children with chronic pulmonary disorders. *Pediatr Infect Dis J* 14:895–899, 1995.)

medicine, based their decisions on unspecified clinical judgment. Thirty-six of the 73 children had asthma, and 26 had other pulmonary disorders.

Results.—The reviewers who used the guidelines were likelier to agree than were the 2 who did not. The respective kappa figures were 0.73 and 0.31. Of 34 children for whom all 4 reviewers recommended vaccination, only 13 (38%) had in fact been vaccinated.

Implication.—Physicians are most likely to agree on the propriety of vaccination in a given case when they have access to a detailed list of pulmonary disorders that may warrant immunization.

▶ Fact: Many high-risk patients do not receive annual influenza immunization.

Fact: Many pediatric care providers, including pediatricians, are not sufficiently familiar with the high-risk conditions that warrant influenza vaccination.

Fact: In many instances, physicians who do have an accurate knowledge of influenza and the influenza vaccine fail to translate this knowledge into clinical practice. Why?

The "why" is probably based on the phenomenon that we don't imprint as well as we should with recommendations that have to do with prevention of diseases that are not uniformly problematic from year to year. Influenza is an important cause of morbidity and mortality in children, especially in those with underlying abnormalities that predispose them to severe influenza. The *Red Book* Committee and the Immunization Practice Advisory Committee of the United States Public Health Service both have made recommendations about the use of influenza vaccine. Both endorse influenza immunization of children at 6 months of age or older who have chronic pulmonary diseases. The *Red Book* Committee targets "children with asthma and other chronic pulmonary diseases,"[1] whereas the Immunization Practice Advisory Committee specifies "children with chronic disorders of the pulmonary system, including children with asthma."[2]

What Hayden et al. have done for us in this report from the *Pediatric Infectious Disease Journal* is to define more specific guidelines about who should and who should not be immunized. Table 1 indicates the entities for which influenza vaccine should be given. Following this table will not lead care providers in a bad direction. For example, if vaccine is available and affordable, it is logistically easier to target all children with asthma rather than having to discriminate between children whose asthma is mild vs. moderate. As resources allow, it is reasonable to extend vaccination even further. Healthy children residing in households of children or adults with asthma (or other chronic pulmonary disorders) can also be targeted for vaccination, to provide an additional wall of immunity surrounding the high-risk patient.

Guidelines should not be intended to be used as rigid rules but rather as flexible ones that can be modified as clinically indicated. How detailed the guidelines should be is a debatable point. Most of us are grateful when we see detailed guidelines rather than vague or nonspecific ones. This is the value of the report abstracted. Detailed guidelines allow us to decide what latitude we should use in applying such guidelines to specific patients whose medical histories and health status may be relatively unique.

To the extent to which committees that make guidelines on vaccinations believe they can provide more specific recommendations, they should. We all know that such recommendations are based on imperfect data. Specific recommendations help practitioners translate the intentions of these committees into practice in a much more effective manner. Such committees worry about tying our hands with highly specific recommendations. On the other hand, the consequence of too vague and too general a set of recommendations is that children will not get immunized. Let practitioners have detailed recommendations, but give them the latitude to use the recommendations as they see fit.

References

1. American Academy of Pediatrics: 1994 *Red Book: Report of the Committee on Infectious Diseases,* ed 23. Elk Grove Village, Ill, American Academy of Pediatrics, 1994, p 275.
2. Advisory Committee on Immunization Practices (ACIP) of the US Public Health Service: *MMWR Morb Mortal Wkly Rep* 43:1, 1994.

Cost-effectiveness Analysis of a Rotavirus Immunization Program for the United States
Smith JC, Haddix AC, Teutsch SM, et al (Natl Ctr for Infectious Diseases, Atlanta, Ga)
Pediatrics 96:609–615, 1995   2–21

Background.—Rotavirus (RV) is the most prevalent cause of severe diarrhea in children throughout the world. Virtually all children are infected in the first 5 years of life. It is estimated that in the early 1980s, RV infection of infants and young children caused at least 65,000 hospital admissions and 125 deaths each year. Live attenuated oral vaccines are under development. They are designed to be administered in 3 doses in the first 6 months of life along with other vaccines.

Objective.—Cost-effectiveness analysis of a national RV immunization program was planned to determine the economic implications of routinely immunizing children younger than 1 year.

Methods.—Health outcomes and costs of RV diarrhea were estimated for a cohort of 4.1 million children followed from birth to age 5 years, with and without an immunization program. Estimates of disease incidence, medical and productivity costs, vaccine efficacy, and vaccine coverage rates were obtained from the published literature and from unpublished vaccine trial reports. Sensitivity analysis was used to gauge the impact of altered estimates of vaccine efficacy and medical costs. Incremental cost-effectiveness was expressed as the savings per case of RV diarrhea prevented.

Results.—During 5 years, vaccination was estimated to prevent more than 1 million cases of RV diarrhea; avoid 433,000 physician visits and 58,000 hospital admissions; and prevent 82 deaths. If vaccine cost $30 per dose, an immunization program would yield a net savings of $79 million in discounted costs. Adding in the productivity gained, society would realize a net savings of $466 million. The incremental cost-effectiveness of immunization was a savings of $78 of health care costs per case prevented. From a societal perspective, the savings per case was $459. The threshold vaccine cost below which immunization saved health care costs was $40 (Fig 2).

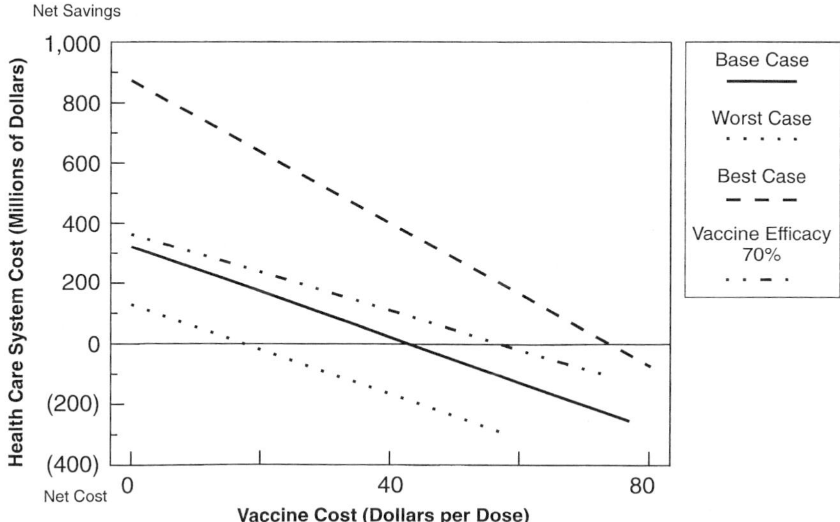

FIGURE 2.—Net savings (cost) of a rotavirus immunization program to the health care system by cost of vaccine (per dose, purchase and administration). Base case, best case, and worst case sensitivity analyses were performed. At the threshold (break-even) vaccine cost, all costs of the vaccine program are offset by reductions in the cost of rotavirus illness (threshold cost: base case, $40; best case, $74; and worst case, $17). With 70% vaccine efficacy, the threshold vaccine cost is $44. (Courtesy of Smith JC, Haddix AC, Teutsch SM, et al: Cost-effectiveness analysis of a rotavirus immunization program for the United States. Reproduced by permission of *Pediatrics,* Vol 96, pp 609–615, Copyright 1995.)

Conclusion.—Immunization of infants against RV appears to be cost-effective from the perspective of both the health care system and society.

▶ Licensure of the RV vaccine took place in 1996. When initially licensed, vaccines do not automatically come with recommendations that would guide the practitioner concerning their use. Such decisions must be based on a combination of demonstrated clinical effectiveness and safety and cost-effectiveness. The latter is what this report is all about.

Rotavirus infection is estimated to cause some 3 million cases of diarrhea, at least 65,000 hospitalizations, and 125 deaths annually among infants and young children. Even if the vaccine is only 50% effective, the investment in a wide-scale immunization program would more than "break even." The figures are pretty straightforward; when cost and probability estimates that would maximally bias against any immunization program are evaluated, a vaccine program remains effective as long as the cost and administration of the vaccine is less than $17 per dose. This cost compares reasonably well with the cost of current routine childhood vaccines, which range from $6.29 per dose (oral polio, vaccine only, weighted public and private sector cost) to $20.31 (measles, mumps, rubella, vaccine only, weighted public and private sector cost). The authors in this report used a 1993 estimate of medical costs resulting from RV infection, a cost of $427 million. Chances are that this is undershooting the true cost of this infection, providing even more margin to the cost-effectiveness of RV immunization program for our country.

To learn more about present and future challenges of a variety of immunizations as related to the health care of children, read the excellent review of this topic by Anne Gershon.[1]

Reference

1. Gershon A: *Pediatr Infect Dis J* 14:445, 1995.

Decay of Maternally Derived Measles Antibody in a Highly Vaccinated Population in Southern Israel

Dagan R, Slater PE, Duvdevani P, et al (Ben-Gurion Univ of the Negev, Beer-Sheva, Israel; Ministry of Health, Jerusalem; Chaim Sheba Med Ctr, Tel-Hashomer, Israel)
Pediatr Infect Dis J 14:965–969, 1995
2–22

Background.—Introducing live attenuated measles vaccine in Israel in 1967 markedly reduced the annual incidence of disease, but outbreaks continued to occur. A number of reports from North America point to a rapid decrease in maternal antibody titers in infants, but there are no accurate data from other highly vaccinated Western populations.

Objective.—Measles antibody titers were monitored in Jewish children born in 1988 and 1989 in southern Israel, where vaccination coverage

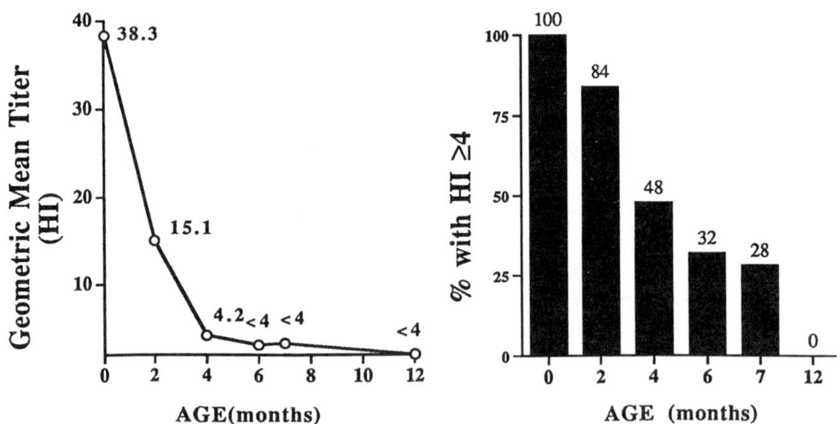

FIGURE 1.—Percent seropositive and geometric mean titer of anti-measles antibodies measured by hemagglutination inhibition during first year of life. Testing was performed on 49 or 50 specimens for each age group. *Abbreviation: HI,* hemagglutination inhibition. (Courtesy of Dagan R, Slater PE, Duvdevani P, et al: Decay of maternally derived measles antibody in a highly vaccinated population in southern Israel. *Pediatr Infect Dis J* 14:965–969, 1995.)

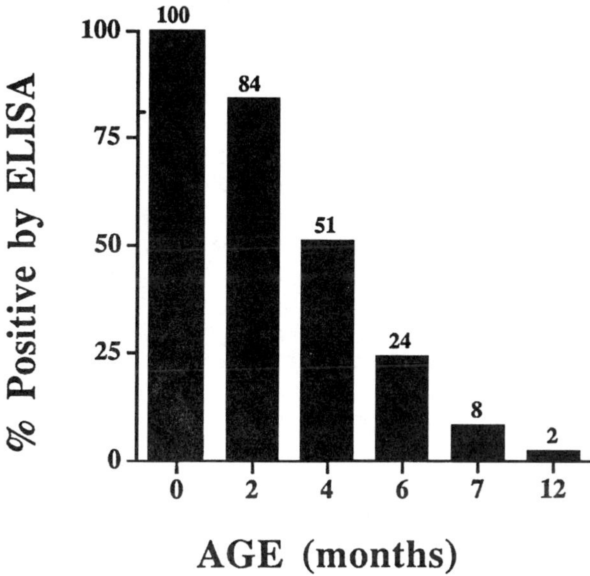

AGE (months)

FIGURE 2.—Percent seropositive for anti-measles antibodies measured by enzyme-linked immunosorbent assay during first year of life. Testing was performed on 47–50 specimens for each age group. *Abbreviation: ELISA, enzyme-linked immunosorbent assay.* (Courtesy of Dagan R, Slater PE, Duvdevani P, et al: Decay of maternally derived measles antibody in a highly vaccinated population in southern Israel. *Pediatr Infect Dis J* 14:965–969, 1995.)

exceeds 90%. All infants studied were born at term weighing at least 2,500 g and had no neonatal or perinatal health problems.

Results.—All cord blood specimens were seropositive by hemagglutination inhibition (HI) testing; the geometric mean titer was 38 (Fig 1). Titers decreased rapidly, and no HI antibody was detected at 6 months of age in 68% of specimens. Similar trends were seen in enzyme-linked immunosorbent assay (ELISA) antibody titers (Fig 2). Only 2 specimens taken at 1 year of age remained positive. In mothers younger than 28 years, maternal age was unrelated to antibody titers and the duration of seropositivity. Only 7% of sera negative by HI and ELISA testing were positive on neutralization testing. All sera were negative by neutralization testing by 1 year of age.

Conclusions.—Most infants become seronegative for measles antibody within a year of birth. The present findings and those from North America suggest that 1-year-old infants receive primary immunization against measles, mumps, and rubella.

▶ Who would have thought that we would still be arguing about the appropriate timing for the measles vaccine? But indeed we are. Measles vaccine traditionally has been given at 15 months of age along with mumps and rubella immunization. There has been concern that immunizing against these viruses earlier would be risky because of the presence of maternal antibody that would interfere with successful immunization, thereby subjecting these kids to the possibility of growing up to be adults with no protection. When determining the age for measles immunization, one must strike a balance between the age at which the risk of infection becomes significant and the age at which optimal seroconversion can be achieved.

Most infants are susceptible to clinical measles infection after the age of 6 months. It's not appropriate, however, to immunize at this young age because there would be many "non-takes." The issue is lowering the age from 15 months to 12 months. This study shows that one can get away with immunizing at 12 months. This could substantially reduce the number of susceptible young children during outbreaks of measles without significantly increasing the risk of vaccine failure. Thus, the American Academy of Pediatrics was correct in its recent recommendation that the measles immunization age be lowered from 15 months to 12–15 months.[1] It's not likely that we'll see a further lowering of this age.

One last comment on the topic of measles. The ever-present dialogue linking vitamin A sufficiency and measles continues to evolve. A report from New York City shows that many children younger than 2 years have low vitamin A levels when ill with measles and that such children seem to have an increased morbidity from their infection.[2] Furthermore, when they recover, they have lower measles-specific antibody levels. This seriously raises the question of whether we as clinicians may wish to consider vitamin A therapy for all children younger than 2 years with severe measles. This would be a relatively innocuous therapeutic tool that could be quite cost-effective.

References

1. Committee on Infectious Diseases: *Red Book: Report of the Committee on Infectious Diseases*, ed 33. Elk Grove Village, Ill, American Academy of Pediatrics, 1994, p 308.
2. Frieden TR, et al: *Am J Dis Child* 146:182, 1992.

Detection of Measles Virus RNA in Urine Specimens From Vaccine Recipients

Rota PA, Khan AS, Durigon E, et al (Natl Ctr for Infectious Diseases, Atlanta, Ga)
J Clin Microbiol 33:2485–2488, 1995   2–23

Introduction.—Despite vaccination programs, there are still occasional outbreaks and epidemics of measles throughout the world, including the United States. Control of these outbreaks now depends more on laboratory tests to confirm the presence of infection than on clinical diagnosis. Reverse transcriptase–polymerase chain reaction (RT-PCR) was used to detect measles virus RNA in urine from recently vaccinated patients.

Methods.—Twelve children aged 15 months and 4 young adults who had received measles immunization were studied. Daily urine samples were

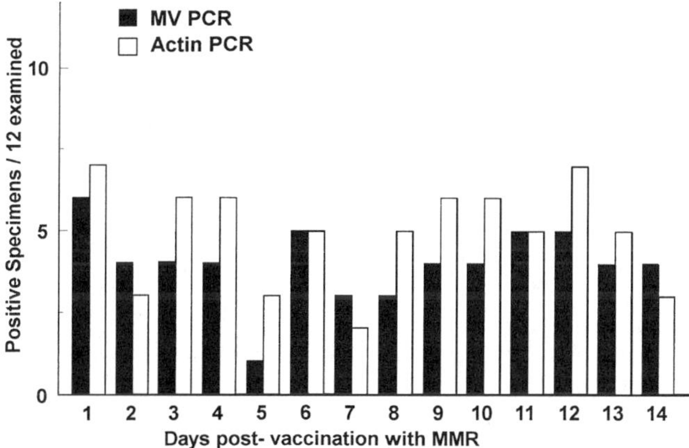

FIGURE 2.—Time course of detection of measles virus RNA in urine specimens from vaccinated children. *Bar heights* indicate numbers (total = 12) of MV-positive and actin-positive samples on each day of sampling. *Abbreviations:* MV, measles virus; *PCR*, polymerase chain reaction; *MMR*, measles-mumps-rubella vaccine. (Courtesy of Rota PA, Khan AS, Durigon E, et al: Detection of measles virus RNA in urine specimens from vaccine recipients. *J Clin Microbiol* 33:2485–2488, 1995, American Society for Microbiology.)

collected from all patients for 2 weeks after immunization and analyzed by RT-PCR for the presence of measles virus RNA.

Results.—The RT-PCR detected measles virus RNA in the urine of 10 of 12 children studied. The identification of measles virus RNA could occur as early as 1 day or as late as 14 days after vaccination (Fig 2). Measles virus RNA was also detected in the urine of all 4 young adults between 1 and 13 days after vaccination. In the adults, there were signs that preexisting immunity may have reduced replication or shedding of the vaccine virus.

Conclusions.—Reverse transcriptase–polymerase chain reaction can detect measles virus RNA in urine samples. It promises to be a quick test for measles infection in a specimen that can be obtained noninvasively from a large number of individuals. Future studies will seek to define the extent of asymptomatic or mild infection of patient contacts during measles outbreaks, to assess the role of these cases in measles transmission, and to define shedding patterns in vaccine recipients.

▶ Another report that shows how powerful a tool PCR is. With the use of PCR and the information provided from the report abstracted, a whole new world of investigation is now possible in examining measles outbreaks. Despite the existence of an effective vaccine, measles virus continues to cause sporadic outbreaks and epidemics of disease in the United States and throughout the world. Most recent outbreaks have involved either children who were too young to be vaccinated or older children and teenagers, most of whom had been previously vaccinated. Because of the sporadic nature of outbreaks in populations with high rates of vaccination, the altered presentation of clinical signs that occurs in "mild" measles infections, and the presence of other exanthem-causing infections, effective public health measures to control measles outbreaks are more dependent on laboratory confirmation of infection than on diagnosis based on clinical presentation. Currently available diagnostic techniques, which include virus isolation, viral antigen detection, and serologic antibody studies, are very sensitive and specific. However, these techniques are labor intensive, require specimen collection by medically trained personnel, and would be inappropriate for screening large numbers of individuals. How wonderful it would be if all one had to do was produce a sample of urine to solve all of these collection and cost problems. This report shows us that it can be that simple. The detection of measles virus RNA in urine using PCR is a rapid means of detecting measles infections with a clinical specimen that is more readily and conveniently accessible than serum or nasopharyngeal aspirates. Collection of urine specimens could be done in the absence of medical professionals, and on-site specimen-processing requirements would be minimal or nonexistent.

The investigators who did this study were able to show that (1) within 24 hours of receiving measles vaccine, we begin to shed viral particles in our urine; (2) during acute natural infection, measles virus is routinely isolated from the urine for as long as 10 days after the onset of a rash; and (3) with the changing epidemiology of measles, we have been missing a lot of clinical cases of measles. Were we to have a cheap, simple urine test, we would be able to find out a great deal more about the total spectrum of natural measles infection.

In summary, PCR has proven to be a rapid and sensitive method to detect measles virus RNA in a variety of clinical specimens including urine. Urine samples will now allow us to detect measles infection from a specimen that can be obtained from large numbers of individuals by inexpensive means. With these technologies, people at the Centers for Disease Control and Prevention are planning to explore the extent of asymptomatic or mild infection in case contacts during outbreaks, to determine the role that these cases play in the transmission of measles, and to determine the shedding pattern of vaccine recipients in healthy and in immunocompromised hosts.

Stay tuned for another round of new information about measles, all of which will be yielded by a new technology—PCR.

Clinical Manifestations Associated With Human Herpesvirus 7 Infection
Torigoe S, Kumamoto T, Koide W, et al (Shingu Municipal Hosp, Wakayama, Japan; Osaka Univ, Japan)
Arch Dis Child 72:518–519, 1995   2–24

Background.—Human herpesvirus 7 (HHV-7), a new herpesvirus recently isolated from CD4⁺ T cells, is a causal agent for exanthem subitum. The clinical manifestations of HHV-7 were reported.

TABLE 2.—Clinical Manifestations in Children Seroconverting to HHV-7

Case No	Past history of exanthem subitum*	HHV-6 antibody	Child's age at HHV-7 seroconversion (months)	Clinical symptoms
1	Yes	Positive	18	Second episode of exanthem subitum*
2	No	Positive	17	Exanthem subitum*
3	Yes	Positive	12	Second episode of exanthem subitum*
4	No	Positive	10	Exanthem subitum*
5	No	Positive	17	Exanthem subitum*
6	Yes	Positive	13	Second episode of exanthem subitum*
7	No	Positive	16	Exanthem subitum*, febrile convulsion
8	No	Positive	20	Exanthem subitum*
9	No	Positive	10	Exanthem subitum*
10	Yes	Positive	31	Second episode of exanthem subitum*
11	No	Negative	18	Exanthem subitum*
12	No	Negative	13	Exanthem subitum*, acute infantile hemiplegia
13	Yes	Positive	15	Skin rash (macular)
14	Yes	Positive	10	No symptoms
15	Yes	Positive	15	No symptoms
16	Yes	Positive	7	Not clear (cough and rhinorrhea?)
17	Yes	Positive	19	Not clear (4 days fever ?)
18	Yes	Positive	23	Not clear (2 days fever ?)
19	Yes	Positive	38	Not clear (macular skin rash ?)
20	Yes	Positive	16	Not clear (2 days fever ?)
21	No	Positive	23	Not clear
22	Yes	Positive	15	Not clear (fever ?)

* Symptoms of exanthem subitum.
Abbreviation: HHV, human herpesvirus.
(Courtesy of Torigoe S, Kumamoto T, Koide W, et al: Clinical manifestations associated with human herpesvirus 7 infection. *Arch Dis Child* 72:518–519, 1995.)

Methods and Findings.—Twenty-two children who seroconverted to HHV-7 were investigated. The mean age of these children was 17.1 months. Twelve children had exanthem subitum around HHV-7 seroconversion. Only 4 children in this group had histories of exanthem subitum associated with the second episode of exanthem subitum with HHV-7 infection. Neurologic complications—febrile convulsion and acute infantile hemiplegia—occurred in 2 patients. Among the 10 children without exanthem subitum around HHV-7 seroconversion, 1 had a skin rash without fever that may have been associated with HHV-7 infection, and 9 had histories of exanthem subitum (Table 2). In the first 12 patients, the mean maximum body temperature was 38.9°C, with a mean duration of 2.08 days. In 58.3% of the children, skin rash appeared 1–1.5 days after defervescence. Mean white blood cell and platelet counts were significantly lower in the acute than in the convalescent phase.

Conclusions.—Human herpesvirus 7 apparently induces exanthem subitum and other symptoms associated with HHV-6 infection. Although neurologic complications occurred in 2 children, more research is needed before HHV-7 infection is concluded to be associated with such sequelae.

▶ Herpesvirus 7 is another causal agent for roseola (exanthem subitum). It is clearly different from HHV-6, which had been previously described to be a cause of roseola. Obviously, more than 1 herpesvirus can produce the same set of clinical findings: temperature higher than 39°C for 1 day or more, followed by a maculopapular rash that appears around the time of defervescence and that disappears within 1–4 days. What this report from Japan tells us is that HHV-7, while mimicking HHV-6 in its clinical presentation vis-à-vis roseola, occurs later than HHV-6 (average age of onset for HHV-7 is 17.1 months vs. 11.5 months for HHV-6). Also, it is well known that HHV-6 is a common cause of febrile seizures in young children. We need to know a lot more about HHV-7 to find out whether the same is true for this virus.[1]

In my computer's literature search database, I looked for every article on HHV-7. There are studies linking it with Kawasaki disease and with a disorder mimicking Epstein-Barr virus infection. Whether it truly causes anything beyond exanthem subitum is something that only additional studies will be able to prove.

Reference

1. Ward KN, et al: *J Med Virol* 42:119, 1994.

California Pediatricians' Knowledge of and Response to Recommendations for Universal Infant Hepatitis B Immunization
Wood DL, Rosenthal P, Scarlata D (Cedars Sinai Med Ctr, Los Angeles; RAND, Santa Monica, Calif; Amgen Corp, Thousand Oaks, Calif)
Arch Pediatr Adolesc Med 149:769–773, 1995   2–25

Objective.—Because pediatricians supervise more than two thirds of primary care visits of children younger than 5 years and give about half of all immunizations to infants, it is necessary to know how aware they are of recent recommendations for universally immunizing infants against hepatitis B. To this end, a questionnaire was sent to 1,030 pediatricians in California, 71% of whom responded.

Respondents.—Nearly half of the 526 eligible respondents practiced alone or in a group. Another quarter practiced in a health center, health department, or public hospital, and one fifth worked in an HMO setting. The average time in practice was about 13 years.

Findings.—All but 6% of respondents were aware of recommendations for hepatitis B immunization. More than half were able to correctly answer questions dealing with hepatitis B virus serology and immunization schedules. Approximately three fourths of the respondents agreed with the recommendations, and 82% presently immunize all infants or plan to do so. Those working in HMOs were likelier to be immunizing all infants (Table 2). Those able to correctly answer questions about screening and prophylaxis also were more likely to report immunizing all infants. The most common reason for disagreeing with the recommendations was concern about the long-term efficacy of hepatitis B vaccine. Cost and an objection to 3 shots at 1 visit also were commonly cited.

TABLE 2.—Comparison Between Pediatricians Who Immunize or Plan to Immunize All Infants Against Hepatitis B Virus and Those Who Do Not

	Universally Immunize Infants?		
	Yes *(n = 402)*	*No* *(n = 90)*	*P*
Practice setting			
Solo/two-physician practice/group practice (n = 240)	79.2	20.8	
Health center/PHD/public hospital/medical school faculty (n =116)	79.3	20.7	0.04
HMO (n =97)	91.8	8.3	
Resident/other (n =34)	79.4	20.6	
Insurance type as proportion of patients in pediatrician's practice*			
HMO			
Low/medium (n =334)	78.7	21.3	
High (n =118)	91.9	8.1	< 0.01
Medicaid			
Low/medium (n =343)	83.1	16.9	
High (n =93)	78.3	21.2	0.29
Privately insured			
Low/medium (n =323)	83.0	12.1	
High (n =119)	79.8	20.2	0.45
Proportion of patients in the practice who have low income*			
Low/medium (n =302)	78.3	21.7	
High (n =103)	88.7	17.2	0.01
Years in practice, mean±SD (n =499)	13.3 ± 8	11.6 ± 9.6	0.01
Physician's primary source of information regarding hepatitis B immunization			
CDC/*MMWR* (n =136)	83.8	16.2	
AAP newspaper (n =261)	84.3	15.7	
Journals (n =37)	67.6	32.4	0.03
Other (n =54)	73.9	26.1	
Maternal hepatitis B screening and infant treatment for hepatitis B antigen-positive mother			
High level of knowledge (n =303)	85.2	14.8	
Incomplete level of knowledge (n =189)	76.2	23.8	0.01
Level of agreement with the recommendations			
Agree (n =351)	90.3	9.7	
Disagree (n =103)	54.4	45.6	< 0.01

* Wilcoxon-Mann-Whitney test used to test differences between groups.

Abbreviations: PHD, public health department; CDC, Centers for Disease Control and Prevention; *MMWR*, Morbidity and Mortality Weekly Report; *AAP*, American Academy of Pediatrics.

(Courtesy of Wood DL, Rosenthal P, Scarlata D: California pediatricians' knowledge of and response to recommendations for universal infant hepatitis B immunization. *Arch Pediatr Adolesc Med* 149:769–773, Copyright 1995, American Medical Association.)

Implications.—The advent of combination vaccines and measures to control costs should help convince all pediatricians of the need to immunize all infants against hepatitis B.

▶ It has been 4–5 years since the Advisory Committee on Immunization Practices of the American Academy of Pediatrics (AAP) issued recommendations calling for hepatitis B immunization of all infants. These recommendations were met with criticism, and their implementation initially was controversial. Several concerns were raised: Why should pediatricians immunize an infant for a disease of adulthood? What is the long-term efficacy of the vaccine? What is the cost-effectiveness of the vaccine, particularly in an era in which our immunization programs are already overburdened?

That was the situation almost half a decade ago. What has happened in the meantime? As this survey shows, virtually every pediatrician, in California at least, is aware of the recommendations. Those who agree with the recommendations implement them. The rub is that 1 pediatrician in 5, at least as of the time of this survey, disagrees with the recommendations. The principal reservation has to do with whether this vaccine will provide lasting immunity. Cost does remain a concern for some.

Candor requires a confession on this editor's part. He, too, had reservations about this vaccine, mostly based on the cost issue. If the amount of money that was to be spent on the hepatitis vaccine could be used for other needs of children, might we not get a better bang for the buck? This confession, however, comes with a penance. The penance is an admission that this editor was wrong. This vaccine is worthwhile and should be administered along the guidelines of the AAP and the Centers for Disease Control and Prevention. It certainly is likely to save as many lives as some of the other vaccines we use these days.

While on this topic, why is orienteering the 513th reason not to exercise? Orienteers may have a higher than anticipated risk of contracting hepatitis B. A little-known fact is that a very large epidemic of hepatitis developed among Swedish orienteers in the early 1960s. In that epidemic, more than 600 competitors became infected with an agent that caused hepatitis. At the time there was no serologic test for hepatitis B, but stored samples that were examined years later showed that the epidemic was caused by hepatitis B virus.[1]

Orienteering is a sport in which runners, with the aid of a map and a compass, try to find control points in the terrain. At the time of the outbreak in Sweden, the cloths worn by the competitors usually consisted of shorts, short-sleeve shirts, socks, and shoes. Competitors rarely used leg shields. During the races, most of the runners received skin scratches on their extremities. Blood contact probably occurred after the competition, when hundreds of orienteers would bathe together in stagnant or slow-moving water. Swedish authorities suspected a communicable agent at the time and insisted that all future orienteering be done with compulsory protective clothing. There has been only one similar outbreak among orienteers after the rules were relaxed in 1981. They are now back in force.

Confucius say: He who runs with map and compass in hand should have head examined.

Reference

1. Berg R, et al: *Acta Pathol Microbiol Scand* 79:423, 1971.

Infectious Mononucleosis in Young Children
Schaller RJ, Counselman FL (Eastern Virginia Med School, Norfolk)
Am J Emerg Med 13:438–440, 1995   2-26

Background.—Infectious mononucleosis (IM) is apparently not as rare in young children as is generally believed. The clinical presentation and diagnosis of IM in a young child were described.

> *Case Report.*—Boy, 2 years, was brought to an emergency department (ED) by his mother, who reported neck swelling. That morning, she had noticed 2 small masses on the right posterior aspect of his neck. Otherwise, the boy was very active, had a good appetite, and was not complaining of a sore throat, earache, or headache. He had no history of fever, nausea, vomiting, diarrhea, or animal bites or scratches. Earlier in the week, he had nasal congestion and occasional nonproductive coughing, which had responded to over-the-counter medication. The boy's immunizations were current, and he had no significant past medical problems. Physical assessment was significant for a blood pressure of 94/40 mm Hg, pulse of 104 beats/min, respiratory rate of 22 breaths/min, and a temperature of 99°F orally. Multiple enlarged, soft, nontender, nonfluctuant lymph nodes were found on the right posterior cervical chain on neck examination. Other findings were normal. After consultation with the child's private pediatrician, it was decided to treat the patient conservatively, and a pediatric appointment was scheduled. The next day, however, the mother returned to the ED with her son because of further neck mass enlargement. A sore throat had also developed. His fever was now 101°F orally. On physical examination, enlarged tonsils and an erythematous posterior pharynx with areas of exudate were noted. A "rapid-strep" test, complete blood cell count, and Monospot were performed. The white blood cell count was 13,500 µL, with a differential of 75% lymphocytes, 20% polymorphonucleocytes, and 5% mononucleocytes. The Monospot was positive. Infectious mononucleosis was diagnosed, and the boy's mother was given precautionary instructions on the management of it. Acetaminophen as needed for fever was prescribed. The patient's symptoms resolved completely within 10 days. When the private pediatrician

was notified of the diagnosis, he expressed surprise that this diagnosis had been considered in a child of that age.

Conclusions.—Patients older than 2 years generally have many of the same signs and symptoms of IM seen in adolescents and young adults. Patients younger than 2 years may initially have minimal or atypical symptoms. The differential diagnosis of young children with fever, lymphadenopathy, sore throat, or nonspecific complaints should include IM.

▶ Although there is nothing new in this report, it is included in the YEAR BOOK OF PEDIATRICS to remind us that even the youngest among us can get IM. Generally speaking, in developed countries, IM usually occurs in older childhood and young adulthood, with a recognized peak incidence in the United States during the teenage years. In contrast to developed countries, IM in Third World countries and developing countries occurs mostly in early life. In the United States we tend to underdiagnose IM in the young child because of its less uniform symptomatology and because the heterophile antibody response is increasingly diminished the younger the child is.

It has now been more than a decade since the classic report by Sumaya and Ench, which articulated the clinical and laboratory findings in children infected with the Epstein-Barr virus (EBV).[1] If you're too young to have been around when this landmark article was published or somehow missed it when it first appeared, it is a study that represents the largest prospective investigation of children with IM. It compared those children younger than 4 years with those 4–16 years old. The incidence of fever, lymphadenopathy, and tonsillopharyngitis was similar in both age groups. However, some signs and symptoms occurred more frequently in younger children. A palpable spleen and enlarged liver were much more frequent in younger children. Signs of an upper respiratory tract infection were 3½ times more common in younger children. Younger children tended to develop rashes, particularly in response to the administration of ampicillin. Evaluation of hematologic findings in the young vs. the older child showed important differences. Young children had a significantly greater total white blood cell count but a smaller proportion of atypical lymphocytes. Although the overwhelming majority of older children had a positive heterophile antibody test, most young children did not. At any age, EBV-specific serologic testing was diagnostic.

A final word on this topic: in the United States, IM is not as rare in young children as we might think. If a child is younger than 4 years, you're going to need to do specific EBV serologic testing; a Monospot or heterophile won't do. Why is 4 years of age the breaking point between atypical and classic IM? Your guess is as good as this editor's.

Reference

1. Sumaya CV, Ench Y: *Pediatrics* 75:1003–1010, 1985.

The Consequences of a Positive Prenatal HIV Antibody Test for Women

Lester P, Partridge JC, Chesney MA, et al (San Francisco Gen Hosp; Ctr for AIDS Prevention Studies, San Francisco; Univ of California, San Francisco)
J Acquir Immune Defic Syndr Hum Retrovirol 10:341–349, 1995   2–27

Background.—Although perinatal HIV screening is associated with medical benefits for seropositive mothers and their infants, it is also associated with socioeconomic and psychological risks, such as denial of health care, loss of confidentiality, alienation from social support, increased psychological stress, and loss of economic resources such as housing, income, and insurance. These potential losses are of particular concern in populations already at risk for discrimination because of ethnicity and poverty, for whom social and health services are often unsatisfactory. The consequences of a positive prenatal HIV antibody test result in a primarily urban, poor population were investigated.

Methods.—Twenty HIV-positive and 20 HIV-negative pregnant women matched for HIV risk, race, income, and delivery date were studied. A semistructured interview was used to assess differences in health care discrimination, economic losses, risk behaviors, changes in relationships, and psychological status.

Findings.—Thirty-five percent of the seropositive women and none of the seronegative women reported health care discrimination because of HIV status. There was no evidence of increased socioeconomic loss in the HIV-positive group (Table 2). Seropositive women reported greater satisfaction with social support from friends and family. However, many women had not told any of their friends or family about their HIV status. Only 56% of seropositive women and 44% of seronegative women knew their partners' HIV status. Many women in both groups reported having

TABLE 2.—Changes in Insurance, Income, and Housing

	HIV+ Women (n = 20) (%)	HIV− Women (n = 20) (%)	
Insurance			
Lost major medical	5 (25)	2 (10)	(p = NS)
Gained major medical	2 (10)	2 (10)	(p = NS)
Gained Medicare	3 (15)	8 (40)	(p = NS)
Insured, no change	10 (50)	8 (40)	(p = NS)
Household income			
Decreased	7 (35)	7 (35)	(p = NS)
Increased	8 (40)	8 (40)	(p = NS)
No change	5 (25)	5 (25)	(p = NS)
Housing			
Lost apartment	1 (5)	1 (5)	(p = NS)
Improved housing	5 (25)	4 (20)	(p = NS)
No change	4 (70)	15 (75)	(p = NS)

(Courtesy of Lester P, Partridge JC, Chesney MA, et al: The consequences of a positive prenatal HIV antibody test for women. *J Acquir Immune Defic Syndr Hum Retrovirol* 10:341–349, 1995.)

sex without condoms after the HIV test. The seropositive women had greater mean standardized anxiety and depression scores than seronegative women.

Conclusions.—Despite increased social support and medical therapy HIV-positive pregnant women had more health care discrimination, personal isolation, and psychological sequelae than HIV-negative pregnant women. Focused medical, social, and mental health services need to be developed to address the needs of HIV-positive women.

▶ There is not another topic of which this editor is aware that has raised a more diverse set of opinions than that of informed maternal consent for HIV antibody testing. In 1991, the Centers for Disease Control and Prevention (CDC) recommended perinatal HIV antibody testing for women living in high-prevalence areas and having a significant risk of infection, including a history of transfusions, sexual risk factors, and IV drug use. Perinatal HIV testing was to be based on targeted epidemiologic research, and an individual informed consent model was instituted in several states. After the report of Protocol 076 of the National Institutes of Health (NIH) appeared showing that if an HIV-positive pregnant woman received zidovudine during pregnancy, her newborn infant would have a two-thirds reduction in the risk of HIV infection, there was a significant push from some for mandatory HIV testing of pregnant women. In 1993, well-publicized legislation calling for mandated, unblinded HIV testing of newborns was proposed in New York State. Although this was subsequently rejected, it served to focus national attention on the increasingly polarized political and public debate over perinatal testing.

What now constitutes the basis of this debate? The debate can easily be framed: mothers' rights vs. infants' rights. On the maternal side, despite increasing evidence of the benefits of early HIV identification in women and infants, perinatal screening represents the same socioeconomic and psychological risks to the mother that have been identified with HIV testing in other settings. These include denial of health care, loss of confidentiality, alienation from social support, loss of economic resources such as housing, income, and insurance, and increased psychological stress. These issues are of particular concern in a population already at risk for discrimination because of ethnicity and poverty, and for whom social and health care services are often inadequate. Perinatal HIV testing is further complicated because the test reflects maternal antibody status for sure but is only a risk factor for HIV infection in the infant. At the core of the debate is the conflict between protection of the woman's right to privacy and the state's obligation to protect the infant. The report abstracted provides further support for those who believe in maternal rights because the study shows that HIV-positive women demonstrate higher levels of health care discrimination, personal isolation, and psychological sequelae.

So what is the right thing to do? This editor has long felt uncomfortable with the current CDC recommendation, which is the same as that of our American Academy of Pediatrics, namely, informed consent rather than universal testing. The concern is that we, as pediatric care providers, may not be doing the most that we can for those under our charge, that is, the newborn infant. Perhaps there is a middle ground between informed consent and maternal testing known as "right of refusal" testing. In essence, this is the kind of testing that gives patients the right to informed refusal without requiring written consent. The pregnant woman would be told that blood is being drawn for various laboratory tests. She would be counseled about what these tests are, including the HIV testing. She would be told that she has a right to refuse to have these tests performed. She would not be required to provide written consent.

Giving patients the right to informed refusal without requiring written consent would result in a de facto deemphasis on both the HIV test and the unique stigmata attached to a positive result. Changing the "exceptional" nature of the consenting process for HIV tests would be significant, because it is not only the fear of social consequences that results in testing rates much lower than those seen with other prenatal tests such as gonorrhea cultures or syphilis serology. The low rates also stem from the requirement that the patient give specific attention to the HIV test and take an affirmative action (written consent) to have that test performed, whereas for other tests it is deferring the test that requires an action (refusal). It is specifically worth noting that a woman is asked to consent to HIV testing after being counseled about modes of transmission—in essence being told that only unsafe sex or needle use would put her at risk. Thus, a patient who might be interested in taking the test but not in sharing her risk-taking background might feel compelled to eschew the test to ensure her privacy. To say all this differently, when an informed refusal approach is used instead of written informed consent, the psychological burden is shifted from those who would choose the test to those who would refuse—in essence requiring a special effort to say no. The confessional nature of the testing (implicitly acknowledging risk behavior through the act of signing consent) would be lessened. Although some patients would choose to opt out of testing even if they had to assert their right to do so, the percentage of individuals tested would undoubtedly rise.

Although the refusal approach noted above does not guarantee universal testing, it does seem a reasonable compromise approach within the current debate. Such a policy that destigmatizes and possibly facilitates the voluntary testing of women for HIV *before* the birth of a child has the greatest chance to save the lives of infants. Also this approach preserves consent and the woman's role as a fetal champion. As importantly, it makes us, the protector of the child, a better defender of that child's rights.

This commentary closes with a thought-provoking query. You moonlight for the public health department in your area. The department is attempting to determine the HIV status of men who frequent prostitutes in your urban area. How would you make this determination if the study is to be totally anonymous and also not require the consent of the individual being tested?

What you would recommend is what investigators in Switzerland recommended when faced with a similar challenge.[2] To explore the possibility of anonymous HIV testing in such a target group, investigators studied the feasibility of testing the seminal fluid in used condoms collected from prostitutes. Eight prostitutes in the eastern region of Switzerland were asked to collect the used condoms of all of their clients over 14 consecutive days. They were offered a reimbursement of 5 Swiss francs per acceptable sample. A minimum of 5 condoms per day were required for participation in the study. To prevent the prostitutes from splitting individual semen samples, reimbursement was granted only for condoms containing more than 1 mL of semen. The women were asked to make a knot in each used condom after removing it from a client, collect the condoms at room temperature, and have them ready to be picked up daily. Some 804 condoms were collected from these 8 ladies during the 2-week sampling period. None of 804 semen samples were reactive on HIV antibody testing.

This Swiss study teaches two things: although the chance of getting HIV is low in Switzerland, condoms should be used on every conceivable occasion; also, at 10 clients a day, prostitutes have an occupational hazard higher than that of lion tamers and bungee jumpers.

References

1. Connor EM, et al: *N Engl J Med* 331:1173, 1994.
2. Vernazza PL, et al: *Lancet* 346:962, 1995.

A Meta-analytic Evaluation of the Polymerase Chain Reaction for the Diagnosis of HIV Infection in Infants

Owens DK, Holodniy M, McDonald TW, et al (Veterans Affairs Palo Alto Health Care System, Calif; Stanford Univ, Calif)
JAMA 275:1342–1348, 1996   2–28

Background.—Serologic diagnosis in HIV infection in the infants of infected mothers is difficult. Because maternal IgG anti-HIV antibodies cross the placenta, conventional HIV antibody tests may be positive for up to 15 months or more after birth regardless of whether the infant is infected. The polymerase chain reaction (PCR), a gene-amplification method, is an important alternative to antibody testing. This method amplifies and detects proviral HIV DNA directly and does not depend on HIV antibody formation. The sensitivity and specificity of the PCR for diagnosing HIV in infants were reported.

Methods and Findings.—Thirty-two studies were included in a meta-analytic examination of the value of PCR in diagnosing HIV infection in infants. These studies, published between 1988 and 1994, were identified in a literature search of 17 databases. Two investigators extracted data independently. The median reported sensitivity and specificity of PCR were 91.6% and 100%, respectively. A summary receiver operating characteristic curve using data from all the studies demonstrated a maximum joint sensitivity and specificity ranging from 93.2% to 94.9%. In a subgroup analysis, the joint sensitivity and specificity was significantly greater in older infants than in neonates. Among low-risk infants, the positive pre-

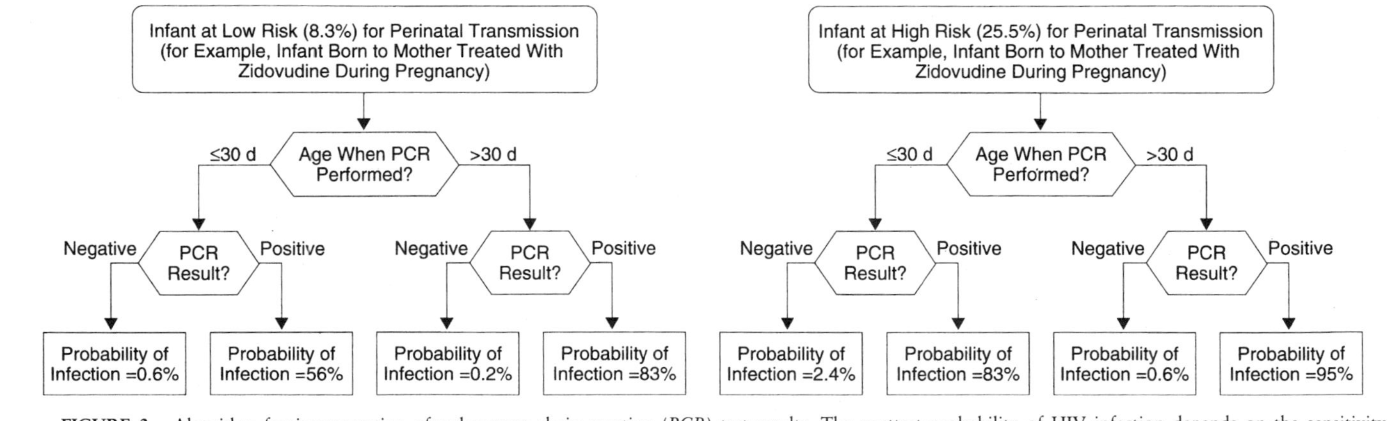

FIGURE 3.—Algorithm for interpretation of polymerase chain reaction (*PCR*) test results. The posttest probability of HIV infection depends on the sensitivity and specificity of PCR and the prior probability of HIV transmission. Sensitivity and specificity depend on the age of the infant and the cutoff chosen for a positive PCR test result. The figure assumes the cutoff is chosen such that PCR had the maximum joint sensitivity and specificity. **Left,** the posttest probability of disease for infants who are at low risk of transmission of HIV. An example of such a clinical situation is infants whose mothers were treated with zidovudine during pregnancy (estimated prior probability of HIV infection, 8.3%). **Right,** the posttest probability of disease for neonates and infants who are at higher risk of infection (prior probability of infection, 25.5%). An example of such a clinical situation is infants whose mothers were not treated with zidovudine. Transmission rates will vary in clinical settings; rates for this example were chosen to coincide with those observed in a randomized trial of therapy with zidovudine during pregnancy. (Courtesy of Owens DK, Holodniy M, McDonald TW, et al: A meta-analytic evaluation of the polymerase chain reaction for the diagnosis of HIV infection in infants. *JAMA* 275:1342–1348, Copyright 1966, American Medical Association.)

dictive value of PCR was 55.8% in newborns and 83.2% in older infants. A negative PCR finding decreased the probability of HIV infection to less than 3% (Fig 3).

Conclusions.—Polymerase chain reaction is one of the best tests available for diagnosing HIV infection in infants, yet it is not definitive. The findings of PCR should be interpreted in the context of careful follow-up assessment. The sensitivity and specificity of PCR are lower in neonates than in older infants, which decreases the positive predictive value. However, negative findings are informative. Test errors can be reduced by delaying the use of PCR until after the neonatal period or repeating PCR on independent samples acquired 30–60 days later.

▶ Although it may be difficult to imagine, if the World Health Organization is correct in its estimates, by the end of this century as many as 10 million children will have become infected with HIV as a result of perinatal transmission.[1] As recently as a year ago, a total of approximately 20,000 children in the United States and 1.5 million children worldwide were infected with HIV.[2] In the United States, 0.17% of all childbearing women are HIV positive, and approximately 7,000 infants are born to HIV-infected women each year. Because we now know that the perinatal administration of zidovudine can substantially reduce vertical HIV transmission, it becomes critical to understand which infants are perinatally infected and which are not. Hence the importance of PCR technology.

In 1989, *Science* selected PCR as the major scientific development of the year.[3] The potential use of DNA PCR for the diagnosis of vertical HIV infection soon became readily apparent because passively transferred maternal HIV antibody makes HIV serologic testing uninformative for diagnosis in the first year to 15 months of life. Culturing HIV is slow, labor intensive, and expensive. This article clarifies the role of PCR. Owens et al. provide a meta-analysis of 32 studies published between 1988 and 1994 to evaluate the sensitivity and specificity of DNA PCR for the diagnosis of vertical HIV infection. The results are supportive of DNA PCR as one of the best available diagnostic tests for vertical HIV infection. The authors warn us, however, that sensitivity and specificity are lower in neonates than in older children and suggest delaying the use of PCR until after the neonatal period or repeating PCR on independent samples obtained 30–60 days after birth. These cautions seem appropriate but should not deter us from early use of this powerful methodology. The diminished sensitivity of DNA PCR found in the neonatal period probably is attributable to differences in the timing of infection and the infrequent sampling intervals in the studies that were cited. Approximately 30% to 50% of infected infants are DNA PCR–positive at birth, suggesting in utero infection, whereas 50% to 70% are DNA PCR–negative at birth but positive after 7 days of age, suggesting intrapartum infection. If a mother were not diagnosed and treated before giving birth, intensive (i.e., at birth and weekly intervals thereafter) sampling within the neonatal period would likely allow earlier diagnosis of vertical infection and hasten the introduction of antiretroviral therapy that could significantly impact infection outcome. In a perfect world, HIV can now be diagnosed in the vast majority of infected infants within weeks of primary infection.

In an interesting editorial on this topic, Luzuriaga and Sullivan suggest that the most important use of PCR has yet to be realized.[4] With the use of perinatal antiretroviral therapy, it may take longer for the virus to be detected in the peripheral blood. Moreover, the introduction of potent combination antiretroviral therapies during the prenatal and early postnatal period may result in infection with little or no detectable replicating virus. In this scenario, the only marker of HIV infection may be the detection of HIV proviral DNA by PCR.

Laboratory quality control is clearly the key to success with PCR technology. With such quality control, the usefulness of DNA PCR in the rapid and accurate diagnosis of HIV-infected infants seems clear. Next step, better therapy and perhaps a vaccine.

References

1. World Health Organization, Global Program on AIDS: *The HIV/AIDS Pandemic: 1994 Overview.* Geneva, World Health Organization, 1994.
2. Stoneburner RL, et al: *Acta Paediatr Suppl* 400:1, 1994.
3. Guyer RL, et al: *Science* 246:1543, 1989.
4. Luzuriaga K, Sullivan JL: *JAMA* 275:1360, 1996.

Disease Patterns and Survival After Acquired Immunodeficiency Syndrome Diagnosis in Human Immunodeficiency Virus-infected Children
Morris CR, Araba-Owoyele L, Spector SA, et al (California Dept of Health Services, Sacramento; Univ of California, San Diego; Stanford Univ, Calif)
Pediatr Infect Dis J 15:321–328, 1996   2–29

Introduction.—The clinical presentations of HIV infection in children vary widely. A better understanding of the natural history of HIV and survival patterns in infected children would have great value in planning future resources and in evaluating new therapies. To contribute to this understanding, the AIDS-defining conditions and survival after AIDS diagnosis were studied in a pediatric HIV-infected population.

Methods.—Data were obtained from a university-based active surveillance program in California. The records of enrolled HIV-infected children were examined to identify the conditions leading to AIDS diagnosis and the length of survival after that diagnosis. Postdiagnosis survival was analyzed in relation to the following variables: sex, race, route of HIV transmission, age at diagnosis of AIDS, treatment, CD4$^+$ T-cell count, and AIDS-defining conditions at diagnosis.

Results.—Of 639 enrolled HIV-infected children, 126 had received a diagnosis of AIDS. There were different disease patterns related to the route of HIV transmission, with more variability in the AIDS-defining conditions among children with nonperinatal than with perinatal HIV transmission. The most common AIDS-defining conditions in the nonperi-

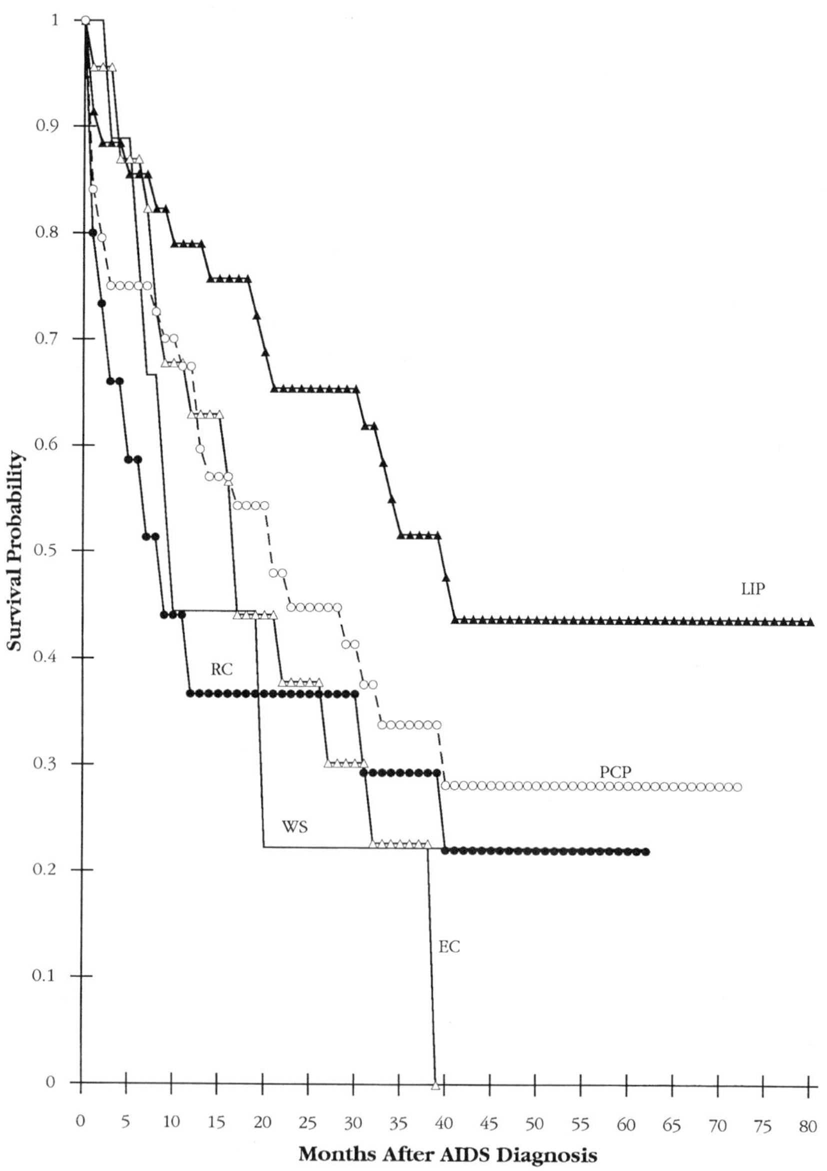

FIGURE 2.—Product-limit probabilities of postdiagnosis survival, (in months) for children with diagnoses of *Pneumocystis carinii* pneumonia (*PCP*), lymphoid interstitial pneumonia (*LIP*), esophageal candidiasis (*EC*), respiratory candidiasis (*RC*), or wasting syndrome (*WS*) as the AIDS-defining condition. (Courtesy of Morris CR, Araba-Owoyele L, Spector SA, et al: Disease patterns and survival after acquired immunodeficiency syndrome diagnosis in human immunodeficiency virus-infected children. *Pediatr Infect Dis J* 15:321–328, 1996.)

natal transmission group were *Pneumocystis carinii* pneumonia (PCP) (42%) and lymphoid interstitial pneumonia (LIP) (30%), whereas the most common conditions in the perinatal transmission group were esophageal candidiasis (31.6%), HIV encephalopathy (21.1%), LIP (21.1%), PCP (18.4%), *Mycobacterium avium* complex (MAC) (18.4%), and wasting syndrome (15.8%).

The cohort had a mortality rate of 54.8% during the study period. The perinatal transmission group had a higher 1-year mortality rate than the nonperinatal transmission group (61.4% vs. 48%). At 2 years after the diagnosis of AIDS, the survival rate was 11.4% in the perinatal transmission group and 40% in the nonperinatal transmission group. Overall, there was a product-limit estimate of median survival of 26 months. Factors associated with a shorter survival in multivariate analysis included a lower $CD4^+$ T-cell count and respiratory candidiasis or wasting syndrome as the AIDS-defining condition at diagnosis (Fig 2). Factors associated with a longer survival included LIP as the AIDS-defining condition at diagnosis and treatment with zidovudine or antiviral drugs.

Conclusions.—Survival was not significantly influenced by gender, race, or route of HIV transmission. Identification of factors associated with increased or decreased survival will help in planning appropriate management strategies, resource use, and therapeutic trials. Further study is needed with larger cohorts and longer follow-up to further elucidate the patterns of disease progression in HIV-infected children and identify additional prognostic factors.

▶ Reliable data on disease and survival patterns of HIV-infected children are invaluable in planning resources for future needs. As newer options for prophylactic or therapeutic management of infected children become available, accurate baseline or retrospective expectation of survival will contribute to evaluating such therapies, thus, the importance of this study that shows the prognostic significance of HIV- or AIDS-related disease patterns.

What we see in California (site of the study abstracted) probably holds for the country as a whole. Previous reports have estimated a median age at development of symptoms among perinatally infected children of between 5 and 10 months. The median age at clinical presentation in California was somewhat higher (13 months), but only AIDS-defining conditions were considered. *Pneumocystis carinii* pneumonia and lymphoid interstitial pneumonia were such conditions. Surprisingly, the mortality rate in California appears to be somewhat higher than expected because the slight majority of children elsewhere are still alive after 5 years of age. The median post-AIDS diagnosis survival time among the children followed in this study was just 26 months.

Reports like this will become increasingly more helpful as antiretroviral therapy evolves and becomes more effective. Current strategies for improving antiretroviral therapy involve using a combination of agents that inhibit different steps in the HIV life cycle. Among the most promising of agents are the HIV protease inhibitors, which reduce the infectivity of chronically infected cells. The latest one to be reported is saquinavir, a hydroxyethylamine transition-state analogue of the HIV protease cleavage site. Saquinavir has potent in vitro inhibitory action against a wide variety of laboratory and clinical isolates of HIV. To learn more about this relatively new agent, see the important article by Collier et al.[1]

Reference

1. Collier AC, et al: *N Engl J Med* 334:1011, 1996.

Cluster of Five Children With Acute Encephalopathy Associated With Cat-scratch Disease in South Florida

Noah DL, Bresee JS, Gorensek MJ, et al (Ctrs for Disease Control and Prevention, Atlanta, Ga; Cleveland Clinic Florida, Fort Lauderdale; Broward County Public Health Unit, Fort Lauderdale, Fla; et al)
Pediatr Infect Dis J 14:866–869, 1995   2–30

Background.—Cat-scratch disease (CSD) is a bacterial zoonosis caused by *Bartonella henselae* that most often consists of a papule developing shortly after a scratch or bite from an infected cat, followed by benign regional node enlargement that lasts 2–4 months. Children and young adults are most often affected. Encephalopathy is one of the most serious complications, usually developing 2–6 weeks after the start of lymphadenopathy and producing seizure activity, combativeness, headache, and coma.

Series.—Five children were seen within 6 weeks of one another at a hospital in South Florida with encephalopathy associated with CSD. They represent the first cluster of such cases to be encountered in the United States.

Clinical Aspects.—Two of the 5 children had lymphadenopathy, and CSD was diagnosed 2 weeks before they were hospitalized. Two other patients were first noted to have adenopathy when hospitalized, and the fifth patient had recently had enlarged cervical nodes. The children were initially seen with status epilepticus, but none had further seizures after being hospitalized. Fever resolved within 48 hours of admission. Computed tomography and MR studies, as well as CSF analyses, were negative. Node biopsy specimens were obtained from 4 patients to exclude other causes. The children were hospitalized for an average of 15 days. None had neurologic sequelae when assessed 2–4 weeks after discharge. The diagnosis was confirmed by an indirect fluorescent antibody test detecting antibody against *B. henselae*.

Epidemiology.—The affected children lived within 7 miles of one another. All had had contact with a pet or stray cat before adenopathy and encephalopathy developed. More than 60% of the 124 cats tested were positive for antibody to *B. henselae*, and 22% of the animals were bacteremic. A questionnaire survey of regional physicians yielded 28 additional cases of CSD occurring in the same period. The encephalitic case patients were younger than the overall group, with a median age of 6 years, but the difference was not significant.

Implications.—Encephalopathy interpreted as being of "unknown origin" may actually be a manifestation of CSD. Infection by *B. henselae* should be considered when a child is seen with an acute onset of seizures or coma.

▶ Before reading this report, this editor was not aware that so many cases of CSD were being reported each year (there are some 22,000 cases) or that serious complications were being noted. Of the serious complications of CSD, 2 are particularly worrisome. One is an entity known as bacillary angiomatosis. This is a vascular proliferation caused by *Bartonella*, most commonly associated with long-standing HIV infection or other significant immunosuppression. The second entity of consequence is the subject of this report: CSD encephalopathy. Common clinical manifestations of this encephalopathy include seizures, combative behavior, headache, and coma. Occasionally the clinical course is severe and protracted, requiring a costly and lengthy diagnostic evaluation. Although all patients recover, recovery can take up to a year.

If it weren't for cats, there would not be such an entity as CSD. Demers et al. recently performed an interesting study of 39 patients with CSD, and of the kittens and cats in their environment.[1] Elevated antibody titers to *B. henselae* were documented in all children with clinical CSD. Blood cultures yielded *B. henselae* and antibody was present in 21 of 29 kittens (less than 1 year of age). From 1 of these kittens, saliva and fleas had *B. henselae* DNA by polymerase chain reaction. Adult cats usually have negative blood cultures but serologic evidence of previous infection. These data corroborate previous observations that CSD appears in those with a close association to flea-infested kittens that had *B. henselae* bacteremia. It is the fleas, not the cat per se, that spread infection between kittens. Apparently the poor little kitten merely infects itself by scratching at fleas, squashing them, and inoculating itself with organisms before it plays with children.

So, is it the flea or the cat that is the real culprit when it comes to *B. henselae*? Should we be renaming this entity as "flea-scratch disease"? Not likely, but a flea collar would probably go a long way toward preventing this troublesome entity.

Because CSD is so common, it is incumbent on us, as pediatric care providers, to keep up with the evolving knowlege base related to cats and the diseases they transmit. The best way to do this is by reading the current kitty literature.

Reference

1. Demers D, et al: *Pediatrics* 127:23, 1995.

3 Nutrition and Metabolism

Breastfeeding and the Working Mother: Effect of Time and Temperature of Short-term Storage on Proteolysis, Lipolysis, and Bacterial Growth in Milk

Hamosh M, Ellis LA, Pollock DR, et al (Georgetown Univ Med Ctr, Washington, DC)

Pediatrics 97:492–498, 1996

3–1

Introduction.—Although a great deal is known about the storage of breast milk donated for use in hospitalized infants, no studies have examined the effects of short-term storage of milk expressed by mothers for later feeding to their own infants. This issue must be examined under the storage conditions available in the workplace. Nutrient stability and bacterial growth in breast milk were studied under suboptimal storage conditions.

Methods.—The study included 16 healthy, breast-feeding mothers, 5 of whom expressed milk for their infants. The women were studied at 1 month or at 5–6 months of lactation. Samples of expressed milk were

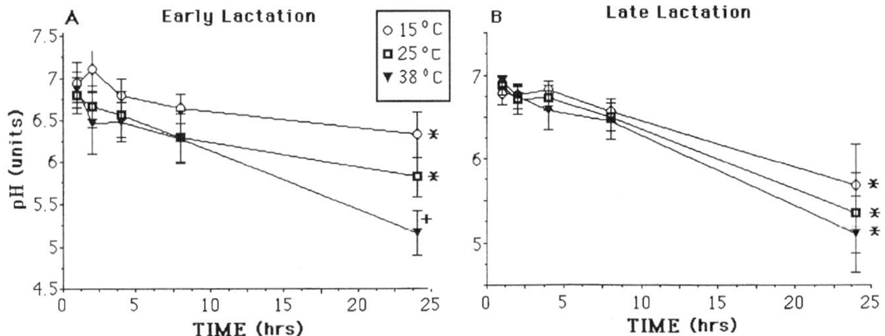

FIGURE 1.—Effect of storage temperature and time on milk pH. **A,** early lactation, **B,** late lactation (1 month and 5–6 months, respectively). *pH was significantly different ($P < 0.05$) between 24 hours and other storage times; +pH was significantly different ($P > 0.05$) between 15° and 38°C. (Courtesy of Hamosh M, Ellis LA, Pollock DR, et al: Breastfeeding and the working mother: Effect of time and temperature of short-term storage on proteolysis, lipolysis, and bacterial growth in milk. Reproduced by permission of *Pediatrics*, Vol 97, pp 492–498, Copyright 1996.)

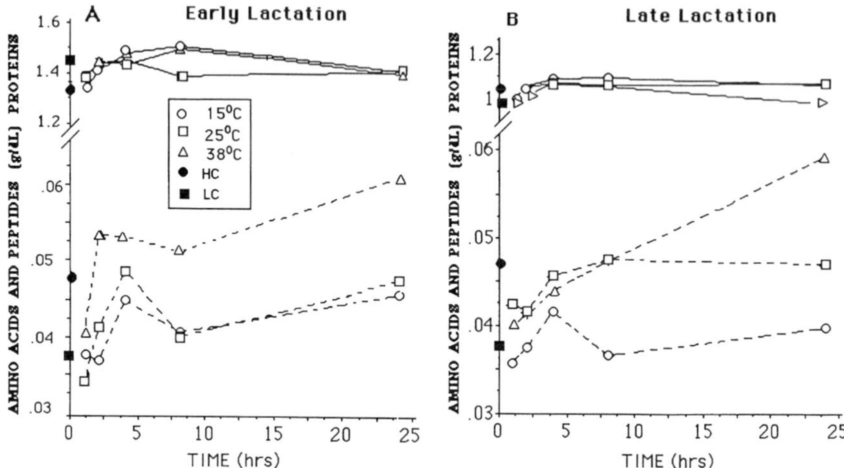

FIGURE 2.—Effect of storage temperature and time on total milk protein (*solid line*) and on acid and peptide (i.e., trichloroacetic acid soluble fraction) concentrations (*dashed line*). **A,** early lactation; **B,** late lactation. *Abbreviations*: *HC,* home control; *LC,* lab control. There were statistically significant differences ($P < 0.05$) in total protein values between milk specimens collected in early and late lactation at 0 time and at all times and temperatures of storage. There was no statistical difference in products of proteolysis (amino acids and peptides) as a function of time, temperature, or stage of lactation. (Courtesy of Hamosh M, Ellis LA, Pollock DR, et al: Breastfeeding and the working mother: Effect of time and temperature of short-term storage on proteolysis, lipolysis, and bacterial growth in milk. Reproduced by permission of *Pediatrics,* Vol 97, pp 492–498, Copyright 1996.)

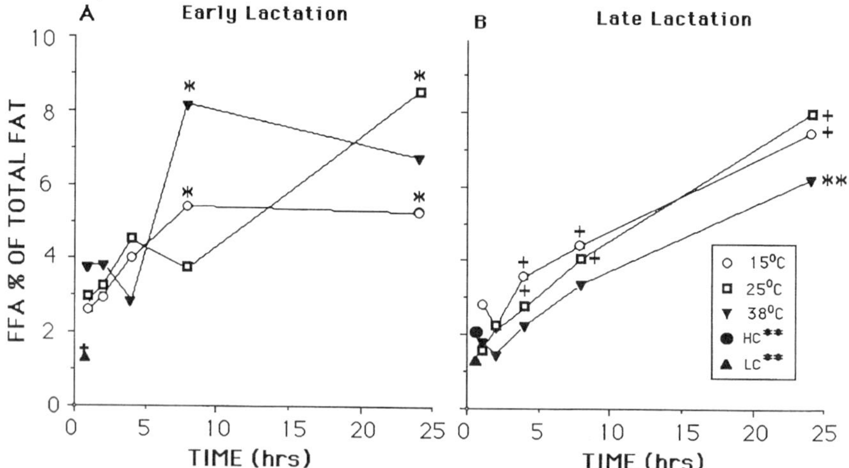

FIGURE 3.—Effect of storage temperature and time on hydrolysis of milk fat. **A,** early lactation; **B,** late lactation. *Abbreviations*: *HC,* home control; *LC,* lab control; *FFA,* free fatty acids. There were statistically significant differences ($P < 0.000-0.05$) between laboratory control specimens and storage times and temperatures in early ($P < 0.05$) and late ($P < 0.002-0.03$) lactation. (Courtesy of Hamosh M, Ellis LA, Pollock DR, et al: Breastfeeding and the working mother: Effect of time and temperature of short-term storage on proteolysis, lipolysis, and bacterial growth in milk. Reproduced by permission of *Pediatrics,* Vol 97, pp 492–498, Copyright 1996.)

TABLE 2.—Effect of Storage Time and Temperature on Bacterial Growth in Fresh Human Milk (CFU $\times$ 10^3) During Early and Late Lactation

Microorganism	No. Mothers Early/ Late	Temper- ature (°C)	Time (h) 0	4 15	25	38	8 15	25	38	24 15	25	38
Gram Negative												
Acinetobacter	1/1		0.2/0	0.4/0	0.4/0	0.2/0	0.2/0	0.6/0	2.2/0	0.1/17	11/17	7.8/17
Bacillus coliformis and Pseudomonas	2/1		0	0	0	0/0.8	0/0.8	0	0.1/17	0/0.4	2.2/0	0/0
Gram Positive												
α-Streptococcus	7/5		0	0	0	0	0	2.9/0	5.9/17	0/0	9.1/10	9.4/38
γ-Streptococcus	1/1		0/0	0/0	0/0	0/0	0/0	0/0	0.9/0	0/0	0/3.3	1.1/8.3
Enterococcus	3/2		0/0.8	0/0.5	0/1.6	0.7/0.8	0/0.8	0.6/8.3	0/0	0.4/0	1.1/0	0/0
Staphylococcus aureus	4/1		0/0	0/0	0/0	1.5/0	0/0	0/0	13.2/1.7	0/0	5.9/5	17.6/3
Staphylococcus epidermis	8/5		0.4/0.1	0.4/0	0.7/0.1	2.7/1.6	0/0	13.4/1.1	7.3/19	0.5/0.3	9.2/13	28.3/27
Lactobacillus	1/1		3.3/0	0/0	3.3/0	4.4/0	0/0	3.3/0	5.6/0	0/0	8.3/17	7.8/17
Total	9/6		3.9/0.9	0.8/0.5	4.4/1.7	9.1/3.2	0.2/1.6	20.8/9.4	35.2/51.7	1/17.3	47.0/62	72.0/120

Note: Milk specimens were collected from 9 women during the first month of lactation. From 6 of these women, milk was also collected at 5–6 months of lactation. Data are group means for early/late lactation. Milk was stored in glass containers. There were no statistical differences in bacterial counts during storage of milk collected in early or late lactation.

Abbreviation: CFU, colony forming units.

(Courtesy of Hamosh M, Ellis LA, Pollock DR, et al: Breastfeeding and the working mother: Effect of time and temperature of short-term storage on proteolysis, lipolysis, and bacterial growth in milk. Reproduced by permission of *Pediatrics*, Vol 97, pp 492–498, Copyright 1996.)

stored at temperatures of 15°C, 25°C, and 38°C for 1 to 24 hours for measurement of pH, proteolysis and lipolysis. Bacterial growth in milk samples was also measured at intervals for a period of 24 hours.

Results.—At all 3 temperatures, the pH of milk decreased 2 units with 24 hours of storage (Fig 1). Proteolysis was not observed until the milk had been stored for 24 hours at 38°C (Fig 2). Lipolysis began shortly after storage, progressing to 8% at 24 hours (Fig 3). After 24 hours of storage at 38°C, there was a 40% increase in proteolysis products along with a 440% to 710% increase in free fatty acid concentration. Most of the bacteria that grew were nonpathogenic. Very little bacterial growth occurred in specimens stored at 15°C for 24 hours, and low growth occurred in specimens stored at 25°C for 4–8 hours. For samples stored at 38°C, significant bacterial growth occurred within 4 hours (Table 2).

Conclusions.—Human breast milk can be safely stored for 24 hours at 15°C and for 4 hours at 25°C, but it should not be stored at 38°C. If the mother does not have access to a refrigerator, it is probably safe to store her expressed milk in a Styrofoam cooler with "blue ice." Milk proteins appear to maintain their structure and function during short-term storage, during which time lipolysis may act to inhibit bacterial growth.

▶ Reports such as this are becoming increasingly important as nursing mothers return to the workplace in ever-increasing numbers at a time when they would like to continue nursing their infants. Many of these mothers are quite successful in doing this, but the logistics can be formidable. Most mothers can express their breast milk during work breaks at their place of employment. In an ideal world, this milk would be picked up and delivered to the care provider for use during daytime feedings and, therefore, would be used as soon as possible. The ideal world and the real world rarely coincide, however. In most cases, women store their expressed breast milk for use the next day, because when they arrive home in the late afternoon, they prefer to directly breast-feed their infants for all of its maternal and infant benefits. Given this approach, the most significant issue is how long breast milk can be stored once expressed. For such women, this report answers that question.

In contrast to the great body of information on the storage of donor milk provided to hospitalized full-term and preterm infants, before this report, little has been known about the effect of short-term storage of a mother's milk for later feeding to her own healthy, full-term infant. If a mother expresses breast milk, the likely storage temperatures include those of a refrigerator (4°C), ambient temperatures (usually 25°C), and in some hot environments, a temperature in the range of 38°C. This report tells us that milk should never be kept at high temperatures (for example 38°C) for any length of time. Room temperature (25°C) is okay, but only for up to 4 hours. This 4-hour limit allows little flexibility for most women and their infants. Thus, a refrigerator would be ideal but is not an option in many workplaces.

To the rescue of these women has come the cooler and blue ice. Insulated storage containers that are refrigerated with solid "blue" ice bars can maintain temperatures at about 15°C. At this temperature, expressed breast milk may be safely stored for at least 24 hours if necessary. So stored, breast milk may undergo significant lipolysis of its fat content (mostly triglycerides), but the products of lipolysis don't harm breast milk's nutritional value. The by-products (fatty acids) are, in fact, bacteriostatic and can be bacteriocidal as well. Thus, a woman in the privacy of her workplace can express her breast milk, toss it into a blue ice–cooled insulated container, take it home, and have it available for use even as long as 24 hours later.

Such an approach relieves the need for considering having a (breast) milk man in a pickup and delivery truck. If you can't afford a cooler and blue ice, and if you live in northern climates, during a good bit of the year you can put your milk container on your outside window sill. Having been a resident of Syracuse, New York, I saw this done all the time with people's lunches. Even in a northern environment such as Syracuse, summer will be a problem. Fortunately, in Syracuse, summer usually occurs 1 day in mid-July.

Effect of the Method of Breast Feeding on Breast Engorgement, Mastitis and Infantile Colic

Evans K, Evans R, Simmer K (Flinders Med Ctr, South Australia)
Acta Paediatr 84:849–852, 1995   3–2

Background.—In theory, prolonged feeding on 1 breast results in less breast engorgement compared with shorter feeding periods using both breasts. Longer intervals between nursing with prolonged feeding on 1 breast should also decrease the rate of milk synthesis. Some authorities have suggested that, with prolonged nursing on 1 breast, infantile colic, overfeeding, and symptoms of lactose malabsorption are partially or completely improved. However, prolonged nursing on 1 breast may also lead to an insufficient milk supply for the infant, and longer intervals between feeding may increase the incidence of mastitis. The effects of 2 methods of breast-feeding on engorgement, mastitis, infantile colic, and feeding duration were investigated.

Methods.—One hundred fifty mothers were assigned to an experimental group, breast-feeding by prolonged emptying of 1 breast at each feed, and 152 were assigned to a control group, in which both breasts were drained equally at each feed. Both groups were prospectively followed up for 6 months after delivery.

Findings.—The incidences of breast engorgement in the experimental and control groups were 61.4% and 74.3%, respectively, in the first week. The incidences of colic during the 6-month study were 12% and 23.4%, respectively. The 2 groups did not differ significantly in mastitis incidence or length of breast-feeding. Sixty-three percent of the women in the experimental group felt they needed to offer the second breast at the end of a feeding to satisfy their infant's hunger. In both groups, perceived insufficient milk supply syndrome was the main reason for quitting breast-feeding.

Conclusions.—During the first week of breast-feeding, prolonged feeding from 1 breast per feed is recommended to prevent engorgement. Thereafter, interventions intended to support the mother-infant dyad should be led by the infant's appetite rather than imposing a rigid structure on breast-feeding. Women should allow their pattern of breast use to change during the day and throughout lactation.

▶ One of the questions most frequently asked by a new mother who is about to breast-feed is whether she should use 1 or both breasts at the time of a feeding. How you respond to that query is probably based more on intuition and personal experience than on objective data from the literature. In fact, there have been few objective data to help you. Theoretically, prolonged emptying of a breast should result in less breast engorgement than the resulting stasis from a shorter feeding period using both breasts, in which the let-down reflex is stimulated but the breasts are not sufficiently emptied. Although the length of a feed may be longer in the prolonged single breast-feeding method, it is known that the interval between feeds is extended in such infants. Further, it has been suggested that with prolonged nursing on 1 breast in which hindmilk is obtained, infantile colic, overfeeding, and symptoms of lactose malabsorption are either partially or completely improved. Hindmilk (the milk that comes toward the end of breast-feeding) has a relatively high concentration of fat, which should delay gastric emptying. Foremilk is low in fat, which may result in more frequent feedings. An increase in feedings can lead to the consumption of more milk and therefore more lactose, possibly contributing to colic. On the other hand, there have been suggestions that the practice of prolonged nursing on 1 breast may lead to an insufficient milk supply for the infant, and that longer intervals between feeds may lead to a higher incidence of mastitis.

Given all these pros and cons, which method of breast-feeding is best? This report provides some important insights that assist us. In the first week of life, feeding on a single breast at each feed is helpful to a new mother. This method of feeding reduces painful breast engorgement. After the first week, it seems reasonable to advise interventions that support a mother-infant relationship without imposing rigid patterns on breast-feeding practices. To say this differently, if an infant's appetite is best satisfied by ultimately using both breasts, so be it. The majority of mothers in this study seemed to find it necessary to use both breasts for the majority of most feeds. It would seem only common sense to suggest that mothers permit their infants to establish their own pattern of breast usage and allow this to vary during the course of the day and throughout lactation. The only exception to this might be advice to mothers whose infants have colic. This study shows that prolonged feeding from 1 breast reduces the frequency of colic.

If you still aren't satisfied that everything is known about the best ways to breast feed, i.e., single vs. both breasts, you're probably in good company, despite the quality of this first-class report. When it comes to topics such as this, common sense and personal experience really aren't all that bad, are they?

Iron Status in Breast-fed Infants

Pisacane A, De Vizia B, Valiante A, et al (Università di Napoli, Italy)
J Pediatr 127:429–431, 1995   3–3

Background.—The high frequency of anemia is the reason for iron supplementation recommendations for breast-fed infants. It is unknown why some infants remain iron sufficient longer than others. There have been no studies of the iron status of infants receiving human milk as the only milk in the first 12 months of life, without other foods containing iron. The iron status of such infants was investigated.

Methods.—Thirty infants breast fed until their first birthday were studied. All had weights appropriate for their gestational age. None had received cow's milk, medicinal iron, or iron-enriched formula or cereals. Iron status was assessed in these children at 12 and 24 months of age.

Findings.—At 12 months, 70% of the infants had a hemoglobin concentration of 110 g/L or more, and 30% had a concentration of less than 110 g/L. Serum ferritin levels were 10 µg/L or more in 57% of the infants. Six of the 9 infants with anemia also had iron deficiency. Duration of exclusive breast-feeding was 6.5 months in nonanemic infants and 5.5 months in anemic infants. None of the infants who had been breast fed exclusively for 7 months were anemic, compared with 43% of those who had received other feedings before 7 months of age (Table 2). Only 1 of 20 infants whose iron status was checked at 24 months had a hemoglobin level lower than the 12-month level.

Conclusions.—None of the infants breast fed exclusively for 7 months or more were anemic, compared with 43% of those breast fed for a shorter time. Infants exclusively breast fed for a prolonged time had a good iron status at 12 and 24 months. Because a very small proportion of infants are breast fed exclusively for a prolonged period, the current policy of iron supplementation in breast-fed infants should not be questioned. However, populations in developing areas, where iron supplementaton is not available or culturally accepted, are gradually losing the tradition of exclusive

TABLE 2.—Influence of Dietary Factors on Iron Status at 12 Months

	Exclusive Breast-feeding for ≥ 7 mo (*n* = 9)	Exclusive Breast-feeding for < 7 mo (*n* = 21)
Hb concentration, gm/L (SD)	11.7 (0.4)	10.9 (0.7)*
No. (%) of Hb concentration < 110 gm/L	0 (0)	9 (43)
Mean serum ferritin, µg/L (SD)	17 (15)	12.3 (11.7)
No. (%) with serum ferritin level < 10 µg/L	2 (22)	11 (52)
No. (%) with Hb > 110 gm/L and serum ferritin level > 10 µg/L	7 (78)	10 (48)

Abbreviation: Hb, hemoglobin.
**t = 3.2; df = 28; P = 0.003.*
(Courtesy of Pisacane A, De Vizia B, Valiante A, et al: Iron status in breast-fed infants. *J Pediatr* 127:429–431, 1995.)

breast-feeding. A policy supporting prolonged, exclusive breast-feeding among such populations could be important to public health.

▶ Score another one for exclusive breast-feeding. Although infants who are exclusively breast fed for a prolonged time represent a very small proportion of all infants, this report is important because it shows us that in such situations, iron supplementation may not be needed. There are populations, mainly in developing countries, in which breast-feeding for prolonged periods is common and iron supplementation is not available or culturally acceptable. With urbanization, these populations are gradually losing the breast-feeding tradition and are then being exposed to the risk of iron-deficiency anemia and infection. A policy supporting prolonged and exclusive breast-feeding among these populations could be important from a public health standpoint and could represent an effective measure to ensure normal iron status.

Despite the importance of these data, real-world situations tell us that few breast-feeding mothers breast-feed exclusively and for long periods. Mothers who breast-feed but also feed other food substances may wind up with iron-deficient infants if such infants are not supplemented with iron. Many solid foods fed to infants contain inhibitors of iron absorption that decrease the bioavailability of iron present in breast milk.

As important as it is to know that exclusive breast-feeding for long periods prevents iron-deficiency anemia, such a feeding practice is so unusual that it seems reasonable to support current policies that recommend iron supplementation to all breast-fed infants, assuming a mother is willing to give the iron and its use is culturally acceptable. See Chapter 13 for a carefully done study showing that most women who breast-feed should give their infants supplemental iron.

One last comment. Although the importance of the report abstracted cannot be underestimated, it really tells us nothing new. Virtually identical data were first reported by McMillan, Landaw, and Oski in 1976.[1] Nonetheless, it is nice to see that modern investigators can successfully reinvent the wheel while continuing to successfully educate us.

Reference

1. McMillan JA, et al: *Pediatrics* 58:686, 1976.

Increased Incidence of Severe Breastfeeding Malnutrition and Hypernatremia in a Metropolitan Area
Cooper WO, Atherton HD, Kahana M, et al (Univ of Cincinnati, Ohio; Univ of Chicago)
Pediatrics 96:957–960, 1995   3–4

Introduction.—Hypernatremic dehydration can occur in newborn infants who are breast-fed. Today many infants are being discharged earlier, and their routine follow-up may not always be appropriately adjusted.

TABLE 1.—Criteria for Diagnosis of Breast-Feeding Malnutrition and Hypernatremia
1. Age >5 days, <6 weeks
2. Predominantly breast-fed with little or no supplementation with infant formula or water
3. Loss of weight 10% or more from birth weight
4. Clinical signs of dehydration at presentation
5. Serum sodium >150 mmol/L at presentation
(Courtesy of Cooper WO, Atherton HD, Kahana M, et al: Increased incidence of severe breastfeeding malnutrition and hypernatremia in a metropolitan area. Reproduced by permission of *Pediatrics*, Vol 96, pp 957–960, Copyright 1995.)

Series.—Five infants with marked breast-feeding malnutrition and profound hypernatremia were referred in a 5-month period to a tertiary care children's hospital from a 3-state region. This represented a significant increase in the number of cases of breast-feeding malnutrition seen at this hospital. The diagnostic criteria are listed in Table 1. Three of the mothers described inverted nipples. Four mothers recalled engorgement, and all 5 reported leakage of milk.

Clinical Aspects.—The infants were discharged 27–48 hours after birth and were nursed every 3–6 hours during the next few days. Most often, feedings were initiated on schedule rather than when the infant appeared to be hungry. The mothers fed their infants for 5–10 minutes per side. In no case was formula or water given more than once before the infant had to be readmitted. The mothers noted fewer wet diapers and a decrease in the number and volume of bowel movements (Table 3). The infants were markedly dehydrated when first seen and had lost an average of 23% of their body weight. The serum sodium averaged 186 mmol/L. Two infants had multiple cerebral infarcts, and 1 required leg amputation because of iliac artery thrombosis.

Hospital Review.—Of 166 infants younger than 6 weeks who were admitted in 1990–1994 with dehydration, hypernatremia, or malnutrition, 16—including the 5 index cases—met all criteria for breast-feeding malnutrition and hypernatremia. The average age at the time of postnatal discharge decreased from 2.4 to 1.7 days during this period.

Conclusions.—Breast-feeding malnutrition and hypernatremia may be increasing in frequency. The optimal follow-up interval remains uncertain, but a follow-up visit in the first week of life might prevent some cases.

▶ Critical malnutrition and hypernatremic dehydration resulting from inadequate breast-feeding has been reported.[1] That there is an association between hypernatremic dehydration and breast-feeding is not the point of this report. The point is that with the rising popularity of managed health care plans, we are possibly seeing more problems related to difficulties experienced by women who breast-feed. The infants involved are usually the product of an uncomplicated pregnancy and delivery and have had a relatively normal but short neonatal stay. The mothers are often not very experienced and fail to clue in on a poor suck in an otherwise contented and

TABLE 3.—Presenting Symptoms and Course of Index Cases

History of decreased urine output (number/volume)	Y	Y	Y	Y	Y
History of decreased bowel movements (number/volume)	Y	Y	Y	Y	Y
"Sleepy" or "irritable"	Y	Y	Y	Y	Y
Age at presentation (d)	9	14	8	12	5
Presenting complaint	Jaundice	Weight check	Blue leg	Decreased feeding	Decreased activity
Percent loss from birth weight	26	32	14	27	16
Sodium (mmol/L)	186	188	176	214	161
BUN (mmol/L urea) (mg/dL)	35.0 (97)	79.5 (222)	46.5 (130)	62.0 (173)	16.0 (44)
Creatinine (µmol/L) (mg/dL)	160 (1.8)	290 (3.3)	160 (1.8)	520 (5.9)	110 (1.3)
Calculated osmolality (mosm/L)	410	468	410	495	342
Complications		Pinpoint cerebrovascular accident	Left leg amputation	Multiple cerebrovascular accidents, seizures	Coagulopathy
Follow-up	Nl	Decreased facial movement	Nl	EEG slowing	Nl

Abbreviations: Y, yes; *N*, no; *BUN*, blood urea nitrogen; *EEG*, electroencephalogram; *Nl*, normal.
(Courtesy of Cooper WO, Atherton HD, Kahana M, et al: Increased incidence of severe breastfeeding malnutrition and hypernatremia in a metropolitan area. Reproduced by permission of *Pediatrics*, Vol 96, pp 957–960, Copyright 1995.)

restful infant. Put that together with the fact that ultra-absorbent diapers give no insight about urinary output, and the necessary ingredients are present for a problem, particularly if a new mother is "rushed" out of the hospital so quickly that adequate instructions about feeding are not given.

This series of newborns, 3 of whom had significant morbidity, including neurologic damage, suggests that the incidence and severity of breast-feeding malnutrition and hypernatremia is indeed increasing and that the needs of some breast-fed infants are not being met. If there is a link between the shortened length of initial hospital stay for newborns and breast-feeding malnutrition, then the current system of follow-up must be adjusted to avert a growing number of tragedies. To say this differently, these data support a recommendation that all infants who are breast-fed should be followed up later in the first week of life to make sure that everything is okay. Failure to do so, particularly when there has been an early discharge, is unacceptable.

Reference

1. Thullen JD, et al: *Clin Pediatr* 27:370, 1988.

Inappropriate Infant Bottle Feeding: Status of the Healthy People 2000 Objective
Kaste LM, Gift HC (Natl Inst of Dental Research, Bethesda, Md)
Arch Pediatr Adolesc Med 149:786–791, 1995   3–5

Background.—Inappropriate infant feeding practices may lead to severe dental caries and other chronic disorders. Early childhood caries has been related to the frequent or protracted use of bottles containing fermentable liquid. The continual use of a sweetened pacifier and at-will breast-feeding also have been implicated.

Objective.—Information on the use of baby bottles was obtained on 1 randomly chosen child from each family with children participating in the 1991 National Health Interview Survey. The data were weighted so that they represented the corresponding United States population. Usable data were available for 5,662 children aged 6 months to 5 years.

Findings.—It was estimated that 17% of United States children of this age are put to sleep with a bottle containing something other than water (Fig 3). About one fourth of Hispanic children and 21% of children from families below the poverty level are managed in this way. Fifty-seven percent of 1,795 bottle users were put to sleep at least once in the 2 weeks preceding the interview with a bottle containing something other than plain water (Fig 4, Table 1). More than 8% of children aged 2–5 years still used a bottle inappropriately either when sleeping or at other times. White and Hispanic children were likelier than black children to continue using the bottle. Parents with less than a high school education also were a factor.

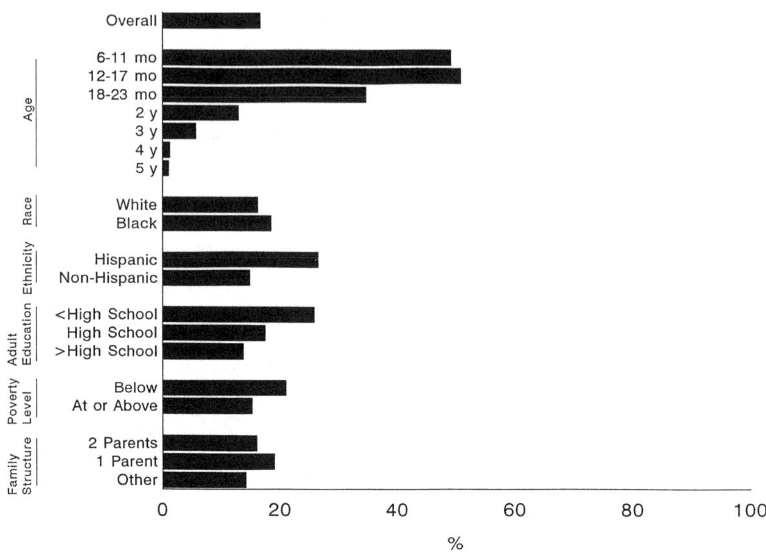

FIGURE 3.—Population prevalence of inappropriate feeding practices among all United States children aged 6 months to 5 years. (From Kaste LM, Gift HC: Inappropriate infant bottle feeding: Status of the Healthy People 2000 objective. *Arch Pediatr Adolesc Med* 149:786–791, Copyright 1995, American Medical Association. Courtesy of the National Center for Health Statistics, 1992.)

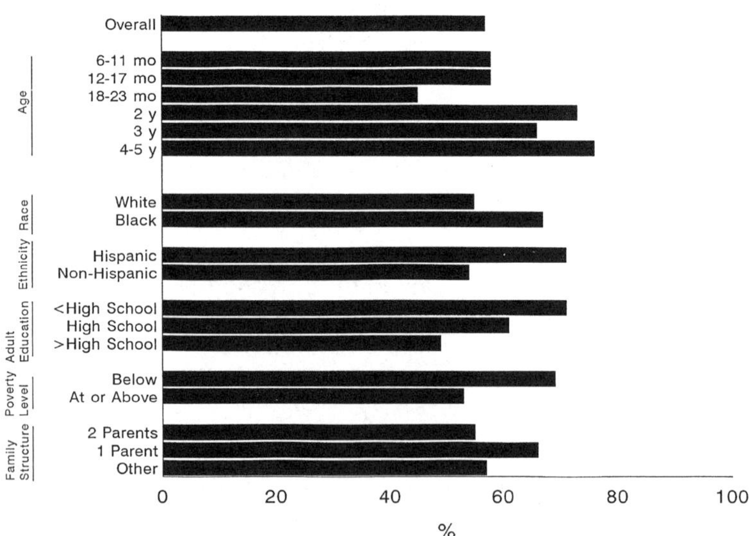

FIGURE 4.—Inappropriate feeding practices among children aged 6 months to 5 years who use a bottle. (From Kaste LM, Gift HC: Inappropriate infant bottle feeding: Status of the Healthy People 2000 objective. *Arch Pediatr Adolesc Med* 149:786–791, Copyright 1995, American Medical Association. Courtesy of the National Center for Health Statistics, 1992.)

TABLE 1.—Percentage of Children Aged 6 Months to 5 Years Who Are Fed With Bottles, by Number of Days Put to Bed With a Bottle in Past 2 Weeks

Variable	Levels	No. of Days* 0	1–13	14
Total, n=1795		42.9	17.2	39.9
Age group				
χ^2=52.25,	6–11 mo	42.2	19.0	38.8
df=10, P<.01,	12–17 mo	42.4	16.0	41.6
n=1795	18–23 mo	54.6	12.0	33.4
	2 y	26.9	24.3	48.8
	3 y	34.0	17.6	48.4
	4–5 y	23.5	32.4	44.1
Ethnicity	Hispanic	28.9	22.3	48.8
χ^2=24.14, *df*=2,	Non-Hispanic	46.3	16.0	37.8
P<.01, n-1795				
Education of adult	<High school	28.7	22.3	49.0
χ^2=21.88,	High school	38.5	17.1	44.4
df=4, P<.01,	>High school	50.5	15.6	33.9
n=1795				
Household income	<$7,000	37.5	22.6	39.9
χ^2=25.8, *df*=6	$7,000–<$14,999	30.4	19.2	50.4
P<.01, n=1582	$15,000–$34,999	42.9	16.6	40.5
	≥$35,000	51.8	14.4	33.8
Poverty-level status	At or above	46.6	15.5	37.8
χ^2=19.97, *df*=2,	Below	31.2	21.8	47.0
P<.01, n=1677				
Region χ^2=20.94, *df*=6,	Northeast	52.3	14.6	33.1
P<.01, n=1795	Midwest	48.2	17.5	34.3
	South	40.8	17.6	41.5
	West	33.8	18.6	47.6

*All values expressed as percentages.
(From Kaste LM, Gift HC: Inappropriate infant bottle feeding: Status of the Healthy People 2000 objective. *Arch Pediatr Adolesc Med* 149:786–791, Copyright 1995, American Medical Association. Courtesy of the National Center for Health Statistics, 1992.)

Implication.—If use of a baby bottle were targeted as inappropriate feeding behavior, early childhood caries and other sequelae might be avoided.

▶ Children who are given a bottle with anything other than water at bedtime are at uniquely high risk for early childhood caries. What is astounding from these data is that 20% of kids in this country are put at such risk by their parents before 1 year of age, and just under 10% of children between the ages of 2 and 5 years still use bottles. Among bottle feeders, about 50% of children in the following groups have a higher risk of inappropriate feeding practices: children of parents with less than a high school education (49%), children within Hispanic families (48.8%), children in a family with an income of $7,000 to $15,000 per year (50.5%), and children from the Western states (47.6%).

As pediatricians, we have the unique opportunity to provide advice, counseling, and follow-up for parents when it comes to appropriate feeding practices and the prevention of dental problems. Read this report in detail to see how we can help.

To update yourself about baby bottle caries, see the excellent editorial by Curzon entitled, "Out of the mouths of babies and sucklings...Do we still care for the oral health of our children?"[1]

Reference

1. Curzon ME: *J Dent Res* 73:714, 1994.

Do Exclusively Breast-fed Infants Require Extra Protein?

Dewey KG, Cohen RJ, Rivera LL, et al (Univ of California, Davis; Liga de la Lactancia Materna, San Pedro Sula, Honduras; Wellstart Internatl, Washington, DC)
Pediatr Res 39:303–307, 1996   3–6

Background.—Some authorities have argued that the growth rate of infants who are exclusively breast-fed may be limited by protein intake. Data on protein intake and growth were obtained in an intervention study conducted in Honduras.

Methods and Findings.—By random assignment, 50 infants were breast-fed exclusively for 6 months, and 91 received preprepared solid foods along with breast milk beginning at 4 months of age. The latter group had a 20% greater protein intake and significantly higher iron, zinc, calcium, vitamin A, and riboflavin intakes. However, the 2 groups did not differ in weight or length gain. Growth rate was also comparable when the 20 infants with the greatest protein intakes in the second group were compared with 20 infants in the first group on the basis of energy intake. The 20 exclusively breast-fed infants with the lowest protein intakes also did not differ significantly in growth from the 20 infants with the lowest protein intake in the solid-food group. In general, infant morbidity was relatively low.

Conclusions.—The protein intake of infants who are breast-fed exclusively probably does not limit growth between 4 and 6 months of age. The difference in growth rates between breast-fed and formula-fed infants at that age apparently is not a function of breast-fed infants' marginal protein intake.

▶ Why breast milk contains less protein compared with other milks is not known. It has been argued that the composition of human milk represents an evolutionary compromise between the needs of the infant and the needs of the mother, and that lower milk protein concentrations may protect the lactating mother from becoming nutritionally depleted. The observation that the breast-fed infant gains weight less rapidly than does a formula-fed infant after 2–3 months of age has led numerous investigators on dead-end trails to figure out why this phenomenon occurs. This study examined whether the lower protein content of breast milk may be the reason for this altered growth. In formula-fed infants, slower growth rates have been observed when such infants are fed formulas with a protein content closer to that of human milk than when they are fed standard, higher protein formulas. This may be due to lower use of protein from formulas than from human milk. What this study does is attempt, once and for all to provide us with a definitive answer to the question of whether breast-fed infants need more protein. Apparently they do not and will not grow better. The results of this study are consistent with those from an observational study of breast-fed infants in an affluent population (DARLING study), in which the protein density of the diet was unrelated to growth throughout the first year of life.[1]

If it's not an altered protein content in breast milk, what is the reason that infants who are breast fed tend to grow more slowly? The answer is not readily forthcoming. The other recent dead-end trail in this regard was the search to determine whether the low zinc content of breast milk might be causative. Investigators in Helsinki recently showed that the diminished zinc intake associated with exclusive breast-feeding does not impair growth.[2]

Because no one has ever shown that otherwise healthy babies who are breast-fed are in any way impaired by being a bit more featherweight, perhaps we should stop paying any attention to the issue of weight gain in relationship to breast-feeding. Because breast-feeding is nature's way, let nature have her way when it comes to infant growth.

References

1. Heinig MJ, et al: *Am J Clin Nutr* 58:152, 1993.
2. Salmenpera L, et al: *J Pediatr Gastroenterol Nutr* 18:361, 1994.

Breastfeeding, Dummy Use, and Adult Intelligence
Gale CR, Martyn CN (Univ of Southampton, England)
Lancet 347:1072–1075, 1996   3–7

Purpose.—There is evidence that breast-fed infants go on to have better scores on intelligence and language tests than their bottle-fed peers, although the significance of this link is uncertain. It could result from the nutritional content of breast milk, from some psychological advantage of breast-feeding, or from some factor in the home environment affecting the decision to breast-feed. The association between breast-feeding and higher social class makes it difficult to assess the influence of breast-feeding on intellectual development. The relationship between feeding method in infancy and adult intelligence was studied among people born when the social connotations of breast-feeding were different.

Methods.—The follow-up study included 994 British men and women born during the 1920s, when breast-feeding was more likely to be practiced by the lower rather than the higher social classes. For each subject, information on feeding method during infancy was available from records of health visits. All subjects took the computerized AH4 intelligence quotient (IQ) test, the results of which were evaluated for relationships with method of infant feeding.

Results.—Two thirds of the subjects were breast-fed exclusively, and only 5% were bottle-fed exclusively. Intelligence quotients were somewhat higher for the subjects who had been breast-fed exclusively than in those who had been breast-fed and bottle-fed exclusively. Subjects who had used a pacifier as infants, whose fathers were manual laborers, and whose mothers were young when the subjects were born had lower IQs. Having more older siblings was also associated with lower IQ scores. After adjustment for other variables on multivariate analysis, feeding method was no longer related to IQ. Pacifier use, number of older siblings, maternal age when the subjects were born, and father's occupational class were still significant predictors of adult intelligence, however.

Conclusion.—The higher IQ scores of adults who were breast-fed at birth do not appear to result from the nutritional qualities of breast milk per se but rather from the child's social environment. Other factors—such as maternal age, father's occupation, and number of siblings—are better predictors of adult intelligence than is breast-feeding. There are several possible explanations for the link between pacifier use and lower intelligence.

▶ This report will be used as an argument to reinforce the convictions of those who believe there is no link between intelligence and breast-feeding. A number of other studies have suggested that breast-feeding in early life affects cognitive development. Children who have been breast-fed are reported to have higher scores on tests of intelligence and language development in comparison to those who are bottle-fed. This beneficial effect is thought to be more pronounced when breast-feeding is continued for extended durations.

The basis for a purported link between higher intelligence and breast-feeding remains unclear. Breast milk does have a higher content of various substances needed for brain development, such as essential fatty acids. Is it possible that children who are bottle-fed may score less well on IQ tests because they lack this nutritional advantage in early life? There is also no question that the act of breast-feeding may confer some psychological advantage, perhaps because of differences in the way mother and baby interact during feeding, or because of the greater control the breast-fed infant has over the pace and duration of feeding. It is also possible that the apparent relationship between IQ and breast-feeding is the result of a parent genetic factor or some other influence in the home environment that affects both the choice of feeding method and the child's cognitive development.

What the report abstracted here does is attempt to shed some light on why current data show a positive relationship between IQ and breast-feeding. Most current studies on the relationship between feeding method in infancy and performance tests of intelligence have investigated infants or children who were born after World War II, a period when the popularity of breast-feeding among mothers in developed countries was declining. Although the popularity of breast-feeding has recently increased a bit, this method of infant feeding still retains strong class connotations. Since World War II, women who breast feed are more likely to be from higher social classes, to have continued their education into college, or to be older at the time of birth. These types of associations between breast-feeding and socioeconomic advantage make it hard to determine whether breast milk affects intellectual development independent of other variables. This report from Great Britain solves the dilemma by going back to the beginning of the 20th century, when the rate and social determinants of breast-feeding were quite different. Then, the majority of infants who were bottle-fed from birth tended to be from the wealthiest classes, the opposite of what we see in more modern times.

So what do we learn from the turn of the century? We learn that those who were breast-fed did not turn out later in life to have higher IQ scores. This suggests that any link between feeding methods and later intelligence may have more to do with a child's social environment than with the nutritional qualities of breast milk ... a hard pill to swallow.

Please do not consider this story as having ended yet. In the long run, nature favors her own ways. A betting person is likely to do better with a wager that sides with Mother Nature.

Weaning Ages in a Sample of American Women Who Practice Extended Breastfeeding

Sugarman M, Kendall-Tackett KA (Massachusetts Gen Hosp, Boston; Perinatal Education Group, Henniker, NH)
Clin Pediatr 34:642–647, 1995   3–8

Objective.—Whereas weaning in the United States typically occurs at 2–4 months, knowledge of the health benefits to mother and child of extended nursing have caused the World Health Organization to recommend breast-feeding for up to 2 years. The weaning ages and practices of women who practice long-term breast-feeding were examined.

Methods.—A total of 179 women who had nursed at least 1 child past the age of 6 months were given a closed-end, self-administered 96-item questionnaire about breast-feeding and weaning.

Results.—Most women who practice long-term nursing do so secretly. The average age of the women was 34.4 years, and their average age at first birth was 27 years. Thirty-seven women had 1 child, 73 had 2, and 69 had 3 or more. There were 14 women who had weaned at least 3 children. The average age of weaning was 3 years 7 months for the youngest child, 2 years 7 months for the middle child, and 2 years 6 months for the oldest child. There was a significant difference between the weaning times for the oldest and youngest children. Most women said weaning was "child-led" and gradual, but a substantial number of women cited subsequent pregnancy as a reason for weaning (Table 2). Women who practiced extended breast-feeding were significantly older than other American mothers. When women were asked to describe their feelings about weaning, most believed weaning should be child-led (75.9%), and they enjoyed the nursing experience (72.3%).

TABLE 2.—Reasons for Weaning and How It Was Accomplished for a Woman's 3 Youngest Children

	Child A* N = 25	Child B N = 125	Child C N = 69
Reasons for weaning (%)			
Lack of information	5.3	4.2	8.7
Lack of support or opposition	2.6	4.2	8.7
Next pregnancy affected taste or supply of milk	7.9	14.3	8.7
Next pregnancy affected mother's motivation	5.3	21.8	24.6
Illness or separation from child	5.3	5.9	11.6
Child-led, happened naturally	63.2	57.1	52.2
Mother's decision that child was ready	15.8	13.4	10.1
Mother's decision based on family circumstance	7.9	5.0	4.3
Other	0	5.9	1.4
How weaning was accomplished (mean %)	1.3	1.4	1.3
Sudden	12.8	7.6	8.8
Gradual	56.4	60.2	45.6
Child-led	53.3	56.7	54.1
Mother deliberately weaned	2.6	11.0	13.2
Mother encouraged weaning by talking to child	23.1	31.4	20.6
Substituted thumb, pacifier	2.6	3.4	1.5
Other	1.7	1.8	1.7
Number of reasons (mean)	1.8	1.8	1.7

*Child A is the youngest.

(Courtesy of Sugarman M, Kendall-Tackett KA: Weaning ages in a sample of American women who practice extended breastfeeding. *Clin Pediatr* 34:642–647, 1995.)

Conclusion.—Long-term nursing is unusual and is typically done secretly in our society. Because of the benefits to mother and child, practitioners can feel comfortable supporting these women.

▶ In this country, women who breast-feed typically rarely do so for more than 4 months. This, of course, is not the norm in many other parts of the world where the average duration of breast-feeding is 2–3 years. There is a renewed interest in the health benefits of prolonged breast-feeding. The health benefits to both mother and infant of extended nursing were the topics of several presentations at a recent meeting of the American Association of the Advancement of Science.[1] Extended breast-feeding is associated with an approximate 30% reduction in risk for premenopausal breast cancer. The health benefits of extended nursing are impressive enough that the World Health Organization's *Innocenti Declaration* has recommended breast-feeding for up to 2 years and beyond for infants worldwide.[2]

This report shows us that there are some women in this country who do believe fully in extended breast-feeding. We also see that they are not typical mothers in many respects. College graduates are overrepresented. Indeed, 25% of extended breast-feeders have graduate degrees. Their average age is older (34.4 years), and they do extend the time of breast-feeding (the first-born child of these mothers was breast-fed for an average of 3 years). One mother in this study fed her child for over 7 years.

If this report teaches us anything, it is that breast-feeding is more than a form of infant nourishment. Infants in this country don't need breast milk for up to 3 years on a nutritional basis. The human infant also requires warmth, love, environmental stimulation, and rest. In a single act, breast-feeding meets all of these needs. Although a bottle-feeding mother can hold and cuddle her infant, it is not the same. Prolonged breast-feeding cannot be considered just a form of nourishment but rather a style of mothering. Not every mother will, or can, do this. The special closeness of a prolonged breast-feeding relationship is not for all mothers. Many women do not want such an exclusive relationship, or are concerned about returning to work or their responsibilities to other children and family members. For these women, there are clearly other options for the feeding and nurturing of their infants that will make them healthy.

What is important for us as medical professionals is to be supportive. Currently, women who breast-feed for extended periods, particularly beyond a year, are considered odd. That's not fair, particularly because such attitudes are fairly unique to nations such as ours. Indeed, the world views us in the United States as being the deviants. We are "short-termers" with respect to the manner in which we breast-feed our infants.

References

1. Poole S: *J NIH Res* 64–66, 1993.
2. UNICEF-WHO: *Innocenti Declaration. On the Protection, Promotion, and Support of Breast-feeding.* New York, UNICEF, 1990.

The Effect of Zinc Supplementation on Pregnancy Outcome

Goldenberg RL, Tamura T, Neggers Y, et al (Univ of Alabama, Birmingham)
JAMA 274:463–468, 1995   3–9

Background.—The role of zinc supplementation as a predictor of pregnancy outcome has not been clearly established. A randomized, double-blind, placebo-controlled study was performed to clarify the association between zinc supplementation during pregnancy and outcome.

Participants and Methods.—Five hundred eighty medically indigent but otherwise healthy black women (mean age, 23 years) were studied. All women had zinc levels below the estimated median for gestational age at enrollment in prenatal care. At 19 weeks' gestation, 294 women were randomly assigned to daily treatment with 25 mg of zinc and 286 to placebo until delivery. All women also received a daily prenatal non–zinc-containing multivitamin/mineral tablet. Birth weight, gestational age at birth, and head circumference at birth were evaluated and compared between groups. Further analyses were performed after subdividing patients into 2 groups based on body mass index (greater or less than 26 kg/m²).

Results.—Infants born to mothers treated with zinc supplementation had significantly greater mean birth weights and head circumferences, at 3,214 g and 34.2 cm, compared with 3,088 g and 33.8 cm among infants delivered to women receiving placebo (Table 1). Zinc supplementation also resulted in a 248-g higher infant birth weight and a 0.7-cm larger head circumference among women with a body mass index less than 26 kg/m^2. A reduction in births occurring at or before 32 weeks' gestation and in very low birth weight infants also was observed among women receiving zinc supplementation, although differences between groups were not significant. Women who received zinc supplementation had significantly higher plasma zinc concentrations than did those given placebo.

Conclusions.—Daily zinc supplementation among women with fairly low plasma zinc concentrations early in pregnancy leads to higher infant

TABLE 1.—A Comparison of the Zinc Supplement and Placebo Groups

	Zinc Supplement Group (*n* = 294)	Placebo Group (*n* = 286)	*P*
Maternal Characteristics			
Age, y*	23.9±5.5	22.8±5.4	.02
Multiparous, %	42.5	46.9	.29
Body mass index, kg/m^2*	28.2±7.5	27.8±7.0	.49
Dietary zinc intake, mg/d*	12.8±5.9	13.1±5.6	.45
Plasma zinc, μmol/L*	9.6±1.5	9.7±1.5	.67
Prenatal care, No. of visits*	12.6±3.0	12.3±3.4	.26
Smoker, %	5.8	4.2	.39
Drug and/or alcohol use, %	12.2	11.0	.63
Pregnancy Outcome			
Birth weight, g*	3214±669	3088±728	.03
Gestational age at birth, wk*	38.8±2.9	38.3±3.5	.06
Preterm birth <37 wk, %	10.2	13.3	.25
Preterm birth ≤32 wk, %	3.4	6.3	.10
Birth weight <2500 g, %	7.8	12.7	.06
Birth weight <1500 g, %	3.1	4.9	.26
Growth retardation, %	5.4	6.3	.66
Neonatal death, %	0.3	0	.32
Fetal death, %	1.7	2.5	.55
Anthropometric Measurements			
Crown-heel length, cm	5.04±3.4	49.8±4.3	.11
Head circumference, cm	34.2±2.0	33.8±2.1	.02
Chest circumference, cm	33.4±2.5	32.9±2.7	.20
Abdominal circumference, cm	33.0±2.8	32.9±2.5	.54
Arm length, cm	9.9±1.0	9.7±1.1	.03
Femur length, cm	10.9±0.9	10.7±1.0	.03
Arm circumference, cm	11.2±1.2	11.0±1.3	.06
Thigh circumference, cm	15.4±1.8	15.3±1.6	.40
Subscapular skinfold, mm	4.0±1.0	3.8±0.9	.01
Triceps skinfold, mm	3.8±0.9	3.7±0.9	.05
Thigh skinfold, mm	4.8±1.3	4.6±1.1	.06
Neonatal Outcome			
Neonatal hospital stay, d	3.6±5.0	4.7±10.0	.11
Respiratory distress syndrome, %	2.0	2.8	.55
Intraventricular hemorrhage, %	0.7	0.7	.98
Necrotizing enterocolitis, %	0.7	0.4	.58
Neonatal sepsis, %	0.3	1.8	.09

* Values are mean ± SD.

(Courtesy of Goldenberg RL, Tamura T, Neggers Y, et al: The effect of zinc supplementation on pregnancy outcome. *JAMA* 274:463–468, Copyright 1995, American Medical Association.)

birth weights and larger head circumferences, particularly among individuals with a body mass index less than 26 kg/m^2. Although the minimum dosage of zinc is not currently known for any population of pregnant women, favorable effects were achieved with a daily dose of 25 mg in this study.

▶ Zinc is an interesting metal. Even more interesting is the story that relates zinc and zinc deficiency to human disease. The first discovery of human zinc deficiency was in the Middle East in the early 1960s, and symptoms included growth retardation, male hypogonadism, anemia, hepatosplenomegaly, and geophagia. Since then, there have been many reports of mild zinc deficiency, including some in the United States. Symptoms in these populations have included decreased growth velocity and loss of appetite in infants and children.

The manner by which zinc supplementation during pregnancy results in increased birth weight, increased fetal growth, and prolonged gestational age is unknown. However, it is likely that a number of complex mechanisms are involved in the improvement of pregnancy outcome associated with zinc supplementation. Zinc is known to play a critical role as a cofactor for numerous enzyme functions, including protein synthesis, nucleic acid metabolism, gene expression, and immune regulation. This element, therefore, is essential for normal growth and development of the fetus.

It's probably going to be some time before we know all the ramifications of this interesting report. One of the implications is that in the United States, there may be numerous pregnant women who would benefit from zinc supplementation. The benefit is the prevention of the birth of some underweight newborns who may have less than ideal head circumferences. Correcting such problems should be a high priority for all of us. All it takes is a touch of element number 105 (atomic number 30).

Are Long-chain Polyunsaturated Fatty Acids Essential Nutrients in Infancy?
Makrides M, Neumann M, Simmer K, et al (Flinders Med Centre, Adelaide, Australia)
Lancet 345:1463–1468, 1995   3–10

Background.—Preterm infants who are breast-fed appear to have advanced neural maturation compared with those who are bottle-fed. Breast-fed infants' higher tissue levels of long-chain polyunsaturated fatty acids (LCPUFAs), especially docosahexaenoic acid (DHA, 22:6w3), may play an important causative role. Whether the disparity in neural maturation between breast-fed and formula-fed term infants could be corrected by adding fish oil, a source of DHA, to formula was investigated.

Methods.—Twenty-six healthy, term infants of mothers choosing to bottle feed were randomly assigned at birth to a supplemented or placebo formula. Twenty-three breast-fed term infants served as a comparison

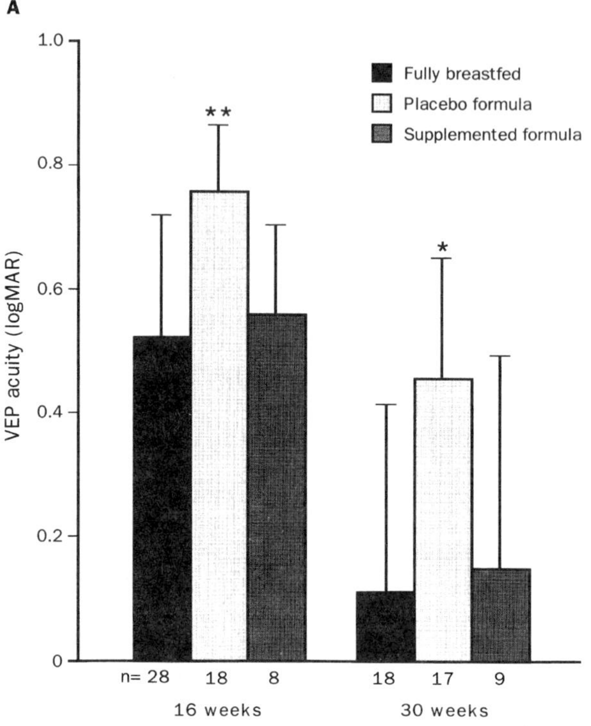

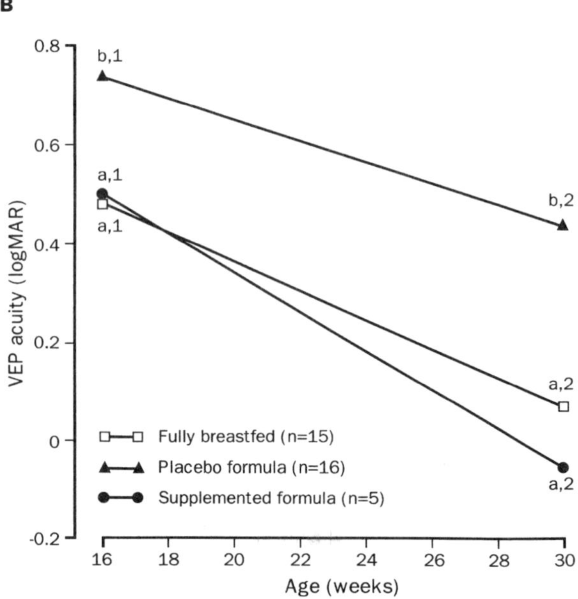

FIGURE 1.—Mean (SD) visual evoked potential (*VEP*) *acuity at 16 and 30 weeks of age (*A), and VEP acuity as a function of age (**B**). *Asterisk* indicates $P < 0.01$; *double asterisk*, $P < 0.001$. Analysis of variance: diet, $P < 0.001$; diet $\times$ age, not significant. *Letters* indicate differences between diet groups at each age. *Numbers* indicate differences between ages for each diet group. (Courtesy of Makrides M, Neumann M, Simmer K, et al: Are long-chain polyunsaturated fatty acids essential nutrients in infancy? *Lancet* 345:1463–1468, copyright by The Lancet Ltd., 1995.)

group. Erythrocyte fatty acids and anthropometric assessments were made on day 5 and at weeks 6, 16, and 30. Visual evoked potential (VEP) acuity was also evaluated at 16 and 30 weeks.

Findings.—At both assessments, the breast-fed and supplemented formula–fed infants had better VEP acuities than the infants given placebo formula (Fig 1). In breast-fed and supplemented formula–fed infants, erythrocyte DHA was maintained near birth levels throughout the 30-week study. In infants given the placebo formula, however, these values declined. In all infants at both ages tested, the only fatty acid consistently correlating with VEP acuity was erythrocyte DHA. Supplemented formula–fed infants had erythrocyte arachidonic acid levels below those of infants given breast milk or placebo formula at 16 and 30 weeks. However, there were no adverse effects. All infants had similar growth.

Conclusions.—Docosahexaenoic acid appears to be an essential nutrient for the optimal neural maturation of term infants. It is still unclear whether formula supplementation with DHA has long-term benefits.

▶ When I first read this report, it struck me as being a bit fishy (pardon the pun) and not worthy of inclusion in the YEAR BOOK OF PEDIATRICS. After reading it a second and third time, however, this editor realized that there could be enormous implications to what these investigators observed. What they observed was that neuronal development, based on observation of VEPs, was markedly enhanced in breast-fed term infants and formula-fed term infants who were supplemented with fish oil in comparison with formula-fed infants. Indeed, all of this does make some sense. Preterm breast-fed infants, for example, are reported to have advanced neuronal maturation compared with bottle-fed infants as assessed by similar VEPs in other studies.[1] It has been proposed that the higher tissue levels of LCPUFAs reported in breast-fed infants may be an important causative factor of this advanced brain development. Breast milk contains much more of such fatty acids than do bottle-milk formulas, which tend to be fortified only with precursor essential fatty acids such as linoleic acid. The main concern about fatty acid nutrition in infancy relates to preterm infants, because the rate of brain growth is known to be greatest in the last trimester of pregnancy and in the first few months of life.

What does all this mean? It means that the best advice to give parents is that their infants should be breast-fed for at least 4 months and possibly a year. Put this in capital letters if one is talking about a preterm infant.

Reference

1. Uavy RD, et al: *Pediatr Res* 28:485, 1990.

Diagnosing Gaucher Disease: Early Recognition, Implications for Treatment, and Genetic Counseling

Sidransky E, Tayebi N, Ginns EI (Natl Inst of Mental Health, Bethesda, Md)
Clin Pediatr (Phila) 34:365–371, 1995   3–11

Objective.—Gaucher's disease, the most frequently inherited disorder of Ashkenazi Jews, results in a deficiency of glucocerebrosidase. Although the disease is easily diagnosed by measuring white blood cell glucocerebrosidase activity, many cases of Gaucher's disease are misdiagnosed. Medical records were reviewed to determine the range of presumptive diagnoses and the means used to determine diagnoses.

Methods.—Records of 25 patients with types 1 and 3 Gaucher's disease were reviewed.

Results.—In 17 patients, the initial diagnosis was not Gaucher's disease (Table 1). Ten patients had hepatosplenomegaly, and many had anemia or thrombocytopenia. In all 17 patients, invasive techniques were used to diagnose Gaucher's disease, including 11 bone marrow biopsies, 4 splenectomies, 1 liver biopsy, and 1 bone biopsy. Ten patients were of Ashkenazi Jewish ancestry. The 7 who were of varied ethnic backgrounds generally had more severe disease. Gaucher's disease is the most common inherited lysosomal storage disease in which abnormal enzymes allow the accumulation of complex macromolecules in lysosomes that lead to a variety of clinical manifestations (Tables 2 and 3). Type 1 disease is most common among Ashkenazi Jews (Table 4).

Conclusion.—A correct diagnosis of Gaucher's disease is important to ensure proper therapy and necessary genetic counseling.

▶ Gaucher's disease may seem like a relatively obscure disorder, but, in fact, it is the most common lysosomal storage disorder. The disease is making the news these days because of cost issues related to its management. Treatment, which is very effective, requires the use of an enzyme replacement therapy (glucocerebrosidase, algulecerase). For a young adult, standard dosing with this enzyme costs an average of $350,000 a year for drugs alone. These extraordinary costs have stimulated a lot of discussion about what's right and what's wrong with health care in the United States and elsewhere.

The article abstracted was specifically written with the intent to help clinicians establish a prompt diagnosis of Gaucher's disease. This is critical, both to avoid misassignment of other illnesses and to consider appropriate therapeutic options. Before enzyme replacement therapy, patients were usually treated by supportive management, including transfusions, orthopedic procedures, and splenectomy. Depending on the type of Gaucher's disease, this was at best palliative treatment, and early death could be expected. Use Tables 1 through 4 to assemble an appropriate set of signs and symptoms that will allow you to make a correct clinical diagnosis, which can be confirmed with a specific enzyme assay, usually performed on white blood cells. The diagnosis can also be made by DNA mutation analysis.

TABLE 1.—Clinical Presentations of Patients With Gaucher's Disease

Patient	Age at diagnosis (years)	Signs/symptoms	Preliminary diagnosis	Means of diagnosis	Ashkenazi Jewish ancestry	Type of Gaucher's disease
1	1	Failure to thrive, hepatosplenomegaly	Childhood tumor	Bone marrow	No	3
2	2	Anemia, thrombocytopenia, splenomegaly	R/O leukemia	Bone marrow	No	1
3	2.5	Thrombocytopenia, left upper quadrant mass	R/O Wilms' tumor	Bone marrow	No	3
4	2.5	Hepatosplenomegaly, petechia, pulmonary infiltrates	Reticuloendotheliosis	Bone marrow	No	3
5	5	Epistaxis, hip pain	Perthes' disease	Bone marrow	Yes	1
6	6	Bone pain	Trauma 2° to ice skating	Bone marrow	Yes	1
7	6	Malaise, anemia, thrombocytopenia	Leukemia	Bone marrow	No	1
8	10	Painless splenomegaly, brother with splenomegaly	Hereditary spherocytosis	Splenectomy	No	1
9	15	Abdominal trauma	Subcapsular hematoma of spleen	Splenectomy	Yes	1
10	18	Leg fracture, hepatosplenomegaly	Bone disease	Liver biopsy	No	1
11	20	Hip pain	Bone tumor	Bone biopsy	Yes	1
12	34	Splenomegaly	R/O lymphoma	Splenectomy	Yes	1
13	37	Abdominal mass during pregnancy	Twin pregnancy	Splenectomy	Yes	1
14	39	Elevated ferritin, borderline thrombocytopenia	R/O malignancy	Bone marrow	Yes	1
15	43	Postsurgical bleeding, prolonged clotting time	von Willebrand's disease	Bone marrow	Yes	1
16	44	Hematuria, bruising	Renal disease	Bone marrow	Yes	1
17	44	Pancytopenia, spleen tip palpated	Myelofibrosis	Bone marrow	Yes	1

(Courtesy of Sidransky E, Tayebi N, Ginns EI: Diagnosing Gaucher disease: Early recognition, implications for treatment, and genetic counseling. *Clin Pediatr (Phila)* 34:365–371, 1995.)

TABLE 2.—Selected Lipid Lysosomal Storage Diseases

Disease	Enzyme deficiency	Enzymatic test	Mode of inheritance	Clinical characteristics
Fabry's disease	α-galactosidase (ceramide trihexosidase) (EC 3.2.1.22)	Enzyme assay in plasma, leukocytes, or tears	X-linked recessive	Angiokeratoma, cardiac disease, episodic pain, hypohidrosis, transient ischemic attacks, strokes, renal failure, acroparesthesias, corneal and lenticular opacities
Farber's lipogranulo-matosis	Ceramidase (EC 3.5.1.23)	Enzyme assay in fibroblasts or WBC	Autosomal recessive	Painful and swollen joints, granulomatous lesions of skin, nodules, muscular atrophy, moderate nervous system dysfunction, failure to thrive, progressive hoarseness
Gangliosidosis GMI Type 1, 2, 3	β-galactosidase (EC 3.2.1.23)	Enzyme assay in WBC or fibroblasts	Autosomal recessive	Three clinical types ranging from acute infantile onset with rapid neurologic decline and severe bony abnormalities to patients with normal intelligence and survival into adulthood, motor weakness, mild or absent bony abnormalities
Gangliosidosis (GM2) (Tay-Sachs disease)	Hexosaminidase A (EC 3.2.1.52) α-subunit (Variant B)	Enzyme assay in WBC or fibroblasts	Autosomal recessive	Four clinical subtypes based upon age of onset. Infantile form is Tay-Sachs disease, motor weakness, hypotonia, dementia, cherry-red macular spot, blindness, deafness, and seizures
Gangliosidosis (GM2) (Sandhoff disease)	Hexosaminidase β-subunit (deficiency of A & B isozymes) (Variant 0)	Enzyme assay in WBC or fibroblasts	Autosomal recessive	Three clinical subtypes; Infantile Sandhoff disease very similar to Tay-Sachs disease
Gaucher disease	Glucocerebrosidase (EC 3.2.1.45)	Enzyme assay in WBC or fibroblasts	Autosomal recessive	See Table 11
Niemann-Pick disease types A & B	Sphingomyelinase (EC 3.1.4.12)	Enzyme assay in WBC or fibroblasts	Autosomal recessive	Type A-neurodegeneration and death by 2 years, with failure to thrive, hepatosplenomegaly, psychomotor retardation, cherry-red macular spots in some patients Type B-variable onset in childhood or adolescence, hepatosplenomegaly, pulmonary involvement

Abbreviation: WBC, white blood cell.
(Courtesy of Sidransky E, Tayebi N, Ginns EI: Diagnosing Gaucher disease: Early recognition, implications for treatment, and genetic counseling. *Clin Pediatr (Phila)* 34:365–371, 1995.)

TABLE 3.—Frequently Encountered Manifestations of Gaucher's Disease

Splenomegaly	• Painless enlargement of spleen is a frequent manifestation • Spleen may be more than 20 times normal size for age • Patients may experience abdominal pain resulting from splenic infarcts • Large organ size may lead to high-output cardiac failure or failure to thrive
Hepatomegaly	• Hepatic enlargement is common • Lipid storage accounts for approximately 20% of total organ mass • Portal hypertension is sometimes seen • Cirrhosis or bleeding from esophageal varices in severe cases
Skeletal involvement	• Although radiographic signs are very common, symptom severity is variable • Pathologic bone fractures may result • Painful bone crises result from bone infarcts • Femoral head necrosis is common • Vertebral collapse may occur • Classic radiologic feature is Erlenmeyer flask deformity of the distal femur
Bruising and bleeding	• Epistaxis is common • Patients may have severe postsurgical bleeding • Bleeding is related both to platelet deficiency and decreased function of clotting factors
Laboratory findings	• Anemia • Thrombocytopenia • Prolonged coagulation times • Elevated acid phosphatase (nontartrate inhibited) • Elevated angiotensin converting enzyme • Abnormal serum immunoglobulins • Elevated ferritin level

(Courtesy of Sidransky E, Tayebi N, Ginns EI: Diagnosing Gaucher disease: Early recognition, implications for treatment, and genetic counseling. *Clin Pediatr (Phila)* 34:365–371, 1995.)

When dealing with Ashkenazi Jewish patients, clinicians should be aware that Gaucher's disease is a relatively common disorder and should be considered in the differential diagnosis of any patient with symptoms such as anemia, thrombocytopenia, splenomegaly, or bony symptoms. Many patients with Gaucher's disease will initially have a bone fracture as their only clinical sign, even though they may have advanced problems.

To learn more about the financial implications of this disorder to patients and to society, read the excellent articles by Hollak et al.[1] and Zimran et al.[2]

References

1. Hollak CEM, et al: *Lancet* 345:1474, 1995.
2. Zimran A, et al: *Lancet* 345:1479, 1995.

TABLE 4.—The Three Types of Gaucher's Disease

	Presentation	Age	Progression	Neurologic manifestation	Genetics
Type 1 (non-neuronopathic)	Very heterogenous	Presents at any age	Variable	None	Autosomal recessive Increased incidence among Ashkenazi Jews
Type 2 (acute neuronopathic)	More stereotypic	Usually presents at 3–6 months Can present in the neonatal period	Death by age 2–3 years	Seizures Strabismus, trimus hyperreflexia Apnea Can present with hydrops fetalis or congenital ichthyosis	Autosomal recessive No ethnic predilection
Type 3 (subacute neuronopathic)	Heterogenous	Usually presents in childhood	Neurologic signs by adolescence	One group has a specific oculomotor abnormality of the horizontal saccades Others have seizures, ataxia, dementia, spasticity	Autosomal recessive Panethnic with a Norrbottnian subgroup

(Courtesy of Sidransky E, Tayebi N, Ginns EI: Diagnosing Gaucher disease: Early recognition, implications for treatment, and genetic counseling. *Clin Pediatr (Phila)* 34:365–371, 1995.)

Enzyme Replacement Therapy for Gaucher Disease: Skeletal Responses to Macrophage-targeted Glucocerebrosidase
Rosenthal DI, Doppelt SH, Mankin HJ, et al (Massachusetts Gen Hosp, Boston; Natl Inst of Neurological Disorders and Stroke, Bethesda, Md; Natl Insts of Health, Bethesda, Md)
Pediatrics 96:629–637, 1995   3–12

Background.—Patients with Gaucher's disease exhibit a wide range of skeletal complications, including generalized osteopenia, bone infarction, osteonecrosis, and pathologic fracture. This, the most common of the lipid storage diseases, reliably responds to infusion of macrophage-targeted glucocerebrosidase. Skeletal responses tend to take place less rapidly than hematologic and visceral responses.

Objective.—Quantitative bone imaging was used to gauge the efficacy of enzyme treatment for reversing skeletal involvement in 8 children and 4 adults with moderate-to-severe type 1 Gaucher's disease. All patients had an intact spleen.

Methods.—The patients initially received macrophage-targeted glucocerebrosidase, 60 units/kg every 2 weeks for 2 years. The dose then was lowered to 30 units/kg for 9 months, and then 15 units/kg for 9 months longer. Bone marrow infiltration was assessed by MRI, radioxenon up-

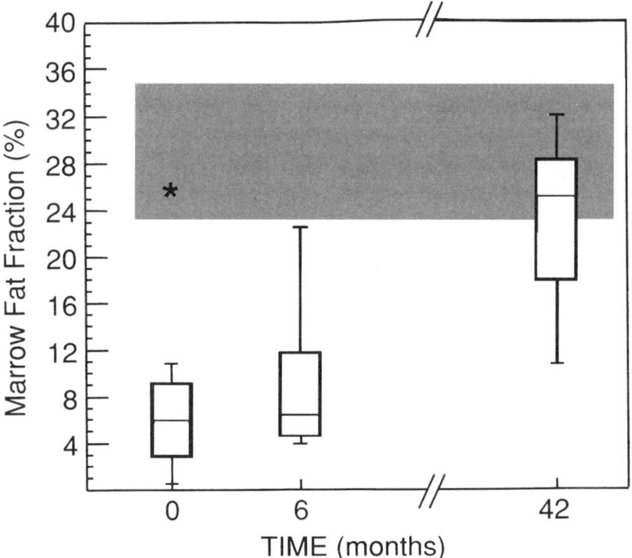

FIGURE 3.—Marrow fat fraction in lumbar spine was measured by quantitative chemical shift imaging. Data are presented as box and whisker plots at time of initial evaluation and after 6 and 42 months of enzyme replacement therapy. *Horizontal line* within each *box* represents median value for data set. The *box* itself depicts inner quartile of values surrounding the mean, and *vertical bars* span range of data. *Asterisk* indicates an outlier. *Shaded area* represents normal range for healthy young adults (29% ± 6%). (Courtesy of Rosenthal DI, Doppelt SH, Mankin HJ, et al: Enzyme replacement therapy for Gaucher disease: Skeletal responses to macrophage-targeted glucocerebrosidase. Reproduced by permission of *Pediatrics*, Vol 96, pp 629–637, Copyright 1995.)

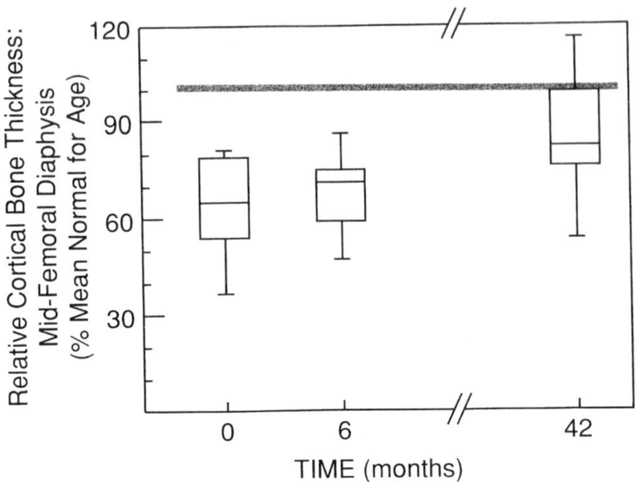

FIGURE 4.—Combined cortical thickness of midfemoral diaphysis was measured and then expressed as a percentage of mean normal value for age. Data are presented as described in Figure 3. *Shaded area* represents a relative value of 100%. (Courtesy of Rosenthal DI, Doppelt SH, Mankin HJ, et al: Enzyme replacement therapy for Gaucher disease: Skeletal responses to macrophage-targeted glucocerebrosidase. Reproduced by permission of *Pediatrics*, Vol 96, pp 629–637, Copyright 1995.)

take, and quantitative chemical shift imaging to estimate the marrow fat fraction. Bone thickness in the spine and lower extremities was determined by dual-energy quantitative CT.

Results.—Serum alkaline phosphatase activity increased significantly in skeletally immature children. Marrow enzyme activity increased substan-

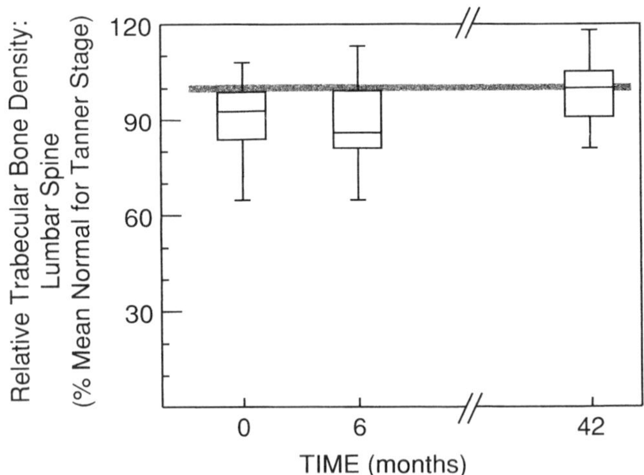

FIGURE 5.—Trabecular bone density of lumbar spine was measured by dual-energy quantitative CT and then expressed as a percentage of the mean normal value for healthy controls of same stage of sexual maturity. Data are presented as described in Figure 3. *Shaded area* represents a relative value of 100%. (Courtesy of Rosenthal DI, Doppelt SH, Mankin HJ, et al: Enzyme replacement therapy for Gaucher disease: Skeletal responses to macrophage-targeted glucocerebrosidase. Reproduced by permission of *Pediatrics*, Vol 96, pp 629–637, Copyright 1995.)

tially over baseline after 6 months of enzyme treatment. Bone mass initially was decreased in all patients in proportion to the overall severity of disease. The marrow fat fraction in the lumbar spine increased slightly after 6 months of treatment but substantially after 42 months of enzyme replacement (Fig 3). Femoral cortical bone thickness also responded significantly after 42 months of treatment (Fig 4). Trabecular bone density in the lumbar spine improved in both children and adults (Fig 5). Five patients had previously had bone marrow infarcts, but no new episodes of acute medullary infarction occurred during treatment. All patients but 1 tolerated the enzyme infusions well.

Conclusion.—Infusion enzyme therapy reverses involvement of the axial and appendicular skeletons in patients with Gaucher's disease, although the response may be delayed. All but 1 of 11 patients studied had a net increase in cortical or trabecular bone mass after 3½ years of enzyme treatment.

▶ Since enzyme replacement was first proposed as a therapeutic option for Gaucher's disease in 1966, the race has been on to initially find an enzyme replacement that was affordable and then to determine which patients with which type of involvement with Gaucher's disease would respond.[1] If one draws the analogy of a marathon to that race, we're probably at about the 22-mile marker with still a little ways to go before the marathon is over. This report brings us a little closer to the finish line.

For some time now, we have known that depending on the dose of enzyme replacement used, one could produce reasonably quick improvements in liver and spleen size and correction of hematologic abnormalities. Early on it was also recognized that there was virtually nothing that could be done about the nervous system involvement in the relatively uncommon type 2 (infantile, acute neuronopathic) and type 3 (juvenile, subacute neuronopathic) variants of Gaucher's disease. Fortunately, in this country, the most common form of Gaucher's disease is type 1 (adult, chronic non-neuronopathic), which is the mildest clinical variant. Type 1 Gaucher's disease is characterized by various degrees of hepatosplenomegaly, anemia, thrombocytopenia, and bone damage, and is defined by sparing of the CNS. The largest population of type 3 is seen among Norbottenian Swedes, whereas type 1 disease is prevalent among those of Ashkenazi Jewish background.

Although type 1 Gaucher's disease is considered mild, it is actually only relatively mild in the sense that affected children and adults can have serious, life-threatening complications. This report shows us one more benefit of enzyme replacement. Until this report appeared, there was little information about whether enzyme replacement could actually improve the skeletal abnormalities so characteristic of Gaucher's disease. Bones have long been known to be less amenable to enzyme replacement therapy, but as this report indicates, prolonged treatment over many years can produce objective reversal of disease in patients with Gaucher's disease.

As has been noted in my commentary for Abstract 3–11, the testy issue regarding enzyme replacement is its cost. A National Institutes of Health consensus conference articulated the many benefits of enzyme replacement but also called for more investigations to determine whether we could find ways to relieve the extraordinary financial burden produced by this disease. Some patients consume in excess of $300,000 per year in financial resources just for enzyme therapy. This is not fair to the individual patient. It's not fair to society. Gaucher's disease is an extremely treatable entity in its most common form. We *must* find affordable, effective ways to manage it.

Reference

1. Brady RO: *N Engl J Med* 275:312, 1966.

Molecular Genetic Analysis in Mild Hyperhomocysteinemia: A Common Mutation in the Methylenetetrahydrofolate Reductase Gene Is a Genetic Risk Factor for Cardiovascular Disease
Kluijtmans LAJ, van den Heuvel LPWJ, Boers GHJ, et al (Univ Hosp Nijmegen, The Netherlands; McGill Univ, Montreal; Municipal Hosp Leyenburg, The Hague, The Netherlands)
Am J Hum Genet 58:35–41, 1996   3–13

Background.—A mild degree of hyperhomocysteinemia is an accepted risk factor for occlusive arterial disease and thrombosis. Classic homocystinuria is accompanied by markedly increased blood homocysteine levels and results from a genetic deficiency of cystathionine β-synthase (CBS). A less common form of severe hyperhomocysteinemia is deficiency of methylenetetrahydrofolate reductase (MTHFR), which helps regulate the folate-dependent remethylation of homocysteine. Studies of 15 unrelated Dutch patients with homozygous CBS deficiency demonstrated the 833T→C mutation in half of alleles. Recently, a common mutation (677C→T; A→V) was identified in the MTHFR gene which, when present in both alleles, is associated with decreased MTHFR activity and increased homocysteine levels.

Objective.—Sixty patients aged 13–68 years with premature cardiovascular disease (myocardial infarction, occlusive cerebral arterial disease, peripheral arterial disease) and 111 control subjects were screened for these mutations.

Findings.—Average fasting and post–methionine-loading homocysteine levels were higher in the patients with premature cardiovascular disease than in control subjects (Table 1). One control subject but none of the patients was heterozygous for 833T→C mutation. Nine of the patients with cardiovascular disease (15%) and approximately 5% of control subjects were homozygous for the 677C→T mutation.

Conclusions.—These findings suggest that a common mutation of the MTHFR gene that produces elevated homocysteine levels is associated with a threefold increase in the risk of premature cardiovascular

TABLE 1.—Fasting and Post–methionine-loading Homocysteine Concentrations in Cardiovascular Disease Patients and Controls

	Cardiovascular Disease Patients	Controls
Fasting homocysteine* (μmol/liter)	14.1 ± 5.1 (n = 58)	12.5 ± 4.0 (n = 111)
Post-methione-loading homocysteine† (μmol/liter)	44.5 ± 18.6 (n = 58)	38.6 ± 13.0 (n = 110)

Note: Results are expressed as mean ± SD.
*Mean difference 1.6 (95% confidence interval (CI), 0.2–3.0).
†Mean difference 5.9 (95% CI, 1.0–10.8).
Abbreviation: CI, confidence interval.
(Courtesy of Kluijtmans LAJ, van den Heuvel LPWJ, Boers GHJ, et al: Molecular genetic analysis in mild hyperhomocysteinemia: A common mutation in the methylenetetrahydrofolate reductase gene is a genetic risk factor for cardiovascular disease. *Am J Hum Genet* 58:35–41, 1996. Published by the University of Chicago.)

disease. There was no evidence that heterozygosity for CBS deficiency is a risk factor.

▶ Twenty years ago, the first reports began to appear linking mild-to-moderate elevations in homocysteine to premature vascular disease in the coronary, cerebral, and peripheral arteries. Most studies to date have concluded that plasma homocysteine is an independent risk factor for cardiovascular disease. Even a modest elevation in homocysteine levels in combination with an elevated serum cholesterol level and elevated blood pressure can have devastating effects.

The report abstracted, although a bit on the heavy-duty side with respect to molecular biology, begins to help us understand which gene mutations that affect homocysteine concentrations are more problematic than others. We as pediatricians should be generally familiar with the overall theories that link homocysteine with early vascular disease.

If you are weak in terms of an organized approach to children in whom you suspect an inborn error of metabolism, see the excellent review of this subject by Lindor et al.[1]

Reference

1. Lindor NM, et al: *Mayo Clin Proc* 70:987, 1995.

Consumption of Soft Drinks With Phosphoric Acid as a Risk Factor for the Development of Hypocalcemia in Children: A Case-control Study

Mazariegos-Ramos E, Guerrero-Romero F, Rodríguez-Morán M, et al (Hosp Gen de Zona No. 1, Durango, Mexico; Hosp de Especialidades Centro Médico Nacional Siglo XXI, Mexico City; Instituto Mexicano del Seguro Social, Mexico City)
J Pediatr 126:940–942, 1995   3–14

Background.—Recent evidence suggests that there is a causal relationship between soft drink consumption and hypocalcemia. Whether consumption of at least 1.5 L of soft drinks with phosphoric acid per week is a risk factor for the development of hypocalcemia in children was studied.

Methods.—Fifty-seven children with serum calcium levels of less than 2.2 mmol/L were compared with 171 children with serum calcium concentrations of 2.2 mmol/L or higher. All of the children and their mothers were interviewed to determine the number of bottles of soft drinks with phosphoric acid consumed per week. Other pertinent information was also elicited (Table).

Findings.—Of the children with low serum calcium levels, 66.7% drank more than 4 bottles of soft drinks per week, compared with only 28% of the children with higher serum calcium levels. Seven percent of the children in the low-calcium group and 0.6% of those in the control group had 1 or more episodes of seizures during the 3 months preceding the interview. Twenty-three percent of the children with low calcium and 5% with normal calcium levels had cramps. Overall, serum calcium levels were significantly, negatively correlated with the number of bottles of soft drinks consumed per week. In 17 children who were followed for 30 days after discontinuation of soft drink consumption, basal serum calcium levels increased from a mean of 2.17 to 2.35 mmol/L, and mean serum phosphorus levels decreased from 1.84 to 1.52 mmol/L.

Conclusions.—Consumption of phosphoric acid–containing soft drinks appears to be strongly associated with hypocalcemia in children. Further research is needed to confirm these findings.

▶ If the data from this report are accurate, those who have been members of the Pepsi generation are growing up to be adults with osteoporosis. Indeed, the leading contenders for this problem are the cola lovers. People who drink 7-Up don't seem to be at significant risk. The status of Dr. Pepper drinkers is not known. The reason is straightforward: certain types of soft drinks contain fairly potent quantities of phosphoric acid. We all know that newborns who are fed formulas with a high phosphate content can have hypocalcemia secondary to the binding of calcium in calcium-phosphate complexes. Apparently, Coca-Cola and Pepsi Cola do the same thing, because the phosphorus content of the former is 19.9 mg/dL whereas that of the latter is 16.1 mg/dL, both being high. Neither of these drinks contains any significant quantities of calcium to offset the effects of the phosphoric acid.

TABLE.—Sex, Age, Number of Bottles of Soft Drinks Consumed Each Week, and Serum Ca, P, and Albumin Concentrations in Case and Control Groups

	Mean ± SD (range)	
	Case	Control
Sex ratio (M/F)*	29/28	87/84
Age (mo)	67.5 ± 29.3 (18–142)	67.5 ± 29.0 (18–142)
Soft drink use (bottles/wk)†	6 ± 8 (0–21)	2 ± 3 (0–9)
Ca (mmol/L; mg/dl)	2.1 ± 0.1 (1.7–2.1); 8.3 ± 0.3 (7.0–8.7)	2.4 ± 0.1 (2.2–2.9); 9.2 ± 0.6 (8.8–11.8)
P (mmol/L; mg/dl)	1.7 ± 0.4 (1.2–3.0); 5.3 ± 1.3 (3.6–9.4)	1.6 ± 0.3 (0.7–2.6); 5.0 ± 1.0 (2.3–7.9)
Albumin (pmol/L; gm/dl)	517 ± 57 (356–620); 4.5 ± 0.5 (3.1–5.4)	528 ± 35 (4.14–666); 4.6 ± 0.3 (3.6– 5.8)

Abbreviations: Ca, calcium; *P*, phosphorus.
*Values expressed as ratio, not as mean ± SD and range.
†Values shown are median (instead of mean) and inner quartile range (instead of SD); case is significantly different from control group (*P* < 0.001, Mann-Whitney U test).
(Courtesy of Mazariegos-Ramos E, Guerrero-Romero F, Rodriguez-Morán M, et al: Consumption of soft drinks with phosphoric acid as a risk factor for the development of hypocalcemia in children: A case-control study. *J Pediatr* 126:940–942, 1995.)

The United States is ranked first among countries with the highest soft drink consumption. The children reported in the abstract are from Mexico, which ranks second in the consumption of soft drinks (142 L/yr). In addition to potentially reducing your calcium levels, this class of soft drinks can also cause enamel erosion, urinary tract stones, and peptic ulcer disease. One wonders what happened to old-fashioned lemonade.

Fruit and Vegetable Intakes of Children and Adolescents in the United States

Krebs-Smith SM, Cook DA, Subar AF, et al (Natl Cancer Inst, Bethesda, Md; US Dept of Agriculture, Riverdale, Md; Management Services Inc, Silver Spring, Md)

Arch Pediatr Adolesc Med 150:81–86, 1996
3–15

Purpose.—Increasing Americans' consumption of fruits and vegetables, and thus of complex carbohydrates and fiber, is a major national health goal. Children who eat a lot of fruits and vegetables are likely to continue to do so as adults, but there are no data on consumption of these foods by

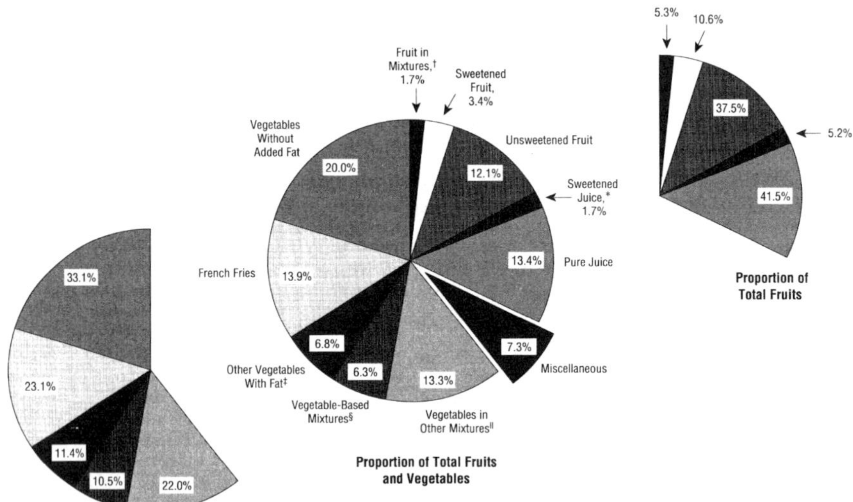

FIGURE.—Ways fruits and vegetables are consumed by children shown as a proportion of total fruits and vegetables and again as a proportion of either total fruits or of total vegetables. The *asterisk* indicates the pure juice contained in sweetened juices and juice-flavored drinks; *dagger,* the fruit in fruit salads, breads, and cereals; *double dagger,* raw and cooked vegetables, other than french-fried potatoes, prepared with butter, margarine, or salad dressing; *section mark,* vegetables contained in mixtures that are mainly vegetables but include other added ingredients, such as cheese sauce; and *parallel symbol,* vegetables contained in meat- and grain-based mixtures, such as stews, soups, pizza, and sandwiches. (Courtesy of Krebs-Smith SM, Cook DA, Subar AF, et al: Fruit and vegetable intakes of children and adolescents in the United States. *Arch Pediatr Adolesc Med* 150:81–86, Copyright 1996, American Medical Association.)

TABLE 2.—Mean Number of Servings of Fruit and Vegetable Subgroups* by Sociodemographic Group Compared With Recommendations†

Mean (SE) No. of Servings per Day

Sociodemographic Group	Citrus, Melon, and Berries	Other Fruit	Green/Yellow Vegetables	Starchy Vegetables‡	Other Vegetables§	All Fruits and Vegetables Excluding Miscellaneous
Recommendations‖	≥1	≥1	≥1	≥1	≥1	5–9
All persons aged						
2–18 y	0.5 (0.03)	0.7 (0.04)	0.2 (0.02)	1.3 (0.04)	0.9 (0.04)	3.6 (0.10)
Age, y						
Males						
2–5	0.6 (0.07)	0.9 (0.09)	0.2 (0.02)	1.0 (0.07)	0.6 (0.04)	3.3 (0.15)
6–11	0.5 (0.04)	0.7 (0.06)	0.2 (0.02)	1.2 (0.08)	0.8 (0.04)	3.4 (0.13)
12–18	0.6 (0.05)	0.5 (0.05)	0.2 (0.03)	1.8 (0.12)	1.2 (0.07)	4.3 (0.20)
Females						
2–5	0.6 (0.07)	1.0 (0.09)	0.2 (0.03)	1.1 (0.08)	0.7 (0.04)	3.6 (0.18)
6–11	0.4 (0.05)	0.9 (0.08)	0.2 (0.03)	1.2 (0.08)	0.8 (0.06)	3.5 (0.18)
12–18	0.5 (0.05)	0.4 (0.05)	0.2 (0.03)	1.2 (0.07)	1.1 (0.08)	3.5 (0.18)
Race/ethnicity						
Non-Hispanic white	0.5 (0.04)	0.8 (0.04)	0.2 (0.02)	1.2 (0.05)	0.9 (0.04)	3.6 (0.11)
Non-Hispanic black	0.5 (0.06)	0.6 (0.08)	0.3 (0.05)	1.5 (0.15)	0.8 (0.11)	3.7 (0.32)
Hispanic	0.6 (0.07)	0.6 (0.12)	0.1 (0.02)	1.2 (0.13)	0.9 (0.10)	3.3 (0.26)
Other	0.9 (0.20)	1.0 (0.14)	0.3 (0.07)	1.1 (0.26)	1.1 (0.12)	4.3 (0.29)
Household income, $						
<10,000	0.4 (0.04)	0.6 (0.04)	0.1 (0.01)	1.4 (0.11)	0.8 (0.05)	3.4 (0.14)
10,000–29,999	0.5 (0.04)	0.7 (0.06)	0.2 (0.02)	1.3 (0.05)	0.9 (0.06)	3.5 (0.14)
30,000–50,000	0.5 (0.04)	0.8 (0.06)	0.2 (0.03)	1.3 (0.07)	0.9 (0.05)	3.6 (0.15)
>50,000	0.7 (0.07)	0.8 (0.08)	0.2 (0.04)	1.2 (0.11)	1.0 (0.10)	3.8 (0.23)

*Excluding miscellaneous fruits and vegetables eaten as part of potato chips, condiments, and candy.
†From the 1989–1991 Continuing Survey of Food Intakes by Individuals. Data are based on 3 days of dietary intake.
‡Starchy vegetables include white potatoes, dried beans and green peas, and corn.
§Other vegetables include tomatoes, lettuce, green beans, cucumbers, onions, cabbage, and peppers.
‖From *The Food Guide Pyramid* and supporting documentation.
(Courtesy of Krebs-Smith SM, Cook DA, Subar AF, et al: Fruit and vegetable intakes of children and adolescents in the United States. *Arch Pediatr Adolesc Med* 150:81–86, Copyright 1996, American Medical Association.)

children. The fruit and vegetable intake of children in the United States, including the ways in which those foods are consumed, was studied.

Methods.—Data were drawn from the U.S. Department of Agriculture's 1989–91 Continuing Survey of Food Intakes by Individuals. The analysis included 3-day dietary information from 3,148 children and adolescents in the United States. The fruits and vegetables eaten were quantified according to a system for disaggregating mixed foods and regrouping their ingredients, and the fruit and vegetable ingredients were weighted to convert quantities to number of servings. The ways in which foods were used, e.g., with or without fat or sugar, were evaluated as well. The analysis sought to identify the forms in which children consume fruits and vegetables, how well their intakes corresponded with recommendations, and what percentage of children met the recommendations.

Results.—Fruit and fruit juices accounted for about one third of total fruit and vegetable intake. About one third of vegetables consumed were prepared with fat, about one third without fat, and the rest as part of a mixture. French-fried potatoes made up nearly one fourth of all vegetables consumed (Fig). The mean number of servings of fruits and vegetables fell well short of current recommendations. Intake was particularly low for citrus, melon, and berries and for dark green and/or dark yellow vegetables. Just 1 in 5 children consumed at least 5 servings of fruits and vegetables per day. Children from higher income families were more likely to consume the recommended number of servings of fruits and vegetables (Table 2).

Conclusions.—The fruit and vegetable intakes of American children and adolescents appear to fall well below recommended levels. Many children consume less than 1 serving of fruit per day, and french fries make up a major portion of their vegetable intake. Children and adolescents should be encouraged to eat more fruits and vegetables, particularly fruits and dark green and/or dark yellow vegetables. The pediatrician can play a key role in encouraging healthier eating by children.

▶ There are probably no surprises in this article for most of us. The slip that has occurred over the years in our children's consumption of fruits and vegetables is merely a reflection of the casualness with which most families dine these days. All too frequently, Thanksgiving dinner is a Quarter Pounder with fries and a large Coke. Add to this the fact that kids have keys to the family car, which can get them to the local fast-food restaurant, and you see the magnitude of the problem.

The Public Health Service (PHS) has recognized the extent of the dietary indiscretion on the part of our teenagers. At the beginning of this decade, it published a report, "Healthy People 2000: The National Health Promotion and Disease Prevention Objectives."[1] In that report, the PHS noted that diets that are abundant in fruits and vegetables are associated with a decreased risk of cancer of the colon, breast, lung, oral cavity, larynx, esophagus, stomach, bladder, uterine cervix, and pancreas. A habit of eating lots of fruits and vegetables, begun during childhood, is a significant positive predictor of fruit and vegetable intake during adulthood. This makes decent eating a social imperative for children. One of the PHS's health objectives for the year 2000 is to "increase complex carbohydrate and fiber-containing foods in the diets of adults to five or more servings for vegetables (including legumes) and fruits." Although this guideline does not specify children and adolescents, the background behind the guidelines concludes that it is "prudent for children age 2 years and older and adolescents to progress toward this kind of dietary pattern as well."

The value of this report is fairly straightforward. It provides baseline data on fruit and vegetable intakes of children, which can be used for comparison purposes during the next decade. Currently a large percentage of our children and teenagers are consuming less than 1 serving of fruit per day and also need to eat more vegetables, including dark green and/or yellow ones. Our school cafeterias aren't doing a much better job with influencing diet either. Overall, the only reasonably healthy eaters of diverse foods including fresh fruits and vegetables are Asian Americans and Native Americans.

This report explains why most children will not finish their dinner if that dinner includes a few servings of vegetables preceded or followed by fresh fruit. To the average youngster, a yellow vegetable is a golden fry from McDonald's or, its southern analogue, a hush-puppy. The closest green vegetable is a jalapeño on a Taco Bell special. The teenage red vegetable of choice, of course, is tomato paste smeared on a pizza. Each of these vittles is close, but no cigar, when it comes to the definition of healthy eating.

Reference

1. U.S. Department of Health and Human Services, Public Health Service. U.S. Department of Health Services Publication PHS 91-50212, September 1990.

Outcomes of a Field Trial to Improve Children's Dietary Patterns and Physical Activity: The Child and Adolescent Trial for Cardiovascular Health (CATCH)
Luepker RV, for the CATCH Collaborative Group (Univ of Minnesota, Minneapolis; New England Research Insts, Watertown, Mass; Univ of California, San Diego, La Jolla; et al)
JAMA 275:768–776, 1996   3–16

Background.—Schools are ideal sites for preventive health programs. The Child and Adolescent Trial for Cardiovascular Health (CATCH), designed to augment the research of the 1980s in cardiovascular disease (CVD) prevention, involved many schools, a multicomponent behavioral health intervention in 3 grades, and children from diverse communities. The major outcomes from the CATCH interventions were reported.

Methods.—A total of 5,106 third-graders from ethnically diverse backgrounds in public schools in California, Louisiana, Minnesota, and Texas were initially enrolled in the study. Interventions were performed at 56 elementary schools, consisting of food service modifications, enhanced physical education (PE), and classroom health curricula at 28 elementary schools, and these interventions plus family education were initiated at the other 28. Forty elementary schools served as controls.

Findings.—At intervention schools, the percentage of energy intake from fat dropped significantly from 38.7% to 31.9% compared with control schools. The intensity of physical activity in PE classes during the CATCH intervention increased significantly at the schools with the intervention compared with those without it. Self-reported daily energy intake from fat among students in the intervention schools declined from 32.7% to 30.3%, significantly different from the reduction of 32.6% to 32.2% in the control schools. Students at the intervention schools also reported significantly more daily vigorous activity than those in control schools. The groups did not differ significantly in blood pressure, body size, or cholesterol levels. The interventions produced no apparent deleterious effects on growth or development.

Conclusions.—The CATCH intervention provides an important model of a school-based health promotion program for the primary prevention of CVD. Through CATCH interventions, the fat content of school lunches was reduced, moderate-to-vigorous physical activity in PE was increased, and eating and physical activity behaviors were modified in children during the third, fourth, and fifth grades.

▶ The CATCH intervention has been successful in meeting several of its goals through the years. At the school level, cafeterias have been able to significantly modify their lunch offerings to approach the national recommendations of a 30% total fat energy intake and a 10% saturated fat energy intake, with much of the reduction coming from saturated fats. Also, the percentage of physical education time devoted to serious exercise has significantly increased. At the individual level, however, the decreases in serum cholesterol levels among students in intervention schools, compared with control students, are not terribly significant.

The results of the CATCH intervention, as reported in this study, lead to several interpretations and recommendations. The CATCH intervention does demonstrate that the policies and practices of schools can be changed without the investment of substantial new resources in terms of school budgets. The changes observed positively affect behaviors and meet national recommendations. These changes, when spread across the entire school-based population, have the potential to produce long-term cardiovascular health benefits. Such benefits can be obtained with minimal training of existing school personnel and only modest follow-up support from other individuals.

As readers of the YEAR BOOK OF PEDIATRICS probably know, this editor is not very enamored by exercise. Exercise can be a waste of the finite number of heartbeats we are born with. This philosophy is not incompatible with the recognized need for youngsters to exercise. Such healthy youngsters will grow up to be healthy adults who, by the time they hit later midlife can enter into "couch potato-ism" with the confidence that they have already achieved extra credit early in life.

4 Allergy and Dermatology

What's New in Pediatric Dermatology?

DANIEL P. KROWCHUK, M.D.
Departments of Pediatrics and Dermatology, Bowman Gray School of Medicine, Winston-Salem, North Carolina

WALTER W. TUNNESSEN, JR., M.D.
Senior Vice-President, The American Board of Pediatrics, Chapel Hill, North Carolina

The Society for Pediatric Dermatology conducted its annual meeting in August 1996. A few highlights of the presentation are abstracted for your interest.

Line Dancing

In 1901, Blaschko presented his collection of distribution patterns of linear skin disorders. These lines, which differ from dermatomes or Langer's lines of cleavage, seem to play true in a number of skin disorders of children. They most likely represent the result of two different clones of cells present early in embryogenesis. Blaschko's lines have received considerable attention in the delineation of a number of disorders primarily involving the skin and, particularly, a number involving lines of hyperpigmentation and hypopigmentation. Over the years, there has been much ado about the significance of these pigmentary abnormalities, especially regarding their association with underlying systemic problems.

Two talks, both from New York University, addressed pigmentary abnormalities following the lines of Blaschko and their association with systemic abnormalities. To investigate whether an association exists between these cutaneous findings and underlying abnormalities, the resident research award recipient, Dr. Kishwer Nehal, reviewed the medical records of 54 children referred to a pediatric dermatology practice with segmental, linear, or swirled hyperpigmentation and/or hypopigmentation following the lines of Blaschko. The literature reports a high association (79% to 94%) of systemic abnormalities in children diagnosed as having a syndrome known as hypomelanosis of Ito, characterized by hypopigmented swirls. A second disorder, descriptively called linear and whorled nevoid hypermelanosis, which as opposed to hypomelanosis of Ito has hyperpigmented swirls and lines, has also been touted to be associated with extra-cutaneous abnormalities, but no large series has been investigated. Nevus depigmentosus, characterized by circumscribed areas of hypopigmentation, has been reported to have similar neurologic and skeletal disorders.

Like a number of associations in the past, many think that the literature has perpetuated the myth of the association of pigmentary changes with systemic abnormalities. Cases tend to be referred and reported that substantiate the literature, and the myth builds. Dr. Nehal's survey supported the charge of overrepresentation of systemic abnormalities with these cutaneous changes. Rather than 79% to 94% of children with hypomelanosis of Ito having systemic abnormalities, only 33% (9 of 27) did. In linear and whorled nevoid hypermelanosis 31% (4 of 13) and in nevus depigmentosus 11% (1 of 9) had systemic findings that were mainly neurologic.

In pediatric practice, it is even more likely that these associations are less prevalent. Normal infants and children are not always referred to pediatric dermatology centers if they have pigmentary disorders. They are more likely to be referred if they have neurologic or skeletal abnormalities in association with the cutaneous changes. Do these infants and children need to have extensive and expensive testing if they have pigmentary changes along the lines of Blaschko? It appears not. Dr. Nehal and her co-investigators found that all systemic abnormalities had been discovered before referral, and, in follow-up ranging from 6 to 42 months, no new abnormalities were found.

These pigmentary changes do not appear to be specific, but rather they represent a collection of heterogeneous disorders. If a child appears normal, physically and developmentally, extensive evaluation does not need to be performed. Do not apply appellations with the potential for misinterpretation. Merely describe what you see and follow the infant or child prospectively. This is particularly true of hypomelanosis of Ito, which has caught the fancy of many. The presence of swirled hypopigmentation should not call forth this diagnosis unless systemic abnormalities are present. There is no need to alarm parents with this name.

Dr. Seth Orlow, Dr. Nehal's pediatric dermatology mentor, reported on disorders with segmental hyperpigmentation. He emphasized again that these pigmentary disorders are much more common than reported, particularly linear and whorled nevoid hypermelanosis, if one chooses to use that term. Like other lesions that follow the lines of Blaschko, these pigmentary changes are signs of cutaneous mosaicism. He noted that incontinentia pigmenti, an X-linked disorder that is lethal in males, with a high percentage of systemic abnormalities, has as its third stage swirled hyperpigmentation. Dr. Orlow stated that this diagnosis can be separated from other swirled pigmentary disorders by the color. In incontinentia pigmenti, the swirls are grayish brown rather than brownish as found, for instance, in linear and whorled nevoid hypermelanosis. He also noted that epidermal nevi may begin as macular areas of pigmentation before they become raised.

Dr. Orlow also discussed another entity that should be recognized by pediatricians called Becker's melanosis. Most of these brown patches with jagged borders develop at puberty, although they can be congenital. They are most common on the shoulders, chest, flank, or thigh, and about 50% become hairy. Associated abnormalities are uncommon. In acquired lesions, males are affected 6 times as frequently as females. The lesions are benign, do not represent a risk for cutaneous cancer, and have no effective therapy. Look for them in your adolescent patients because they are not uncommon.

Ring Around the Collar

Most pediatricians are familiar with the entity known as acanthosis nigricans (AN). It seems to be an increasingly recognized and written about disorder and, perhaps with the increasing incidence of obesity in the United States, more frequent in occurrence. It can be found in 7.1% of unselected populations. There is a higher prevalence in black, Latino, and white populations.

Acanthosis nigricans is characterized by velvety, rugated, hyperpigmented hypertrophy of skin affecting primarily flexural areas, particularly the neck, groin, axillae, and skin under the breasts. Various classifications of AN have been proposed. The most common association, by far, is with obesity. Dr. Lawrence Eichenfield of the University of California at San Diego reviewed the systemic disorders associated with AN as a lead-in to a report on his study of children referred to an endocrine clinic for obesity. Some interesting findings were teased out. Obese children with AN had higher insulin levels, higher hemoglobin A_1C levels, higher serum triglycerides, and lower high-density lipoprotein levels than obese children without AN. There was a significant trend toward increased severity of AN and fasting insulin levels, body mass index (weight/height), and hemoglobin A_1C levels. The higher these findings, the more severe the AN.

It appears that AN follows the obesity, but its presence should be a red flag for adult disorders, including coronary artery disease, hypertension, lipid disorders, type II diabetes mellitus, and polycystic ovary disease in women. Examine your patients for AN and keep your eye on the literature for future associations and reports. Insulin resistance seems to be a marker for a number of problems. If we could only find a good way to effectively and reliably help our patients to lose weight!

Kawasaki Syndrome: Searching for a Cause

Dr. Cody Meissner, Associate Professor of Pediatrics and Chief of Pediatric Infectious Diseases at Tufts University School of Medicine, provided an update on Kawasaki syndrome (KS) with an emphasis on its possible etiology. As many readers are aware, KS has surpassed acute rheumatic fever as the leading cause of acquired heart disease among children. Dr. Meissner observes that 4 lines of evidence support an infectious cause: the syndrome is acute and self-limited, there is geographic clustering of cases, the age distribution is similar to that of other childhood infections, and the symptoms are characteristic of an infectious disease. The failure to identify a responsible organism and the apparent lack of person-to-person transmission, however, argue against this hypothesis. Immunologic abnormalities, including increased numbers of CD4 T lymphocytes and decreased numbers of CD8 T cells, polyclonal B-cell activation, increased cytokine production, and the formation of antibody directed against endothelial cells, are commonly observed in KS and offer yet another etiologic explanation.

One way in which the evidence supporting the role of infection and immunologic dysfunction in causing KS can be linked is through superantigens, a class of proteins that, unlike conventional antigens, are able to stimulate a large proportion of circulating T lymphocytes. Dr. Meissner believes that the vasculitic changes characteristic of KS may result when there is mucosal colonization by *Staphylococcus aureus* that is capable of producing superantigens. In the absence of neutralizing antibodies, these superantigens cause immune activation and cytokine production. New antigenic molecules are expressed on endothelial cells, resulting in leukocyte infiltration and subsequent vascular injury. Although this unifying hypothesis remains to be proven, it offers an intriguing explanation for the cause of this perplexing syndrome.

The Skin and Child Abuse

As pediatricians are aware, the skin may offer valuable clues to a child's having been physically or sexually abused. Dr. Bernard Cohen, Associate Professor of Pediatrics and Dermatology at Johns Hopkins University, reviewed the subject of child abuse from the dermatologic perspective. Of particular interest were Dr. Cohen's observations about primary cutaneous disorders that may mimic abuse. For example, Schönlein-Henoch purpura, idiopathic thrombocytopenic purpura, macular hemangiomas, and mongolian spots all may be confused with bruising resulting from physical abuse. Insect bites, especially those that blister, bullous impetigo, or immune bullous disorders produce lesions that mimic cigarette burns. At times, the erosions seen in staphylococcal scalded skin syndrome or immunologically mediated blistering disorders may be confused with scald burns. In the genital area, lichen sclerosus et atrophicus, linear IgA dermatosis, or bullous pemphigoid may produce blisters or erosions that may be erroneously interpreted as signs of sexual abuse.

An issue of some controversy is whether the presence of genital warts indicates that sexual abuse has occurred. Research performed by Dr. Cohen and his colleagues suggests that the majority of children with these lesions apparently have not been victims of abuse, although this possibility must always be entertained. Dr. Cohen believes that nonvenereal modes of transmission may be considered when there is no associated evidence of sexual abuse, the child is younger than 3 years of age, warts are present in caretakers, or the child has extragenital warts.

You're Gonna Need an Ocean of Calamine Lotion

Poison ivy and related plants are well-known causes of allergic contact dermatitis in children and adolescents, but many primary care providers are unaware that a host of other agents may produce this condition. William Weston, M.D., Professor and Chairman of the Department of Dermatology of the University of Colorado School of Medicine, attempted to dispel the myths that have led to this misunderstanding.

* The myth about new exposures: Asking what new products (e.g., soaps, etc.) have been used is useful only if one is seeking a cause for urticaria. With the exception of plant dermatitis, in contact allergy the problem results from prolonged exposure to weak antigens that eventually, not acutely, sensitize the patient.

* The myth of immunologic immaturity: In contrast to what is often taught, newborns and young infants can be sensitized to allergens, and lymphocyte proliferation is excellent. For 15 of the most common contact allergens, the majority of children are sensitized by age 5 years.

* The myth of limited exposure of infants to contact allergens: Many clinicians believe that sensitization does not occur early in life because infants are not exposed to contact allergens. In fact, infants are exposed to a variety of common sensitizers, including nickel (present in earrings), preservatives (contained in many infant care products), and topical antibiotics (e.g., neomycin present in topical preparations).

* The myth that infants may be allergic to disposable diapers: The cotton, superabsorbent gelling material, and cellulose contained in disposable diapers are inert and do not sensitize infants.

* The myth that the use of "baby" products protects against the development of contact allergy: Many infant care products, including shampoos, conditioners, and soaps, contain preservatives (e.g., thimerosal, formaldehyde, benzalkonium, and Kathon CG) that may cause contact sensitivity.

* The myth that children with atopic dermatitis (AD) are more likely than others to experience contact dermatitis: Studies suggest that children with atopic dermatitis are no more likely than their unaffected counterparts to have allergic contact dermatitis develop.

Dr. Weston then reviewed some of the most common agents producing contact dermatitis in infants and children. Neomycin is present in a variety of first-aid creams and ophthalmologic and otic antibiotic preparations. By age 5 years, 7% of children have developed a sensitivity to neomycin and, because of cross-reactivity, often will be sensitive to gentamicin or tobramycin. The common practice of combining neomycin with other agents may cause sensitization to an antibiotic that otherwise would not occur;

such is the case with bacitracin. Contact sensitization to silver sulfadiazine, mupirocin, or erythromycin, however, has not been reported in children and is rare in adults.

Shoe dermatitis is caused by chemicals used to prevent rubber from breaking down or by leather tanning agents such as potassium dichromate. Although uncommon in children, shoe dermatitis involves the dorsum and, occasionally, the lateral aspects of the forefoot and toes but spares the instep. If a child is allergic to potassium dichromate, leather-free shoes, of which many varieties exist, can be recommended. If the culprit is a rubber allergy, rubber-free shoes are harder to find, although Birkenstock's, leather moccasins, plastic jellies, and some tennis shoes manufactured by Puma or Nike are satisfactory alternatives.

Allergies to formaldehyde or formaldehyde releasers (e.g., Quarternium 15 [Dowicil 200, 100, 50], Bronopol, DMDM hydantoin, Kathon CG [MCI/MI], and imidazolinyl urea) are on the rise. These agents are preservatives that, as noted previously, are incorporated into a host of lotions, over-the-counter corticosteriods and antifungals, and sunscreens used by children. If you believe that a child may be allergic to a sunscreen, however, it may not be the preservative. Remember that a photocontact allergy may result from the active screening agent (e.g., octyl methyl PABA, benzophenones or dibenzylmethones).

For children with a long-standing dermatitis, Dr. Weston notes that patch testing and allergen avoidance can be quite valuable in reducing the disease duration, activity, and severity.

The Itch That Rashes

Atopic dermatitis affects approximately 4% of children and is characterized by a recurrent, pruritic eruption. John Harper, M.D., F.R.C.P., Consultant in Pediatric Dermatology at the Great Ormond Street Hospital for Sick Children in London, provided an update on this affliction. Approximately 70% of children with AD have a family history of atopy, and studies of identical twins reveal a concordance rate of more than 50%. Recent investigations suggest a link between atopy, specifically asthma and allergic rhinitis, and chromosome 11q13, and a potential locus for atopy has been found on this chromosome. Other chromosomal loci that may have an impact on atopy have also been identified. In addition, it appears that maternal influences on the inheritance of an atopic tendency are particularly important.

Patients with AD are more likely than normal individuals to be colonized with *S. aureus* at affected and normal skin sites. Dr. Harper explains that this may be the result of increased adherence of the organism to the skin and mucous membranes of those with AD. The role of *S. aureus* in AD can be inferred from the clinical improvement that often follows antibiotic therapy. From the standpoint of pathogenesis, it is intriguing that certain *S. aureus* phage types found on the skin of individuals with AD are toxin-producing organisms that can act as superantigens. These antigens, in turn, may induce immune activation that leads to the development of symptoms.

Dr. Harper reviewed two forms of therapy that have received considerable attention in Europe. In the United Kingdom, cyclosporin is licensed to treat atopic dermatitis in adults. Preliminary studies in children with severe disease reveal that the drug is effective, safe, and well tolerated in short-term use, and that the severity of recurrences after discontinuation of the drug is less than expected. Although this is encouraging information, cyclosporin has the potential for causing serious toxicity and careful monitoring is required. Traditional Chinese medical practitioners often prescribe a tea, composed of 10–12 plants, to treat AD in children. Although the exact mechanism of action has not been defined, the plants have been found to contain chemicals that possess anti-inflammatory, sedative, and antimicrobial effects (sound familiar?...corticosteroids, antihistamines, antibiotics). A number of studies have demonstrated a potential benefit of these preparations, although some concern exists about potential hepatotoxicity. Dr. Harper reports that a freeze-dried product of a specific formulation of plant materials has been undergoing clinical trials.

Hormones: All Things in Moderation

Acne is a multifactorial disorder that reflects the combined influences of infection, abnormal keratinization, immunologic activity, and hormones. Dr. Anne Lucky, Adjunct Professor of Dermatology at the University of Cincinnati College of Medicine, discussed the endocrine aspects of acne and hirsutism in young women and the hormonal treatment of these related conditions. Androgens play a central role in the production of acne lesions, changing the way epithelial cells are shed from pilosebaceous follicles and increasing sebum production, both of which contribute to obstruction and the creation of acne lesions. There are 3 sources of androgens in women: the ovaries, the adrenals, and the skin. Normally, the ovaries contribute approximately 50% of circulating androgens. Ovarian tumors or the polycystic ovary syndrome, however, may produce excessive androgens resulting in hirsutism or unusually troublesome acne. The adrenal glands contribute the remaining 50% of androgens, although age is a determinant of glandular activity. Interestingly, the neonatal adrenals secrete androgens at levels typically seen during puberty, thus explaining the transient appearance of acne in infants. From the age of 1 year until approximately 6–8 years, the time of adrenarche, the glands produce low levels of these hormones. With adrenarche, adrenal androgen production rises and acne lesions begin to appear. The skin's role in androgen metabolism relates to its ability to convert relatively nonandrogenic precursors to more potent agents that exert a local effect.

In view of the impact that androgens have in causing acne, it seems logical to ask whether patients with acne have elevated levels of these hormones. As it turns out, there is no simple correlation between androgen levels and acne severity. Recent work by Dr. Lucky and her colleagues suggests, however, that dehydroepiandrosterone sulfate (DHEAS) levels, although within the normal range, are higher in girls with acne than in those without lesions. When is an endocrine evaluation warranted in a patient with acne? Dr. Lucky suggests that a measurement of free testosterone, DHEAS, follicle-stimulating hormone, and luteinizing hormone levels be obtained when children are seen with acne before the age of 8 or 9 years, when acne does not improve with standard therapies, or when acne has its onset or persists into the late teens or early twenties. A primary reason for performing these tests is to identify an adrenal or ovarian tumor that is secreting high levels of androgens. The possibility of polycystic ovary disease is suggested by a luteinizing hormone:follicle-stimulating hormone ratio of greater than 3.

Dr. Lucky notes that hormonal treatment of acne may be beneficial, although conventional therapies should be used initially. Combined oral contraceptives are often used adjunctively because the estrogen increases sex hormone–binding globulin levels, thereby reducing the level of free testosterone, and suppresses ovarian androgen production. As an aside, Dr. Lucky reminds clinicians that not all contraceptive agents offer such benefits. The progestins contained in Norplant and Depo Provera, for example, are quite androgenic and may worsen acne or cause hirsutism or male pattern alopecia. In contrast, desogestrel, gestodene, and norgestimate—the progestins contained in "newer" oral contraceptives—have minimal androgenic effect.

Review of Prescribed Treatment for Children With Asthma in 1990

Warner JO (Univ of Southampton, England)
BMJ 311:663–666, 1995   4–1

Background.—An international pediatric asthma consensus group published guidelines for the management of childhood asthma in 1989, which sought to enable affected children to participate in sports, reduce school absence, prevent daytime and nighttime symptoms, normalize lung function and reduce diurnal variation, and prevent exacerbations. The guidelines recommended preventive treatment to reduce the need for β-agonists and other bronchodilators. Treatment practices in Great Britain during the 12 months after publication of the guidelines were studied to assess the impact of the guidelines on prescription patterns and to evaluate the effectiveness of asthma control with guideline compliance.

Methods.—Prescribing data for 1990 were gathered from 398 general practices and from some practices for the first 6 months of 1991. Treatment for asthma was prescribed for 9.6% of the children between the ages of 4 and 17 years. A subgroup of children who were regularly using preventive treatment was defined as those prescribed at least 6 corticosteroid inhalers or at least 9 sodium cromoglycate inhalers during 1990. The use of bronchodilators was examined in this subgroup and compared with their use in the group as a whole.

Results.—In the study group of 17,846 children who received asthma treatment, 52.5% were prescribed preventive treatment, 90.8% were given bronchodilators, and 9.3% were given oral steroids (Figure). Of the

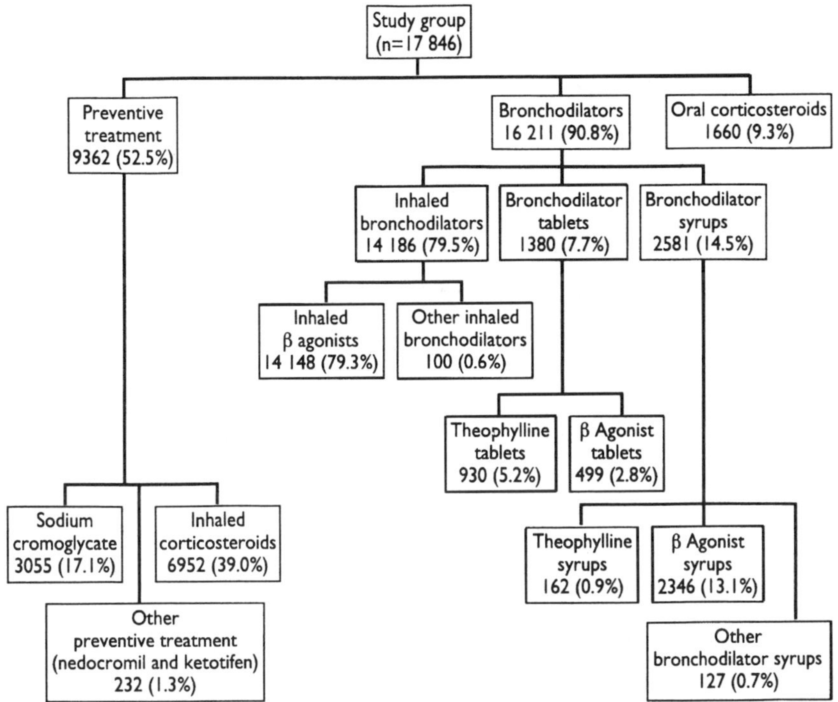

FIGURE.—Numbers (percentages) of children aged 4–17 years receiving at least 1 presciption for asthma treatment from January to December 1990. (Courtesy of Warner JO: Review of prescribed treatment for children with asthma in 1990. *BMJ* 311:663–666, 1995.)

preventive treatments, 17.1% of the patients were given sodium cromoglycate and 39% were given inhaled steroids. During the study period, the proportion of patients receiving sodium cromoglycate decreased and the proportion receiving inhaled steroids increased significantly. The rate of prescription repetition suggested consistent prophylaxis in only 14.5% of the children receiving asthma treatment, including 15.3% of those taking inhaled steroids and 6.1% of those taking sodium cromoglycate. There were no significant differences between the group regularly using preventive treatment and the rest of the patients in the amount of salbutamol prescribed. Salbutamol prescription also did not vary with the type of preventive treatment prescribed.

Conclusions.—Almost 10% of the children between the ages of 4 and 17 years were given treatment for asthma in 1990. Although about half of these children were prescribed preventive treatment, only about 15% demonstrated compliance. However, compliance with preventive therapy was not associated with a reduced need for bronchodilator therapy.

▶ If there is any medical entity that benefits from having a treatment protocol in hand, it is asthma in children. There are many such protocols around. In 1989, guidelines for the management of childhood asthma were published by an international pediatric asthma consensus group.[1] When these European guidelines were published, they were used subsequently in many countries around the world as a basis for management protocols, and they were widely publicized and distributed to pediatric practitioners in Great Britain. They were revised a second time in 1992 with the intent to enable children (1) to participate in normal activities during sports; (2) to avoid excessive absence from school; (3) to be free of symptoms during the day and night; (4) to have normal lung function with no excess diurnal variation; and (5) to have fewer exacerbations of asthma.[2]

The National Heart and Lung Institute's International Statement on Asthma is very similar to the European statement.[3] After several years of the availability of these kinds of protocols, what Dr. Warner (the author of the study abstracted as well as the senior author of the first European consensus conference statement) has done is to see how well these protocols are working. He finds that nearly 10% of all children in Great Britain continue to receive prescriptions for the treatment of asthma. Only about 15% of these children were totally compliant with their treatment protocol. Worse yet, the use of regular preventive treatment was not found to be associated with a reduced use of short-acting inhaled β-agonists. Time for a similar, well-constructed study on our shores.

So much for the treatment of asthma. As far as prognosis is concerned, at least for acute attacks, look to the blood eosinophil count. The child with a low eosinophil count in the presence of an acute attack of asthma is more likely to experience a severe episode of reactive airway disease. Why this happens isn't entirely known, but presumably in a severe asthma attack, eosinophils will sequester in the lungs. A very significantly positive correlation has been documented between a decrease in the eosinophil count and a decrease in arterial oxygen tension. Exactly how eosinophils are recruited into the lung structure in bronchial asthma is not known, but once there, these cells produce intense inflammation and damage, as was shown recently by Spallarossa et al.[4]

References

1. Warner JO, et al: *Arch Dis Child* 64:1065, 1989.
2. Editorial comment. *Arch Dis Child* 67:240, 1992.
3. Editorial comment. *Clin Exp Allergy* 22:1S, 1992
4. Spallarossa D, et al: *Arch Dis Child* 73:333, 1995.

Theophylline in Acute Childhood Asthma: A Meta-analysis of Its Efficacy

Goodman DC, Littenberg B, O'Connor GT, et al (Dartmouth Med School, Hanover, NH)
Pediatr Pulmonol 21:211–218, 1996   4–2

Background.—Theophylline has been widely used for treating children with acute and chronic asthma, although few randomized clinical studies

TABLE 3.—Pooled Results From 4 Studies Comparing the Effect of Theophylline With Placebo in Acute Childhood Asthma

Measure	Degrees of freedom	Test of homogeneity (χ^2)	Mean effect difference*	Pooled effect size† (95% confidence intervals)	P value
FEV_1 or PEFR	2	1.2‡	+3.9% of predicted	+1.6 SD (−2.6, +5.9)	0.25
Albuterol treatments	2	< 1‡	−2.1 treatments	−0.18 SD (−0.3, −0.1)	0.02
Hospital stay	2	< 1‡	−0.31 days	−0.18 SD (−0.3, −0.05)	0.03

Note: Positive effect difference signifies that aminophylline group had a better outcome.
* Effect difference is difference in means of theophylline and comparison group (expressed in units of measurement).
† Effect size equals effect difference divided by the standard deviation.
‡ $P > 0.05$.
Abbreviations: FEV$_1$, forced expired volume in 1 second; *PEFR,* peak expiratory flow rate; *SD,* standard deviation.
(From Goodman DC, Littenberg B, O'Connor GT, et al: Theophylline in acute childhood asthma: A meta-analysis of its efficacy. *Pediatr Pulmonol* 21:211–218, Copyright 1996 by Wiley-Liss, Inc. Reprinted by permission of John Wiley & Sons, Inc.)

have evaluated its efficacy in this population. The published randomized clinical trials of theophylline in children hospitalized with acute asthma were identified and the results were pooled for meta-analysis.

Methods.—Six published randomized, controlled clinical trials of theophylline or aminophylline in hopitalized children with acute asthma were identified with a MEDLINE search of articles published between 1966 and 1994. There were data on 164 patients, aged 1.5–18 years. Effect differences and percent effect differences were calculated, comparing the treatment and control groups.

Results.—Only 1 of the 6 clinical trials showed a statistically significant benefit associated with theophylline treatment. The results of another trial showed no statistically significant differences between aminophylline or albuterol treatment. In 4 clinical trials, the theophylline group required more albuterol treatment and had a longer average hospitalization compared to the control group (Table 3).

Conclusions.—There are no significant benefits of theophylline treatment in children hospitalized with acute asthma. In addition, there is some evidence of a slight detrimental effect of theophylline treatment.

▶ This article is not just a nail in the coffin of theophylline, it's a giant stake right through its heart. In this meta-analysis, which reviewed 1,854 citations in the medical literature dealing with the effects of theophylline in children with asthma, there were only 6 randomized clinical trials of this drug involving just 164 children. The results of the meta-analysis indicate with a fairly high degree of certainty that any beneficial effects on the pulmonary function of patients with asthma as a result of theophylline use are small, if any.

If you are not yet turned off by all the negative rhetoric having to do with theophylline, read the superb review of theophylline in asthma that appeared just a few months back in *The New England Journal of Medicine.*[1] Weinberger et al. believe that there remain 3 indications that can be identified for which theophylline still provides a useful alternative to other available maintenance medications: primary therapy in cases in which the administration of an inhaled corticosteroid is difficult or cumbersome, such as in toddlers or preschool-aged children; primary therapy in any patient more likely to adhere to a regimen of oral medication than an inhaled regimen; and additive therapy for patients whose asthma is not adequately controlled with conventional doses of an inhaled corticosteroid. These indications are far fewer than most of us learned as residents 20 and more years ago.

Theophylline has been an old friend to many of us. Its passing will be mourned and not forgotten. Long live steroids and albuterol.

Reference

1. Weinberger M, et al: *N Engl J Med* 334:1380, 1996.

Use of Health Services by African-American Children With Asthma on Medicaid

Lozano P, Connell FA, Koepsell TD (Univ of Washington, Seattle; Group Health Cooperative of Puget Sound, Seattle)
JAMA 274:469–473, 1995

4–3

Background.—Black children have a higher prevalence of asthma, higher asthma-related death rates, and higher hospitalization rates than do white children. These differences may be related to differences in socioeconomic status or may reflect failures of preventive and outpatient care. Detailed utilization profiles of black and white children with similar socioeconomic and insurance status were examined.

Methods.—Data were obtained from the Washington State Medicaid Management Information System. Black and white children between the ages of 3 and 17 years with a diagnosis of asthma were identified and were compared for the type and frequency of use of medical services. Utilization rates were then compared in the 2 races, controlling for age, sex, insurance status, area of residence, and predominant office provider type.

Results.—A total of 576 black children and 1,369 white children were identified. The 2 groups were similar for mean age, gender distribution, and the number of months on Aid to Families With Dependent Children. The utilization profiles revealed that, compared with the white children, the black children had significantly higher rates of emergency department and inpatient services and lower rates of office visits for asthma. Multivariate analysis showed that, compared with white children, black children had odds ratios of 1.70 for emergency department visits, 1.42 for hospitalization, 0.48 for office visits, and 0.87 for prescriptions for asthma care, whereas rates of well-child care were very similar in the 2 groups (Table 3).

Conclusions.—Black children have disproportionately fewer office visits and more emergency and inpatient admissions for asthma, although utilization of well-child care was similar to that of white children. It appears that sociodemographic factors influence the use of office services differ-

TABLE 3.—African-American Race as a Predictor of Use

Type of Service	African-American Race as a Predictor of Percentage of Children Who Used Services		African-American Race as a Predictor of Use Rate Among Users	
	Adjusted OR*	95% Confidence Interval	Adjusted RR†	95% Confidence Interval
Asthma care				
Emergency				
department visit	1.70	1.34–2.15	1.15	1.04–1.27
Hospitalization	1.42	1.03–1.96	1.07	0.92–1.26
Office visit	0.48	0.26–0.85	0.96	0.88–1.05
Prescription	0.87	0.44–1.72	1.08	0.95–1.23
Well-child care	0.96	0.72–1.28	0.93	0.87–1.00

* OR indicates odds ratio for African-American children compared with white children. Covariates include age, sex, area of residence, predominant office provider type (for asthma and well-child care), and person-years contributed to the study.

† RR indicates rate ratio for African-American children compared with white children. Covariates include age, sex, area of residence, and predominant office provider type (for asthma and well-child care). Individual, not pooled, rates were used in this model.

(Courtesy of Lozano P, Connell FA, Koepsell TD: Use of health services by African-American children with asthma on Medicaid. *JAMA* 274:469–473, Copyright 1995, American Medical Association.)

ently than they influence well-child care utilization. Further study is required to identify the institutional, cultural/behavioral, and societal factors that influence the relationship between race and health service use.

▶ Why African-American race should influence utilization of medical services is not adequately answered by this report. Future studies of black children with asthma should attempt to discern which institutional, cultural, behavioral, and societal characteristics mediate the influence of African-American race on the use of health services.

Read Abstract 4–4 to learn more about the role of steroids used early in the course of an asthma attack.

Independent Parental Administration of Prednisone in Acute Asthma: A Double-blind, Placebo-controlled, Crossover Study

Grant CC, Duggan AK, DeAngelis C (Johns Hopkins Univ, Baltimore, Md)
Pediatrics 96:224–229, 1995
4–4

Introduction.—Because asthma is now regarded as an inflammatory disease, corticosteroids are used as first-line therapy for asthmatic attacks. Characteristically, the longer it takes to initiate treatment for an asthmatic attack, the longer it takes to resolve. Previous studies have shown that giving a single dose of prednisone in the emergency department can reduce the need for hospital admission for children with acute asthma. The effectiveness of a single dose of prednisone given by a parent at the onset of an asthmatic attack was examined.

Methods.—The randomized, double-blind, placebo-controlled, crossover study included 86 children with asthma. The children were 2–14 years of age, and all had made at least 2 outpatient visits for acute asthma in the previous year, either to an emergency department or primary care clinic. Seventy-eight children completed 1 year of study enrollment: 6 months with prednisone and 6 months with placebo. Prednisone was supplied in capsules containing a dose of 2 mg/kg, to a maximum of 60 kg. If the child had an asthma attack that did not improve with his or her regular medicine for acute asthma, the parents were to give a single prednisone or placebo capsule. The parents were interviewed every 3 months, and the information they provided was checked against computerized patient records and chart reviews. The effects of prednisone vs. placebo on the numbers of outpatient visits and on hospitalizations for acute asthma were assessed.

Results.—The 2 arms of the study were similar in terms of the total number of attacks and the number of attacks for which medicine was used. The mean number of attacks resulting in outpatient visits was 1.1 when the children were receiving prednisone vs. 0.59 when they were receiving placebo. When the analysis was limited to attacks for which the medicine was given, the mean number of outpatient visits was 0.58 vs. 0.35, respectively. There were no significant differences in the number of attacks leading to admission or in the number of hospital days.

Conclusions.—Giving prednisone at home for use during the early phases of asthmatic attacks in children appears to increase, rather than reduce, the number of outpatient visits for acute asthma. Parental administration of prednisone is therefore not recommended for children with asthma. The results should be confirmed in different patient populations, especially those who are taking optimal anti-inflammatory and inhaled β-agonist therapy.

▶ Asthma is a curious disease. There is a characteristic inertia to an asthma attack, i.e., the longer it takes to initiate therapy, the more difficult it is to effect resolution. Several controlled clinical trials have shown that steroids are effective when administered in the emergency department or outpatient clinic, or immediately after admission to the hospital. When used in these settings, steroids can reduce the number of admissions, the duration of admission, and the time to improvement in clinical scores and pulmonary function tests. A single dose of prednisone administered on presentation to the emergency room has been shown to reduce the need for admission, and, in those children admitted, to result in a more rapid improvement in pulmonary function and a reduced need for any additional doses of prednisone.

Thus, the trick with asthma is, among other things, to give steroids as quickly as possible after the start of an asthmatic attack. Thus, it makes sense to do what these authors have hypothesized, which is to give steroids even before a doctor is seen. Obviously this means a parent would make the decision to institute steroid therapy. Unfortunately, at least in the population studied, steroids given under such conditions did not do what they were supposed to do.

Why steroids did not work within the tight design of this clinical trial is anyone's guess. It would seem important that this study be repeated in different populations of asthmatic children, particularly in those who are using more optimal anti-inflammatory and inhaled β-agonist therapy.

Many pediatricians in their own practices do exactly what this study found to be noneffective. This does not mean that those who recommend that steroids be given at home are wrong. In fact, this editor believes that they are probably quite correct in what they are doing. The problem with this study and its outcome should not deter care providers from using steroids early to abort asthmatic attacks. Hopefully there will be another study along soon that allows steroids to show their optimal benefit.

A Major Outbreak of Asthma Associated With a Thunderstorm: Experience of Accident and Emergency Departments and Patients' Characteristics
Wallis DN, for the Thames Regions Accident and Emergency Trainees Association (Newham Gen Hosp, London; et al)
BMJ 312:601–604, 1996   4–5

Background.—Localized outbreaks of asthma after thunderstorms have been reported. In London in 1994, an epidemic occurred the night of a severe thunderstorm that was notable for the large number of people who were affected and the broad area in which it occurred. The time course of this epidemic, the characteristics of the patients, and the demand on emergency medical resources were investigated.

Methods and Findings.—Data were collected on all patients seen at 12 emergency departments with asthma or other airway diseases on the night of the thunderstorm. The onset of the epidemic was sudden. Six hundred forty patients were assessed during a 30-hour period, which was almost 10 times the number expected. More than half the patients were aged 21–40 years. A history of hay fever was documented for 403 patients. For 283, that attack of asthma was their first. Twelve patients had a history of chronic obstructive airway disease. One hundred four patients were hospitalized, including 5 admitted to an ICU. Several departments ran out of equipment or drugs or called in more physicians to assist with the case load. The sudden drop in air temperature associated with the thunderstorm and the sudden increase in grass pollen concentration were independently correlated with the increase in patients with asthma or airway obstruction seen in emergency departments. Also, several environmental changes occurring just before and during the thunderstorm were significantly temporally associated with the epidemic.

Conclusions.—Thunderstorms can precipitate an asthma epidemic under certain conditions. The factors associated with nonepidemic asthma apparently differ from those associated with that seen in epidemics. Thus, patients with thunderstorm-related reversible airway obstruction seeking care in emergency departments may comprise a different population sensitive to different environmental stimuli.

▶ Nothing is safe anymore, not even the "fresh" air you breathe after a thunderstorm. In recent years, environmental epidemiologists have conducted numerous studies investigating the relationship between asthma and environmental pollutants. Apparently, there is a very complex environmental relationship between what happens during a thunderstorm and asthma, a phenomenon known as "thunderstorm-associated asthma." This phenomenon was recognized more than a decade ago, first in England and then elsewhere.[1] Studies to date consistently suggest that this phenomenon occurs in late spring, is associated with thunderstorms or a drop in temperature, and is followed by a rapid increase in the number of visits to hospital emergency rooms by people with asthma. We now know that thunderstorm-induced asthma is not a result of true air pollution. Several studies have documented no changes in air pollution as a result of a storm. Here in the United States, some have attributed such reactive airway disease to the release of highly reactive oxygen particles, such as ozone or singlet oxygen.

If this report from England is to be believed, the real culprit is plain old pollen. The pollen concept is also supported by the data of Celnza et al., who also found marked increases in the amount of airborne pollen concurrent with the onset of a thunderstorm.[2] Apparently, as the wind whips up, pollen is driven up into the air and acts as a trigger for wheezing. A few hours after such storms, pollen counts are usually at their lowest. The rain deposits the pollen back down to earth. This editor suspects that this article and related ones will get a fair amount of attention in the press. One can see it now—"Asthma Weather Alerts" on television.

Fresh air is supposed to be refreshing and frankly, air is never fresher than right after a storm. If you have asthma, however, when the lightning strikes, reach for your inhaler. That will be the best chance you have for a breath of air that refreshes. Lastly, those with asthma should remember that it's always quietest before the storm. Use the quiescent period to take shelter from the pollen.

References

1. Packe GE, et al: *Lancet* 2:199, 1985.
2. Celnza A, et al: *BMJ* 312:604, 1996.

Genetic Susceptibility to Asthma: Bronchial Hyperresponsiveness Coinherited With a Major Gene for Atopy
Postma DS, Bleecker ER, Amelung PJ, et al (Univ Hosp, Groningen, The Netherlands; Univ of Maryland, Baltimore; Johns Hopkins Univ, Baltimore, Md; et al)
N Engl J Med 333:894–900, 1995   4–6

Background.—The bronchial hyperresponsiveness characteristic of asthmatic individuals is thought to be partly heritable. Children whose bronchoconstrictor responses to various stimuli are heightened are at increased risk of becoming asthmatic. This condition is closely related to the serum IgE level. A major locus regulating serum IgE recently was found on chromosome 5q31-q33.

Objective and Methods.—The relationship between bronchial hyperresponsiveness to histamine and atopy was examined in 303 children and grandchildren of 84 asthmatic probands. Sibling pairs were analyzed for linkage between bronchial hyperresponsiveness and genetic markers on chromosome 5q31-q33. Hyperresponsiveness was expressed as the provocation concentration of histamine producing a 20% reduction in 1-second forced expiratory volume.

Findings.—Bronchial hyperresponsiveness was identified in 34% of first-degree offspring and 36% of second-degree offspring of the asthmatic probands, as well as in 19.5% of spouses. Serum IgE levels correlated in 35 sibling pairs who were concordant for bronchial hyperresponsiveness. There was, however, no significant correlation of bronchial hyperresponsiveness with the serum IgE level. Linkage analyses indicated an association between bronchial hyperresponsiveness and a number of genetic markers on chromosome 5q.

Conclusions.—It appears that a disposition to elevated serum total IgE levels is coinherited with a trait for bronchial hyperresponsiveness. The findings are consistent with the presence of 1 or more genes on chromosome 5q that make carriers susceptible to asthma.

▶ These investigators and others have recently identified a major locus regulating serum IgE levels on chromosomes 5q31-q33. This chromosomal region is rich in genes that regulate IgE production either directly or indirectly and affect the activation and proliferation of cells involved in inflammatory processes associated with reactive airway diseases such as asthma and a variety of allergies. The study abstracted mapped bronchial hyperresponsiveness to a region of chromosome 5 previously reported as 1 site of regulation of total serum IgE. These data provide strong and potent evidence of 1 or more loci on chromosome 5 that contribute to the pathogenesis of asthma. These data will generate many new questions about the molecular basis of susceptibility to asthma.

We are what our genes and our environment make us, including the fact that some of us wheeze. It is likely that in the near future we'll be hearing a lot more about chromosome 5, perhaps explaining why some children who ultimately become asthmatic have more difficulty when they are infected with respiratory syncytial virus for the first time. Perhaps these investigators from Johns Hopkins should look up twins in the Danish registry of twins to see what percentage of identical twins who wheeze do so on the basis of chromosome 5q identity. To say all this differently, now that we know the chromosome that is at least partially responsible for reactive airway disease, the light is green to pursue further what all this really means.

Breastfeeding as Prophylaxis Against Atopic Disease: Prospective Follow-up Study Until 17 Years Old

Saarinen UM, Kajosaari M (Univ of Helsinki)
Lancet 346:1065–1069, 1995   4–7

Background.—Atopic disease, already common, is becoming increasingly prevalent. Environmental exposure to antigens in early infancy may promote both sensitization and the later development of atopy, presumably because of a functionally immature immune system. It also is possible that the intestinal absorption of macromolecules is defective in atopic individuals. Prolonged breast-feeding appears to prevent atopic disease up to 3 years of age.

Study Plan.—The long-term influence of breast-feeding on atopic disease was examined in a longitudinal follow-up study of 236 healthy infants first seen in the initial year of life. One hundred fifty were followed to age 17 years, and the occurrence of atopy related to whether breast-feeding had continued for less than 1 month, 1–6 months, or more than 6 months.

Observations.—The prevalence of atopy increased from 20% at age 1 year to 47% at 17 years of age, when 29% of those followed had substantial atopy. All but 2 of the 70 individuals considered to be atopic at age 17 years had positive skin-prick reactions. Including those with latent atopy, two thirds of the group were atopic at last follow-up. Atopy was most frequent in those who had not been breast-fed for more than 1 month. A positive family history of atopy also was a factor. Eczema was most frequent during the infant years, whereas food allergy peaked at age 3 years, and respiratory allergy during the school and adolescent years (Fig 4).

Conclusion.—Breast-feeding can protect against atopic disease at least into early adulthood.

▶ Another report that shows the benefits of breast-feeding. Breast-feeding for 6 months or longer is an excellent prophylaxis against atopic eczema, a prophylaxis that lasts for the first 3 years of life. Exclusive breast-feeding for longer than just 1 month already is known to prevent most food allergy and respiratory allergy.

There are many good reasons to breast-feed. Prevention of the onset of allergy is just one of them. If you know of a mother who is about to give birth

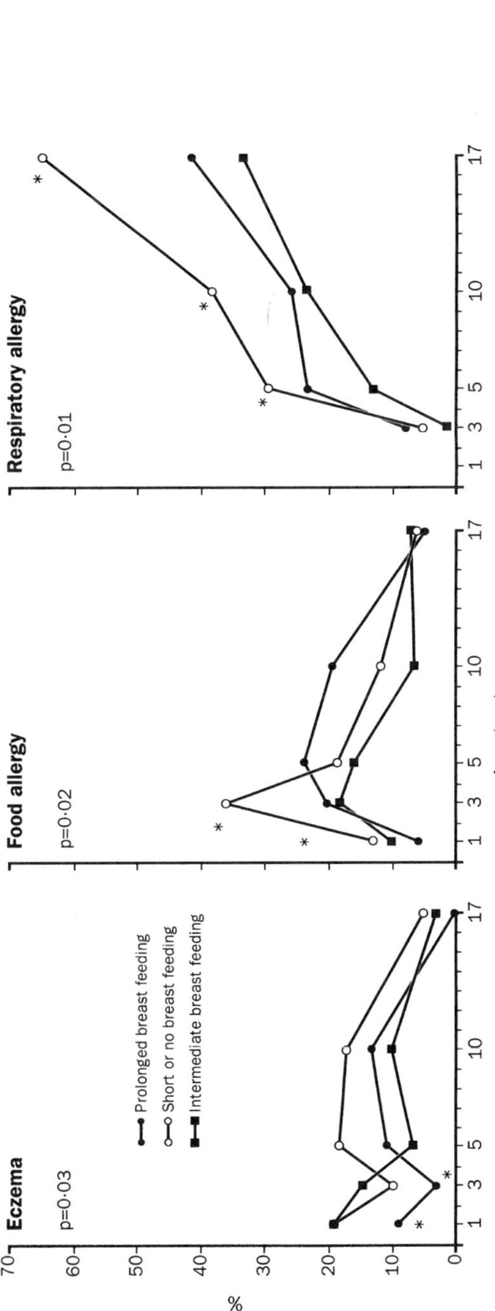

FIGURE 4.—Prevalence of atopic eczema, food allergy, and respiratory allergy in infant feeding groups during follow-up for 17 years. Tests for differences during the appropriate age periods—marked with *asterisks* (eczema 1–3 years, food allergy 1–3 years, respiratory allergy 5–10–17 years)—were done by analysis of variance and covariance with repeated measures. (Courtesy of Saarinen UM, Kajosaari M: Breastfeeding as prophylaxis against atopic disease: Prospective follow-up study until 17 years old. *Lancet* 346:1065–1069, 1995, Copyright by The Lancet Ltd.)

who has severe allergies herself or whose husband has problems with hay fever, eczema, or asthma, show her this report. The long-term payoff will be a rich reward for just a minor investment.

On the other hand, there are relatively few contraindications to breast-feeding. As we all know, HIV infection is one of these. The report of the Committee on Pediatric AIDS, which provides guidelines about breast-feeding in the presence of a maternal risk of HIV infection is well worth your time to read.[1] That committee report reminds us that in addition to the risk that breast milk from an HIV-infected mother poses for her infant, health care workers in neonatal ICUs who handle expressed human milk for nutrition of neonates are theoretically at risk and should wear gloves when exposed to breast milk, even though current Occupational Safety and Health Administration standards do not require this.

Reference

1. Scott GB, et al: *Pediatrics* 96:977, 1995.

Isolated Rice Intolerance: Clinical and Immunologic Characteristics in Four Infants
Cavataio F, Carroccio A, Montalto G, et al (Ospedale "Di Cristina," Palermo, Italy; Univ of Palermo, Italy)
J Pediatr 128:558–560, 1996   4–8

Introduction.—Many infants will have problems with food allergies during the first few months of life. However, rice intolerance is an unusual problem, except in patients with multiple food allergies. Four infants with intolerance to rice only were reported.

Patients.—All 4 infants had clinical manifestations such as shock, vomiting, and diarrhea in response to rice ingestion. All patients tested positive for occult blood in stools. Immunologic testing yielded negative results, including radioactive immunosorbent tests for the major food allergens. The patients were maintained on a rice-free diet for 6 weeks, with no other dietary changes. None had any clinical manifestations during this time; there were no hypersensitivity reactions to other foods, such as cow's milk or other cereals. When the patients were given a rice challenge in the hospital, 3 of the 4 had continuous vomiting, intense sweating, skin pallor, and hypotension within 30 minutes, and the fourth vomited after about 40 minutes. Intestinal biopsy specimens showed various histologic alterations after rice ingestion. Rice challenge was also associated with reduced xylose absorption, positive tests for occult blood in stool, and increased circulating leukocytes. All 4 patients have done well on a rice-free diet. Two had reactions when attempts were made to reintroduce rice.

Conclusions.—Isolated intolerance to rice in infants may be an unusual condition with severe clinical manifestations. This is an unexpected finding, because rice is often used in elimination diets in patients with food allergies. The reactions in these cases are consistent with rice-induced enteritis; the reactions do not appear to represent allergic or anaphylactic reactions.

▶ This editor was concerned when this article first appeared. The concern was that a report may have crept into the literature that had little scientific basis, calling into question a perfectly good food substance that is often relied on as the food of last resort in a child with dietary allergies. Read this report in detail, however, and see that it summarizes a problem that is likely to be real, albeit rare. To be certain of a specific food intolerance, all other sources of potential food intolerance must be excluded. Ideally radioactive immunosorbent testing for the common food allergens should be negative, particularly regarding milk proteins. A child should improve when the offending food is removed and have a recurrence of symptoms when rechallenged. This study meets all of these criteria. On rice rechallenge, in particular, continuous vomiting, intense sweating, skin pallor, and hypotension occurred—pretty impressive. Of equal importance, when rice was removed from the diet, small intestinal biopsies were normal. With rice, the histology demonstrated a variety of findings ranging from simple lymphocytic infiltration with thickening of the mucosa to a marked shortening and fusion of the intestinal villi. Also, while consuming a rice-containing diet, these children had a reduced D-zylose absorption and positive occult blood tests in their stools.

Frankly, however, these data are unsettling. Rice indeed is the food of last resort for food-intolerant children, but apparently this is no longer true for some. Unfortunately the abstracted report fails to tell us when rice can be reintroduced to these children's diets. We do learn that rice is not a perfect food. Intolerance to it can be a serious isolated allergy, associated with significant clinical manifestations.

The observation that rice can be a food allergen is sad news for many of us who have become accustomed to using it for allergic children. Also unhappy are the attendees of the world-famous Duke Rice Diet Center, a renowned weight reduction program; sad news also for Rice-A-Roni and Uncle Ben.

Double-blind Controlled Trial of Effect of Housedust-mite Allergen Avoidance on Atopic Dermatitis

Tan BB, Weald D, Strickland I, et al (Univ of Liverpool, England)
Lancet 347:15–18, 1996   4-9

Background.—Atopic dermatitis, which affects up to 1 in 10 children, can persist into adulthood and greatly impair quality of life. *Dermatophagoides pteronyssinus*, the house dust mite (HDM), is thought to be an important factor in the pathogenesis of atopic dermatitis, but its role has not been established definitively. It was hypothesized that atopic dermatitis would improve if HDM allergens were reduced in the home.

Methods.—Twenty-four adults and 24 children participated in the 6-month study. Their mean ages were 30 and 10 years, respectively. In the homes of 28 patients, Gore-Tex bedcovers, benzyltannate spray, and a high-filtration vacuum cleaner were used. In the homes of the remaining 20 subjects, cotton bedcovers, water spray, and a conventional vacuum cleaner were used. Dust levels were sampled monthly.

Findings.—The weight of dust collected from Gore-Tex–covered mattresses decreased by 98% at 1 month, after which there were no changes. Reductions in dust load were smaller with placebo covers. At 6 months, the difference between active and placebo covers was very significant. Both treatments significantly decreased Der p1 concentrations in bedroom and living room carpets. Between-group differences were nonsignificant. The severity of eczema declined in both groups. However, the active treatment group had significantly greater improvements in severity score and area affected. Most of the active treatment effect resulted from mattress dust and carpet Der p1 reductions.

Conclusions.—Subjects in the active treatment group had significantly greater clinical improvement overall than those in the control group. Symptom relief was dramatic in some patients, who experienced a substantial improvement in quality of life. Children seemed to benefit the most.

▶ The contribution of HDM allergy to the etiology of atopic dermatitis is accepted as certain in the lay press, debated among allergists, and viewed with skepticism by dermatologists. Allergic reactivity to mite antigens can be detected by prick-test challenge in virtually all patients with atopic dermatitis. The real issue is the clinical significance of these responses.

In this study, a combination of anti-HDM measures appeared to decrease the severity of eczema fairly significantly. The measures used included Gore-Tex bed coverings, a spray to kill live mites, and a high-filtration vacuum cleaner to prevent dispersion of mite antigens into the air. Of the 3 measures, it appears that Gore-Tex bed covers have the most effect. This makes sense because the mere killing of mites doesn't solve the problem. It is the mites' doo doo that is the antigen (DER p1) that causes the allergy, not the mite itself.

It has been known for some time that the density of mites in the mattresses of patients with atopic dermatitis is higher than in the mattresses of those without this skin disorder; but what is the chicken and what is the egg? To say this differently, does eczema develop because you have a high mite concentration in your mattress, or are the mites there because you have atopic dermatitis? Colloff recently solved this puzzle.[1] The density of mites in the beds of patients with atopic dermatitis relates to differences in the lipid composition of shed skin cells on which the mites feed. Individuals with atopic dermatitis shed more cells than their nonallergic counterparts and thereby actually feed the mites in their beds—incredible, but true. One wonders whether mites enjoy the shed squames better with mustard or with ketchup.

The topic of eczema and what causes it wouldn't be much of an issue except for the magnitude of the problem that atopic dermatitis causes. A rough estimate suggests that the annual total national expenditure for treatment of childhood atopic dermatitis is $364 million, a conservative estimate. Of this amount, $49 million is spent on hospitalizations. The total cost of the office visits is $107 million. Emergency departments see a fair amount of atopic dermatitis and charge out about $87 million per annum. The largest single category of expenditures, however, is the cost of prescriptions at $121 million. Grand total: $364 million. A third of a billion dollars here, a third of a billion dollars there, and soon you're talking about real money.[2]

References

1. Colloff MJ: *Br J Dermatol* 127:322, 1992.
2. Lapidus CS, et al: *J Am Acad Dermatol* 28:699, 1993.

Comparison of 1% and 2.5% Selenium Sulfide in the Treatment of Tinea Capitis
Givens TG, Murray MM, Baker RC (Univ of Cincinnati, Ohio)
Arch Pediatr Adolesc Med 149:808–811, 1995   4–10

Objective.—Tinea capitis is a common dermatophytic infection in children. Whether an over-the-counter shampoo containing 1% selenium sulfide is as effective an adjunct as the prescribed lotion of 2.5% selenium sulfide was studied prospectively.

Study Plan.—Fifty-four children, 1–15 years of age, who had culture-documented tinea capitis infection caused by *Trichophyton tonsurans* were enrolled in a randomized but nonblinded trial. All patients received griseofulvin, 15 mg/kg daily. In addition, the patients were assigned to shampoo twice weekly with 2.5% selenium sulfide lotion, the 1% shampoo (Selsun Blue), or a nonmedicated placebo shampoo. The scalp was cultured every 2 weeks for dermatophytes.

Results.—Among 37 patients who were evaluated at 2 weeks, none of 7 using the control shampoo had negative cultures for *T. tonsurans.* Only 2 of 12 patients using the 2.5% lotion and 1 of 18 using the proprietary shampoo had negative cultures at this time. Subsequent conversions occurred at varying intervals, but both active preparations were effective in 5 weeks on average, whereas the control shampoo took 7½ weeks. Viable spores were eliminated significantly more rapidly by each of the active products.

Conclusion.—A commercial shampoo of 1% selenium sulfide is as effective as the conventionally prescribed 2.5% product in clearing tinea capitis, and it is less costly.

▶ Times have changed when it comes to tinea capitis. In the middle of this century, the most common organism causing scalp infection was *Microsporum audouini.* Now it is *T. tonsurans. Trichophyton tonsurans* does not produce characteristic yellow-green fluorescence under examination with a Wood's light, making screening for this agent difficult. As many as 10% to 20% of kids who live in impoverished inner cities are infected with this organism. From a public health standpoint, it then becomes critical to find simple and cheap ways to treat the infection. Although systemic griseofulvin is highly effective in treating patients with tinea capitis, it is not sporicidal. Viable spores continue to be shed from affected patients until complete regrowth of new hair can occur. Thus, from a public health standpoint, it is beneficial to provide adjunctive therapy with a sporicidal agent to control the spread of infection. Selenium sulfide shampoos do the trick in this regard.

The problem with selenium sulfide shampoos is that current recommendations require a prescription for the strength (2.5%) that we are accustomed to using. What this report tells us is that you can get away with 1% selenium sulfide and still achieve the same benefits. The latter preparation requires no prescription. Because the recommended application of these shampoos is twice a week, expense becomes a concern with prolonged use. At the time the study abstracted was undertaken, 2.5% selenium sulfide lotion was available only by prescription in a 4-oz bottle at a cost of $13.70. Even at an uptown pharmacy, over-the-counter Selsun Blue, containing 1% selenium sulfide, costs half as much and comes in an 11-oz bottle.

Try Selsun Blue. It cures tinea capitis. If you happen to have dandruff, it'll work well on that, too.

Systematic Review of Clinical Efficacy of Topical Treatments for Head Lice

Vander Stichele RH, Dezeure EM, Bogaert MG (Univ of Ghent, Belgium)
BMJ 311:604–608, 1995   4–11

Introduction.—Although there are numerous products for the treatment and prevention of head lice, epidemics still occur regularly. All trials of topical treatments for head lice were reviewed and evaluated to determine the clinical efficacy of the various treatments.

Methods.—Twenty-eight trials of topical treatments of head lice were identified, using MEDLINE and reference searches. The trials were evaluated for quality using 8 general criteria and 18 criteria specific for head lice treatment. Of the 14 trials considered to have acceptable methodology, 7 that assessed the cure rate by examination of the scalp 14 days after treatment were reviewed.

Results.—The 7 selected trials compared the efficacy of placebo with that of 8 compounds: lindane, bioresmethrin, chlorphenamide, δ-phenothrin, pyrethrin, malathion, carbaryl, and permethrin. The cure rates for all the natural pyrethrines were lower than 90%. Only permethrin 1% creme rinse, tested in 5 studies, including 2 high-quality studies, demonstrated cure rates of close to 100%. The odds ratio of treatment failure with lindane, compared with permethrin, was 15.11.

Conclusions.—Permethrin was the most effective topical treatment for head lice. There was insufficient evidence of the efficacy of other less expensive treatments, including malathion, carbaryl, lindane, and the natural pyrethrines, to justify their use.

▶ Head lice engender more endogenous adrenaline on the part of parents than just about anything else. The human head louse, an ectoparasite, isn't a vector of serious disease and in many cases doesn't even cause symptoms. Yet, problems such as fear of insects, fear of stigmatization, and denial of infection by patients and schools may cause undertreatment, overtreatment, and sometimes unnecessary prophylaxis. With all the sound and fury surrounding the treatment of head lice, it's a relief to see a study like this one, which takes time out to review the published randomized trials of recent years that deal with the clinical efficacy of topical treatments for head lice.

Treatment with natural pyrethrines has been known for more than 100 years, and lindane has been used since World War II. The synthetic pyrethrines were marketed in the 1950s, malathion and carbaryl in the 1960s, and permethrin in the 1980s. What we see from these clinical trials is that only 1 in 4 have been well done, and that of 8 different compounds evaluated, only permethrin 1% cream rinse shows efficacy in more than 2 studies. Less expensive treatments such as malathion and carbaryl need more evidence of efficacy, whereas lindane and the natural pyrethrines are not sufficiently effective to truly justify their use. When it comes to head lice, old drugs are not like old wine, they don't get better with age. Stick with permethrin if you want the best results.

As far as lice are concerned, many parents *do* have a fear of insects, a fear that at times is both unfocused and unneeded. One of your obligations as a practitioner is to stamp out unneeded entomophobia wherever you see it.

Acute Hemorrhagic Edema of Infancy
Lantner RR, Ros SP (Loyola Univ, Maywood, Ill)
Pediatr Emerg Care 12:111–112, 1996   4–12

Introduction.—The combination of fever and a petechial skin rash can occur with a wide variety of diseases, making diagnosis difficult. Most of these conditions have a viral or bacterial cause. Recently, a patient with fever and petechiae was found to have acute hemorrhagic edema of infancy (AHEI).

> *Case Report.*—Girl, 7 months, was brought to the emergency department with irritability, decreased appetite, and a rapidly spreading skin rash, which began on the face and spread to the ears, buttocks, and extremities. The infant also had edema of the hands, feet, gums, and eyelids. Her history included otitis media, recently treated with amoxicillin, and exposure to varicella. She

was alert and did not appear ill, had a rectal temperature of 38.7°C, heart rate of 160 beats/min, respiratory rate of 50 breaths/min, and blood pressure of 80/50 mm Hg. She was given IV ceftriaxone, clindamycin, and gentamicin and was hospitalized for 3 days. She maintained hemodynamic stability. Blood, urine, and cerebrospinal culture were all negative. A diagnosis of AHEI was made, and she was discharged home.

Discussion.—Acute hemorrhagic edema of infancy typically occurs in infants between the ages of 4 months and 2 years and is usually associated with a recent history of respiratory infection or medication. There is a striking contrast between the dramatic cutaneous manifestations and the general healthy state of the patient. The general health status includes hemodynamic stability and a typically low fever. The rash usually appears on the face and extremities only, beginning with small, erythematous, maculopapular lesions, evolving into large, purpuric plaques. There is only rarely visceral involvement. Diagnosis cannot be established with laboratory tests. Differential diagnosis includes Henoch-Schönlein purpura, urticaria, urticarial vasculitis, erythema multiforme, Kawasaki disease, and meningococcemia. There is no specific treatment that is effective with AHEI, which resolves spontaneously within 1–3 weeks and has no long-term complications.

▶ The patient who is seen with fever and a petechial rash does indeed present a diagnostic challenge. Meningococcemia immediately jumps to mind, but a wide variety of diseases can cause the very same set of findings. In fact, most studies, including the large one by Baker et al.,[1] have shown that only a small percentage of children with fever and petechiae will be documented to have invasive bacterial disease. What Lantner and Ros tell us is that there is a very dramatic, although benign, subset of the fever and petechiae syndrome known as acute hemorrhagic edema of infancy (AHEI). Acute hemorrhagic edema of infancy was described first about 25 years ago and has carried with it a number of names over the years including the terms "Finkelstein disease," "Seidlmayer syndrome," and "purpura en cocarde avec oedema." The typical patient with AHEI is 4 months to 2 years of age, has a history of a recent respiratory tract infection, has dramatic skin changes consisting of purpura and edema of the cheeks, eyelids, earlobes and extremities, and a low-grade fever. Rash with involvement of the trunk is uncommon. The rash usually starts as small erythematous, maculopapular lesions, which rapidly evolve into large (up to 5 cm in diameter), round, sharp-edged, purpuric plaques. Melena, bloody diarrhea, intussusception, and transient renal impairment with microscopic hematuria and mild proteinuria have been reported. The latter set of findings obviously mimic those seen in Henoch-Schönlein purpura. Overall, AHEI and Henoch-Schönlein purpura are distinct entities. The differential diagnosis of AHEI includes urticaria, urticarial vasculitis, erythema multiforme, Kawasaki disease, and purpura fulminans as caused by meningococcemia.

Despite their appearance, youngsters affected by AHEI really are not ill. The disorder resolves spontaneously in 1–3 weeks, and no long-term complications are to be expected. Antibiotics do not change the clinical course.

Acute hemorrhagic edema of infancy is something that most of us will not run across every day. In fact, one can wager that many of us had not even heard of the entity until this report appeared. If you had not, now you have.

Reference

1. Baker RC, et al: *Pediatrics* 84:1051, 1989.

Estimation of the Age of Bruising

Stephenson T, Bialas Y (Univ Hosp, Nottingham, England)
Arch Dis Child 74:53–55, 1996   4–13

Objective.—In cases involving suspected nonaccidental injury, the pediatrician will commonly be called as an expert witness to provide an opinion as to the age of a soft-tissue injury. Forensic textbooks describe the color changes occurring in bruises over time. This information does not appear to be based on research in children, however, and, in any case, there is no general agreement on the exact pattern of color changes in bruises (Table 1). The sequence of color changes of accidental bruises in children was investigated.

Methods.—Photographs were taken of 50 accidental bruises of known age in 23 children. The bruises ranged in age from 1.5 hours to 14 days. All photographs were made by the same medical photographer using the same equipment and lighting. A physician experienced in nonaccidental injury cases evaluated each photograph in blinded fashion, recording the colors present in each bruise and estimating the age of the injury.

Results.—Red was seen in 15 of 37 bruises that were less than 1 week old and yellow in 10 of 42 bruises that were more than 1 day old (Figure). The observer provided an age estimate in 44 of the 50 bruises. The estimate was correct in 24 cases and incorrect in 20. Although no bruise older than 48 hours was classified as fresh, misclassifications occurred for

TABLE 1.—Schemes for the Aging of Bruises

	Adelson	Rentoule and Smith	Camps	Polson and Gee	Spitz and Fisher
Initial	Red/blue	Violet	Red	Red, black	Blue/red
1–3 days	Blue/brown	Dark blue	Purple, black	Purple, black	Dark purple
1 week	Yellow/green	Green	Green	Green	Green/yellow
8–10 days		Yellow	Yellow		Brown
2 weeks		Normal	Normal	Yellow	Normal

(Courtesy of Stephenson T, Bialas Y: Estimation of the age of bruising. *Arch Dis Child* 74:53–55, 1996.)

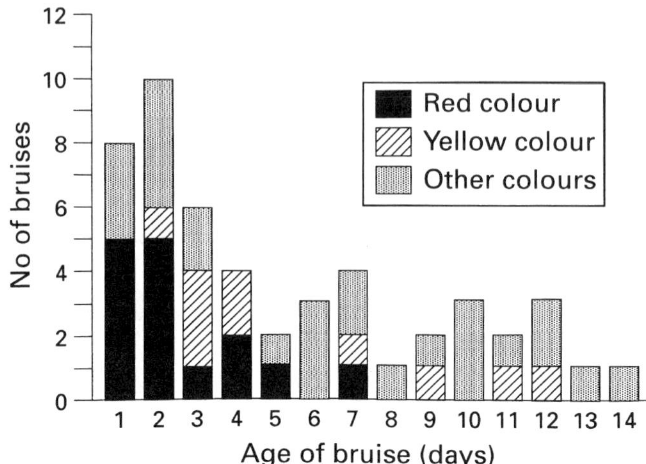

FIGURE.—The height of the bars shows the total number of bruises at each age. (Courtesy of Stephenson T, Bialas Y: Estimation of the age of bruising. *Arch Dis Child* 74:53–55, 1996.)

all other permutations of aging. The accuracy with which bruises were aged was unrelated to the patient's age, the presence of fracture, or the site of the bruise.

Conclusion.—Bruises in children cannot be reliably aged from medical photographs, the results suggest. The exception is that injuries older than 48 hours are unlikely to be classified as fresh. An experienced physician's eyewitness opinion as to the age of an injury may be more reliable than a retrospective opinion based on a photograph.

▶ You can bet that this report will surface time and time again in the courtroom. Pediatricians are often requested to give an opinion on the age of bruises. Unfortunately, forensic textbooks, which frequently give detailed information about the appearance of bruises as related to their age, are relatively silent on research done in children. The purpose of this study was to document the sequence of color changes in photographs taken after accidental bruising in children. Expert witnesses are usually asked to look at such photographs and tell the court when injury occurred.

What we see from this study is that it is really tough trying to time the occurrence of a bruise from a still photograph. All that one can say is that many bruises which appear "fresh" are, in fact, old. On the other hand, old-looking bruises rarely are fresh. Redness does not imply a young bruise and yellow an old one, but the distinctions blur fairly significantly. The next time you see someone who is black and blue, recognize that the easiest way to find out how old the bruises are is to ask the patient, if he or she is old enough to answer. Even non–color-blind physicians are more likely to be right taking this approach.

A Pregnancy-prevention Program in Women of Childbearing Age Receiving Isotretinoin

Mitchell AA, Van Bennekom CM, Louik C (Boston Univ)
N Engl J Med 333:101–106, 1995   4–14

Background.—Although isotretinoin treatment is effective in patients with severe acne, it is also teratogenic. In 1988, the drug manufacturer and the Food and Drug Administration together began a multicomponent Pregnancy Prevention Program to minimize pregnancies among women exposed to isotretinoin. An ongoing survey was conducted to determine program compliance.

Methods.—A total of 177,216 women enrolled in the survey between 1989 and 1993 were assigned randomly to telephone or mail follow-up. Telephone interviews were done at treatment initiation, midway through treatment, and 6 months after treatment completion. Mail questionnaires were filled out 6 months after treatment completion. The duration of therapy was a median of 20 weeks.

Findings.—During phone interviews within 1 month of survey enrollment, 99% of the 24,503 women said they had been told to avoid pregnancy. About 54% said they were not sexually active at that time. Thirty-seven percent of this group used contraception. Of the 42% who were sexually active, 99% used contraception. Four percent of the women were infertile. Four hundred two pregnancies occurred during therapy among 122,582 women with completed telephone or mail survey data who had taken isotretinoin for less than 1 year (Fig 1). Seventy-two percent had elective abortions. Spontaneous abortions occurred in 16%, and ectopic pregnancies in 3%. Eight percent of the pregnant women had live births.

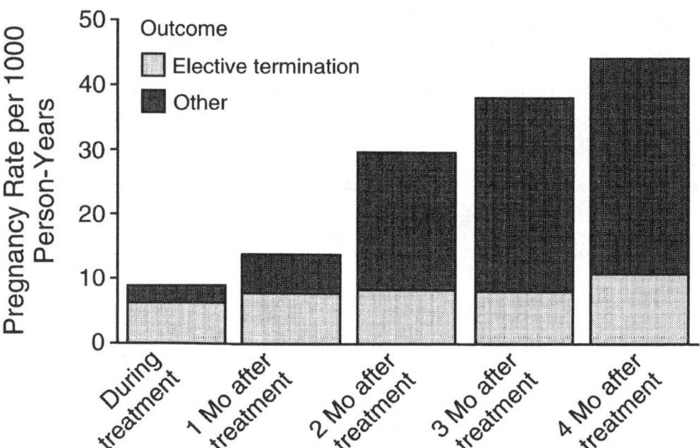

FIGURE 1.—Pregnancy rates and outcomes during and after therapy with isotretinoin in 122,582 women, 1989–1993. (Reprinted by permission of *The New England Journal of Medicine* from Mitchell AA, Van Bennekom CM, Louik C: A pregnancy-prevention program in women of childbearing age receiving isotretinoin. *N Engl J Med* 333:101–106, Copyright 1995, Massachusetts Medical Society.)

Conclusions.—These isotretinoin-treated women had a substantially lower pregnancy rate than that in the general population. Virtually all the women understood the teratogenic risks associated with isotretinoin and the need to avoid pregnancy.

▶ Accutane (isotretinoin) has been available in the United States since 1982 as part of the treatment of severe, recalcitrant cystic acne. It was found early on that live-born infants exposed to Accutane in utero had a 25% to 30% risk of birth defects—the so-called Accutane embryopathy, consisting of craniofacial, heart, and CNS defects. Despite warnings to physicians in direct mailings, advertisements, and in the package insert, reports of pregnancies in exposed women continued to accumulate. By 1989, approximately 78 malformed infants had been reported. The Food and Drug Administration (FDA) became so concerned that it created an advisory committee to make recommendations as to whether Accutane should be removed from the market. Dermatologists and others asserted that its unique efficacy in the treatment of severe acne, together with its relatively short treatment course (15–20 weeks), warranted its continued availability. The FDA chose a middle ground. As an alternative to removing the drug from the market or to formally restricting its use, the FDA accepted a manufacturer proposal: an aggressive program designed to reduce the risk of pregnancy among women taking the drug. What resulted was a Pregnancy Prevention Program, which commenced in the fall of 1988.

This program was targeted at prescribers and patients. Materials were distributed to every dermatologist and to all nondermatologists identified as prescribers of Accutane in this country. These materials included guidelines for physicians (instructing them, for example, to warn patients of risks, to obtain negative pregnancy tests, and to delay therapy until the second or third day of the next normal menstrual period). They also included a patient-qualification checklist and an information brochure for patients. The manufacturer would even reimburse patients for a visit to another physician for contraceptive counseling. In addition, the manufacturer replaced traditional medication bottles with a 10-capsule blister pack that contained information directed specifically at women: the package included warnings about the risks of becoming pregnant while taking Accutane or during the month after treatment, and an "avoid pregnancy" icon behind each capsule. The program was reinforced by periodic communications directed to prescribers and pharmacists.

Did all of this work? Yes, pretty much so. Among American women 15–44 years of age, the pregnancy rate is approximately 109 per 1,000 person-years. For women in the same age group who were taking Accutane, the rate during Accutane exposure was 8.8 per 1,000 person-years, or approximately 8% of that of the general population.

Dai et al.[1] examined in great detail the "epidemiology" of Accutane exposure during pregnancy. They found that 33% of women who were exposed to Accutane during pregnancy were already pregnant when they started Accutane. Some 16% became pregnant in the first 3 weeks of drug use. Of 409 Accutane-exposed pregnancies, 54% ended in elective abortion and 7%

in spontaneous or missed abortion. Of live births, 48% were normal, 47% had congenital malformations, and 5% had abnormalities unrelated to Accutane. As little as 1 capsule was enough to result in a deformed infant.

What all of this means is straightforward. Accutane continues to represent an extraordinary risk for the unborn fetus. At the same time, if a full-court press is maintained to inform potential Accutane users about the risks of this drug, dire outcomes can be avoided. Despite its downsides, Accutane is a marvelous drug for those who need it. It should be made available, but every precaution possible must be taken.

This chapter of the YEAR BOOK OF PEDIATRICS, which deals with the skin, closes with a query: How did the Michelin Tire mascot get his name, and what does this have to do with dermatology? The answer to this query is pretty straightforward. There is an entity characterized by excessive redundancy known as the Michelin Tire syndrome. The latter name was applied to this dermatologic condition because the mascot of the Michelin Tire Company, "Bib," has the appearance of many layers of skin. Dr. M.F. Fridberg, of Elton, Maryland, recently informed this editor of the manner by which Bib got his name. She says: "The full name of the Michelin Tire mascot is 'Bibendum', from the Latin verb 'to drink'." The analogy is that Michelin tires "drink up" road hazards. Early advertising posters showed the Michelin Tire man quaffing a goblet of broken glass, nails, etc. Of course, his visual appearance is that of a stack of animated innertubes. His appearance is also one that would qualify for the topical application of retinoic acid. All this should be easy for pediatricians to remember. The object that mothers put around their babys' necks, a bib, has the same Latin origin as the "Bib" of Michelin Tire fame. Both drink up hazards.

Reference

1. Dai WS, et al: *J Am Acad Dermatol* 26:599, 1992.

5 Miscellaneous

Evaluation of Clinical Competence: The Gap Between Expectation and Performance
Joorabchi B, Devries JM (Henry Ford Health System, Detroit; St Joseph Mercy Hosp, Pontiac, Mich)
Pediatrics 97:179–184, 1996   5–1

Objective.—The Objective Structured Clinical Examination (OSCE) has been widely used in Europe to evaluate the clinical skills of medical students. The test has seen limited application in the United States. A 3-year experience with the OSCEs in the United States comparing validity, reliability, and faculty expectations vs. performance was reported.

Methods.—The 4-hour test was administered in 3 consecutive years to 126 pediatric residents in a community-based program. Monitors graded residents as they interacted with real or simulated patients, interviewing or counseling, examining, perfoming procedures, handling telephone calls, and interpreting results. The patients evaluated the residents' communication skills and attitudes. Residents were also asked open-ended and multiple-choice questions. Results were compared with other measures of performance.

Results.—Content, construct, concurrent validity, and reliability were comparable to those of other measures of performance. In all 3 tests, there was a significant difference between faculty expectations and resident performance at all levels. The percentage of residents scoring below the minimum pass level was 41% at 1 year of training, 55% at 2 years, and 96% at 3 years. These results compare with other studies of clinical competence. The difference between faculty expectations and resident performance could be the result of poor caliber of the residents, poor quality of the test, unrealistic expectations of the faculty, inadequate observations of clinical performance, inaccurate data gathering, or unrealistic standards of the faculty.

Conclusion.—The difference between faculty expectations and resident performance suggests that a change in educational philosophy toward a more clinically oriented, learner-directed, problem-based approach is needed.

▶ Educators have forever been looking for the best way to determine whether medical students and residents have the requisite clinical skills and

"

attitudes, as well as cognitive knowledge, to be good physicians. The authors of this report have used the OSCE to see whether this would help them determine which residents in their house officer training program were doing well and which were not. The OSCE method uses real or simulated patients in a multistation format that evaluates a variety of clinical skills and knowledge of medicine. In half of the stations, the examinees, provided with specific instructions, carry out clearly defined tasks, such as patient interviewing or counseling, focused physical examination, performance of a procedure, telephone management, and interpretation of test results. While performing these tasks, an observer evaluates the students using a detailed checklist that contains all possible actions that the students should take and some they should avoid. Additionally, the real or simulated patients complete their own rating scales, evaluating communication skills and attitudes. In the other half of the stations, the students answer open-ended or multiple-choice questions based on the results of the clinical task just completed. They may be asked to generate a differential diagnosis list, to interpret clinical findings, to propose treatment plans, and to write admission orders.

This form of examination is gaining a fair degree of acceptance in Europe and in the Commonwealth countries. Its use in the United States has been limited to a relatively tiny number of medical schools and university residency training programs. The reasons for this are several and include a lack of a tradition for clinical evaluation in this country, historical reliance on paper-and-pencil tests, the high cost of faculty time, and the commitment and expertise required.

What the authors of this report have found was that although their residents scored well on the yearly in-training examination provided by the American Board of Pediatrics and also did well on their monthly clinical evaluations, a very high percentage of the residents actually scored below the minimum passing levels established by those overseeing the OSCEs. Whether the residents were actually performing poorly or whether their observers had unrealistically high standards was not answered in this report.

We need better ways to evaluate our residents in training. We need better ways to determine who truly is competent. Residency program directors need additional tools to evaluate resident performance. Currently, very few of our almost 10,000 pediatric residents in training are deemed inadequate by their program directors. Clinical testing tools such as the OSCE should be considered by some program directors as tools that they can use to help make good judgments about their house staff.

One last comment. Someone once said that the only real test in life is life itself. In some respects this is true of professional competency. Perhaps we should reserve final judgment about competency until one has experienced the test of professional life for a period after residency. In essence, this is probably what we are doing now. Managed care physician profiling and recertification are intended to keep the oversight process an indefinite one. The curtain does not fall on assessment of our competencies until our professional shingle is taken down.

Stress in Pediatric Faculty: Results of a National Survey

Barton LL, Friedman AD, Locke CJ (Univ of Arizona, Tucson; St Louis Univ)
Arch Pediatr Adolesc Med 149:751–757, 1995   5–2

Objective.—A random survey of 252 full-time pediatric faculty at 26 medical school–based programs throughout the United States was undertaken to learn how much stress they are experiencing, what contributes to it, and its consequences.

Study Population.—Respondents had an average age of 44 years; two thirds were males. More than 80% of the group were subspecialists, and a majority were in tenure-track positions. The mean interval since completion of training was 12½ years.

Findings.—Nearly half the respondents characterized their customary level of stress as being high or very high, and only 11% indicated that it was low or very low. Women reported higher levels of stress than men, as did those on the tenure track. Nearly two thirds of pediatric faculty reported frequently being stressed beyond an "energizing" level. Internal and external stresses were cited with similar frequency. The most prevalent specific stresses were pressure to do research, family needs, and trouble finding time for personal activities (Table). The most common sources of satisfaction were the family, providing patient care, and teaching. The respondents generally felt more valued—and respected—by their patients than by any other group. Nearly three fourths had seriously considered making a major change in their work life in the past 12 months. A majority of respondents, however, would make the same career choices again.

TABLE.—Sources of Stress and Satisfaction

Sources	Percent Citing as 'Most Important' *
Stress	
Need to do research	49
Family needs	48
Lack of personal time	40
Patient care complexity	34
Financial needs of department	33
Administrative responsibilities	27
Patient load	24
Personal compensation	18
Financial issues in patient care	11
Teaching commitments	10
Satisfaction	
Family	83
Patient care	74
Teaching	54
Research	44
Hobbies, personal interests	29
Departmental activities	7
Other personal relationships	6
Personal compensation	4

*Respondents could cite up to 3 sources.
(Courtesy of Barton LL, Friedman AD, Locke CJ: Stress in pediatric faculty: Results of a national survey. *Arch Pediatr Adolesc Med* 149:751–757, Copyright 1995, American Medical Association.)

Conclusion.—Pediatricians teaching in medical school programs have a substantial degree of stress that may importantly influence their long-term commitment to academic medicine.

▶ It's a strange world of academia when stress from a perception of a need to do research exceeds a faculty member's perception of stress related to family needs. Then again, in academia, the most potent instinct is that of survival, the old "publish or perish" imperative. Despite all the negative connotations of this report, respondents to the survey did take solace in sources of satisfaction that are familiar to all of us: family, patient care, and teaching. Add to that satisfying peer support, and in the end everything probably turns out well. Please note that feeling respected and valued by the chairperson of a department not only is inversely related to the amount of stress a faculty person experiences, but the absence of such respect and value is the surest reason for a faculty member wanting to exit.

Some have said that stress is good for you, the impetus for excellence. Others have said that stress is good for you because it's like hitting your head against the wall...it feels good when you stop. What is important, however, is to realize that it isn't likely that stress will diminish in the future. The faculty of our academic departments are being expected to pull more of their own share, both in research and in clinical activities, to support their salaries. Additionally, in an era in which residents work less than they did 10 years ago, it is the faculty who must take up the slack.

Whatever the level of dissatisfaction as it is perceived by some in academia, the grass is not necessarily greener on the opposite side of the fence. Those involved in clinical practice outside of medical centers have their own share of concerns these days. Nonetheless, for all of us, what we have chosen as a career is still likely to be the choice we would make again. Dissatisfaction is the main ingredient in the formula for self-inspection. Out of self-inspection comes a renewed commitment, if we want it to.

Professional Liability of Residents in a Children's Hospital

Grupp-Phelan J, Reynolds S, Lingl LL (Northwestern Univ, Chicago)
Arch Pediatr Adolesc Med 150:87–90, 1996   5–3

Introduction.—During the past 2 decades, professional liability has been a growing concern for physicians. Residents can be involved in malpractice cases as well as attending physicians. Residents' risk of professional liability suits was evaluated in a pediatric hospital setting.

Findings.—In a 20-year retrospective study, 49 malpractice suits involving residents—with or without the involvement of attending physicians—were identified. The study included 886,000 hospital admissions or emergency department visits. The risk of being involved in a malpractice case was 5.5 in 100,000 patient encounters for residents compared with 20.5 in 100,000 for attending physicians. The rate of malpractice cases was 1.8 in 100,000 in the emergency department compared with 13.9 in 100,000 in

TABLE.—Areas and Allegation

	No. (%) of Complaints
Area	42
Inpatient unit	15 (36)
Operating room	13 (30)
Emergency department	9 (21.5)
NICU/PICU	4 (10)
Cardiac catheterization laboratory	1 (2.5)
Allegation	49
Technique	13 (27)
Failure to diagnose	12 (25)
Failure to diagnose and treat	8 (16)
Medication error	7 (14)
Failure to monitor	5 (10)
Treatment failure	4 (8)

Abbreviations: NICU, neonatal intensive care unit; *PICU*, pediatric intensive care unit.
(Courtesy of Grupp-Phelan J, Reynolds S, Lingl LL: Professional liability of residents in a Children's hospital. *Arch Pediatr Adolesc Med* 150:87–90, Copyright 1996, American Medical Association.)

all other areas put together. The most common categories of allegation were a problem with technique (e.g., a retained foreign body) and failure to diagnose a condition (e.g., meningitis) (Table). Patients with preexisting chronic medical conditions were involved in more than half the cases. An out-of-court settlement was reached in 49% of cases, 22% were dismissed, and 2% were decided in favor of the plaintiff; the remaining 27% were still pending at the time of the reviews. The mean award increased from $580,000 from 1968 through 1979 to $760,000 from 1980 through 1992. Median payments increased from $163,000 to $275,000, respectively.

Conclusions.—About one fourth of malpractice cases in the pediatric hospital setting may involve residents. These cases pose financial risk for the hospital, even though the majority of cases are either settled out of court or dismissed. Risk management training for residents would likely reduce residents' and institutions' involvement in malpractice cases.

▶ It doesn't take a rocket scientist to reach the same conclusion that these authors reached. Everyone involved with the care of patients should have risk management training of the highest quality. Every dollar invested in risk management will produce a significant return. If this editor's math is even remotely close, it's likely that about 1 resident out of every 15–20 became caught up in a malpractice lawsuit. Such a resident has about 2 chances out of 3 of being on the losing side (either in court or in an out-of-court settlement). Imagine exiting a residency knowing that you had been involved in a malpractice claim in which the average award was somewhere between $580,000 and $760,000.

As difficult as all this is for residents, it's an equally difficult problem for teaching institutions. One hospital alone paid out well over $1 million a year in malpractice claims based on suits that involved residents. Given the fact that residents were involved with only 26% of all lawsuits at this particular institution, you can see the magnitude of the malpractice problem, at least as it impacts a single pediatric hospital.

Frequently lost in all these types of discussions is the patient. Many of these claims, presumably, were legitimate claims. Those involving residents may or may not have been the result of the fact that a trainee, rather than an attending, was providing the care. Medical education is an imperfect science, one in which there will be some risks. If we want physicians trained, such risks have to be taken. The challenge is to minimize these risks.

The Initial Employment Status of Physicians Completing Training in 1994

Miller RS, Jonas HS, Whitcomb ME (American Med Assoc, Chicago; Assoc of American Med Colleges, Washington, DC)

JAMA 275:708–712, 1996   5–4

Objective.—The career status of physicians who completed residency training in the 1993–1994 academic year was examined.

Background.—According to most academics and policymakers, there will soon be an oversupply of physicians in the United States. It has been reported that physicians who complete residency in some specialties have difficulty finding suitable work, and that the number of patients that some established physicians treat has declined significantly.

Methods.—A survey was completed by 3,090 directors of residency programs. The survey included questions about total number of graduates, number of physicians working full time in their specialty, and number of physicians who had trouble finding employment.

Results.—Of almost 16,000 physicians who completed residency in 1 of 26 specialties, 63% were seeking employment. Of those not seeking employment, 93% were pursuing additional training. The percentage of physicians who did not find a full-time job in their specialty ranged from 0% in urology to almost 11% in pathology, and was 5.5% in rheumatology. The total percentage of physicians who did not find a full-time job in their specialty was 3%. Approximately 70% of graduates seeking employment obtained a position in their specialty. Physicians in more general specialties, such as family practice and internal medicine, had less trouble finding a position in their field. Program directors in nongeneral specialties believed that it will become more difficult to find a full-time position.

Conclusions.—The full-time employment opportunities for physicians in some specialties are becoming more limited in some regions of the United States. These findings may be helpful to medical students and to members of the academic medical community who make decisions about the supply of physicians and the relationship to graduate medical education.

▶ If there is one report to read in your pile of untouched journal articles, it is this one. Carefully understood, this survey of graduating residents provides enormous insights into what the market effects are these days that impact workforce issues in medicine. The data are directly attributable to 2 stars that have now come together in the constellation of factors that influence our need for physicians: growth in managed care and a continued growth in the numbers of individuals exiting residency training.

From this report, several things are crystal clear. There are several specialties of medicine that have quickly gotten themselves into difficulty. Some internal medicine subspecialties (such as gastroenterology), along with pathology, radiology, and anesthesiology, are on the ropes. More than 80% of program directors in anesthesiology anticipate that their residents will have difficulty finding career opportunities. More than half of radiology program directors feel similarly. Pediatrics is not totally off the hook, because as many as 11% of program directors of general pediatric training programs anticipate some problems placing their residents. The figure for family practice is just 3%.

Where is all this leading? Clearly, the primary care disciplines will be among the last to be oversupplied in this country. What the balance will be between family practice, general pediatrics, and internal medicine isn't entirely clear. Our family medicine colleagues are pushing strongly to gain support for more and more people going into family practice (as opposed to internal medicine or pediatrics). A companion article to the one abstracted surveyed all family physicians who graduated from residency training programs since 1969 and found that 91% are still in primary care.[1] Fewer than half of those exiting internal medicine training programs practice primary care, and approximately two thirds of those exiting pediatric residency do similarly. These types of data are touted to imply that family practice residency training is more likely to produce a generalist physician for the nation's needs than is residency training in pediatrics and internal medicine.

So where is the truth in all this? The truth, as usual, lies somewhere in the middle. Pediatrics, family practice, and internal medicine residency training programs do train primary care physicians who are competent. Chances are that even though there may be shortages in these primary care disciplines, such shortages are probably not as great as rhetoric would have one believe. If the pipeline stays open the way it currently is, all disciplines, primary care included, will be in trouble. This editor's bet is that family practice may be in trouble sooner rather than later. The numbers of residents going into family practice residency training programs has increased each year for the past several years at double digit numbers. Take these numbers and add to them Canadian family practitioners who are streaming south and one can envision that family medicine will be oversupplied quickly.[2] More than one third of the 1996 graduates of the University of Toronto's 1995 family medicine residency training program have moved or are in the process of moving to the United States. For the 1996 group, approximately 80% have indicated a desire to seek the warmer and less physician-populated climate of the United States. They are doing this because of the surplus of family physicians in certain areas of Canada.

It truly is time to pay attention to the Pew Commission Report and also the findings of the Institute of Medicine. Both organizations tell us, in an unbiased way, that medicine in the United States is on a collision course with disaster, a disaster catalyzed by an oversupply of physicians, potentially even including primary care–trained individuals. There isn't a lot of time left to make midcourse corrections. We're well beyond the point of no return. The situation, however, is not hopeless for us in primary care *if* we accept the admonishment that the handwriting that is currently on the wall is not a forgery in terms of oversupply.

References

1. Kahn NB, et al: *JAMA* 275:713, 1996.
2. Korcok M, et al: *Can Med Assoc J* 154:893, 1996.

The Effect of Gaps in Health Insurance on Continuity of a Regular Source of Care Among Preschool-aged Children in the United States
Kogan MD, Alexander GR, Teitelbaum MA, et al (Ctrs for Disease Control and Prevention, Natl Ctr for Health Statistics, Hyattsville, Md; Univ of Alabama, Birmingham; Children's Defense Fund, Washington, DC; et al)
JAMA 274:1429–1435, 1995   5–5

Rationale.—It has been suggested that a lack of adequate health care coverage delays children's access to both acute and preventive care services. Such children are less immunized and may not receive needed treatment in a timely manner. It is less clear that gaps in insurance coverage influence the continuity of primary or preventive care.

Objective.—Whether gaps in health insurance coverage preclude regular care was examined in a follow-up survey of a nationally representative sample of 3-year-old children. Information on 8,129 children was obtained by phone or personal interview. The mothers previously had been interviewed for the 1991 Longitudinal Follow-up to the National Maternal and Infant Health Survey.

Findings.—Twenty-three percent of the children had a period of 1 month or longer without any health insurance coverage. Nearly 60% of these children were without insurance for longer than 6 months or had never been covered. A majority of children had been cared for at more than 1 pediatric site by age 3 years (Table 1). Gaps in coverage were relatively likely and were longer for children from poorer working-class families. At family incomes below $30,000, whites were likelier than blacks to have had a gap in insurance coverage; the reverse was the case at higher income levels (Figure). Children who never had a coverage gap and those who were never covered were relatively likely to have had a single site of care. After adjusting for sociodemographic and health-status factors, a gap in insurance coverage did influence the continuity of care received from a regular source of care.

Implications.—Gaps in health insurance coverage for children may well start a pattern of irregular health care that continues into adult life. A

TABLE 1.—Percentage of Women Reporting Any Gap in Their Children's Health Insurance, Length of Insurance Gap, and Number of Pediatric Care Sites

Variable	Weighted %
Any insurance gap	
Yes	22.6
No	77.4
Length of insurance gap*	
No gap	77.4
1–6 mo	8.2
≥ 7 mo	10.2
Never covered	3.8
No. of Pediatric care sites	
1	44.3
2	36.2
3	13.8
≥4	5.8
No. of pediatric care sites with emergency care as secondary site	
1 Site	44.3
2 Sites (second site for emergency services)	15.0
2 Sites with no emergency services or more than 2 sites	40.7

*Percentages vary slightly between length and presence of a gap because of missing data on length of gap.

(Courtesy of Kogan MD, Alexander GR, Teitelbaum MA, et al: The effect of gaps in health insurance on continuity of a regular source of care among preschool-aged children in the United States. *JAMA* 274:1429–1435, Copyright 1995, American Medical Association.)

failure to provide regular coverage to all children compromises their health care during the years when they are most vulnerable.

▶ The statistics that emerge from the Centers for Disease Control and Prevention and the National Center for Health Statistics show a problem

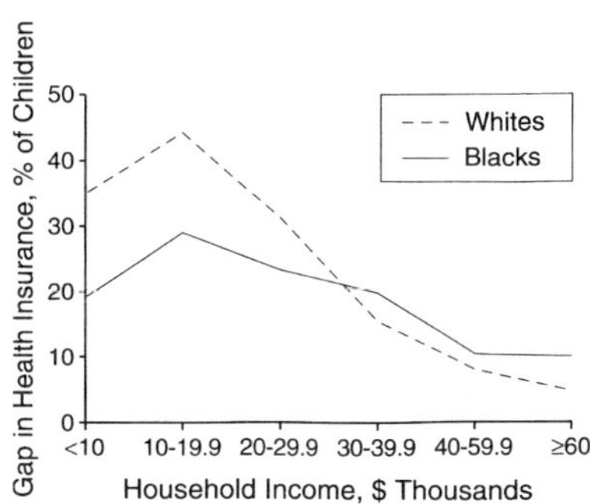

FIGURE.—Percentage of preschool-aged children not having health insurance for at least 1 month by interaction of race and income. (Courtesy of Kogan MD, Alexander GR, Teitelbaum MA, et al: The effects of gaps in health insurance on continuity of a regular source of care among preschool-aged children in the United States. *JAMA* 274:1429–1435, Copyright 1995, American Medical Association.)

whose magnitude seems to elude our federal legislators. Almost 15% of children have a health insurance gap of 7 months or more or are never covered in any way for their health needs. The poor are affected the most, but astoundingly it is the children of the working poor (families with $10,000 to $20,000 per-year income) who have the highest levels of gaps in health insurance coverage.

Congress seems to be caught on the horns of a serious dilemma. Our legislators see that the number of individuals on Medicaid has increased by 60% in the past 8 years. Nonetheless, Medicaid still only covers 58% of poor Americans. Children are critically dependent on it because half of all Medicaid enrollees are kids. The program finances health care for 1 in every 4 children in this country.

In the past, children have fared poorly in battles over budget allocations at the state and federal levels. Before the current brouhaha, early in the Reagan administration there was an 8% decrease in real per capita public social welfare spending for children that occurred at a time when spending continued to increase for other population groups. Today, the stakes for children are even higher. More children live in poverty now than have at any other time since the Kennedy era.

Why can't we view pediatric health care system reform as a long-term investment in children rather than as a means of short-term deficit reduction? The payoffs well into the next century would more than justify such an approach.

Influence of Referring Physicians on Interventions by a Pediatric and Neonatal Critical Care Transport Team

Kronick JB, Frewen TC, Kissoon N, et al (Children's Hosp of Western Ontario, London, Ont, Canada; Univ of Western Ontario, London, Ont, Canada)
Pediatr Emerg Care 12:73–77, 1996   5–6

Background.—Authorities disagree on the best composition of transport teams for interhospital transport of critically ill neonates and children. The role played by the referring physician in pediatric critical care transport has not been studied adequately. The effects of pediatrician vs. nonpediatrician referrals on the transport team's treatment interventions, as well as the effects of the referring physician's year of graduation on interventions performed by the team, were prospectively investigated.

Methods.—Between 1987 and 1989, 213 newborn and 149 consecutive pediatric transports were prospectively studied. All patients were admitted to an ICU. More than 80% in both age groups received assisted ventilation.

Findings.—Significantly more procedural interventions were needed in newborns referred by nonpediatricians than in those referred by pediatricians. However, children referred by pediatricians received more frequent interventions than those referred by nonpediatricians. The referring physician's year of medical school graduation was inversely related to the

TABLE 2.—Total and Procedural Interventions in Each Age Group: Effect of the Referring Physician

Interventions	Newborn (%)			Pediatric (%)		
	Pediatrician $n = 171$	Nonpediatrician $n = 42$	$P*$	Pediatrician $n = 89$	Nonpediatrician $n = 60$	$P*$
Total interventions per patient, mean ± SD	3.40 ± 2.65	4.23 ± 3.24	NS	3.00 ± 2.78	2.82 ± 3.30	NS
At least one intervention required (%)	86.6	97.6	0.042	88.8	71.7	0.008
Procedural interventions per patient, mean ± SD	1.91 ± 1.74	2.64 ± 1.74	0.016	1.30 ± 1.60	1.43 ± 1.88	NS
At least one procedural intervention required (%)	73.7	97.6	0.001	64.0	53.3	NS

*P determined by χ^2, pediatrician vs. nonpediatrician within each age group. Total interventions include both procedural and pharmacologic.
Abbreviation: NS, not significant.
(Courtesy of Kronick JB, Frewen TC, Kissoon N, et al: Influence of referring physicians on interventions by a pediatric and neonatal critical care transport team. *Pediatr Emerg Care* 12:73–77, 1996.)

number of treatment interventions and procedural interventions. Medical training influenced the number of interventions provided. Children were likely to receive more interventions if the referring physician had not been trained recently (Table 2).

Conclusions.—Newborns referred by nonpediatricians underwent more interventions during transport than those referred by pediatricians. Critically ill patients of more recently trained physicians needed fewer interventions by the transport team than the patients of physicians trained earlier. Continuing medical education focused on neonatal and pediatric resuscitation and stabilization is warranted.

▶ This study raises an interesting issue. If one looks at all the data about whether it's important to have physicians involved with pediatric and neonatal critical care transports, one is left in a state of confusion. Some say a physician is not always required on such a team. Others say that only a physician can perform major procedures and administer and monitor the effects of certain drugs. Rubenstein and colleagues argue that the majority of pediatric transports do not objectively require the presence of a pediatrician with extensive experience in acute stabilization of children to provide optimal care.[1] These findings are supported by a study by Beyer et al. in which the authors concluded that, under proper medical guidance, well-trained nonphysician personnel can provide low-risk transport of intubated pediatric patients.[2] The findings of such studies are not supported by a previous report, which states that the presence of a tertiary care pediatrician significantly decreases the frequency of secondary insults during transports when compared with a group of patients transported by a team with extensive pediatric training but sans a pediatrician.[3]

The question posed by this study was does the past experience and training of the referring physician influence the requirements for transport team intervention. Not surprisingly, significantly more newborns referred by nonpediatricians received at least 1 subsequent intervention when compared with those referred by pediatricians. On the other hand, among critically ill older pediatric patients, there was no increase in transport team interventions among patients referred by nonpediatricians. This suggests that in spite of the wider variety of disease processes leading to critical care illness in the pediatric age group, nonpediatricians appear to stabilize pediatric patients as well as pediatricians do.

Whether you are a referring pediatrician or a nonpediatrician, time from graduation in medical school varies inversely with one's ability to properly prepare a patient for transport. No surprise here. The authors suggest that anyone caring for children needs to develop and maintain neonatal and pediatric advanced life support skills, and also to have their board certification updated via periodic recertification. These approaches, together with the concept of our Academy's continuing medical education and other continuing medical education courses would go a long way toward helping pediatricians and nonpediatricians maintain their technical skills, expand their knowledge base, and increase their comfort level when managing neonatal and pediatric resuscitation, stabilization, and transport situations.

References

1. Rubenstein JS, et al: *Crit Care Med* 20:1657, 1992.
2. Beyer AJ III, et al: *Crit Care Med* 20:961, 1992.
3. MacNab AJ: *J Trauma* 31:205, 1991

Physician Experience With Pediatric Inpatient Care in Washington State
Melzer SM, Grossman DC, Rivara FP (Univ of Washington, Seattle)
Pediatrics 97:65–70, 1996   5–7

Objective.—Whether the number of primary care physicians is adequate to meet health care demands is problematic. Hospital discharge data in Washington State were retrospectively reviewed to determine who provides care for pediatric patients.

Methods.—The Comprehensive Hospital Abstract Reporting System (CHARS) was reviewed for records of patients, younger than 18 years, with a medical diagnosis in which the attending physician was identified, who discharged the patient between January 1, 1989, and December 31, 1990.

Results.—Of the 181,581 discharges in the study, pediatricians were listed 61% of the time and family physicians 28% of the time as the attending physician. Statewide, 97% of all pediatricians, 86% of all family practitioners, and 22% of other physicians were listed as attending physicians to at least 1 inpatient, including newborns. Pediatricians discharged an average of 78 patients per year, whereas family practitioners discharged 14.5 patients per year. Excluding healthy newborns, the numbers of discharges were 25 and 3, respectively. The mean age of patients discharged differed significantly, from 2.7 years for pediatricians to 4.1 years for

TABLE 3.—Annual Discharges (Excluding Healthy Newborns) by Physician Specialty and Hospital Locations, Washington State, 1989 and 1990

| | Attending Specialty | | | |
| | Pediatrics | | Family Medicine | |
	Median	Range	Median	Range
Urban hospital discharges (n = 57 976)	25*	1–834	3†	1–187
Rural hospital discharges (n = 6 180)	25*	1–187	4.5†	1–213

*P = nonsignificant.
†P < 0.0001.

(Courtesy of Melzer SM, Grossman DC, Rivara FP, et al: Physician experience with pediatric inpatient care in Washington State. Reproduced by permission of *Pediatrics*, Vol. 97, pp 65–70, Copyright 1996.)

family practitioners. Five percent of attending physicians cared for 50% of all hospitalized patients with the exception of healthy newborns, and 50% of attending physicians cared for 95% of these patients. Most children were cared for at urban hospitals (Table 3). Only 21% of family practitioners and 7% of pediatricians worked at rural hospitals. In rural hospitals, pediatricians cared for 37% of the children.

Conclusion.—Annually, a large number of physicians cared for few hospitalized children. This calls into question the emphasis on inpatient training in many pediatric and family practice residency programs.

▶ The times, they are a changing. This report clearly indicates this. The problem set forth in this study is a timely one, to say the least. One of the issues currently being debated is how to increase the number of primary care and generalist physicians practicing in the urban and rural areas of our country. Medical schools have come under increasing scrutiny and criticism for their perceived failure to supply primary care physicians who meet health care demands adequately. One of the solutions to this problem that has been proposed is the development of primary care as an ambulatory specialty while developing separate, smaller cadres of physicians to care for hospitalized patients. Presumably, with this approach there would be a better recognition of different skills needed for inpatient and outpatient practice. Some have suggested that this would require substantial changes in postgraduate training, including development of a dual-track system of training, resulting in a group of office-based practitioners and a separate cohort of hospital-based physicians. There has been strong resistance to such changes based on the belief that continuity of care epitomized by the primary care practitioner demands that the same physician have the ability to provide both inpatient and outpatient care, especially in rural areas. The dilemma is obvious: in what direction should residency training move? Given the paucity of existing data on the types of physicians who provide care for hospitalized children and how often they actually provide such care, it's obvious that a report such as the one abstracted must be paid attention to.

This report tells us the types of pediatric patients who are admitted in 1 large state (Washington), the characteristics of the individuals who provide care to these children, and the overall frequency with which this care is provided. The results are most interesting:

• Of all pediatric admissions (younger than 18 years), normal newborn infants comprise 64.3% of pediatric hospital discharges.

• Ninety-seven percent of all pediatricians, 86% of all family physicians, and 22% of other physicians serve as attending physicians for pediatric inpatients on other than surgical services.

• Sixty-one percent of hospitalized patients are cared for by pediatricians, 28% by family physicians, and 11% by nonpediatrician/non–family physician providers.

• The average annual number of pediatric inpatients per pediatric attending physician is 78; this number drops to 14.5 for family physicians.

- After a subtraction of healthy newborns, the average number of pediatric inpatients is 25 for pediatricians and 3 for family physicians. Therefore, pediatricians serve as inpatient physicians 5 times more often than family physicians and 8 times more often for patients with diagnoses other than healthy newborn.

- Adolescents older than 10 years of age constitute 22% of the family physician's inpatients compared with 11% of the pediatrician's inpatients.

- Five percent of all attending physicians care for 50% of all hospitalized pediatric patients with diagnoses other than healthy newborn, whereas 50% of attending physicians cared for 95% of patients in this group.

- Eighty-nine percent of all pediatric inpatients receive care at urban hospitals; 11% are treated at rural hospitals.

- Pediatric patients in rural hospitals are 3.3 times (44% vs. 14%) more likely to have a family physician attending than patients in urban hospitals.

- Even in rural areas, where the total number of pediatricians working is low, this group still provides care for 37% of children discharged from rural hospitals.

All of these data are critically important for understanding where primary care and generalist training are going in this country. Clearly only the sickest children are being hospitalized. Are we spending a disproportionate amount of time training pediatric and family medicine residents to treat hospitalized patients, when many of these physicians (especially those in generalist practice) will spend very little, if any, of their clinical time in this activity? On the other hand, our residency training programs are charged with training physicians to work in a wide variety of practice settings with vastly different responsibilities. For example, rural hospitals are highly reliant on family physicians to care for pediatric inpatients; these physicians must be prepared to care for ill children with a variety of common diagnoses in this setting. The flip side is that inpatient services in many urban settings are moving toward the model of care in Canada and Great Britain, in which inpatients are cared for by a relatively few hospital-based generalist and subspecialist physicians.

It's up to all of us to read the tea leaves correctly. We must address whether training in inpatient care should be reorganized to reflect the reality of today's practice environments. Specifically, the content of training needs to be targeted such that the time spent rotating on inpatient medicine services is focused on the care of patients with the most common pediatric diagnoses, with a sprinkling of the rare ones.

Lastly, and not the most minor issue in this whole debate, is the question of who picks up the tab for a redesigned curriculum. To date, residents have paid a fair share of their own educational costs by the care they provide on inpatient services. This is less likely to be true when teaching is done in the ambulatory setting. The average residency training program that obtains Medicare funding for resident education receives about $70,000 per year, per resident trainee. Are we making best use of these dollars?

Children's and Women's Ability to Fire Handguns

Naureckas SM, for the Pediatric Research Group (Northwestern Univ, Chicago; Univ of Chicago)
Arch Pediatr Adolesc Med 149:1318–1322, 1995   5–8

Introduction.—No satisfactory safety devices preventing children from triggering handguns have been made widely available. It is not clear whether it is feasible to make such devices dependent on differences in hand strength between children and adults.

Study Plan.—Whether children actually can fire available handguns was studied in a sample of healthy children 3–10 years of age and their mothers who visited pediatric practices. Siblings of emergency department patients also were studied. Trigger-pull strength using 1 index finger or both was measured for 64 commercially available handguns. The device uses a load cell configured from strain gauges to measure the force applied to a simulated trigger.

Results.—Using the fifth percentile 1-finger trigger-pull strength for adult women as a reference, an estimated one forth of children aged 3–4 years had a greater 2-finger trigger-pull strength. The same was the case for 70% of children aged 5–6 years and 90% of those aged 7–8 years (Fig 2). More than 90% of the guns tested had a trigger-pull set at 10 lb or less. At least 85% of the youngest children could fire the 40 models having a

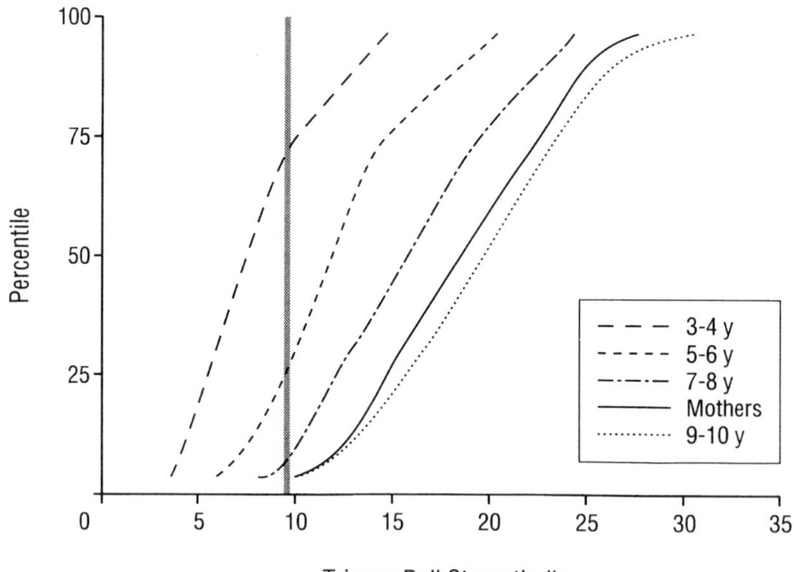

FIGURE 2.—Trigger-pull strength of children and women. Children pulled the "trigger" with both index fingers, mothers with 1 index finger. (Courtesy of Naureckas SM, for the Pediatric Research Group: Children's and women's ability to fire handguns. *Arch Pediatr Adolesc Med* 149:1318–1322, Copyright 1995, American Medical Association.)

setting less than 5 lb, and at least one fourth of these children could fire the 19 handguns set at 5–10 lb.

Implications.—Even young children are able to fire many handguns. Therefore ways should be found of keeping guns away from children, rather than relying solely on making handguns less dangerous.

▶ This brief report contains many alarming statistics about firearms. One family in 5 has a handgun in the house. One in 10 of these families leaves the gun sitting around loaded, ready for a youngster to pick it up. Fifteen hundred people are killed each year by unintentional firearm discharge injuries. That number seems fairly small, but recognize that this represents just 1% of all such injuries. To say this differently, 150,000 people are so traumatized every 365 days. One in 10 of these occurrences will have a child younger than 6 years as the shooter.

Wouldn't it be wonderful if a childproof safety device for handguns could be designed based on differences in cognition between children and adults, a safety device that would engage automatically, not requiring the owner to remember to set it each time the gun was used? To be marketable, such a safety device would have to be easy for adults to disengage so they wouldn't have the temptation to remove or disable it permanently. No such device is currently marketed. The only alternative is something that was tried some years back, i.e., to make handguns known as "lemon squeezers." These guns required an incredibly strong pull to fire, so strong that they could not be unintentionally fired by young children. They are not being sold currently for one simple reason: no one buys them.

Thus we're left with studies such as this. This study shows that a high percentage of even the smallest of children can squeeze a relatively firm trigger. Therefore, if you satisfy an adult woman's needs, you're going to also create guns that children can fire as well.

No more hair-trigger guns. All they're good for is for some hair-raising consequences.

The Ongoing Hazard of BB and Pellet Gun–related Injuries in the United States
McNeill AM, Annest JL (Natl Ctr for Injury Prevention and Control, Atlanta, Ga)
Ann Emerg Med 26:187–194, 1995   5–9

Introduction.—There is increasing recognition of the injury potential of BB and pellet guns. Data from the National Electronic Injury Surveillance System (NEISS) were analyzed to determine the 1-year estimates of injuries caused by BB and pellet guns and the characteristics of these injuries.

Methods.—Data on BB and pellet gun–related injuries were obtained from the 91 emergency departments (EDs) comprising the NEISS sample.

TABLE 1.—National Estimates of BB and Pellet Gunshot Injuries Treated in United States Hospital EDs, June 1992 Through May 1993

| | Patients With BB and Pellet Gunshot Injuries | | |
Patient Characteristics	No. (%)*	Rate	95% CI
Total	31,547 (100.0)	12.3	10.4 – 14.2
Sex			
Male	26,292 (83.3)	21.0	17.7 – 24.3
Female	5,255 (16.7)	4.0	2.9 – 5.1
Age (yr)			
0 – 9	4,983 (15.8)	13.1	9.5 – 16.7
10 – 14	13,007 (41.2)	71.4	57.4 – 85.4
15 – 19	7,229 (22.9)	42.1	31.4 – 52.8
20 – 24	2,928 (9.3)	15.3	10.2 – 20.4
25 – 34	1,701 (5.4)	4.0	2.2 – 5.8
35 or order	1,699 (5.4)	1.4	0.7 – 2.1
Race/ethnicity			
White†	17,576 (55.7)	8.2	6.7 – 9.7
Black	4,663 (14.8)	14.6	10.3 – 18.9
Hispanic‡	1,563 (5.0)	6.4	3.4 – 9.4
Other§	2,591 (8.2)	—	
Not stated	5,154 (16.3)	—	

*Percentages may not add up to 100 because of a rounding error.

†Number of injured persons excludes those of Hispanic origin; injury rates were calculated with "white, non-Hispanic" population estimates.

‡Excludes weighted data for 2 cases, 1 coded "white/Hispanic" and the other coded "black/Hispanic," to avoid double-counting. Remainder is based on 41 cases; interpret results with caution.

§Rates could not be calculated because of the small numbers of people of other races in the study.

Abbreviation: ED, emergency department.

(Data source: US Centers for Disease Control and Prevention (CDC) Firearm Injury Surveillance Study: June 1, 1992–May 31, 1993. Courtesy of McNeill AM, Annest JL: The ongoing hazard of BB and pellet gun–related injuries in the United States. *Ann Emerg Med* 26:187–194, 1995.)

These data were weighted, and the injury rates per 100,000 population were calculated using United States Census data for the same period (1992–1993). The NEISS abstracted information on the characteristics of the victim, the injury, and the injury incident were analyzed.

Results.—It was estimated that 32,997 patients were treated with injuries related to BB or pellet guns during the study, with 95.6% treated for BB or pellet gunshot wounds. On average, 86 BB or pellet gunshots were treated daily in EDs. Analysis of demographic data revealed that gunshot wounds were most common in males, children between the ages of 10 and 14 years, and blacks (Table 1). Arms and legs were most frequently injured (55.3%), and 30.6% of the injuries were to the eye, face, or head and neck (Table 2). Hospitalization was required for 6.5% of the injuries. The injuries were self-inflicted in 30.7% of the cases and inflicted by friends, acquaintances, or relatives in 31%. Most injuries (62.4%) were unintentional, but 13.7% were assaults. Assault injuries most frequently involved male victims between the ages of 10 and 24 years.

Discussion.—Injuries from BB and pellet gunshots are a significant public health problem. These guns have the potential for causing widely varying penetrating injuries and even death. Only 14 states regulate the sale or possession of nonpowder guns, and only 1 state, New Jersey, treats nonpowder guns as conventional firearms (Table A2). Further research is

TABLE 2.—National Estimates of BB and Pellet Gunshot Injuries Treated in United States Hospital EDs, by Selected Characteristics, June 1992 Through May 1993

Characteristics	No. of Patients (%)*
Total	31,547 (100.0)
Mode of transport	
to the ED	
Private vehicle	18,729 (59.4)
Walked in	6,359 (20.2)
EMS/fire rescue/	
ambulance	3,106 (9.8)
Police vehicle	365 (1.2)
Other/not stated	2,988 (9.5)
Primary body part	
Extremity	17,450 (55.3)
Trunk	4,353 (13.8)
Face	4,057 (12.9)
Head/neck	3,790 (12.0)
Eye	1,811 (5.7)
Other	86 (0.3)
ED discharge	
disposition	
Not hospitalized	29,500 (93.5)
Hospitalized	2,047 (6.5)
Victim-offender	
relationship	
Self	9,696 (30.7)
Friend/acquaintance	5,824 (18.5)
Relative other than	
spouse/ex-spouse	3,954 (12.5)
Stranger	952 (3.0)
Spouse/ex-spouse	120 (0.4)
Other/offender not seen	1,655 (5.2)
Not stated	9,346 (29.6)
Locale of injury incident	
House/apartment/	
condominium	12,994 (41.2)
Street/highway	1,541 (4.9)
Other property	777 (2.5)
School/recreation area	764 (2.4)
Farm	34 (0.1)
Not stated	15,437 (48.9)
Type of injury	
Unintentional	19,680 (62.4)
Assault	4,326 (13.7)
Suicide attempt	787 (0.2)
Law enforcement	34 (0.1)
Not stated	7,430 (23.6)

*Percentages may not add up to 100 because of a rounding error.
Abbreviation: ED, emergency department.
(Data source: CDC Firearm Injury Surveillance Study: June 1, 1992–May 31, 1993. Courtesy of McNeill AM, Annest JL: The ongoing hazard of BB and pellet gun–related injuries in the United States. *Ann Emerg Med* 26:187–194, 1995.)

needed to characterize the circumstances of these injuries, the extent of nonpowder gun use in assaults, and the association of injury with access to BB and pellet guns. In addition, interventions need to be proposed and evaluated.

TABLE A2.—State Laws Pertaining to Nonpowder Guns, 1993

State	Restrictions Pertaining to Nonpowder Guns
California	Purchase restrictions: No sale to minors younger than 18 years without parental consent.
Connecticut	Possession/use: A permit is necessary to cary pellet/BB gun. No age restrictions on possession or use.
Delaware	Purchase restrictions: No sale to minors younger than 16 years without parental consent. Possession/use: Possession prohibited for minors younger than 16 years without adult supervision.
Florida	Possession/use: Use prohibited by minors younger than 16 years without adult supervision.
Illinois	Restrictions for BB/pellet guns fall within the definition of firearms for guns with muzzle velocities of 700 feet/second or more. For guns with muzzle velocities of less than 700 feet/second, the following restrictions apply: Purchase restrictions: No sale to minors younger than 13 years. Possession/use: Prohibited to minors younger than 13 years except on private property or shooting ranges.
Massachusetts	Purchase restrictions: No sales to minors younger than 18 years without parental consent. Possession/use: Prohibited to minors younger than 18 years in public space unless minor is accompanied by an adult or possesses a sporting or hunting license.
Michigan	Possession/use: BB/pellet handguns limited to minors younger than 18 years within the property boundaries of their home unless minor is accompanied by an adult.
Minnesota	Purchase/restrictions: No sales to minors younger than 18 years without permission of parent/guardian.
North Carolina	Purchase restrictions: No sale to minors younger than 12 years without consent of parent. Possession/use: Prohibited to minors younger than 12 years without adult supervision.
New Hampshire	Purchase restrictions: No sales to minors younger than 18 years without parental consent. Possession/use: Prohibited to minors younger than 18 years except within the property boundaries of their homes or at designated shooting range with supervision by parent or responsible adult.
New Jersey	Restrictions for BB/pellet guns fall within the definition of firearms. Purchase restrictions: Must be at least 18 years old. Background check and permit required for purchase. Possession/use: Must be at least 18 years old. Background check and permit required to carry and use.
New York	Purchase restrictions: No sales to minors younger than 16 years. Possession/use: Prohibited to minors younger than 16 years without supervision at a shooting range or unless the minor possesses a hunting/sporting license.
Pennsylvania	Purchase restrictions: No sales to minors younger than 18 years without parental consent. Possession/use: Prohibited to minors younger than 18 years without adult supervision.
Rhode Island	Purchase restrictions: No sales to minors younger than 18 years without parental consent. Possession/use: Prohibited to minors younger than 18 years without adult supervision.

(Data source: LEXIS database search, August 1994. Courtesy of McNeill AM, Annest JL: The ongoing hazard of BB and pellet gun–related injuries in the United States. *Ann Emerg Med* 26:187–194, 1995.)

► This is not the first report to show that modern technology has elevated the BB gun from a toy to a weapon. Often appearing trivial, BB and pellet gun injuries must be considered in the same class as those from small-calibre low-velocity powder firearms. A patient with a nonpowder firearm injury must be evaluated with a high index of suspicion for injuries that are not apparent during a general physical examination. Why this is so is readily seen from a description of what BB guns and pellet guns really are. These terms refer to nonpowder guns that use compressed air or gas to propel lead pellets or steel BBs. They encompass pistols and long guns with smooth-bore and rifled barrels. The force with which the guns propel the projectiles is known as "muzzle velocity," usually measured in feet per second. Velocity depends largely on the type of propulsion and the mass of the ammunition. There are 3 propulsion systems used in BB and pellet guns. These are spring-loaded compression, manual pump compression, and pressurized carbon dioxide (CO_2) stored in disposable cartridges. Spring-loaded guns typically have muzzle velocities of 250–350 ft/sec, although some new models have velocities of up to 900–930 feet/sec. Pressurized CO_2-powered guns possess muzzle velocities of 400–450 ft/sec. Manual compression guns can yield velocities of up to 900 ft/sec because most models enable users to increase the level of pressurized air through multiple pumps.

Why must we consider these types of "toys" to be in a similar league to gunpowder weapons? Because several studies have illustrated that over short distances, many of these guns can propel BBs and pellets at the same speeds at which conventional gunpowder firearms discharge their ammunition.[1,2] Although rifles and shotguns propel ammunition at much greater velocities than nonpowder BB and pellet guns, pistols such as the .45, .38 revolver, .38 automatic, and .32 have muzzle velocities of 860, 750, 970, and 800 ft/sec, respectively. It's no wonder some BB and pellet guns shoot a projectile that can penetrate the human body at close range.

Read this report in detail. It should convince you that if you don't live in a state that has restrictions on purchase pertaining to nonpowder guns, you ought to start lobbying for one. It only takes a muzzle velocity of 150 ft/sec to penetrate skin; 200 ft/sec will penetrate bone. A little more than that can penetrate brain tissue, as was noted recently in a child who sustained a severe brain injury after being shot in the head with a BB gun.[3]

If you are uncertain what your state's laws are pertaining to nonpowder guns, see Table A2. New Jersey has the toughest restrictions (must be 18 years of age, undergo a background check, and obtain a permit). Michigan doesn't allow minors to use these things unless they are within their own home's property boundary (unless accompanied by an adult). Illinois is even more sophisticated; its restrictions are based on an actual determination of muzzle velocities.

References

1. Harris W, et al: *J Trauma* 23:566–569, 1983.
2. Reddick EJ, et al: *Ann Emerg Med* 14:1108–1111, 1985.
3. Ford EG, et al: *Pediatrics* 6:278–279, 1990.

Penetrating Abdominal Air Gun Injuries: Pitfalls in Recognition and Management

DiGiulio GA, Kulick RM, Garcia VF (Univ of Cincinnati, Ohio)
Ann Emerg Med 26:224–228, 1995   5–10

Introduction.—The public and emergency care personnel underestimate the injury potential of air guns. Although the potential for eye injury is recognized, the potential for head, thoracic, and abdominal injury is typically not understood. The case histories of 4 patients with abdominal air gun injuries (all of whom recovered uneventfully) and the published reports of similar cases were reviewed.

Case 1.—Boy, 6 years, was shot from a distance of 3 feet with a multiple-pump air gun (MPAG). After taking the patient's history, the attending physician and the surgical resident delayed emergency management. Examination revealed an entrance wound in the right upper quadrant and peritoneal irritation. Radiographs located the pellet near the right kidney. Laparotomy revealed multiple injuries to the colon, duodenum, and proximal jejunum, requiring immediate closure or resection. The pellet was located 1 cm from the vena cava.

Case 2.—Girl, 3 years, had been shot from a distance of 3 feet with an MPAG. Examination revealed an entrance wound in the right upper quadrant, a soft abdomen, and the presence of bowel sounds. Radiographs revealed an intraperitoneal pellet at the level of the third lumbar vertebra. Laparotomy revealed 1 colon perforation, which was closed.

Case 3.—Boy, 9 years, was admitted with a 24-hour history of worsening abdominal pain, vomiting, anorexia, and fever. His examination revealed a possible penetrating wound in the right lower quadrant, hypoactive bowel sounds, and diffuse tenderness. He then reported being shot with an MPAG. The pellet was located radiographically. The laparotomy revealed 4 enterotomies that were closed and the pellet located in the mesoappendiceal wall.

Case 4.—Boy, 4 years, was shot with an MPAG from a 6-inch distance. The entrance wound was 3 cm above the umbilicus, and he had diffuse tenderness. Laparotomy revealed a laceration in the left lobe of the liver and a perforation in the gallbladder, which were closed.

Literature Review.—There were 12 additional reports of abdominal injuries from air guns, yielding a series of 16 cases. Of the 16 patients, 15 had intraperitoneal injury, although only 7 had signs of peritoneal irritation and only 1 had hypotension. The injuries included at least 1 bowel perforation in 13 patients and liver laceration in 4 patients.

Discussion.—Air guns have a substantial potential for serious intraabdominal injury, which is often underestimated by emergency care providers. It is recommended that all patients with abdominal air gun injuries should be given emergency triage and trauma management, including assessment of airway and cardiovascular status, radiographic location of the pellet in stable patients, and immediate laparotomy in patients with hypotension or likely intraperitoneal or hollow viscus injury. Exploratory celiotomy is recommended when radiographs locate the pellet intraperitoneally, even in patients without peritoneal signs. Preventive measures are also recommended, including modifying the impact velocity of all toy firearms, regulation of MPAGs similarly to regulation of firearms, and pediatric counseling of parents about the dangers of toy firearms.

▶ In case Abstract 5–9 failed to give you enough powder to arm yourself to do battle with your state legislature about the risks of air gun injuries, a second article dealing with penetrating abdominal air gun injuries is included in this YEAR BOOK. Although it seems somewhat un-American to think about removing BB guns from our youngsters' hands, or at least significantly restricting them (even this editor had his Daisy rifle while at a single-digit age), the world is a lot more complex than it was almost half a century ago.

Children Who Are Shot: A 30-year Experience

Laraque D, Barlow B, Durkin M, et al (Columbia Univ, New York; Harlem Hosp, New York; New York Med College; et al)
J Pediatr Surg 30:1072–1076, 1995   5–11

Purpose.—Gunshot injuries in children, especially adolescents, represent a growing national problem. Patterns of gunshot injuries in children during the past 3 decades were assessed using a number of different databases.

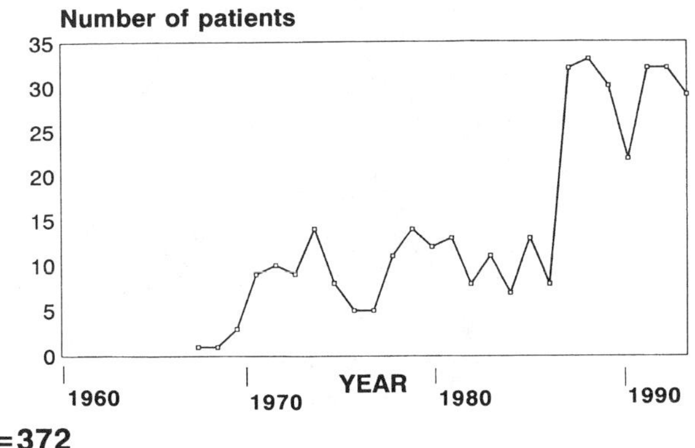

FIGURE 1.—Pediatric gunshot wound admissions (birth to 17 years of age) to Harlem Hospital from 1960 to 1993. Data from the Harlem Hospital Pediatric Trauma Registry. (Courtesy of Laraque D, Barlow B, Durkin M, et al: Children who are shot: A 30-year experience. *J Pediatr Surg* 30:1072–1076, 1995.)

Methods.—The 3 databases used were the Harlem Hospital Pediatric Trauma Registry (HHPTR), the population-based Northern Manhattan Injury Surveillance System (NMISS), and the National Pediatric Trauma Registry (NPTR). The information in these databases was used to examine changes in the pattern of gunshot injuries to children from 1960 to 1993. In addition, a small case-control study was performed to compare the characteristics of children who were shot with those of a matched community control group.

Results.—Gunshot injuries were rarely seen in children in Harlem before 1970. The number of children admitted for such injuries began to increase the next year, peaking at 33 in 1988 (Fig 1). The population-based data of the NMISS found that the rate of gunshot injuries among 10- to 16-year-old children in Central Harlem increased from 65 per 100,000 in 1986 to 268 per 100,000 in 1987. From 1960 to 1993, 3% of children admitted to Harlem Hospital for gunshot injuries died. Most of these children died of brain injury, usually before hospitalization (Fig 2). During the same period, the number of felony drug arrests in Harlem increased by 163%. A similar increase in admissions for pediatric gunshot injuries and in felony arrests was noted in the neighboring South Bronx, according to the NMISS. Furthermore, the NPTR data suggested a similar pattern in communities across the United States.

The case-control study included 26 pediatric gunshot injury patients treated during 1993 and 1994. Compared with controls, the injured children were more likely to be school dropouts, to have lived in a household without a biological parent, to have had a parent die, and to know a friend or relative who had been shot. The incidence of pediatric gunshot wounds decreased somewhat from 1990 to 1992. This corresponded to the institution of the Harlem Injury Prevention Program, a coalition of school,

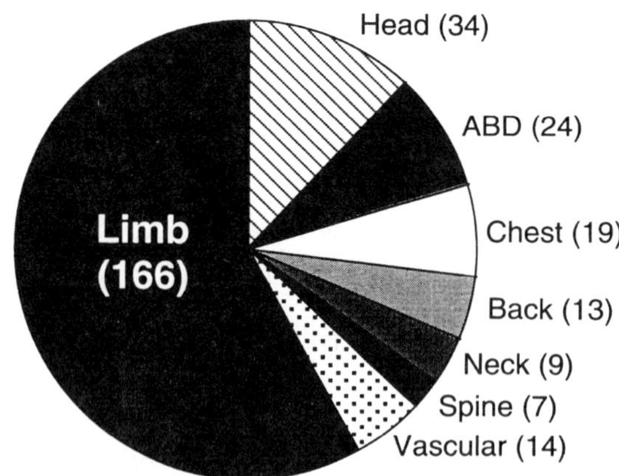

FIGURE 2.—Pediatric gunshot wound injury sites for children admitted to Harlem Hospital from 1982 to 1993. The first series of children (1971–1981) was reported by Barlow B, et al: *J Pediatr Surg* 17:927, 1982. (Courtesy of Laraque D, Barlow B, Durkin M, et al: Children who are shot: A 30-year experience. *J Pediatr Surg* 30:1072–1076, 1995.)

community, and law enforcement organizations that sought to eliminate drug selling from schools and playgrounds and to provide safe, supervised activities for children.

Conclusions.—In Harlem as in other United States communities, pediatric gunshot injuries are a growing problem. Primary prevention through gun control is the only method that seems likely to reduce child deaths from gunshot wounds. The presence of a parental figure and the availability of school and extracurricular activities may have protective effects.

▶ Harlem Hospital, located in northern Manhattan, is the only hospital in Central Harlem. It has a level I trauma center that provides the majority of care for local residents. This report shows how dangerous it is to be a youngster in this neighborhood. From 1990 to 1993, 115 children were admitted to the hospital with gunshot wounds. This averages out to slightly under 1 child admitted with a gunshot wound every week. If being shot were a disease, the rate of increase in pediatric gunshot injuries would qualify it as an epidemic, as defined by the Centers for Disease Control and Prevention. The only slightly positive aspect of this report is that the death rate from being struck by a bullet was as low as it was in kids.

Bullets are made for one purpose only. They were not invented to bite on. They were not invented to merely injure. They were specifically designed to kill. We are lucky that 97% of the time when they find a childhood target, there isn't a lethal outcome.

Tobogganing Injuries in Children

Kim PCW, Haddock G, Bohn D, et al (The Hosp for Sick Children, Toronto)
J Pediatr Surg 30:1135–1137, 1995   5–12

Background.—Despite the popularity of tobogganing in Canada, there is little information on injuries sustained in tobogganing accidents. One experience with tobogganing-related injuries was reviewed.

Patients and Findings.—Twenty-two children with toboganning-related injuries treated between December 1991 and December 1993 were studied. The patients were 13 boys and 9 girls, aged 3–17 years. Nine patients had struck a tree, 8 had struck other objects, and 5 had fallen from the toboggan. Only 1 child was wearing protective headgear at the time of the accident. In 13 children, the initial site of impact was the head; in 5, the trunk; and in 4, the extremities. Major injuries occurred in all systems of the body. Fifty-nine percent of the children needed surgery. Two children died, 1 of cerebral edema and 1 of acute renal failure and subsequent multiorgan failure.

Conclusions.—Injuries sustained while tobogganing comprise a small percentage of all injuries in hospitalized children. However, these injuries can be serious. Significant morbidity and mortality can result. Public awareness of the risks associated with tobogganing needs to be increased. Several precautions should be stressed. Tobogganing where there are trees, posts, and other stationary objects is dangerous and should be avoided. Tobogganing in the prone, head-first position should also be avoided. Wearing protective headgear seems a reasonable precaution. Towing toboggans behind a motor vehicle, a very dangerous practice, should be banned. Children tobogganing need close supervision, especially when the hill is crowded.

▶ Tobogganing injuries don't occur often in children, mainly because most children don't go tobogganing, but when they do occur they can be doozies. Lessons from this report on tobogganing can be equally applied to the more common pastime, sledding.

The authors of this report teach us that the prevention of tobogganing injuries is truly based on common sense. They recommend the following to the public:

* Tobogganing where there are trees, posts, or other stationary objects that could result in a collision is hazardous and should be avoided.
* Tobogganing in the prone, head-first position should be discouraged.
* Protective headgear, although not proven to be of value (no studies have been done), would seem a reasonable precaution and should be encouraged.
* Towing toboggans behind a motor vehicle is extremely dangerous and should be abandoned, for such toboggans rarely follow straight paths.
* Children on toboggans must be closely supervised, particularly when a hill is crowded with other sledders.

Severe Dog Bites in Children

Brogan TV, Bratton SL, Dowd MD, et al (Univ of Washington, Seattle; Univ of Missouri, Kansas City)
Pediatrics 96:947–950, 1995

5–13

Objective.—Although dogs have a prominent place in our culture, providing cheer and practical help to many, there may be as many as 2 million dog bites per year, and a majority of the victims are children. Experience with severe bite injuries—those resulting in hospital admission or death—was reviewed at 3 large city hospitals. Forty children aged 16 years and younger were reviewed.

Epidemiology.—Thirty-eight patients were admitted to the hospital. Two of the 3 deaths took place in the emergency department. Sixty percent of patients were boys; the average age was 58 months. A majority of the dogs were large breeds, German shepherds and Rottweilers in particular. Nearly all the dogs implicated were from the immediate household or neighborhood; only 3 were strays. Most attacks occurred at a place familiar to the victim.

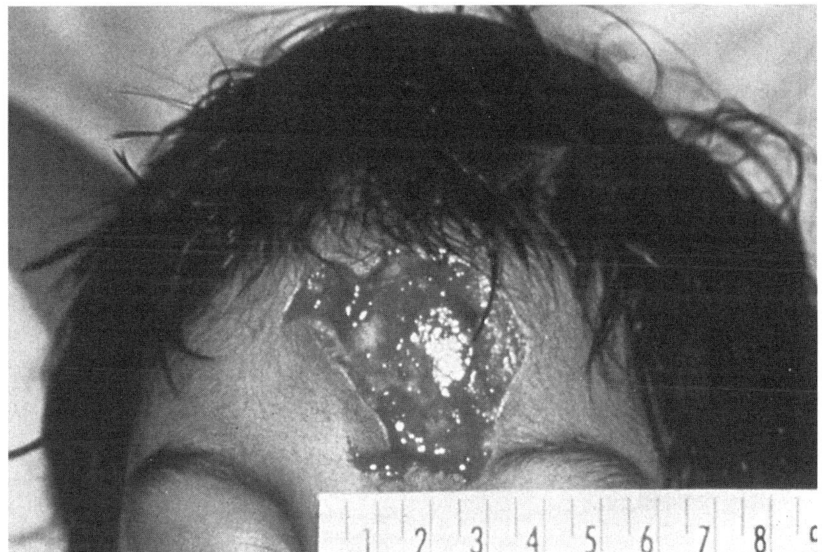

FIGURE.—Face of a toddler who had soft-tissue avulsion as a result of a dog bite. (Courtesy of Brogan TV, Bratton SL, Dowd MD, et al: Severe dog bites in children. Reproduced by permission of *Pediatrics*, Vol. 96, pp 947–950, Copyright 1995.)

Injuries and Outcome.—The 37 surviving children were hospitalized for 6 days on average. Twelve of them required intensive care. The head, face (Figure), and neck were the most common sites of injury. Soft-tissue injuries were universally present and, in addition, 16 children incurred fractures—most often of the skull or facial bones. All children required débridement and repair of their lacerations, and a number of patients required other procedures. Six surviving children had long-term complications.

Prevention.—Most severe dog bite injuries are produced by large animals. These dogs may incorrectly interpret human gestures relating to dominance signals. Aggressive behavior of this sort usually takes place in relation to a known person and in familiar surroundings. Children always must be adequately supervised in the presence of dogs—even the family dog. Aggressive or dominant behavior must be recognized at an early stage because retraining is difficult.

▶ Dog bite reports are so common that it's not likely you'll want to pick up such a report unless it starts, "Man bites dog." Nonetheless, dog bites can be serious, as this report indicates. Each year, 10–20 children are literally murdered by dogs. Of the serious dog bites, most involve the head and neck, including bites that result in fractures of the skull. Most of these biting dogs are well known to the victim and to the victim's family. Stray dogs are usually wary of humans and are rarely aggressive. Strays are more likely to be misconstrued as being aggressive. Because of this misperception, parents tend to be less diligent in supervising their children in the presence of a familiar dog, although it is the latter animal that is more likely to bite.

Why some dogs bite and others don't remains a mystery. The most important rule to remember is that any dog that perceives itself to be threatened is capable of biting. Most biting dogs are medium and large breeds. Large dogs are primarily responsible for the more severe injuries. A number of studies have attempted to define the most frequently aggressive breeds. Gershman et al. showed that German shepherds and Chows predominate as biting dogs, particularly if they have not been neutered.[1] In all fairness to Rin Tin Tin, it is almost impossible to get accurate prevalence figures for which dogs bite because of shifting frequencies in the popularity of different breeds of dogs.

Approximately 1% of the 500,000 to 2 million children bitten by dogs this year will show up in emergency departments. If the amount of money spent on such visits were used to purchase collars and leashes, or perhaps fences and doghouses with padlocks (where needed), perhaps we would all be better off.

While on the topic of bites inflicted by pets, here's a question for you. Is it possible that someone can develop *Pasteurella multocida* infection from a cat without being bitten by the cat? The answer to this query is, as with so many things, it depends. It depends on whether you are an individual with a poorly differentiated rhabdomyosarcoma who has had a cat who chews on your Hickman catheter. The case of such a patient, who was sleeping at home and who woke up to find fresh blood on his chest, was recently reported. His Hickman catheter was damaged and had bite marks on it. It appeared to have been chewed. The patient had a cat who resided in the room where he had been sleeping. The patient went to the emergency department, was admitted, and had the Hickman catheter removed. During the second day of his hospitalization, he spiked a high fever, and blood cultures grew *P. multocida*. *Pasteurella multocida* is a common organism that is found in the mouths of cats and dogs. With a lot of penicillin, the patient did well.

If cats can't get you one way, they'll surely try another.[2]

References

1. Gershman KA, et al: *Pediatrics* 93:913, 1994.
2. Majeed H, et al: *N Engl J Med* 332:338, 1995.

Are Patients Pleased With Computer Use in the Examination Room?
Solomon GL, Dechter M (Northridge Hosp Found, Calif)
J Fam Pract 41:241–244, 1995   5–14

Objective.—The use of computers by physicians to keep patient records is growing. However, there are still concerns that having a computer in the examining room could interfere with the patient-physician relationship. Patient satisfaction with physicians who used either written or computerized note-taking was prospectively assessed.

Methods.—The 2-phase crossover study included 60 patients attending a 2-physician family practice office. In the first phase, 15 patients were randomly selected to be seen by a physician who took traditional written notes and 15 to be seen by the other physician, who took notes on a laptop computer. In the second phase, the 2 physicians switched note-taking methods. Patient satisfaction was assessed by a questionnaire administered after the examination.

Results.—Patient satisfaction was no different when the physicians made handwritten or computerized notes. The method of note-taking had no impact on the patients' assessments of physician distraction or listening. No interactions were noted between method of note-taking and physician, and the patients' level of satisfaction was unrelated to their previous exposure to computers.

Conclusions.—Physician use of a computer for note-taking does not appear to have a negative impact on patient satisfaction. The results offer reassurance that the trend toward computerized record keeping will not have an adverse effect on the patient-physician relationship.

▶ Any new technology is going to be viewed with some degree of suspicion and curiosity on the part of a patient. It would not be unreasonable to ask the questions this article poses: do patients believe that the quality of medical care is changed when a physician uses a computer in their presence?; will a patient encounter become more impersonal because of a computer?; will a physician divert attention from the patient to the computer?; do patients feel that the computer will reduce the confidentiality of the medical record? The results of this survey show that the answers to all of these questions favor the computer.

This isn't the first study to examine the use of computers in patient examining rooms. Several earlier studies confirm the impression that if handled properly, the use of a computer does not interfere with the normal physician-patient interaction. These data come at a time when everyone is looking for ways to reduce paperwork. Even the federal government is interested in this issue. The Institute of Medicine called for automated medical records as long ago as 1991.[1] In 1992, Congress considered mandating automated record keeping for hospitals receiving federal funds.

We in the United States are behind the curve when it comes to figuring out how to use computers in the examination room. For years, Europeans have done this and have studied the effects on patient-physician relationships. Pick up any issue of the *British Medical Journal* and you will see an article on the role of computers in the office setting. Such a topic is now a regular feature of many European journals.

Please note that this study was done in a family practice office that dealt mostly with adult patients. Chances are that a pediatric practice would have no greater difficulty, and probably less, integrating computers into the examination room. Although infants might not be turned on by computers, children past this age are into the electronic age. So should we all be.

Reference

1. Committee on improving patient records, Institute of Medicine; Dik RS, Steen EB (eds): *The Computer-based Medical Record: An Essential Technology For Health Care.* Washington, DC, National Academy Press, 1991.

Characteristics of Frequent Pediatric Emergency Department Users

Yamamoto LG, Zimmerman KR, Butts RJ, et al (Univ of Hawaii, Honolulu; Kapiolani Med Ctr for Women and Children, Honolulu, Hawaii)
Pediatr Emerg Care 11:340–346, 1995   5–15

Introduction.—Emergency departments (EDs) are often used as the only source of medical care. The medical and demographic characteristics of frequent users of emergency care at a pediatric ED were examined.

Methods.—The database of the ED in a medical center for women and children was searched to find pediatric patients using the ED 10 or more times during the 4.6-year study. The outpatient and inpatient medical records of these frequent users were reviewed, with attention to chronic and acute medical conditions and demographic features. The characteristics of these patients were compared with those of a control group of 47,983 pediatric patients treated in the ED fewer than 3 times.

Results.—During the study, 79,049 pediatric patients were treated in the ED, and 357 patients were treated in the ED at least 10 times. Of these 357 frequent users, chronic disease conditions were present in 265 patients (74%), of whom 223 had good functional status, 25 had mild or moderate functional impairment, and 17 had severe functional impairment. Medicaid or state assistance was the predominant source of medical insurance (in 60%), followed by private insurance (38%), no insurance (1.4%), and military insurance (0.3%). There were significantly more Polynesian ethnic groups represented in the frequent user group than in the control group, although there were no differences in pediatric primary care providers or insurance status between Polynesians and the cohort as a whole. Pulmonary conditions, particularly recurrent wheezing, represented the most common chronic conditions among the frequent users, followed by neurologic conditions, particularly seizure disorders (Table 3). Among the frequent users without chronic conditions, trauma, fever, respiratory tract infections, and otitis media were the most common acute conditions treated (Table 5).

Conclusions.—The frequency of emergency medical care for fever, respiratory tract infections, and otitis media indicates a need to educate populations of frequent ED users how to seek more appropriate medical care. However, because several chronic conditions, including recurrent wheezing, will require emergency care, training for pediatric emergency physicians should include the chronic management of these conditions.

▶ This report emanates from the Kapiolani Medical Center in Honolulu. As such, it has certain limitations in terms of its data being extrapolated to the

TABLE 3.—Chronic Conditions Among Frequent Emergency Department (ED) Users

	No.	Total patient visits	ED visits/ patient/year	Mean age (yr)
No chronic conditions	92	1149	2.7	2.4
All chronic conditions	265	4029	3.3	3.7
Pulmonary conditions	231	3409	3.2	3.4
Recurrent wheezing	226	3330	3.2	3.3
Recurrent pneumonia	8	132	3.6	5.3
Chronic large airway problems	5	75	3.3	1.3
Chronic aspiration	1	19	4.1	1.5
Cystic fibrosis	1	12	2.6	15.3
Neurologic conditions	33	589	3.9	4.5
Seizure disorders	21	413	4.3	5.0
Psychomotor retardation	17	316	4.0	3.8
CNS injury and/or cerebral palsy	11	170	3.4	3.1
Hydrocephalus with ventricular shunt	9	136	3.3	3.3
Paraplegia or quadraplegia	4	67	3.6	4.0
Noncorrectable vision problem	3	75	5.4	3.7
Hearing problem	3	45	3.3	4.2
Gastrointestinal conditions	13	181	3.0	4.3
Malabsorption condition	6	81	2.9	3.7
Liver disease	2	25	2.7	8.4
Recurrent flux	2	31	3.4	1.5
Inflammatory bowel disease	1	10	2.2	0.8
Cardiac conditions	12	170	3.1	2.1
Noncyanotic (left-to-right) shunt	8	114	3.1	2.1
Cyanotic (right-to-left) shunt	3	43	3.1	2.6
Recurrent supraventricular tachycardia	1	16	3.5	0.6
Endocrine conditions	9	168	4.1	7.9
Diabetes mellitus	4	89	4.8	11.5
Recurrent hypoglycemia (nondiabetic)	1	10	2.2	9.5
Thyroid conditions	1	20	4.3	6.3
Corticosteroid deficiency	1	25	5.2	2.1
Other endocrine conditions	4	54	2.9	4.8
Hematology/oncology conditions	8	139	3.8	6.6
Hemophilia A or B	3	72	5.2	6.7
Leukemia	2	21	2.3	6.2
Other malignancy	2	32	3.5	6.2
Chronic thrombocytopenia	1	14	3.0	6.9
Renal conditions	5	81	3.5	2.0
Renal or collecting system anomalies	4	57	3.1	1.7
Nephrosis	1	27	5.9	2.7
Recurrent infection	1	19	4.1	1.5
Orthopedic conditions	5	61	2.7	3.3
Severe scoliosis	3	40	2.9	3.4
Hip or lower extremity dysfunction	2	21	2.3	5.3
Arthrogryposis	1	14	3.0	2.4
Upper extremity dysfunction	1	11	2.4	2.7
Psychiatric conditions	2	30	3.3	10.5
Depression	1	14	3.0	5.4
Eating disorder	1	16	3.5	14.9

(Courtesy of Yamamoto LG, Zimmerman KR, Butts RJ, et al: Characteristics of frequent pediatric emergency department users. *Pediatr Emerg Care* 11:340–346, 1995.)

rest of the United States. The percentage of Asians is substantially higher and the percentages of whites and blacks are lower than in the mainland United States. For this reason, there is a paucity of ED users with conditions such as cystic fibrosis and sickle cell disease. Despite these limitations, we learn that there are some who show up in EDs not because of a lack of a

TABLE 5.—Frequency of Acute Conditions Among 92 Healthy Frequent ED Users

	No. of patients	Hospitalization rate (%)	Ambulance use rate (%)	Private insurance (%)	Medicaid insurance (%)	Mean age (yr)
All healthy frequency ED users	92	4	2	30	65	2.4
Trauma						
>25%	12	3	2	42	58	1.9
Pulmonary conditions						
>25%	15	8	2	53	40	1.5
Neurologic conditions						
>25%	3	0	3	33	67	2.7
Acute intoxications						
>25%	1	10	10	0	100	15.1
Fever						
>25%	84	4	2	30	67	1.9
>50%	51	5	2	27	71	1.6
>75%	14	6	4	21	71	1.5
Respiratory infection (upper or lower)						
>25%	70	4	2	31	64	2.0
>50%	27	4	2	30	63	1.5
>75%	3	7	0	0	100	0.9
Otitis media						
>25%	60	4	2	30	65	1.7
>50%	18	5	1	39	56	1.5
>75%	3	3	0	0	100	1.8

(Courtesy of Yamamoto LG, Zimmerman KR, Butts RJ, et al: Characteristics of frequent pediatric emergency department users. *Pediatr Emerg Care* 11:340–346, 1995.)

primary care provider or medical insurance, but rather because of a cultural tradition of seeking medical care in EDs. Samoans represent such an example. Fortunately for such patients, high-quality emergency services have provided adequate immunizations and preventive services. One other aspect of this report is particularly revealing. A fair number of children with chronic management conditions, such as asthma, receive a huge percentage of their medical care in EDs. See Tables 3 and 5 that accompany this article for the list of both acute and chronic diagnoses that inhabit our EDs.

Two conclusions are obvious. First, we must do more to determine ways of providing optimal care without EDs. They are too expensive and inherently ill designed to provide any continuity. Second, because the likelihood of accomplishing this goal is relatively low, our emergency medicine fellowships must have curricular elements that include chronic diseases. Emergency medicine training involves a great more than the care and treatment of emergent problems. Emergency departments are a microcosm of all of pediatrics. It takes a highly trained individual to function in such an environment.

Preferences of Parents for Pediatric Emergency Physicians' Attire

Gonzalez del Rey JA, Paul RI (Univ of Cincinnati, Ohio; Univ of Louisville, Ky)
Pediatr Emerg Care 11:361–364, 1995   5–16

Introduction.—Typically, pediatric emergency care involves interaction among the physician, parents, and patients. Previous studies of inpatient pediatric units and outpatient pediatric clinics have shown that parents of the patients clearly preferred and attributed more competence to physicians wearing formal dress. The physician's attire preferred by parents in the pediatric emergency department and variables affecting preferences were investigated.

Methods.—During the 6-month study, 344 parents or guardians of patients seeking treatment in the pediatric emergency department were shown a set of 8 photographs of a male and female physician wearing varying attire (Fig 1). The parents were asked to choose which physicians they would most and least like to treat their child and why they made their choices. Information was also collected on the patient's age, sex, and type of medical insurance; the participant's age, sex, and relationship to the patient; time of the visit; severity of the illness; and the type of visit.

Results.—The photograph showing the physicians dressed most formally was most frequently chosen by parents of patients in all triage categories treated in all 3 shifts, although parents visiting the pediatric emergency department between 11 PM and 7 AM were somewhat less likely to prefer the formal attire. The photograph showing the physicians wearing formal pants or skirt, casual shirt, no tie, no laboratory coat, and

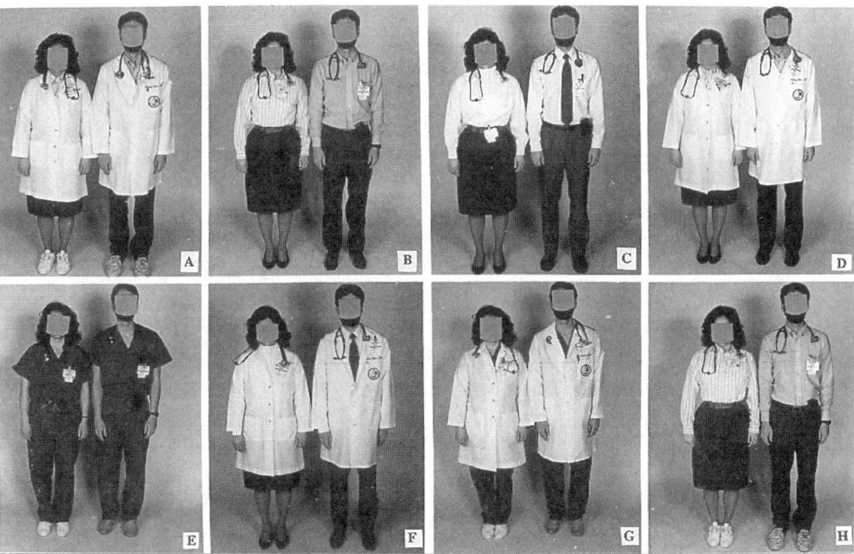

FIGURE 1.—Photographs of physicians in different levels of attire used during the study survey. (Courtesy of Gonzalez del Rey JA, Paul RI: Preferences of parents for pediatric emergency physicians' attire. *Pediatr Emerg Care* 11:361–364, 1995.)

TABLE 1.—"Most Liked Dress Code"

Photograph	Parent/Guardian	Preferences (%)
F	158/360	44
D	61/360	17
E	39/360	11
C	35/360	9.9
G	33/360	9.2
A	18/360	5
B	7/360	2
H	6/360	1.9

(Courtesy of Gonzalez del Rey JA, Paul RI: Preferences of parents for pediatric emergency physicians' attire. *Pediatr Emerg Care* 11:361–364, 1995.)

tennis shoes was most frequently selected as the physicians least preferred in each group of parents (Table 1). However, most of the parents reported that they did not associate attire with capability or really care how the physicians were dressed. No variables significantly influenced the selection of physicians, but there was a trend toward a greater preference of the physicians wearing surgical scrubs among the parents of children with surgical emergencies.

Conclusions.—Although most parents report not caring about physicians' attire, they did prefer physicians wearing formal attire with a white laboratory coat, tie, and dress shoes and did not like casual dress with tennis shoes and no tie. Therefore, it is recommended that pediatric emergency physicians follow a dress code of formal attire designed to make a positive first impression on the patients' parents.

▶ This is an interesting report. Although it would be fair to say that most kids and their parents would prefer not to see an emergency department physician at all, when they have to, they will give the nod toward the more nicely dressed doctor. In a sense these are not new findings. After reviewing 386 teenagers in 1985, Neistein et al.[1] found that although dress styles ranging from very informal to very formal appear to have little or no impact on the comfort level of adolescent patients, as far as inpatients are concerned, parents are twice as likely to attribute competence to the physician wearing formal dress as compared with the physician wearing operating room attire, and Taylor published similar findings.[2] Similarly, parents of children attending outpatient clinics have a strong positive preference for the physician dressed in a "short lab coat and tie."[3] No prior studies have been solely oriented toward the pediatric emergency department setting. Thus, this report is a first.

So what do we learn? We learn that even though most parents say they don't care what the physician caring for their kids is wearing, when specifically asked they will state a preference. Their preference is for "formal" attire, not an evening jacket and bow tie, but rather a white laboratory coat and dress shoes, certainly not tennis shoes. On the other hand, if there is a wound to be sutured, the parents prefer to see emergency department physicians in scrubs.

This study was completed before "Chicago Hope" and "ER" had any potential impact on this type of issue. Given the way George Clooney et al. dress, there is indeed hope for decently attired physicians in emergency departments, at least on TV.

This is an age where casual dress is more the norm than not. There is nothing wrong with such dress *except* if it interferes with the way in which the perception of care is understood by patients and their parents. Because either directly or indirectly they are the payer of a health care bill and certainly are its recipient, it is probably most appropriate to suggest that the personal preferences of physicians, including emergency department physicians, should be left at the locker room door unless they are in line with what is expected of us by those whom we serve. In any debate about what to wear, the default setting should be "puttin' on the Ritz."

References

1. Neistein L, et al: *J Adolesc Health Care* 64:456, 1985.
2. Taylor PT: *Am J Dis Child* 141:426, 1987.
3. Marino RV, et al: *J Dev Behav Pediatr* 12:98, 1991.

Physicians' Children Are Treated Differently in the Emergency Department

Diekema DS, Cummings P, Quan L (Univ of Washington, Seattle; Children's Hosp and Med Ctr, Seattle)
Am J Emerg Med 14:6–9, 1996   5–17

Introduction.—Previous studies have suggested that physicians and their relatives receive medical care that differs from that received by other patients. To further investigate possible differences in the delivery of medical care, the treatment received in a pediatric emergency department (ED) at a teaching hospital was compared between children with and without a physician parent.

TABLE 2.—Number of Nonconsulting Physicians Seen During Emergency Department (ED) Visit

Number of ED Physicians	Physician Parents $n = 92$ (%)	Nonphysician Parents $n = 181$ (%)	Crude Relative Risk (95% CI)*	Adjusted Relative Risk (95% CI)†‡
0	10 (11%)	7 (4%)	2.81 (1.11–7.14)	2.23 (0.86–5.77)
1	19 (21%)	21 (12%)	1.78 (1.01–3.14)	1.76 (0.99–3.12)
2	59 (64%)	137 (76%)	0.85 (0.71–1.01)	0.86 (0.72–1.03)
3	4 (4%)	16 (9%)	0.49 (0.17–1.43)	0.52 (0.18–1.48)

*Relative risk of a child with a physician parent seeing given number of ED physicians compared with a child with nonphysician parents.
† P value for linear trend in proportions = 0.005.
‡ Adjusted for urgent vs. nonurgent final diagnosis.
(Courtesy of Diekema DS, Cummings P, Quan L: Physicians' children are treated differently in the emergency department. *Am J Emerg Med* 14:6–9, 1996.)

Methods.—The ED registry over a 28-month period was searched to identify 92 children with at least 1 parent who was a physician. The next 2 children without a physician parent seen served as controls. Because none of the children with physician parents were hospitalized, only non-hospitalized children were used as controls. The ED records of the 92 children with a physician parent and the 181 control children were reviewed. Data were collected on the length of the ED stay, the number of laboratory tests performed and radiographs obtained, and the identity of all of the physicians seen by the patient. The severity of illness was categorized by the nursing acuity level and the final diagnosis, which was retrospectively classified as either urgent or nonurgent.

Results.—There were no clinically or statistically significant differences in the characteristics of the patients in the 2 groups. Compared with the control children, the children with physician parents were only slightly more likely to have a radiograph obtained (34% vs. 30%), slightly less likely to have a laboratory test performed (23% vs. 29%), and had a slightly shorter length of ED stay (94 vs. 105 minutes). The children with physician parents had a higher proportion of urgent final diagnoses (66% vs. 44%) and surgical problems (54% vs. 31%). There were significant differences in the physicians seen by the patients in the 2 groups, with children with physician parents seeing significantly more consultant physicians and physicians with greater experience than did the control children, even after adjustment for the urgency of the final diagnosis. The children with physician parents typically saw fewer physicians overall (Table 2).

Conclusions.—Although there was little difference in the diagnostic testing performed or in the length of stay, the children of physicians were more likely than other patients to see consultants in the ED and less likely to see medical students or residents.

▶ This article is well worth reading in detail. If you are anticipating an exposé on how physicians' children receive elitist care, you may be a bit disappointed, however. More than two thirds of the children in this report who had a physician parent were evaluated in the ED by a resident or medical student. It is also reassuring that children with a physician parent appear to have similar lengths of visits and similar rates of laboratory studies and radiographs as other children. Nonetheless, statistically speaking, children of a physician parent *are* less likely to see a resident or medical student. One could not tell from reading this article whether the difference in how a child with a physician parent is treated relates to the desires of the child's parent or to the ED staff.

The increased frequency with which children with a physician parent bypass medical students and residents raises several issues. The child who is directly triaged to a specialist benefits in terms of convenience and comfort. Such a child will face fewer questions and will have fewer examinations, but it is also possible that such direct referrals may not serve a child's best interest. For example, a direct referral to a surgeon for abdominal pain benefits the child if the problem is ultimately determined to be surgical but shortchanges the child otherwise.

The privilege of practicing medicine has been granted to physicians only after an education that relies on the willingness of patients to allow medical students and residents to care for them. The real issue may well be that such occurrences are potentially unfair to others who seek care in EDs. When an ED staff physician is busy caring for a physician's child, trainees may not have ready access to the person with whom they must discuss their patients. Emergency staff physicians may be unable to devote as much attention to the patients being cared for by the house staff.

This report teaches us that the motto "Do as I say, not as I do" applies to doctors and their children in the ED. Maybe it's possible that what goes on in Seattle doesn't go on throughout the rest of the United States. Such fanciful thinking aside, physicians who require different care for their own children in the ED are not very good role models for those who may follow in their footsteps.

The Preparedness of Pediatricians for Emergencies in the Office: What Is Broken, Should We Care, and How Can We Fix It?
Flores G, Weinstock DJ (Boston Univ; Shady Grove Adventist Hosp, Rockville, Md)
Arch Pediatr Adolesc Med 150:249–256, 1996   5–18

Background.—Although children with life-threatening medical emergencies are regularly brought to pediatricians' offices, few studies have examined the preparedness of office pediatricians for handling such emergencies. The frequency of pediatric practice emergencies, the level of office preparedness, and pediatricians' reasons for lack of preparedness were investigated.

Methods and Findings.—Data were obtained from 51 pediatric practices in Fairfield County, Connecticut. In total, these offices reported handling more than 2,400 emergencies annually. The median number of emergencies per practice per year was 24. Fourteen percent of eligible staff were certified in basic life support and 17% in pediatric advanced life support. Many offices lacked emergency equipment. Twenty-seven percent of the offices surveyed had no oxygen; 27%, no IV catheters; 29%, no bag-valve mask; 33%, no nebulizers; 53%, no epinephrine 1:10,000; and 55%, no IV fluids. Seventy-three percent of the offices had the minimum recommended equipment and training for status asthmaticus management. Only 33% of the offices had similar preparation for each of 6 other emergencies. Few offices were well prepared for emergencies. Pediatricians believed that office emergencies were rare. Also, these busy, cost-conscious pediatricians believed that high-level emergency preparedness was difficult to achieve.

Conclusions.—Emergencies occur commonly in pediatric practices. Unfortunately, achieving adequate levels of preparedness is difficult. Pediatricians must be made more aware of the need for such preparedness.

▶ It's hard to argue that the concept of "semper fidelis" should not apply to the pediatric office setting. Nonetheless, a number of pediatricians are not adequately prepared, nor are their environments adequately prepared, to handle true emergencies that might show up on their office doorsteps. Why is this?

* Is it because emergencies are rarely seen? Hardly. This report documents median of 24 emergency visits per pediatric practice annually, averaging 2 per month. At least 1 emergency occurs per month in 82% of pediatric practices. Some practices have a black cloud (25% had more than 50 emergencies per year; 12% of practices had more than 100 emergencies per year).

* Is it because we are too busy? Everyone is busier than they would like. Have you ever, however, run into somebody who is too busy to attend their own funeral? To say this differently, some things are too important to be left unattended to.

* Is it that we can't afford to have the required equipment? It's hard to imagine that we can afford not to because all it takes is an initial investment of about $550 to stock an office with the minimum equipment and medications necessary for initial stabilization and management of the most common emergencies. If you're in an office setting that sees a lot of heavy-duty emergencies, an initial investment of about $6,000 would cover all the equipment and medications necessary, including pulse oximeters and defibrillators.

* Is it possible that we don't have time to maintain our skills in life support and emergency care? Basic life support certification does require a 1-day course and 1 day each year for annual recertification. Pediatric advanced life support certification requires 2 days, and recertification consists of a 1-day course every 2 years. These are significant commitments, but they do payoff.

The punch line of this report is obvious. The office setting in which we practice needs to be ready for most any emergency. Not only does the office have to be ready, we need to be ready. Of course, not every pediatrician in a multigroup practice needs to maintain these skills, but those who don't probably ought not to allow themselves to be in situations where the lack of such skills (or equipment/medications) will result in adverse patient care. To learn more about what the Committee on Pediatric Emergency Medicine of our Academy says about all this, obtain the published guidelines that the American Academy of Pediatrics provides.[1] The Institute of Medicine has also recently published extensive guidelines and includes short lists of recommended equipment and training for pediatric emergency care.[2]

References

1. *Emergency Medical Services for Children: The Role of the Primary Care Provider.* Elk Grove Village, Ill, American Academy of Pediatrics, 1992.
2. Committee on Pediatric Emergency and Medical Services. Division of Health Care Services, Institute of Medicine: *Emergency Medical Services for Children.* Washington, DC, National Academy Press, 1993

Adults in the Pediatric Emergency Department: A Fish Out of Water?
Hayes A, Reynolds S, Davis AT (Children's Mem Hosp, Chicago)
Pediatr Emerg Care 11:170–172, 1995   5–19

Background.—Adults occasionally come to the pediatric emergency department (PED) with acute problems. It is unknown whether PED staff physicians have adequate training to manage adult problems. An evaluation of adult patients who initially came to one PED was presented.

Methods.—All patients older than 17 years of age who were seen in the PED of 1 children's hospital during a 1-year period were studied. The patients were classified as new—having no previous medical care association with the hospital—or chronic—adult patients receiving follow-up care in hospital clinics for chronic problems. The spectrum of illness of these patients was evaluated. Quality of care and patient satisfaction were assessed by a follow-up telephone call or written survey.

Results.—Three hundred eighty-four adult patients, representing 0.9% of patients seen during the study year, were identified. The median patient age was 21 years, and 49% of the patients were men. Most were seen between 3 PM and 11 PM, and 84% were triaged as urgent or emergent care patients. One hundred forty patients were classified as new and 230 as chronic; the remaining 14 were unclassifiable.

In the new patient group, the mean age was 33 years. Fifty-three percent of these patients were hospital employees, and 40% had pre-existing illnesses. Cardiac or hypertensive problems were the most common problem type in this group (27%). Other common problems included blunt trauma in 22% of patients, eye splash in 13%, and lacerations in 9% (Table 2). Transfer to an adult hospital was made for 48% of patients, and

TABLE 2.—New Patient

Diagnosis category	%
Cardiac/hypertension	27
Minor trauma	22
Eye injury/splash	13
Lacerations	9
Asthma	5
Obstetrics/Gynecology	4
Other*	20

*Gastroenterology, neurology, psychology, metabolic disorder, and dermatology.
(Courtesy of Hayes A, Reynolds S, Davis AT: Adults in the pediatric emergency department: A fish out of water? *Pediatr Emerg Care* 11:170–172, 1995.)

20% of those transferred were admitted. The chronic patients were younger, with a mean age of 21 years. Fever or infection accounted for 37% of the problems in this group, followed by minor trauma in 17%, and gastrointestinal problems in 12%. Thirty-six percent of the chronic patients were admitted. New patients spent an average of 70 minutes in the PED, and chronic patients spent 202 minutes. The adult patients generally perceived their care as adequate.

Conclusions.—The problem of adults initially coming to the PED was studied. The chronic-type adult patients seen in this setting have problems similar to those of pediatric patients, and PED physicians have the preparation to manage them. In contrast, new patients have adult problems, such as chest pain and hypertension, that the PED physician should be prepared to manage.

▶ One of the scariest things for a highly trained pediatric resident, and even someone who has completed residency training, is the sudden appearance of an adult seeking care that must be provided. As a house officer, this editor recalls being called to the emergency department to see a hospital employee who was having a seizure. Although he got the correct management (he turned out to be a diabetic with hypoglycemia), the experience was unnerving.

This report shows how frequently adults do initially come to a PED. This busy PED in a children's hospital in Chicago sees about 10 adult patients per month. Obviously, many of these are patients who have been followed in their own institution since childhood, but many are not.

The conclusion of this report suggests that pediatric emergency medicine residents must become skilled in the care of the most commonly encountered adult problems that might be seen in a PED. This editor agrees with this conclusion but assumes that acquiring such familiarity and skill does not require becoming an adult emergency medicine specialist. There just isn't enough time in the curriculum to do that. Furthermore, one must realize that the experience summarized in the abstract is hardly typical. The Children's Memorial Hospital in Chicago is a free-standing children's hospital that is more than 2 miles from its adult affiliate institution. Most PEDs are in hospitals that have adult services. Even those children's hospitals that do not are usually a stone's throw away from such facilities. Take, for example, the Children's Hospital of Philadelphia. There, adults (older than 18 years, not followed in their institution) account for only 0.01% of all PED visits, even though the Children's Hospital of Philadelphia is a free-standing pediatric hospital. The hospital of the University of Pennsylvania, an adult facility, is just around the corner.

Pediatric emergency departments will always be instruments of care, on infrequent occasions, for adults. Common sense would indicate that the infrequency of these contacts should not drive pediatric training programs to produce adult emergency medicine–qualified individuals. Trainees should be as comfortable as possible, however, with the type of care that they are providing. Yes, adults in the PED are fish out of water. As pediatricians, we need to know something about adult care so we won't get in hot water; we just don't need to go overboard in learning how to do it.

"Adult" Trauma Surgeons With Pediatric Commitment: A Logical Solution to the Pediatric Trauma Manpower Problem

D'Amelio LF, Hammond JS, Thomasseau J, et al (Robert Wood Johnson Med School, New Brunswick, NJ)
Am Surg 61:968–974, 1995   5–20

Background.—The medical community has recently recognized the need for organized pediatric trauma care. Most guidelines stipulate that a pediatric surgeon should direct efforts in pediatric trauma care. However, there are currently not enough pediatric surgeons. Mortality, discharge disposition, and operative frequency were investigated in one series of children cared for by nonpediatric surgeons at a level I trauma center.

Methods and Findings.—Four hundred twenty-four children were studied. Their mean age was 10 years, and mean Injury Severity Score was 11.5. The critical care surgeons involved treated Major Trauma Outcome Study (MTOS)–comparable patients with outcomes similar to MTOS. Neurosurgeons were the only other specialists who treated an MTOS-comparable population. For all patients, the z statistic was $+0.17$, and the m statistic, 0.908. Eighteen children died, resulting in an actuarial survival of 95.8%. Two children expected to die did not, and 1 expected to live did not. Seventy-three percent of the survivors had age-appropriate locomotion.

Conclusions.—Outcomes among children with traumatic injuries treated by nonpediatric surgeons compare favorably with national standards. Because of these outcomes and the paucity of available pediatric trauma surgeons, the recommendation that pediatric trauma care be directed by pediatric surgeons should be modified.

▶ This report teaches us how to make do in a less-than-perfect world, characterized by the presence of relatively few pediatric surgeons. The 1996 American Board of Medical Specialties Directory of Certified Physicians lists just 532 board-certified pediatric surgeons in this country. Compare this number with the number of pediatric deaths from trauma (25,000) that occur annually in the United States. Additionally, there are more than 600,000 children hospitalized with trauma every year. To say this differently, every pediatric surgeon in the United States would be operating on 3 children with trauma every day of the year just to keep up with the load. It would be impossible.

What this study tells us is that "adult" surgeons can provide pediatric trauma care at at least level I center activities.

It does seem reasonable that not every child requiring surgery as a result of trauma needs the care and expertise of a pediatric surgeon. If one is available, terrific. If not, others will have to do their best to fill the void. Given the limited number of pediatric surgery fellowships available, there may not be any alternative but to accept the conclusions of this report.

Economic Comparison of a Tissue Adhesive and Suturing in the Repair of Pediatric Facial Lacerations

Osmond MH, Klassen TP, Quinn JV (Univ of Ottawa, Ontario)
J Pediatr 126:892–895, 1995

5–21

Background.—Children are commonly seen in the emergency department (ED) for facial lacerations. The 3 methods most widely used to repair these injuries in children are with nondissolving sutures, dissolving sutures, and tissue adhesive. The relative cost-effectiveness of these methods was investigated.

Methods.—The costs of equipment, pharmaceuticals, health care worker time, and parental loss of income for follow-up visits were included in the cost calculation for each method. The preferences and willingness to pay for each wound closure method were determined in a convenience sample of 30 parents in the ED.

Findings.—The cost per patient of switching from the standard nondissolving sutures to tissue adhesive was reduced by $49.60 and to dissolving sutures, $37.90, in Canadian dollars (Table 2). Ninety percent of the parents surveyed preferred adhesive, and 10% preferred dissolving sutures. Almost all parents ranked nondissolving sutures as third among the 3 wound closure methods. If only dissolving sutures were provided, parents were willing to pay a median of $40 for adhesive and $25 for dissolving sutures.

TABLE 2.—Estimated Cost per Patient in Each Treatment Group

| | Cost per patient ($) | | |
	Nondissolving sutures	Dissolving sutures	Tissue adhesive
ED physician	7.80	7.80	3.95
ED assistant	2.60	2.60	1.32
Pharmacy	0.14	0.14	3.00
Supplies	5.13	9.76	0.33
Follow-up physician visit	16.25	—	—
Parental costs	26.28	—	—
Total*	58.20	20.30	8.60
Incremental cost†	—	($37.90)	($49.60)
Cost per year‡	36,084	12,586	5,332
Incremental cost per year†	—	(23,498)	(30,752)

* Excluding costs of emergency department (*ED*) registration and overhead and parental wages lost during the initial ED visit.

† Values in parentheses indicate that by changing treatments, fewer resources would be consumed.

‡ Based on 620 simple facial lacerations per year.

(Courtesy of Osmond MH, Klassen TP, Quinn JV: Economic comparison of a tissue adhesive and suturing in the repair of pediatric facial lacerations. *J Pediatr* 126:892–895, 1995.)

Conclusions.—The use of tissue adhesive for children with facial lacerations results in the most cost-effective use of resources. Also, most parents prefer this wound closure method over nondissolving and dissolving methods.

▶ Nothing argues for success like success. Gluing a laceration together is cheaper and more acceptable to parents than traditional suturing. In fact, it is $49.60 cheaper than traditional suturing if you figure in incidentals such as lost wages on the part of a parent. The institution from which this report comes estimates that the use of tissue glue would save patients receiving care at their facility some $30,752 each year (extrapolated to all of Canada, this would amount to about $1 million countrywide).

Please note that this is not the first report that shows how beneficial the use of wound adhesives is. A report from Guy's Hospital in London[1] shows that cyanoacrylate glue is a satisfactory agent to close relatively minor (not deep) lacerations. In this early report, the investigators demonstrated that after appropriate cleansing and drying, all you need to do is approximate the edge of a wound with your fingertips and then glue the wound together. In a group of 50 children with lacerations less than 3 cm, instead of suturing or "Steri-stripping," the physicians simply applied glue to the skin edges. The majority of children had very good responses, did not require dressings, and healed within just a few days. When these British reports first appeared, the Food and Drug Administration (FDA), upon learning of the medical application of this type of adhesive, became "unglued" and initially stated that cyanoacrylate glues should not be approved for use in the United States. Fortunately, the FDA has seen the light, and "crazy glue" is here to stay.

For what it's worth, orthopedic surgeons have long been using methacrylate cement to stabilize the spines of patients with metastatic cancer involving bone. It has mended broken bones. Broken hearts are next.

Reference

1. Watson DP: *BMJ* 299:1014, 1989.

Factors That Influence an Anesthesiologist's Decision to Cancel Elective Surgery for the Child With an Upper Respiratory Tract Infection
Tait AR, Reynolds PI, Gutstein HB (Univ of Michigan, Ann Arbor)
J Clin Anesth 7:491–499, 1995
5–22

Purpose.—The question of whether to administer anesthesia for an elective surgical procedure in the child with an upper respiratory infection (URI) has always been a vexing one. Usual practice has been to postpone surgery for fear of increasing intraoperative respiratory complications and postoperative morbidity, although there are few outcome data on this issue. Factors considered by anesthesiologists as they decide whether to cancel elective surgery for children with URIs were studied.

Methods.—A questionnaire was mailed to 400 members of the Society for Pediatric Anesthesia across the United States. They were asked about the factors they considered in deciding to cancel elective surgery for pediatric patients with URIs. The response rate was 54%.

Results.—Thirty-five percent of anesthesiologists reported that they seldom canceled pediatric surgery because of URI (i.e., no more than 25% of the time) and 21% that they usually did (i.e., more than 75% of the time). One percent of respondents said that they never canceled a surgery for this reason, and 3% said that they always did. Most of the anesthesiologists used IV hydration for pediatric surgical patients with URIs, and nearly half occasionally used regional rather than general anesthesia (Fig 2). Although the respondents' type of practice had no effect on their likelihood of cancellation, those who had been in practice for longer than 10 years were significantly more likely to cancel.

The most important factors in making the decision to cancel were the urgency of the operation and the presence of asthma. Concern about complications and personal experience in anesthetizing children with URIs were also cited as important considerations, but factors related to economics and inconvenience were not (Table 3).

Conclusions.—Pediatric anesthesiologists differ in their opinions as to whether elective surgery should be canceled for the child with a URI. The approach to this issue may be changing, as younger anesthesiologists seem

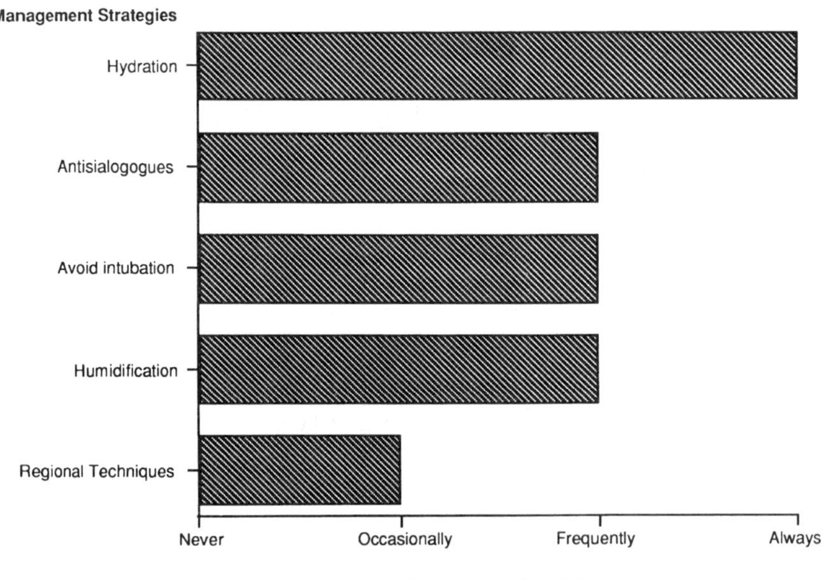

FIGURE 2.—Types and frequencies of management techniques used by anesthesiologists when anesthetizing the patient with an upper respiratory infection. (Reprinted by permission of the publisher from Tait AR, Reynolds PI, Gutstein HB: Factors that influence an anesthesiologist's decision to cancel elective surgery for the child with an upper respiratory tract infection. *J Clin Anesth* 7:491–499, Copyright 1995 by Elsevier Science Inc.)

TABLE 3.—Degree to Which Anesthesiologists Consider Different Factors in Making Decisions Regarding Cancellation of the Patient With a URI

		Never	Occasionally	Frequently	Always
			n (%)		
a.	Distance travelled by patient/family	62 (30.1)	120 (58.3)*	22 (10.7)	2 (0.9)
b.	Urgency of surgery	2 (0.9)	20 (9.7)	84 (41.0)	10 (48.8)*
c.	Length of surgery	53 (26.1)	93 (45.8)*	52 (25.6)	5 (2.5)
d.	Pressure to complete cases expediently	136 (66.0)*	69 (33.5)	1 (0.5)	0 (0.0)
e.	Site of surgery	24 (11.6)	92 (44.4)*	76 (36.7)	15 (7.3)
f.	Procedure requiring intubation	26 (12.6)	67 (32.4)	93 (44.9)*	21 (10.1)
g.	Patient has asthma	5 (2.4)	47 (23.0)	72 (35.1)	81 (39.5)*
h.	Number of times the surgery has been cancelled previously due to URI	45 (21.8)	103 (50.0)*	51 (24.8)	7 (3.4)
i.	Cost of rescheduling a patient with a URI	119 (57.2)*	74 (35.6)	12 (5.8)	3 (1.4)
j.	Fear of perioperative complications	6 (2.9)	52 (25.0)	85 (40.9)*	65 (31.2)
k.	Fear of potential litigation	88 (42.7)*	82 (39.8)	24 (11.7)	12 (5.8)
l.	Attitude of patient/family	48 (23.3)	109 (52.9)*	36 (17.5)	13 (6.3)
m.	Inpatient versus outpatient	100 (48.5)*	81 (39.3)	22 (10.7)	3 (1.5)
n.	Past experience anesthetizing patients with a URI	13 (6.3)	54 (26.1)	85 (41.0)*	55 (26.6)
o.	Results from published studies	15 (7.2)	95 (45.7)*	74 (35.6)	24 (11.5)

*Indicates the most frequently reported responses (mode).
Abbreviation: URI, upper respiratory infection.
(Reprinted by permission of the publisher from Tait AR, Reynolds RI, Gutstein HB: Factors that influence an anesthesiologist's decision to cancel elective surgery for the child with an upper respiratory tract infection. *J Clin Anesth* 7:491–499, Copyright 1995 by Elsevier Science Inc.)

less likely to cancel. By identifying the important factors in this decision, the study may help to provide a more standardized approach to the decision-making process and to reduce the potential for unnecessary cancellations.

▶ Most of us were trained to believe that elective surgery should be canceled when a child has a cold on the day of surgery. The concern is that URI may be associated with complications of anesthesia. Unfortunately, there is very little information regarding outcome in patients with URIs who undergo elective procedures. Do such patients have an increased risk of laryngospasm, bronchospasm, atelectasis, or postoperative desaturation? Upon reviewing all the data, there is no convincing evidence that a common cold is a reason for canceling surgery. Because children have an average of 3–8 URIs per year, it is sometimes impossible to avoid elective surgery just because of a cold. Once an elective surgical procedure is canceled, it will be rescheduled most likely in 3 or 4 weeks...in time for another cold.

What this report does is tell us, absent any information about real risks of anesthetic complications, what anesthesiologists do with all these ambiguities. It seems that the older you are as an anesthesiologist, the more cautious you are. Younger anesthesiologists are much more comfortable with "putting a child under" even though he or she has a cold.

Chances are that even though you as a practitioner don't do much in the way of surgery, you do get calls from parents of a child with a cold 1 or 2 days before elective surgery asking you whether you think the surgery should still go on. Although you obviously pass this query off to the anesthesiologist or the surgeon, you should be able to predict, based on the results of this study, what the answer will be. If the anesthesiologist is younger than 35 years of age and your patient simply has a cold, odds are the patient shortly will be under the knife, cold or no cold.

The Cost of Implementation of the Clinical Laboratory Improvement Amendments of 1988: The Example of Pediatric Office-based Cholesterol Screening
Tershakovec AM, Brannon SD, Bennett MJ, et al (Children's Hosp of Philadelphia; Pennsylvania State Univ, University Park; Univ of Texas Southwestern Med Ctr, Dallas)
Pediatrics 96:230–234, 1995   5–23

Introduction.—The Clinical Laboratory Improvement Amendments of 1988 (CLIA '88)—stimulated in part by reports of inaccurate results of office laboratory testing—include performance of proficiency testing criteria for office-based laboratories. Cholesterol testing is a source of potential inaccuracies in some extra-laboratory settings. The example of cholesterol screening for children was used to assess the additional costs of implementing CLIA '88 in the office-based laboratory.

Methods.—The study included 7 pediatric practices that screened 4- to 10-year-old children for hypercholesterolemia during well-child visits. Data on the volume of testing were used to calculate the average number of screenings per day and days per month. Information on nurses' and technicians' time in the screening process and on salary and fringe benefit rates was used to assess personnel costs. The cost estimates included the costs of supplies, analysis of control samples, instrument calibration, and instrument depreciation. Relevant proficiency testing and laboratory inspection programs were then used to calculate the costs of implementing CLIA '88.

Results.—Six of the practices performed a low volume of tests, screening a total of 2,807 children during the 4-month study period, or 5 or 6 per week. The seventh practice screened a total of 414 children—about 25 per week—after implementing universal screening. The cost of screening per child was $10.60 at the low-volume practices and $5.47 at the high-volume practice. The additional costs of CLIA '88 implementation were estimated at $3.20 per test at the low-volume practices and $0.71 per test at the high-volume practice.

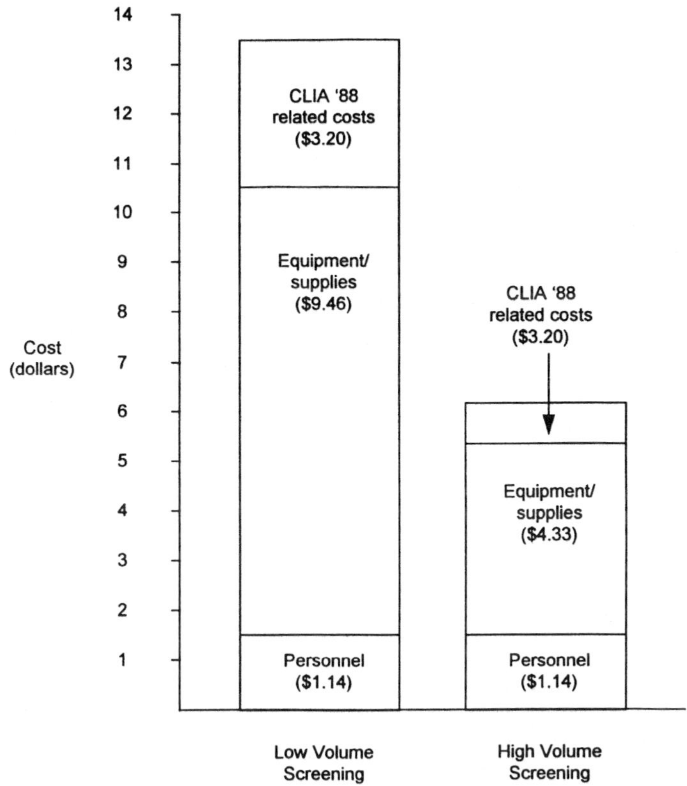

FIGURE.—Contributing costs of high- and low-volume cholesterol screening. *Abbreviation: CLIA* '88, Clinical Laboratory Improvement Amendments of 1988. (Courtesy of Tershakovec AM, Brannon SD, Bennett MJ, et al: The cost of implementation of the Clinical Laboratory Improvement Amendments of 1988: The example of pediatric office-based cholesterol screening. Reproduced by permission of *Pediatrics,* Vol 96, pp 230–234, Copyright 1995.)

Conclusions.—The example of pediatric office-based cholesterol screening shows that implementation of CLIA '88—including additional proficiency testing and laboratory inspection—will make a significant addition to the costs of office-based laboratory testing. However, the cost of testing remains reasonable, even with the additional expense. The impact of implementing CLIA '88 is very sensitive to the volume of tests performed (Figure).

▶ With all of the CLIA bashing that goes on these days, it's almost (but not quite) refreshing to see a report in a legitimate journal that suggests that CLIA isn't all that bad. In fact, the authors of this article probably have stuck their necks out by saying as much as they did in support of the CLIA recommendations, at least with respect to the modest cost involved with implementing CLIA requirements regarding cholesterol screening.

The American Academy of Pediatrics and the American Medical Association have recommended repeal or significant modifications of the CLIA '88 regulations. These recommendations were largely based on the anticipated cost of implementing these regulations. One study supported by the American Hospital Association, the American Medical Association, the Health Industry Manufacturers Association, and the Health Industry Distribution Association concluded that the nationwide cost of the first year of implementation of CLIA would be $409 million.[1] Based on information provided by the Health Care Financing Administration, the cost to a medical practice of individual laboratory implementation for relatively simple tests, such as cholesterol levels, has been estimated at over $4,200 for the first year alone. If the report abstracted truly has validity, these estimates may have been exaggerated.

In prior commentaries, this editor has expressed his dismay (more like disdain) for CLIA. The only reason CLIA has existed is because many practice medicine, and carry out laboratory testing, without decent quality assurance. If quality assurance procedures had been in place in office laboratories, there would probably be no CLIA right now. Unfortunately, CLIA swings the pendulum too far the other way. Maybe the solution is simply to stop the clock, at least for awhile, and let things settle down. After all, if nothing else, deregulation is in.

References

1. Fleischman D: *AAP News* June 1992.

Pediatric Emergency Physician Interpretation of Plain Radiographs: Is Routine Review by a Radiologist Necessary and Cost-effective?
Simon HK, Khan NS, Nordenberg DF, et al (Emory Univ, Atlanta, Ga)
Ann Emerg Med 27:295–298, 1996   5–24

Background.—There is wide variation in the radiologic services available in the pediatric emergency department. More than one third of programs may not have overnight access to interpretation by a radiologist or radiologic resident. Pediatric emergency physicians' interpretations of plain radiographs in children were compared with those of pediatric radiologists.

Methods.—The prospective study included 707 plain radiographic examinations in children performed in the emergency department of an urban tertiary care children's hospital. All films were read by a pediatric emergency physician, then reviewed within 24 hours by a pediatric radiologist. The 2 sets of interpretations were analyzed for concordance. The impact of incorrect interpretations on patient management was assessed, together with the necessity of cost-effectiveness of having a radiologist review all plain radiographs.

Results.—The most common types of radiographs were chest, 56%; skeletal, excluding the spine, 20%; and abdomen, 12%. The interpretations of the pediatric emergency physicians and pediatric radiologists agreed in 90% of cases, and clinical management was unchanged in 97%. Forty-eight of 69 discordant readings were considered clinically significant, and 22 led to changes in management. The pediatric emergency physicians made 9 false negative interpretations, including 5 fractures, 2 cases of pneumonia, and 1 case each of sinusitis and cardiomegaly. The pediatric emergency physicians also made 10 false positive interpretations: 5 fractures, 4 cases of pneumonia, and 1 case of sinusitis. They made 3 false positive interpretations: 1 case each of C2 spine subluxation, 1 retropharyngeal abscess, and 1 case of necrotizing enterocolitis. However, the misreadings did not lead to any adverse outcomes for the patients. It cost an estimated $210,000 per year to have all films reviewed by a radiologist.

Conclusion.—Pediatric emergency physicians are generally accurate in interpreting plain radiographs, and there are few management changes or adverse outcomes when misreadings do occur. The interpretation of children's radiographs in the emergency department setting is probably aided by the fact that the interpreter has performed a clinical assessment. Pediatric emergency care might be made more cost effective through judicious consultation with a radiologist during initial evaluation of high-risk patients, at the discretion of the pediatric emergency physician.

▶ When one recognizes that, on average, 1 patient in 5 who visits a pediatric emergency department will eventually have an x-ray study made before discharge from the facility, one can readily see the magnitude of the issue surrounding the necessity of having a trained radiologist look at each film. The trick would be to figure out which patient among the many who undergo x-ray examination are the ones who really need a radiologist as a backup to a board-certified/board-eligible pediatric emergency-trained physician. The latter are quite good at reading x-ray films as their interpretations were correct over 90% of the time in this series. Where overreading or underreading was done, no adverse clinical outcomes actually resulted.

So is it worth $210,000 per year to have a radiologist read all the films for a pediatric emergency department? Given that 4 eyes are better than 2 and given the potential negative consequences of just 1 seriously bad outcome as a result of underinterpretation or overinterpretation by an emergency department physician, the answer is likely to be "yes." Even though we are currently doing an excellent job in training emergency department physicians, more attention should be paid to reading x-ray films. It is patently obvious that the eyes cannot interpret what the mind is unprepared to.

Quiz: What is the true marginal cost when a nonurgent patient is seen in the emergency department setting? The answer to this query is not available, as yet, for pediatric emergency departments. For adult emergency departments, the true marginal cost of a nonemergent/nonurgent emergency department visit is just $24. A marginal cost is the extra cost of seeing an additional patient in an emergency department that is already staffed and waiting and is seeing other patients at the same time.[1]

Reference

1. Williams RM: *N Engl J Med* 334:642, 1996.

Physical and Mental Development in 4–6-year-old Triplets

Åkerman BA, Hovmöller M, Rådestad A, et al (Karolinska Hosp, Stockholm)
Acta Paediatr 84:661–666, 1995   5–25

Objective.—The incidence of triplet births has increased, as have the chances of good obstetric and neonatal outcomes. However, these infants can still cause problems because of their prematurity and need for neonatal care, and because of the strain on the family. The physical and mental development of triplets were assessed when the children were 4–6 years old.

Patients.—Twenty-one families with complete sets of triplets born within 200 km of Stockholm between 1986 and 1989 were invited to participate in the study. After 4 families declined to participate, 17 sets of triplets born at 11 different hospitals were studied. Seven of the mothers had undergone fertility treatments. Average gestational age at birth was 35 weeks, and 13 of the women were delivered by cesarean section. The mean birth weight was 2,104 g in 28 boys and 1,882 g in 23 girls. Eleven of the infants were small for gestational age (SGA). None of the children had asphyxia or other major complications at the time of delivery.

Methods.—At a mean age of 4 years 5 months, the triplets underwent a complete neurologic examination and assessment on the Griffiths mental developmental scales (GMDS). These assessments were performed in the homes of the families.

Findings.—None of the children had any major physical disabilities or malformations. Visual problems were present in 9 children. Nineteen of the triplets had a history of treatment for otitis media, often repeated. Mental development was not significantly affected by birth order or sex, although quotients tended to be lower for triplets with birth weights of less than 2,000 g. The lack of a significant difference by sex was in contrast to previous studies of singletons and twins. For the triplets who were SGA at birth, total GMDS score and most subscale scores were significantly lower than those of their siblings. Mental development was no different for the triplets from assisted conceptions vs. those from spontaneous conceptions.

Conclusions.—At 4–6 years of age, most triplets appear to have similar physical and mental development to twins and singletons of the same birth weight (Table 7). Triplets who are born SGA may not have the same level of mental development as their siblings. The results of interviews with the triplets' parents will be published in another paper, and the authors plan further follow-up of the triplets once they reach school age.

▶ Having triplets is not as unique as it once was. This is largely a reflection of the increase in assisted pregnancies. The importance of this study from Sweden is that it puts together a very large series of triplets and tells us how well these youngsters do half a decade after birth. They seem to do very well. The only disclaimer is that those who are SGA do not appear to have the same level of mental development as their peers. This aside, physically and intellectually, triplets seem to be faring okay. Additionally, they don't

TABLE 7.—Comparison Between Performance (GMDS) in Singletons, Twins, and Triplets With Birth Weights < 2,500 g

Scale	Triplets (n = 47)		Twins* (n = 37)		Singletons† (n = 11)		T/diff.
A (locomotor)	100.0	(15.3)	94.4	(13.2)	93.8	(14.9)	ns
B (personal-social)	98.3‡	(12.5)	101.4	(13.7)	107.6‡	(13.4)	‡(Tr<S)
C (hearing and speech)	97.5	(12.6)	105.6	(17.0)	94.6	(13.4)	ns
D (eye and hand coordination)	100.9	(14.0)	96.2	(16.0)	101.9	(18.8)	ns
E (performance)	101.3	(13.0)	95.7	(14.8)	104.6	(19.1)	ns
F (practical reasoning)	94.1	(10.7)	98.1	(15.7)	97.7	(14.9)	ns
Total	98.9	(8.9)	98.5	(12.5)	100.0	(10.7)	ns

Note: Values are mean (SD).
*From a 4-year follow-up study of twins published in 1991.
†From a 4-year follow-up study of singletons published in 1994.
‡$P < 0.05$.
Abbreviation: GMDS, Griffiths mental development scales.
(Courtesy of Åkerman BA, Hovmöller M, Rådestad A, et al: Physical and mental development in 4–6-year-old triplets. *Acta Paediatr* 84:661–666, 1995.)

even seem to suffer from the entity that has become known as "deprivation of individuality." to the degree that has been seen in the past.[1] The latter entity refers to the fact that when a parent or parents have more than 1 infant of the same age, it's harder for them to relate to each infant individually, which is necessary for normal personal-social development. Fortunately, triplets do get enough individual attention to turn out all right, even though they probably have to compete for attention, stimulation, and love. One very positive spin of being a triplet is that your parents are not likely to get divorced (there was only 1 divorce in this entire series). The likely explanation for the low divorce rate is that the parents probably can't afford to get divorced.

The fact that triplets in Sweden thrive physically and intellectually invalidates the old saying that two's company, three's a crowd. Three infants at one time are a handful, but apparently parents and infants survive the stress, and survive it very nicely.

Reference

1. Rowland C: Family relationship, in: Harvey D, Bryan R (eds): *The Stress of Multiple Births*. London, Multiple Births Foundation, 1991.

Dimeric Inhibin A as a Marker for Down's Syndrome in Early Pregnancy

Aitken DA, Wallace EM, Crossley JA, et al (Duncan Guthrie Inst of Med Genetics, Glasgow, Scotland; Univ of Edinburgh, Scotland; Ctr for Reproductive Biology, Edinburgh, Scotland, et al)
N Engl J Med 334:1231–1236, 1996   5–26

Purpose.—Markers commonly used in screening for Down syndrome in the second trimester of pregnancy include α-fetoprotein, β–human chorionic gonadotropin, and intact human chorionic gonadotropin. Efforts to improve biochemical screening for Down syndrome focus on finding better markers and the possibility of first-trimester screening. Dimeric inhibin A was studied as a potential new marker of Down syndrome in early pregnancy.

Methods.—Serum samples were obtained between the seventh and eighteenth week of gestation from 3 groups of pregnant women: 58 whose fetuses had known Down syndrome, 32 whose fetuses had known trisomy 18, and 438 whose fetuses were normal. Concentrations of α-fetoprotein, β–human chorionic gonadotropin, intact human chorionic gonadotropin, and dimeric inhibin A were measured in each sample. The values for each marker were converted to multiples of the median at a given length of gestation in normal pregnancies. Multivariate analysis was performed to determine the ability of inhibin A screening to detect Down syndrome, in combination with the various other markers.

Results.—Serum inhibin A concentrations in women with Down syndrome pregnancies were 2.06 times higher than the median value in women with normal pregnancies. By comparison, values in the Down syndrome group were 2.00 times the normal median for β–human chorionic gonadotropin, 1.82 times the median for intact human chorionic gonadotropin, and 0.72 times the median for α-fetoprotein. Serum inhibin A concentrations in the Down syndrome pregnancies did not rise above normal until the end of the first trimester. In the trisomy 18 pregnancies,

TABLE 4.—Detection Rates for Down Syndrome at a Constant 5% False Positive Rate for Various Combinations of Serum Markers and Maternal Age

VARIABLES	DETECTION RATE (%)	95% CI
Alpha-fetoprotein and age	33	19–48
Intact human chorionic gonadotropin and age	41	26–57
β Subunit of human chorionic gonadotropin and age	47	32–63
Inhibin A and age	48	32–63
Alpha-fetoprotein, intact human chorionic gonadotropin, and age	54	38–69
Alpha-fetoprotein, β subunit of human chorionic gonadotropin, and age	53	37–68
Alpha-fetoprotein, inhibin A, and age	57	41–72
Intact human chorionic gonadotropin, inhibin A, and age	57	41–72
β Subunit of human chorionic gonadotropin, inhibin A, and age	68	52–81
Intact human chorionic gonadotropin, β subunit of human chorionic gonadotropin, and age	40	25–56
Alpha-fetoprotein, intact human chorionic gonadotropin, inhibin A, and age	72	57–84
Alpha-fetoprotein, β subunit of human chorionic gonadotropin, inhibin A, and age	75	60–87
Alpha-fetoprotein, intact human chorionic gonadotropin, β subunit of human chorionic gonadotropin, and age	52	36–67

Abbreviation: CI, confidence interval.

(Reprinted by permission of *The New England Journal of Medicine* from Aitken DA, Wallace EM, Crossley JA, et al: Dimeric inhibin A as a marker for Down's syndrome in early pregnancy. *N Engl J Med* 334:1231–1236, Copyright 1996, Massachusetts Medical Society.)

inhibin A values were similar to those in the normal group. The combination of α-fetoprotein, β–human chorionic gonadotropin, and maternal age detected 53% of Down syndrome cases, with a false positive value of 5%. When inhibin A was added to this combination, the detection rate reached 75%, with the same false positive rate (Table 4).

Conclusion.—Adding serum inhibin A concentration to other markers used for second-trimester screening permits detection of 75% of cases of Down syndrome. This finding must be confirmed in larger studies. Inhibin A measurement does not improve the detection of trisomy 18, however.

▶ If you haven't kept close tabs on the literature having to do with maternal screening techniques for detecting pregnancies involving fetuses with Down syndrome, read this report in detail. Since the observation that serum levels of α-fetoprotein were reduced in women with fetuses affected by chromosomal anomalies, numerous other fetoplacental markers in maternal serum that mark pregnancies with affected fetuses have been found. There are several such markers: intact human chorionic gonadotropin, the β-subunit of human chorionic gonadotropin, unconjugated estriol, and α-fetoprotein.

The problem with individual serum markers is the overlap between affected and unaffected populations, so the ability to use any single marker in isolation to detect an affected pregnancy is marginal. The most effective approach to screening is the use of a combination of markers. Most protocols use α-fetoprotein and either intact human chorionic gonadotropin or its β subunit, with or without unconjugated estriol. If you put these markers together with maternal age as a risk factor, you should be able to pick up about two thirds of pregnancies affected by Down syndrome.

The report abstracted here adds to our knowledge of the breadth of markers that can be used to detect Down syndrome in early pregnancy. Dimeric inhibin A appears to be elevated in a high percentage of women carrying affected fetuses. When added to other markers, it adds a significant 22% increase in the rate of detection of Down syndrome. Not bad.

Physician Malpractice: Does the Past Predict the Future?
Taragin MI, Martin K, Shapiro S, et al (Univ of Medicine and Dentistry of New Jersey, New Brunswick; Rutgers Univ, New Brunswick, NJ)
J Gen Intern Med 10:550–556, 1995   5–27

Introduction.—It is still is not clear whether malpractice rates correlate with physician competence. If such an association exists, physicians who have had a high malpractice rate should continue to have a high rate.

Methods.—Rates of malpractice claims were determined for 12,730 physicians who were insured in New Jersey from 1977 to 1991. Physicians insured for 7 years or longer were included in the primary analysis. Physicians having the highest 1%, 5%, or 10% rate of malpractice claims were identified.

TABLE 3.—Physician Claims Experience for Selected Specialties—The First 4 Years vs. the Next 3 Years

Specialty	Physicians	High during First Four Years	Remain High during Next Three Years	Odds Ratio (95% Confidence Interval)
Anesthesiology	352	24	4	1.4 (0.5–4.3)
Dermatology	157	26	3	1.2 (0.3–4.5)
Emergency medicine	121	6	0	—
General surgery	386	42	7	2.2 (0.9–5.2)
Head, eyes, ears, nose, and throat	108	15	3	1.7 (0.4–6.8)
Internal medicine	1,235	207	14	1.0 (0.5–1.7)
Neurosurgery	44	9	4	8.5 (1.7–43.1)
Obstetrics/gynecology	384	44	15	4.4 (2.2–8.5)
Ophthalmology	324	69	10	1.4 (0.7–3.1)
Orthopedics	319	57	12	4.7 (2.2–10.3)
Pathology	121	10	0	—
Pediatrics	486	73	3	0.3 (0.1–0.8)
Plastic surgery	64	14	5	2.9 (0.8–10.8)
Psychiatry	63	8	0	—
Radiology	346	57	6	0.9 (0.3–2.1)
Thoracic/vascular surgery	53	9	3	1.9 (0.4–9.3)
Urology	166	18	2	0.7 (0.2–3.1)
ALL PHYSICIANS	6,300			1.4 (1.1–1.7)

(Courtesy of Taragin MI, Martin K, Shapiro S, et al: Physician malpractice: Does the past predict the future? *J Gen Intern Med* 10:550–556, 1995.)

Results.—Of 55 physicians having the highest malpractice claims rates (representing 1% of the insured population) in the first 4 years, 2 (3.6%) continued in the highest group during the next 3 years. Another 9% were in the very high (5%) group and 20% were in the high (10%) group. Of 260 physicians initially in the very high group, 4% were subsequently in the highest group; 10% were in the very high group; and 18% were in the high group. Of 947 physicians in the high group in the first 4 years, 2.5% were in the highest group, 7% in the very high group, and 12.5% in the high group during the next 3 years. A breakdown by specialty is presented in Table 3.

Implications.—Because most physicians with high malpractice rates subsequently improve, those found to have high rates in any given period should not face disciplinary action. Nevertheless, close scrutiny of those who continue to have high rates will help identify problem physicians.

▶ There is no rhyme or reason to much of what happens in the realm of physician malpractice. This report clearly shows that a history of malpractice claims does not predict a future full of similar problems. Physicians are usually not sued when malpractice does occur and are often sued in circumstances in which they are not at fault. No wonder, then, that this report shows that most physicians who have high malpractice rates over a 4-year period are unlikely to continue to be in a high-risk group subsequently.

One must be cautious when interpreting study results such as these. It is important to identify physicians who do not practice good medicine. A history of malpractice claims does not appear to be a good marker of the problem physician. It's unlikely that the National Practitioner Data Bank will ease the identification of such physicians. As we see in this report, only 0.03% of physicians who are in a high-risk malpractice category remain in such a category during 2 consecutive periods. There must be better ways to identify high-quality and poor-quality practice of medicine. Predicting quality based on malpractice claims is *not* a good way to do this.

This chapter closes with a quiz. According to the *1996 American Board of Medical Specialties Directory of Medical Specialists,* name in rank order the 10 most common surnames of board-certified physicians. The answer to this comes with a list that is not very surprising. It is as follows:

1.   Dr. Smith (2,824)
2.   Dr. Miller (1,956)
3.   Dr. Johnson (1,912)
4.   Dr. Brown (1,534)
5.   Dr. Lee (1,484)
6.   Dr. Jones (1,318)
7.   Dr. Williams (1,313)
8.   Dr. Davis (1,211)
9.   Dr. Cohen (1,070)
10.   Dr. Martin (847)

6 Neurology and Psychiatry

Delayed Central Cord Syndrome After a Handstand in a Child: Case Report
Lee KS, Doh JW, Bae HG, et al (Soonchunhyang Univ Chonan Hosp, Korea)
Paraplegia 34:176–178, 1996   6–1

Introduction.—Pediatric spinal cord injuries account for 1% to 10% of all spinal cord injuries, and pediatric central cord syndrome without radiographic abnormality accounts for less than 1% of all spinal cord injuries. These injuries usually occur with significant trauma. However, a child was seen who experienced delayed central cord syndrome after only trivial trauma. This case study joins only 8 cases previously reported of central cord syndrome resulting from trivial trauma (Table 1).

Case Report.—Girl, 7 years, was brought to the emergency department with sudden respiratory difficulty. Earlier in the day, she had performed several headstands without falling. After 2–3 hours, she had sudden upper thoracic back pain and leg weakness, followed by vomiting and severe dyspnea. She had no other history of trauma. She required immediate resuscitation with intubation and ventilation upon arrival in the emergency department. Although she recovered consciousness, she remained apneic and tetraplegic. There were no abnormal findings on plain cervical radiographs and CT scans of the cervical spine and brain and no CSF abnormalities. She was kept on the ventilator until weaning on the 13th day and extubation on the 15th day. She began moving her legs on the second day, with progressive improvement. She began moving her fingers on the 8th day but had persistent upper extremity weakness. She was able to walk on the 24th day and was discharged from the hospital on the 28th day.

Discussion.—Anatomical and biomechanical characteristics predicting susceptibility to spinal cord injury without radiographic abnormalities in children include hypermobility of the spine associated with lax ligaments, open ossification centers, horizontally oriented articular facet joints, immature joints of Luschka, wedge-shaped vertebral bodies, and a large head

TABLE 1.—Summary of Central Cord Syndrome After Trivial Trauma in Children

Case	Authors	Year	Sex/Age	Type of trauma	Onset	Outcome (FP)
1	Ahman, *et al*	1975	F/4 years	fell from swing	several hours	death (48 days)
2	Ahman, *et al*	1975	M/22 months	fell to floor	4 h	death (6 months)
3	Cheshire	1977	M/26 months	fell backward	overnight	limited ambulation (18 months)
4	Chen, Blaw	1986	F/2 years	fell from crib	1 h	normal (3 months)
5	Chen, Blaw	1986	F/7 years	jumped on bed	overnight	weak UE (6 months)
6	Riviello, *et al*	1990	F/3 years	somersault/fell	30 min	spastic gait (2 years)
7	Riviello, *et al*	1990	F/2 years	fell from sofa	2 h	mild quadriparesis (2 years)
8	Bondurant, Oro	1993	M/27 months	fell from porch	5 min	weak UE (30 months)
9	Lee, *et al*	1995	F/6 years	handstand	2–3 h	weak UE (18 months)

Abbreviations: FP, follow-up period, *UE*, upper extremities.
(Courtesy of Lee KS, Doh JW, Bae HG, et al: Delayed central cord syndrome after a handstand in a child: Case report. *Paraplegia* 34:176–178, 1996.)

associated with underdeveloped neck muscles. These factors may contribute to the development of delayed neurologic deficits caused by a vascular injury with progressive thrombosis after a relatively trivial trauma. Because the progression of these neurologic deficits is rapid, they require prompt diagnosis and respiratory management for patients with apnea.

▶ Who would have ever believed that a 7-year-old standing on her head would experience a central cord syndrome, characterized by clinical evidence of quadriplegia? Before this case was reported, the majority of cases of central cord syndrome had been reported in the elderly with arthritic changes of the spine. In young children, spinal cord injury of the type this child experienced usually results from significant trauma, such as a motor vehicle accident or a fall. Failure in a somersault can cause this as well.[1]

The pathophysiology of this injury includes a primary neuronal or vascular injury or a secondary impairment of spinal cord blood flow. It is also possible that a self-reducing transient subluxation of a juvenile spine can cause neurologic injury and compression of the cord. In all such cases, radiographs of the spine show no abnormalities, giving no clue to the underlying problem—thank goodness for the MRI.

What to do about this problem is unclear. Surgery may be beneficial in a few cases, but conservative management with proper immobilization is the usual route of therapy. The outcome of central cord syndrome in general is good, especially in childhood. An MRI can be quite predictive of outcome. An MRI that shows major cord hemorrhage or cord discontinuity obviously implies a poor prognosis. Good recovery is expected if the MRI shows evidence of edema with or without minor cord hemorrhage. If the initial MRI findings are normal, complete recovery can be expected.

The case of a 7-year-old experiencing a central cord syndrome as a result of a headstand might be considered an oddity were it not for a similar phenomenon reported recently. Take the case of a 31-year-old woman (a dance teacher) who was admitted to the hospital because of acute vertigo preceded by a headache and pain in the neck for a week. A severe throbbing left-sided headache and ipsilateral neck pain developed 48 hours after she rode on a new roller coaster ("Space Mountain" in Disneyland near Paris). This attraction has a loop (360 degrees), a spiral, and an abrupt U-turn. During the ride, this patient's entire body, including her head, was properly protected and she experienced no direct trauma. The pain did not subside, and she suddenly experienced vertigo, nausea, and vomiting. She then experienced the sensation that her body was being pulled to the left. On MRI of the head, a left cerebellar infarct was noted along with dissection of the left vertebral artery. It seems likely that the acceleration and abrupt changes of direction of the roller coaster induced an uncontrolled twisting of the neck and stretching of the cervical blood vessels causing the arterial dissection.[2,3]

So what is the lesson from all this? The lessons are pretty straightforward when it comes to central cord lesions and headstands. Consider such entities the 501st reason not to engage in sporting activities. The head is meant to sit on top of the body, not vice versa. As far as Space Mountain is concerned, avoid it like the plague. When in Paris, try the Eiffel Tower.

References

1. Noguchi T: *Paraplegia* 32:170, 1994.
2. Abbasy BO, et al: *N Engl J Med* 332:1585, 1995.
3. Biousse V, et al: *Lancet* 346:767, 1995.

Twenty-year Experience With Early Surgery for Craniosynostosis: II. The Craniofacial Synostosis Syndromes and Pansynostosis—Results and Unsolved Problems

McCarthy JG, Glasberg SB, Cutting CB, et al (New York Univ)
Plast Reconstr Surg 96:284–295, 1995   6–2

Background.—Recently, fronto-orbital advancement cranial vault remodeling has been performed when patients with craniofacial synostosis are younger than 18 months. However, early surgery has not prevented the midface hypoplasia and class III malocclusion associated with the craniofacial synostosis syndromes. The results and unsolved problems seen in a series of patients who underwent early surgical treatment for pansynostosis and the craniofacial synostosis syndromes were reviewed.

Methods.—The operative experience and photographic and radiographic records were reviewed of 180 patients who underwent surgery before the age of 18 months for the treatment of pansynostosis (7), craniofrontonasal dysplasia (8), Apert syndrome (24), Crouzon syndrome (15), Pfeiffer syndrome (15), and other craniofacial synostosis syndromes.

Results.—In the patients with pansynostosis, the primary procedures, addressing only functional problems (radical vertex craniectomies or strip craniectomy with morcellation), were performed at a mean age of 3.9 months. Six of the 7 patients underwent secondary cranial vault remodeling procedures at a mean age of 8.3 months. Craniofacial form was good or satisfactory in 5; 2 had residual trigonocephaly and scaphocephaly.

In the patients with craniofrontonasal dysplasia, primary procedures, including fronto-orbital advancement (6) and coronal strip craniectomy (2), were performed at a mean age of 5.8 months. Only 1 patient required a secondary fronto-orbital advancement. Of the 8 patients, 5 had good and 1 had acceptable craniofacial form, 1 had residual hypertelorism and poor frontal bone form, and 1 required minor remodeling of the frontal bone.

In the 24 patients with Apert syndrome, primary procedures were performed at a mean age of 6.4 months. Secondary procedures were performed in 9 patients at a mean age of 38.4 months. Midface hypoplasia was evident by the age of 3 years in 16 of these patients, and 9 had a class III malocclusion. A Le Fort III advancement procedure was performed in 10 patients and recommended for 5 more. The results were good or satisfactory in 17 patients; 6 patients had postoperative turricephaly.

There were serious complications in this group, including respiratory obstruction and intracranial pressure problems.

In the 15 patients with Crouzon syndrome, primary procedures were performed at a mean age of 6.8 months. Five patients underwent secondary procedures at a mean age of 30.5 months, and 2 underwent tertiary procedures at a mean age of 76.7 months to improve craniofacial form. There was evidence of midface hypoplasia in 9 patients by 3 years of age and of class III malocclusion in 9 patients; a Le Fort III advancement was performed in 7 patients and recommended in 2 more. Craniofacial form was good or satisfactory in 12 patients and poor in 3. This group also had follow-up complications relating to airway obstruction and intracranial pressure.

In the 15 patients with Pfeiffer syndrome, primary procedures were performed at a mean age of 5.8 months, but postoperative craniofacial form tended to be unsatisfactory, requiring secondary procedures in 9 patients at an average age of 18.2 months and tertiary procedures in 3 patients at an average age of 34.4 months. Midface hypoplasia occurred in 10 patients and class III malocclusion in 5. The Le Fort III advancement was performed in 6 patients and recommended in 3 more. This group had the most severe complications and least satisfactory results. However, 10 of 15 had satisfactory results in the upper third of the face.

Of the 7 patients with other syndromes, the primary procedures were performed at a mean age of 5.8 months and secondary procedures were performed in 3 patients at a mean age of 22.5 months to improve craniofacial form. Six of the 7 patients had excellent, good, or satisfactory results.

Conclusions.—Early surgical treatment of severe craniofacial synostosis deformity is relatively safe, with a perioperative major complication rate of 11.3% and a long-term complication rate of 44.7%, with follow-up as long as 20 years. Unsolved problems include cranial vault maldevelopment (anterior turricephaly), midface hypoplasia, and reduced frontal sinus development.

▶ The results of this report are amazing. Most of us have seen or otherwise heard of the technical tour de force that is necessary to surgically correct the deformities seen with craniosynostosis. Such surgery should be performed only in centers that are highly skilled in the techniques necessary to produce a satisfactory result. The Institute of Reconstructive Plastic Surgery at New York University Medical Center is one such facility. There, 363 patients have been operated on with these problems in the past 20 years. About half of the patients had isolated craniofacial synostosis, and the remainder had this problem in conjunction with some syndromes such as Crouzon or Pfeiffer syndromes. Incredibly, the majority of all children achieved a normal or near-normal appearance.

To give you a sense of what these children go through, what follows is the current New York University treatment protocol for the patient with craniosynostosis:

Neonatal period: First, tracheotomy if there is severe respiratory distress unresponsive to conservative measures. Gastrostomy should be considered for severe feeding problems refractory to conservative measures. Second, ultrasound and/or CT scan to evaluate intracranial pressure status. Ventriculoperitoneal shunt placement if necessary. Calvariectomy for severe hydrocephalus/increased intracranial pressure as in pansynostosis. Third, eye lubricants, eyelid taping, mist cups, or lid occlusal sutures for corneal exposure secondary to exorbitism.

Age 6–9 months: Fronto-orbital advancement and/or cranial vault remodeling (more extensive in the parieto-occipital region in the syndromal patient). Parents should be forewarned of the possible need for a secondary procedure (e.g., Apert, Pfeiffer).

Age 4 years: Le Fort III midface advancement for respiratory and aesthetic problems. Parents should be forewarned of the need for secondary midface advancement in the adolescent period.

Adolescence: Jaw surgery (if necessary), i.e., Le Fort I or Le Fort III advancement, maxillomandibular osteotomies, or genioplasty.

Pediatric Basilar Skull Fracture: Do Children With Normal Neurologic Findings and No Intracranial Injury Require Hospitalization?
Kadish HA, Schunk JE (Univ of Utah, Salt Lake City)
Ann Emerg Med 26:37–41, 1995   6–3

Background.—Because patients with basilar skull fractures (BSFs) may have complications including CSF leakage, cranial nerve palsies, hearing impairment, meningitis, and delayed intracranial hemorrhage, patients with this diagnosis are usually admitted. However, the necessity of admission was examined in a subgroup of pediatric patients with BSF who had normal neurologic examinations, Glasgow Coma Scale (GCS) scores of 15, and no CT evidence of intracranial pathology.

Methods.—The charts were reviewed of all pediatric patients with a diagnosis of BSF seen between 1991 and 1993 in the emergency department. Data were collected on patient demographics, mechanism of injury, GCS score, neurologic examination findings, signs of BSF, CT scan findings, and complications. A subgroup of patients with normal neurologic findings, GCS scores of 15, and no CT evidence of intracranial pathology was identified and specifically analyzed.

Results.—There were 239 pediatric patients with BSF, of which 21% were younger than 3 years, 42% were 3–9 years old, and 37% were 10–17 years old (Table 1). Falls and motor vehicle accidents were the most common mechanisms of injury. Of the 239 patients with a diagnosis of BSF, 51 (21%) had no clinical signs and diagnosis was based only on CT findings. Of the 188 patients with clinical signs, 50% had CT evidence of BSF. The most common clinical sign was hemotympanum, occurring in 65%, followed by CSF otorrhea, Battle's sign, CSF rhinorrhea, and cranial

TABLE 1.—Age Distribution and Mechanisms of Injury for 239 Pediatric Patients With Basilar Skull Fracture

Age distribution (yr)	
Less than 3	50 (21%)
3 to 9	101 (42%)
10 to 17	88 (37%)
Mechanism of injury	
Fall of more than 5 feet	49 (20%)
Fall of less than 5 feet	47 (20%)
Motor vehicle accident	47 (20%)
Pedestrian versus vehicle	34 (14%)
Bicycle	27 (11%)
Fall from horse	12 (5%)
Sledding	8 (3%)
Motorcycle	6 (3%)
Boating	3 (1%)
Skiing	2 (1%)
Assault	2 (1%)
Nonaccidental trauma	2 (1%)

(Courtesy of Kadish HA, Schunk JE: Pediatric basilar skull fracture: Do children with normal neurologic findings and no intracranial injury require hospitalization? *Ann Emerg Med* 26:37–41, July 1995.)

nerve involvement (Table 2). There were 114 patients with normal neurologic examination findings, GCS scores of 15, and no CT evidence of intracranial pathology. This subgroup did not differ from the rest of the patients in sex, age, or mechanism of injury. Vomiting was the most common complication in this group, occurring in 7 patients (6%). Meningitis was the only major complication; it occurred in 1 patient. In addition, a late CSF fistula developed in 3 patients, 2 patients had unexplained fever, and 2 patients had iatrogenic complications related to drug administration (Table 4).

Conclusions.—A subgroup of patients with BSF who had a normal neurologic examination, GCS score of 15, and no intracranial pathology on CT had a low incidence of complications and may represent a group of patients with BSF who do not require hospitalization. A larger cohort of patients should be studied to determine the safety of outpatient management in patients with these characteristics.

TABLE 2.—Clinical Findings in 188 Pediatric Basilar Skull Fractures

Hemotympanum	122 (65%)
CSF otorrhea	32 (17%)*
Battle's sign	26 (14%)
CSF rhinorrhea	24 (13%)*
Cranial nerve involvement	1 (.8%)

* In 46 patients (19%), both CSF otorrhea and rhinorrhea were present.
(Courtesy of Kadish HA, Schunk JE: Pediatric basilar skull fracture: Do children with normal neurologic findings and no intracranial injury require hospitalization? *Ann Emerg Med* 26:37–41, July 1995.)

TABLE 4.—Complications in 114 Patients With Simple Basilar Skull Fractures

Complication	No. of Patients (%)
Vomiting during hospitalization	7 (6%)
"Late" CSF fistula*	3 (3%)
Fever without source	2 (2%)
Iatrogenic	2 (2%)
Meningitis	1 (1%)

* CSF fistula developed after patient was admitted to the hospital.
(Courtesy of Kadish HA, Schunk JE: Pediatric basilar skull fracture: Do children with normal neurologic findings and no intracranial injury require hospitalization? *Ann Emerg Med* 26:37–41, July 1995.)

▶ To admit or not admit the child with a BSF: that is the question. Anytime a child is struck by a car or otherwise has a serious head injury, and is seen with a hemotympanum or bleeding in the ear canal, an alarm should go off to alert you to the possibility of a BSF. Such skull fractures are associated with a much higher risk of CSF leak, cranial nerve paralysis, hearing impairment, meningitis, and delayed intracranial hemorrhage. For these reasons, the natural reflex is to hospitalize all children with BSFs. The validity of this response to such an injury is the subject of this report.

This Utah study shows that about 20% of children with BSFs have a CSF leak. On the other hand, only 0.4% have meningitis as a consequence of such a leak. As importantly, 21% of patients with a normal neurologic examination and an acceptable GCS score were found to have intracranial injuries when a CT scan was performed. The most important issue raised by this study was whether there was any evidence of delayed intracranial hemorrhage in a child who has a normal CT scan. None was seen.

Although most authorities recommend admission for all patients with BSFs, this report suggests that something different might be able to be done for some patients. There is a subset of patients with a simple BSF who have a normal neurologic examination, an acceptable GCS score, and no intracranial pathology on CT scan. This group appears to have no risk of delayed intracranial hemorrhage. One in 114 patients did have meningitis secondary to a CSF leak. The latter frequency is sufficiently low that in selected cases, in-hospital observation may not be necessary.

This editor is not sure that we ought to hang our hats on the results of this study. Further investigation with a larger cohort of patients is needed to support the safety of outpatient management of patients with simple BSF.

Variability in Brain Death Determination Practices in Children
Meija RE, Pollack MM (George Washington Univ, Washington, DC)
JAMA 274:550–553, 1995

6–4

Introduction.—The Task Force for the Determination of Brain Death in Children published specific guidelines for defining brain death in infants and children in 1987 (Table 1). These guidelines were widely disseminated

---

TABLE 1.—Guidelines for the Determination of Brain Death in Children

---

Historical criteria
  Determination of the
    proximate cause of coma*
Physical examination criteria
  Coexisting coma and apnea†
  Absence of brain-stem
    function
  Absence of hypothermia or
    hypotension
  Flaccid tone or absence of
    spontaneous or induced
    movements (except spinal
    cord events)
  Consistent examination
    findings throughout observation
    and testing periods
**Observation periods and laboratory
  testing**
  7 d to 2 mo; two clinical
    examinations and apnea tests
    and two electroencephalograms
    48 h apart
  2 to 12 mo; two clinical examinations
    and apnea tests and two electroen-
    cephalograms at least 24 h apart‡
  >12 mo; two clinical examinations
    and apnea tests 12 h apart§

---

* Absence of remediable or reversible conditions: toxins, drugs (sedatives, hypnotics, paralytics), metabolic disorders, surgically correctable conditions, hypotension, and hypothermia.

† Apnea test using standardized methods.

‡ Repeat examination and electroencephalogram obviated by absence of flow on cerebral radio-nuclide angiography.

§ If hypoxic-ischemic encephalopathy is suspected, the observation period should be extended to 24 hours. Laboratory testing is not required if there is absence of a remediable or reversible condition.

(Courtesy of Meija RE, Pollack MM: Variability in brain death determination practices in children. *JAMA* 274:550–553, Copyright 1995, American Medical Association.)

---

to aid in end-of-life decision-making and organ procurement. Adherence to these guidelines and factors relating to the success and impediments in organ procurement were investigated in a national sample of pediatric ICUs (PICUs).

Methods.—A random selection of 16 PICUs collected data on consecutive admissions between 1989 and 1992 until there was information on 15 deaths. Descriptive data and data related to the determination of brain death and to solid organ procurement were obtained from the medical records and analyzed.

Results.—Of the 5,415 admissions, 4.6% of the patients died and 37% of the deaths were secondary to brain death. Compared with patients who died of other causes, brain-dead patients had significantly greater evidence of physiologic derangement, were more likely to have had traumatic injuries, and were less likely to have had chronic conditions (Figure). Among the brain-dead patients, 75% underwent at least 1 apnea test and 12% had at least 2 apnea tests. However, apnea testing was inappropriate in 22% of the patients. Apnea tests were performed in all brain-dead patients at 7 sites, in none of the brain-dead patients at 1 site, and in 50%

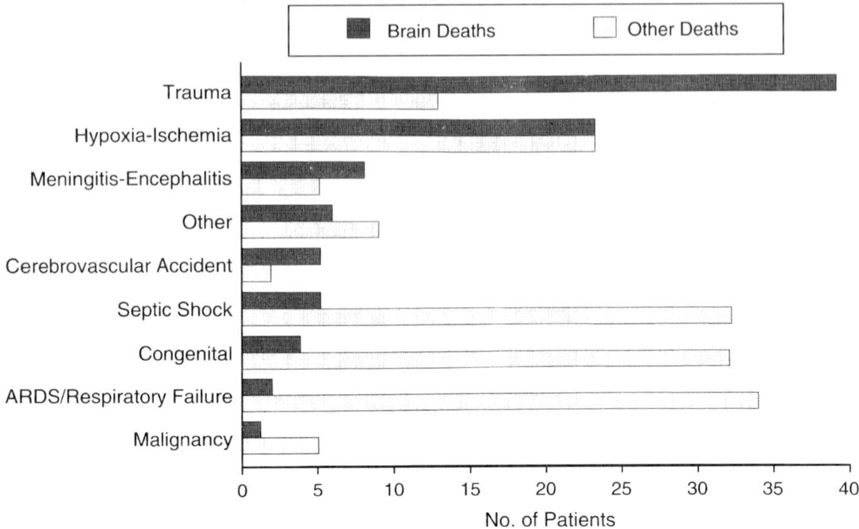

FIGURE.—Diagnosis classified according to primary reason for admission to the pediatric ICU. *Abbreviation: ARDS,* adult respiratory distress syndrome. (Courtesy of Meija RE, Pollack MM: Variability in brain death determination practices in children. *JAMA* 274:505–553, Copyright 1995, American Medical Association.)

to 80% of the patients at 8 sites. Confirmatory tests were performed in 84% of the patients overall (Table 4), including all brain-dead patients at 10 sites, none of the patients at 1 site, and in 63% to 90% of the patients at 5 sites. Organs were harvested from 32% of the brain-dead patients. The reasons for nonprocurement included medical examiner's case (22%), parental refusal (12%), disease state (12%), no recipient (1%), and indeterminate reasons (21%).

Conclusions.—There were many deviations from the guidelines, including controversial apnea testing practices, the lack of clinical examinations

TABLE 4.—Brain Death Diagnosis by Age Groups and Tests

| | | Confirmatory Tests* | | | | |
| | | ≥1 | | | | |
Age Groups	Total No. (%)	Coma Examinations, No. (%)	Apnea Tests, No. (%)	EEG, No. (%)	Flow Study, No. (%)	EEG and Flow Study, No. (%)
7 d to 24 mo	6 (6)	6 (100)	5 (83)	3 (50)	1 (17)	2 (33)
2 to 12 mo	24 (26)	22 (92)	19 (79)	6 (25)	8 (33)	
>12 mo	63 (68)	60 (95)	46 (73)	22 (35)	17 (27)	13 (21)
Total	93 (100)	88 (95)	70 (75)	31 (33)	24 (26)	23 (25)
P†	...	.73	.92	.43	>.99	.40

* Coma examinations consistent with brain death documented by physicians in physician section of medical record.
† Comparison among age groups.
Abbreviation: EEG, electroencephalogram.
(Courtesy of Meija RE, Pollack MM: Variability in brain death determination practices in children. *JAMA* 274:550–553, Copyright 1995, American Medical Association.)

and apnea testing, and the lack of ancillary confirmatory testing, indicating that the guidelines have not become a national standard. The most common impediment to organ procurement was the need for the medical examiner to safeguard forensic evidence, suggesting that changes in the coroner's office protocols could significantly increase organ procurement.

▶ When 3% of all deaths in PICUs are brain deaths (body functions continue, but the brain is dead), we see the magnitude of the importance of this report. To more fully understand it, some background information is in order. In 1981, the American Bar Association, the American Medical Association, the National Conference for Commissioners on Uniform State Laws, and the President's Commission for the Study of Ethical Problems in Medicine and Biomedical and Behavioral Research proposed a model statute (the Uniform Determination of Death Act) and guidelines for the determination of death. The intention here was to unify the language of the existing state-to-state statutes regarding brain death. The Uniform Determination of Death Act states:

"An individual who has either sustained (1) irreversible cessation of circulatory and respiratory functions, or (2) irreversible cessation of all functions of the entire brain, including the brain stem, is dead. A determination of death must be made in accordance with accepted medical standards." *These guidelines excluded children younger than 5 years, based on the assumption that children's brains have increased resistance to insults and injuries.*

The lack of standards regarding the determination of brain death in young children became the catalyst for the formation of a task force. In 1987, the Task Force for the Determination of Brain Death in Children, formed by representatives from well-respected societies including the American Bar Association, the American Academy of Neurology, the American Neurological Association, the American Academy of Pediatrics, and the Child Neurology Society, endorsed the Determination of Death Act and published and disseminated throughout medical literature specific guidelines for the determination of brain death in infants and children (see Table 1). The objective of these guidelines and their dissemination was to facilitate end-of-life decisions and organ procurement in infants and children.

The point of this report was to see whether these uniform guidelines were being followed. They are not. Even though the guidelines for the determination of brain death in children had been widely disseminated, they are not a national standard as this study documents. The major deviation that is seen relative to these guidelines is inadequate apnea testing. If you are not familiar with apnea testing for death, the patient is given 100% oxygen for a fairly extended period, followed by turning off the respirator. The patient will accumulate carbon dioxide before significant hypoxia occurs. If the patient's partial pressure of carbon dioxide reaches 60 mm Hg without a respiratory effort, the patient has failed the apnea test. It is critical that apnea testing be done and that it be done properly. Apnea testing has been considered the most important criterion for brain-death diagnosis.[1]

The second important finding in this report was the observation that the major reason organ procurement isn't possible in more brain-dead cases has nothing to do with parental refusal or a disease state precluding procurement: it has to do with medical examiners. The violent or suspicious nature of many deaths in PICUs frequently leads to involvement of the medical examiner. The medical examiner's obligation to safeguard forensic evidence is in conflict with the obligation to release potential donor organs that fall under his or her jurisdiction. The increasing number of medical examiner denials has had major repercussions on the organ recovery process nationwide and is the basis of significant friction between the organ procurement agencies and medical examiners. The data from this report are chilling in that if the medical examiners had released all of these patients for potential donations, and if the parents had agreed to donate the same percentage of organs as other parents, approximately one third more organs would have become available to other children.

Two things are clear at this point. We need to know more about why pediatric care providers do not uniformly adhere to the guidelines for the determination of brain death in children. Second, we need to get our medical examiners to figure out a way to solve their problem and the problem of children who need donor organs. Is it too much to ask medical examiners to attend to organ harvesting as the first step in an autopsy, rather than forfeiting any ability to use an organ by transporting a body to the autopsy room of the medical examiner?

Reference

1. Ashwal S, et al: *Adv Pediatr* 38:181, 1991.

Natural History and Treatment Effects in Guillain-Barré Syndrome: A Multicentre Study
Korinthenberg R, Mönting JS (Albert-Ludwigs-Univ, Freiburg, Germany)
Arch Dis Child 74:281–287, 1996   6–5

Purpose.—Children are more likely than adults to recover from the immune-mediated acute polyradiculoneuritis Guillain-Barré syndrome. Still, ventilatory insufficiency and even death may occur during the acute phase of the syndrome. Few studies have looked at the effectiveness of immunomodulatory treatments in children with Guillain-Barré syndrome. The natural history and effectiveness of treatment for children with this syndrome were assessed.

Methods.—Information on children treated for acute Guillain-Barré syndrome during a 5-year period was gathered by a questionnaire sent to 155 pediatric hospitals. All patients had to meet internationally accepted diagnostic criteria. The responses included information on the signs and symptoms, degree of disability, immunomodulatory therapy, and time course of recovery.

TABLE 6.—Time Course of Recovery

Days from first symptoms to	No	Median	Minimum	Centiles 10th	90th	Maximum
First sign of recovery	168	17	1	7	34	61
Leave bed	85	23	3	14	63	107
Walk unaided	108	37	4	16	85	199
Leave hospital	174	28	2	10	68	256
Be free of symptoms	105	66	2	22	181	790

(Courtesy of Korinthenberg R, Mönting JS: Natural history and treatment effects in Guillain-Barré syndrome: A multicentre study. *Arch Dis Child* 74:281–287, 1996.)

Results.—Information on 175 patients with Guillain-Barré syndrome was received from 69 hospitals. The patients were 98 boys and 77 girls aged 11 months to just under 18 years. Peak disease severity varied substantially—although 26% of patients were able to walk throughout the course of disease, 16% required artificial ventilation. The initial signs of recovery occurred a median of 17 days after symptom onset. The median time to unaided walking was 37 days, and the median time to freedom from symptoms was 66 days (Table 6). The course was fairly benign in a large proportion of patients, but a minority had a protracted course. Of 106 patients with long-term follow-up, 98 were symptom-free and all were able to walk without help. The best prognostic factor was the maximum extent of disability. Immunoglobulins seemed to hasten recovery for children who were unable to walk but were not tetraplegic. Corticosteroids were less helpful, and only a few severely affected patients received plasmapheresis.

Conclusion.—The course of Guillain-Barré syndrome in children is variable but appears to be more benign than in adults. Patients who cannot walk should be considered for immunoglobulin therapy; there are not data on the benefits of early immunoglobulin treatment. Corticosteroids should not generally be used, except for patients with a prolonged course and suspected chronic inflammatory demyelinating polyneuropathy.

▶ Data on the course of recovery in the patients in this series are better than in the literature. The mean time for freedom from symptoms in most studies has ranged from 120 to 180 days. The patients in this report were free of symptoms at a mean of 64 days. A significant finding here is the observation that there are a large number of patients with a favorable prognosis and a much smaller cluster of patients who will have a protracted course. No matter which group a child falls into, all can be expected to walk unaided given enough time.

This study also confirms the treatment effect of IV immunoglobulin. Unfortunately, the study does not tell us the indications for this treatment. The impression given is that the benefit of IV immunoglobulin is greatest in children who are unable to walk independently but who are not yet paralyzed and ventilated. Even a few days' advantage offered by IV immunoglobulin would more than pay for this treatment in terms of shortened hospital stays and required physical therapy. Intravenous immunoglobulin is expensive, but Guillain-Barré syndrome does appear to be a disease for which cost-benefit analysis favors early therapy for most, if not all.

Cerebrospinal Fluid Values in the Term Neonate

Ahmed A, Hickey SM, Ehrett S, et al (Univ of Texas, Dallas)
Pediatr Infect Dis J 15:298–303, 1996   6–6

Background.—Although lumbar punctures are frequently included in the evaluation of febrile neonates, interpretation of the data is complicated by the variability of reference values for this age group. This variability may be related to the variability of definitions of noninfected infants, with some data on CSF cellularity derived from infants with traumatic lumbar punctures, systemic bacterial disease, or CNS viral disease. In addition, there appear to be significant age-related variations in CSF values among newborns. To clarify CSF reference values for newborns, strict inclusion and exclusion criteria were used to identify noninfected neonates, in whom the CSF values were analyzed in groups defined by age in weeks.

Methods.—A total of 108 infants in the first 30 days of life were identified from 2 prospective studies on aseptic meningitis. All of these infants had complete data on CSF values; atraumatic lumbar puncture; no history of antibiotic therapy; negative blood, urine, and CSF bacterial cultures; negative CSF viral cultures; and negative polymerase chain reaction (PCR) assays for CSF enteroviruses. The differences in CSF values were determined within each 1-week age group.

Results.—For the complete group of 108 noninfected neonates, the mean total CSF white blood cells (WBC)/mm^3 was 7.3, the median was 4, and the range was 0 to 130. Most (90%) had a total CSF WBC/mm^3 of no greater than 11. The age groups did not show significant variations in mean CSF WBC counts, absolute neutrophil counts, or CSF glucose concentration. There was a significantly higher CSF protein concentration in the first 2 weeks of life than in the 3rd and 4th week of life.

Conclusions.—The strict inclusion and exclusion criteria used to define the noninfected neonate population ensured a more accurate representation of normal CSF values among infants younger than 1 month and produced clinically useful reference values for the evaluation of febrile neonates.

▶ One of the more difficult things we have to do as care providers of children is figure out whether the results of a lumbar puncture performed on a newborn are within normal limits. Reference values for CSF in noninfected infants may be found in a variety of reference sources, but few studies are internally consistent with each other in terms of the criteria used to define noninfected or "normal" CSF. Many reports include so-called "normal" infants with traumatic lumbar punctures. Viral disease of the CNS is not entirely excluded in some studies. The real value of the report abstracted is that rigorous inclusion criteria were established. Better yet, rigorous exclusion criteria were used to make certain that no CNS bacterial or viral disease-infected patients were included in the database. Polymerase chain reaction enteroviral technology has made it possible to exclude infants with viral disease who might previously have been considered noninfected.

So what did the authors find? As noted in the abstract, the mean ± SD total WBC/mm³ in the population of noninfected infants was 7.3 ± 14. Recognize, however, that there was not a normal distribution of the CSF WBC values. Thus, the median may be a better comparative measure of noninfected CSF. The median value in this report was just 4 WBC/mm³. Ninety percent of infants in this report had a total CSF WBC count of ≤ 11/mm³. This is a lower value than that seen in any previous study.

One last point: The total CSF WBC isn't the only thing that one looks at when a lumbar puncture is done. All of us look to see if there are "polys" in the CSF. A single polymorphonuclear cell in the CSF of an adult is enough to buy an adult a tentative diagnosis of bacterial meningitis. In infants, Ahmed et al. found that the median normal CSF poly count was 0, with 88% of noninfected infants having no polys whatsoever in their CSF. As can be seen in the tables, the CSF:blood glucose ratios and CSF protein concentrations in this report are similar to the findings reported in earlier studies.

There is no question that the CSF WBC count is important in attempting to tell one febrile neonate from another with respect to infection. More importantly, recognize that an abnormal CSF WBC count does not always imply infection. Even more importantly, viral meningitis and occasionally bacterial meningitis may be present without evidence of pleocytosis. In the population of neonates studied in Texas, 22% of those identified by culture and 39% of those identified by PCR had what otherwise would be called "normal" CSF WBC counts. This should teach us a lesson. There is no better substitute for diagnostic purposes than experience and common sense. Laboratory data help, but don't hang your hat on a hook that isn't entirely screwed in—such is the tenuous nature of the hooks we call laboratory results.

Discontinuation of Antiepileptic Drug Treatment After Two Seizure-free Years in Children With Cerebral Palsy

Delgado MR, Riela AR, Mills J, et al (Texas Scottish Rite Hosp for Children, Dallas; Univ of Texas, Dallas)
Pediatrics 97:192–197, 1996

6–7

Objective.—There is a 25% to 35% incidence of epilepsy in patients with cerebral palsy (CP). Although antiepileptic drug (AED) treatment can be discontinued successfully in some patients, the seizure remission rate in children has not been well studied. Because epileptic children with neurologic deficits or mental retardation are at increased risk for seizures, it is important to have more information about relapse rates. Prognostic fac-

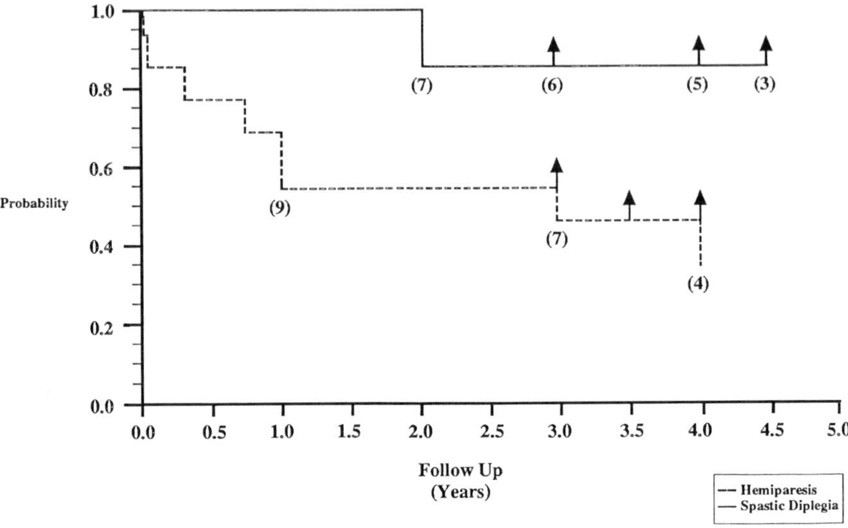

FIGURE 3.—Probability of remaining seizure-free after antiepileptic drug discontinuation according to type of cerebral palsy (spastic diplegia vs. hemiparesis). *Arrows* indicate children who were last seen in remission, with the length of follow-up indicated on the *horizontal axis*. *Numbers in parentheses* are the numbers of children at risk for relapse at that time. (Courtesy of Delgado MR, Riela AR, Mills J, et al: Discontinuation of antiepileptic drug treatment after two seizure-free years in children with cerebral palsy. Reproduced by permission of *Pediatrics*, Vol 97, pp 192–197, Copyright 1996).

tors for seizure relapse, as well as the relapse rate after AED discontinuation, were determined prospectively in children with CP who had been seizure-free for 2 years.

Methods.—Treatment with AEDs was stopped in 65 epileptic children (32 boys), aged 2–16 years, with CP who had been seizure-free for 2 years. Patients were followed for at least 2 years or until seizures recurred to determine factors associated with relapse.

Results.—In 41.5% of children, seizures recurred after an average of 1.11 years, with 13 children having a relapse within 6 months. After 4 years, 26 patients were seizure-free. Differences in relapse rates based on seizure type, frequency, seizure-free time, therapy, family history, sex, or mental development were not significant. Patients with spastic hemiparesis had a relapse rate of 62%; with spastic quadriparesis, 40%; with hypotonic quadriparesis, 27%; and with spastic diplegia, 14% (Fig 3). Three of four patients with mixed motor deficits relapsed. No correlate of relapse was found.

Conclusion.—Although most patients with CP do not have a 2-year seizure-free period even while on medication, children should be given the opportunity to discontinue AEDs when possible. Patients with spastic hemiparesis appear to have the highest risk of relapse.

▶ Many of us have had a sense over the years that there is more art than science involved with the "correctness" of ways to discontinue seizure medication. This report brings such decision-making more into the world of rationality. As far as children with CP who have seizures are concerned, if they have been free of seizures for 2 or more years, the risk of relapse off antiepileptic drugs is not very different than for children without CP who have a seizure disorder.

Please read this article in detail before concluding that all is rosy for children with CP and seizure disorders. In fact, the majority of patients with CP and epilepsy do not have a 24-month period in which they remain free of seizures, even while on medication. In this report, only 13% of such children were free of seizures for 2 years and were then able to be removed from medication. The subsequent seizure relapse rate in the latter group was 41.5%. By this editor's math, this means that perhaps 7% of all children with CP and seizures will be able to discontinue seizure medications without a recurrence of their convulsive disorder.

Children with CP who have seizures should be given the opportunity to discontinue medications if the opportunity presents itself. Those with hemiparesis will have a higher recurrence rate than those with other forms of CP. Children with spastic diplegia will have the best prognosis off medication (a relapse rate of only 14%). Mental subnormality does not correlate with the recurrence of seizures, nor do electroencephalogram findings before antiepileptic therapy is discontinued. What all this means is that a trial off drugs is the most correct test to determine who will and who will not do well. Give it a try.

High-dose Corticotropin (ACTH) Versus Prednisone for Infantile Spasms: A Prospective, Randomized, Blinded Study
Baram TZ, Mitchell WG, Tournay A, et al (Univ of Southern California, Los Angeles; Southern California Permanente, Los Angeles)
Pediatrics 97:375–379, 1996   6–8

Background.—Corticotropin (ACTH) and prednisone have been shown to be effective for infantile spasms (IS). The efficacy of a 2-week course of high-dose ACTH was compared with that of prednisone in suppressing clinical spasms and hypsarrhythmic electroencephalograms (EEGs) in IS.

Methods.—Twenty-nine of 34 eligible infants were enrolled in the prospective, randomized, single-blinded study. The median patient age was 6 months. Twenty-two infants were symptomatic, with known or suspected cause. The remaining 7 were cryptogenic.

Findings.—Thirteen of 15 infants randomized to ACTH (86.6%) responded on the basis of both EEG and clinical findings. In another infant, seizures stopped, but the EEG remained hypsarrhythmic. By contrast, only 4 of 14 infants given prednisone (28.6%) responded according to EEG and clinical criteria. The differences between these response rates were significant.

Conclusion.—A 2-week course of high-dose ACTH is more effective than 2 weeks of prednisone in the treatment of IS. Further research establishing the mechanisms by which ACTH acts would be useful in the development of more direct treatments for age-specific epilepsies such as IS.

▶ For this editor, one of the great enigmas of medicine is why IS respond to ACTH and corticosteroids. It has been almost 40 years since Sorel first showed the usefulness of ACTH and prednisone, which have subsequently become the standard therapy for IS.[1] There is no controversy regarding whether these agents work. The residual controversy has been whether ACTH is better than glucocorticoids. Quite conclusively, these authors seem to show the selective advantage of high-dose ACTH over standard prednisone therapy (2 mg/kg/per day), each given for 2 weeks. Other studies have shown that lower doses of ACTH (such as 20 or 30 μ/day), although somewhat effective, have a much lower response rate.[2]

Infantile spasms are a form of epilepsy that is age specific to infancy. They are triggered at a vulnerable developmental stage in the setting of a previously stressed or injured CNS. Whether the spasms per se or the ongoing hypsarrhythmic EEG activity is the cause of the poor cognitive outcome is not clear. It is fair to say that whatever therapy is chosen, the goal should be to eliminate the EEG findings, not merely to stop the seizures.

Your guess is as good as anyone's regarding exactly how glucocorticoids and ACTH help to control IS. Some have said that ACTH may function as a promoter of adrenal glucocorticoid secretion: High-dose ACTH may result in higher, more sustained plasma cortisol. Many, however, believe that ACTH exerts its therapeutic effects directly on the CNS, in addition to or independent of cortisol release. Analogues of ACTH that are devoid of steroidogenic effects, however, are not effective for IS. It is not likely that the generalist physician, pediatric or otherwise, will be taking on the task of treating a youngster with IS. Nonetheless, it is important to remember that effective therapy must be given as soon as possible.

If the individual who ultimately receives these referrals is still in the mode of low-dose steroids or ACTH, give that person a reprint of this paper. These youngsters do not have a lot of time to undergo inadequate therapeutic trials. Go for the gold as expediently as possible. A bronze or a silver may very well mean a loss of IQ points.

References

1. Hrachovy RA, Frost JD Jr: Infantile spasms: A disorder of the developing nervous system, in Kellaway P, Noebels JL (eds): *Problems and Concepts in Developmental Neurophysiology.* Baltimore, Johns Hopkins University Press, 1989, pp 131–147.
2. Hrachovy RA, et al: *Epilepsia* 32:212, 1991.

Effect of Acetaminophen and of Low Intermittent Doses of Diazepam on Prevention of Recurrences of Febrile Seizures

Uhari M, Rantala H, Vainionpää L, et al (Univ of Oulu, Finland)
J Pediatr 126:991–995, 1995

6–9

Background.—Long-term medication has been used to prevent the recurrence of febrile convulsions. However, the efficacy of the medications used has not been established definitively. The value of diazepam in unselected patients was determined, and the effects of acetaminophen alone or combined with diazepam were investigated.

Methods.—In this placebo-controlled, double-blind trial, children having had 1 febrile seizure were assigned to placebo or to 1 dose of rectal diazepam followed 6 hours later by oral diazepam, 0.2 mg/kg, administered 3 times daily for the first 2 days if the patient's temperature continued to exceed 38.5°C. In addition, each febrile episode was assigned randomly to acetaminophen treatment or placebo. Of 180 children enrolled in the study, 161 were followed for 2 years.

Findings.—Final analysis included data on 153 children who had at least 1 recurrent febrile episode during follow-up. Six hundred forty-one fever events occurred. Thirty-eight children, or 21.1%, had 55 recurrences of febrile seizures. Recurrence rates were unaffected by acetaminophen. Seizures recurred at least once in 28.4% of the children given diazepam and in 21.5% of the children given placebo (Figure).

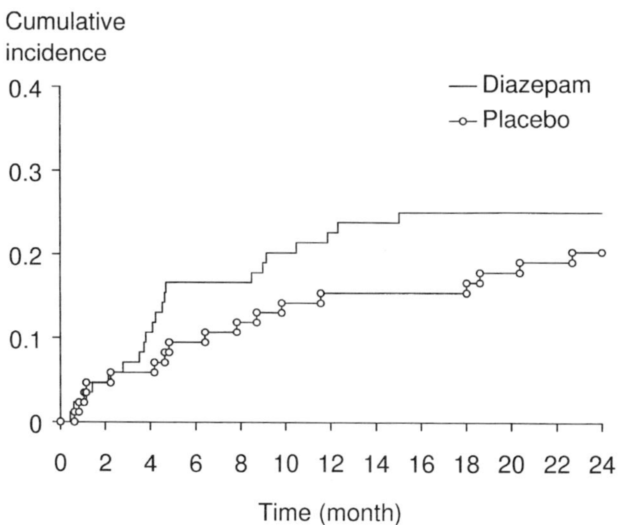

FIGURE.—Cumulative incidence of recurrent febrile seizures, by treatment group. Difference between curves was not significant ($P = 0.4138$). (Courtesy of Uhari M, Rantala H, Vainionpää L, et al: Effect of acetaminophen and of low intermittent doses of diazepam on prevention of recurrences of febrile seizures. *J Pediatr* 126:991–995, 1995.)

Conclusions.—The recurrence of febrile seizures is unaffected by low-dose acetaminophen, diazepam, or both in these children. Antipyretic agents combined with anticonvulsant medication did not decrease febrile seizure recurrences.

▶ In an absolutely wonderful editorial that accompanied this article, Camfield et al.[1] stated: "Disorders of high prevalence but low morbidity rates, such as febrile seizures, are rich sources of controversy." They are absolutely right, and the article abstracted confirms their suspicions. The most common medical treatment aimed at reducing febrile seizure recurrences is the use of an antipyretic agent. Unfortunately, it doesn't work. Alternatively, the second most common approach is the prescription of an anticonvulsant medication to be given prophylactically with the onset of fever. That doesn't work either.

A febrile seizure, by and large, should be considered a benign disorder with only rare complications. Because there is no effective way to easily prevent an occurrence of a febrile seizure, it's best for everyone to stop worrying. Let nature have her way.

Reference

1. Camfield PR, et al: *J Pediatr* 126:929, 1995.

Long Term Outcome of Prophylaxis for Febrile Convulsions
Knudsen FU, Paerregaard A, Andersen R, et al (Glostrup Univ Hosp, Denmark)
Arch Dis Child 74:13–18, 1996   6–10

Background.—Major cohort studies have shown that long-term outcomes are normal for most children with febrile convulsions. As a result, long-term prophylaxis with antiepileptic agents has been abandoned for the most part. However, febrile convulsions may be associated with more subtle adverse outcomes in motor, neurologic, intellectual, or cognitive functions. Whether medical intervention in early childhood affects long-term prognosis, including the occurrence of subsequent epilepsy, was investigated in a randomized, controlled, long-term follow-up study.

Methods and Findings.—Follow-up data were collected from 289 children 12 years after randomization to intermittent prophylaxis or no prophylaxis. All had had febrile convulsions in early childhood. The mean ages in the 2 groups were 14 and 14.1 years, respectively, at follow-up. Body weight, height, and head circumference were also comparable between groups. The groups also had very similar findings on neurologic assessment, the Stott motor test of fine and gross motor development, the Wechsler Intelligence Scale for Children (including verbal intelligence quotient [IQ], performance IQ, and full-scale IQ), a neuropsychologic test battery (including short- and long-term, auditory, and visual memory), and visuomotor tempo, computer reaction time, and reading tests. Scholastic

TABLE 7.—Long-term Outcome After Simple and Complex Febrile Convulsions Given Prophylaxis or No Prophylaxis: Intellectual, Scholastic, and Motor Abilities

| | Simple febrile convulsions | | | | Complex febrile convulsions | | | | |
| | Prophylaxis | | Controls | | Prophylaxis | | Controls | | |
	No of children	Mean (SD)	No of children	Mean (SD)	No of children	Mean (SD)	No of children	Mean (SD)	P Value
WISC	72		57		14		15		
Verbal IQ		104 (16)		104 (16)		110 (16)		110 (16)	NS
Performance IQ		113 (14)		111 (19)		120 (12)		111 (22)	NS
Full scale IQ		109 (13)		107 (15)		115 (12)		111 (17)	NS
Scholastic achievement									
(school score)	105	4·4 (2·5)	96	4·2 (2·1)	17	5·7 (2·4)	22	5·1 (2·3)	NS
Stott motor test	73		59		14		15		
Fine motor		1·4 (1·5)		1·6 (1·6)		1·0 (1·5)		1·5 (1·7)	NS
Gross motor		3·1 (3·5)		3·6 (3·4)		2·6 (2·3)		3·1 (4·0)	NS
Total motor		4·5 (4·6)		5·2 (4·7)		3·6 (2·9)		4·1 (5·6)	NS

Abbreviations: WISC, Wechsler Intelligence Scale for Children; *NS*, not significant.
(Courtesy of Knudsen FU, Paerregaard A, Andersen R, et al: Long term outcome of prophylaxis for febrile convulsions. *Arch Dis Child* 74:13–18, 1996.)

achievement was also comparable between groups. The incidences of epilepsy in patients receiving and not receiving prophylaxis were 0.7% and 0.8%, respectively (Table 7).

Conclusions.—The type of treatment of febrile convulsions in early childhood did not affect the occurrence of subsequent epilepsy or long-term neurologic, motor, intellectual, cognitive, and scholastic ability. Thus, in the long term, preventing new febrile convulsions appears to be no better than abbreviating them.

▶ Continuous prophylaxis with anticonvulsants to prevent recurrence of febrile seizures has largely been abandoned. When this editor picked up this article to read it in detail, he was concerned that these investigators from Denmark might be reopening Pandora's box. The results of this study, however, leave that box securely sealed.

There has been concern for some time that febrile convulsions may presage neurologic, motor, intellectual, or cognitive dysfunction. We see in this study that simple and complex febrile convulsions have a similar long-term prognosis in all aspects of neurologic function. This study also showed that children with complex febrile convulsions who are given prophylaxis do not fare any better in the long run than when given acute anticonvulsant treatment. We also see that prevention of true epilepsy is not a realistic target of prophylaxis. It is impressive that not even a single case of temporal lobe epilepsy caused by underlying hippocampal sclerosis has emerged after 12 years of observation among some 300 children with prior febrile convulsions, confirming that this sequence of events is rare.

We must pay attention to the conclusions of this report: prevention of new febrile convulsions appears to be no better in the long run with respect to sequelae than modifying them as they occur. The authors suggest that it is reasonable to recommend that all families with children who have had febrile seizures be equipped with 1 or 2 doses of rectal diazepam in solution, or other rapidly acting benzodiazepines, for abbreviating new febrile seizures. Intermittent, short-term prophylaxis with such drugs given at times of fever, which effectively reduces the recurrence rates in most studies, should probably be reserved for a few selected cases. These treatment recommendations are not totally devoid of side effects, but at least now we know from this study that such an approach to young children at time of fever has no detrimental effect on later neurologic, motor, intellectual, cognitive, or scholastic achievement.

Randomised Comparative Monotherapy Trial of Phenobarbitone, Phenytoin, Carbamazepine, or Sodium Valproate for Newly Diagnosed Childhood Epilepsy

de Silva M, MacArdle B, McGowan M, et al (King's College Hosp, London; Inst of Child Health, London; Inst of Public Health, Cambridge, England)
Lancet 347:709–713, 1996   6–11

Background.—The medical treatment of epilepsy in children is greatly influenced by the results of clinical trials involving adults. There has been only 1 randomized comparative trial involving children with newly diagnosed epilepsy. The efficacy and toxicity of 4 standard antiepileptic drugs used as monotherapy in children with newly diagnosed epilepsy were compared in a long-term, prospective, randomized, unmasked trial.

Methods.—One hundred sixty-seven children aged 3–16 years participated in the study between 1981 and 1987. All had had at least 2 previously untreated tonic-clonic or partial seizures, with or without secondary generalization. By random assignment, they received phenobarbitone, phenytoin, carbamazepine, or sodium valproate.

Findings.—Overall outcomes with all 4 drugs were good, with 73% of children achieving 1-year remission and 20% free of seizures after 3 years of follow-up (Table 4). The efficacy of the drugs did not differ significantly at 1, 2, or 3 years of follow-up. Overall, the frequency of adverse effects that required withdrawal of a drug was 9%. Treatment had to be withdrawn from 6 of the first 10 children assigned to phenobarbitone, after which no more children were given this drug. Of the remaining drugs, phenytoin was more likely to be stopped than carbamazepine or sodium valproate.

Conclusion.—These 4 antiepileptic drugs were equally effective in the treatment of the seizure types studied. The choice of first drug will be

TABLE 4.—Actuarial Percentages Seizure-free by Selected Times From Randomization

	Number of children			Actuarial % seizure free			
	Random-ized	With seizure recurrence	Seizure free	6 mo	12 mo	24 mo	36 mo
Treatment							
Phenobarbitone	10	8	2	40*	40*	20*	20*
Phenytoin	54	42	12	46	39	27	25
Carbamazepine	54	47	7	30	28	21	12
Sodium valproate	49	39	10	37	30	24	24
Total	167	136	31	38	33	24	20

* Number at risk small.

(Courtesy of de Silva M, MacArdle B, McGowan M, et al: Randomised comparative monotherapy trial of phenobarbitone, phenytoin, carbamazepine, or sodium valproate for newly diagnosed childhood epilepsy. *Lancet* 347:709–713, copyright by The Lancet Ltd., 1996.)

largely determined by toxicity and cost. Carbamazepine and valproate had the lowest withdrawal rates.

▶ In an era of fairly widespread acceptance of polypharmacy by some, it is nice to see a report that reinforces the use of single-drug therapy. There have been few prospective, comparative studies of the efficacy and toxicity of 2 or more standard drugs in newly diagnosed seizure patients, and only 1 has been undertaken in children. With this caveat, it is important to understand that single-drug therapy, in and of itself, is as likely to be effective in comparison with a mixture, or gruel, of various therapies. In fact, if the results of this study are accepted, it does not matter which of the 4 standard initial therapies (phenobarbital, phenytoin, carbamazepine, or sodium valproate) is used. All would be equally effective as the initial management of generalized tonic-clonic seizures or partial seizures. Thus, you can base your treatment as much upon which drug you think is less likely to produce side effects as on which is more likely to be effective. Given the flagging interest in phenobarbital these days (given its frequency of unacceptable cognitive and behavioral side effects), alternative therapies are being sought.

It is not likely that the results of this study will be totally embraced by all care providers. Most who have treated children with seizures tend to become comfortable with one form of therapy or another. For example, here in the United States, some believe in a greater efficacy of carbamazepine than valproate for partial seizures. If there is any message from the study abstracted, it is that whatever our own individual preferences, we should recognize that all commonly used drugs seem to work reasonably well.

While on the topic of childhood seizures, a form of seizure that is not often reported, reading epilepsy, was recently described. Reading epilepsy is a fairly unusual form of reflex epilepsy in which seizures are induced by reading. These were first recognized in 1956. In its classic form, reading epilepsy is characterized by jerking movements of the jaw during reading that may evolve into generalized tonic-clonic seizures if reading continues. Baseline electroencephalograms are normal, but seizure activity is noted during reading. The pathogenesis of reading epilepsy remains obscure despite more than 60 cases now in the literature.[1] Reading seizures are poorly responsive to treatment with anticonvulsants such as phenobarbital and phenytoin. Valproate or clonazepam may be needed. When nothing works, it's time for books on tape.

Reference

1. Singh B, et al: *Neurology* 45:1623, 1995.

Hyponatremia as the Cause of Seizures in Infants: A Retrospective Analysis of Incidence, Severity, and Clinical Predictors

Farrar HC, Chande VT, Fitzpatrick DF, et al (Univ of Arkansas, Little Rock; Children's Hosp of Pittsburgh, Pa; Rainbow Babies and Childrens Hosp, Cleveland, Ohio)
Ann Emerg Med 26:42–48, 1995

6–12

Introduction.—Managing infants with seizures introduces difficulties in both diagnosis and therapy. Because the duration and cause of seizures are the most important predictors of patient outcome after status epilepticus, it is important to identify the underlying cause as quickly as possible. Hyponatremia is diagnosed increasingly frequently in infants with seizures, particularly in infants younger than 6 months. The incidence of hyponatremic seizures, the severity of seizures and outcomes associated with hyponatremia, and the utility of clinical indicators in diagnosing hyponatremic seizures were investigated retrospectively.

Methods.—The charts were reviewed of all patients younger than 2 years who were admitted to Rainbow Babies and Childrens Hospital through the emergency department (ED) during a 5-year period with a diagnosis of seizures and/or electrolyte imbalance of unknown cause. The patients were divided into 2 groups determined by the presence or absence of hyponatremia. The demographic characteristics, historical factors, and physical features of the 2 groups were compared. Seizure severity (reflected in duration of seizures in ED, incidence of status epilepticus, and treatment required to control the seizures) and outcome were also compared. The diagnostic value of findings available at or shortly after admission in the identification of hyponatremic seizures was analyzed.

TABLE 3.—Predictors of Hyponatremia as the Cause of Seizures

Test	*OR (95% CI)*	*P*
Exact univariate logistic regression		
Temperature 36.5°C or lower*	64 (7.8–1,026)	<.0001
History of excess water intake	24 (4–280)	<.0001
Generalized seizures	5.3 (.9–41)	.08
No. of anticonvulsants (0, 1, 2, 3)	3.7 (1.3–13)	.008
Exact multivariate logistic regression		
Model 1		
Temperature 36.5°C or less	39.4 (3.6–2,121)	.005
History of excess water intake	12.4 (.9–709)	.07
Model 2		
Temperature 36.5°C or lower	71.4 (9.4–20,767)	<.0001
No. of anticonvulsants	10.3 (1.2–549)	.03
Model 3		
Temperature 36.5°C or lower	76.3 (7.1–4,486)	<.0001
Generalized seizures	9.5 (.4–748)	.24

* Temperatures of 36.3°C or less could not be evaluated because all normonatremic patients had temperatures over 36.3°C, resulting in an unstable statistical model.
(Courtesy of Farrar HC, Chande VT, Fitzpatrick DF, et al: Hyponatremia as the cause of seizures in infants: A retrospective analysis of incidence, severity, and clinical predictors. *Ann Emerg Med* 26:42–48, July 1995.)

TABLE 4.—Clinical Findings in Acute Symptomatic Hyponatremia: Comparison of the Numbers of Patients in 4 Series

Parameters	This study	Medani	Keating	Short
Total no. of patients	33	19	31	15
Age 6 to 24 mo	0	4 (21%)	2 (6%)*	Not stated†
Generalized seizures	30 (91%)	15 (79%)	28 (90%)	Not stated
Status epilepticus	24 (73%)	Not stated	Not stated	15 (100%)
Intubation	12 (36%)	5 (26%)	15 (48%)	9 (60%)
Intubation for more than 24 hr	4 of 12	Not stated	1 of 15	2 of 9
Temperature 36.5°C or less	29 (93%)	15 (79%)	27 (87%)	Not stated§
Hypothermia (35.5°C or less)	15 (48%)	9 (47%)	18 (58%)	Not stated

* These authors also reported patients 2, 3, and 8 years of age who were not included in the group of 31 reported patients.
† Mean age, 3.4 ± 1.8 years.
‡ Mean temperature, 35.4 ± 1.0°C.
(Courtesy of Farrar HC, Chande VT, Fitzpatrick DF, et al: Hypnoatremia as the cause of seizures in infants: A retrospective analysis of incidence, severity, and clinical predictors. *Ann Emerg Med* 26:42–48, July 1995.)

Results.—Of 59 patients without a suspected cause for seizures, 33 (56%) were hyponatremic. Among infants younger than 6 months, the incidence of hyponatremia was 70%. Compared with normonatremic infants, hyponatremic infants had significantly lower core body temperatures and significantly higher serum glucose levels. The hyponatremic patients had longer seizures, a higher incidence of status epilepticus, and a lower incidence of brief seizures (shorter than 10 minutes). Their seizures required more anticonvulsant medication to control than did the seizures in normonatremic infants. Emergency intubation for respiratory failure was required in 36% of the hyponatremic infants and none of the normonatremic infants. Four hyponatremic infants (12%) and 1 normonatremic infant (7%) had mechanical ventilation for at least 24 hours. There were complications in 12% of the hyponatremic and none of the normonatremic infants. Hypothermia was the strongest clinical predictor of hyponatremic seizures; a need for increased anticonvulsant therapy was also a statistically significant independent predictor (Table 3). Although other studies have occasionally reported hyponatremic seizures in patients older than 6 months, no patients in this study older than 6 months had hyponatremia (Table 4).

Conclusions.—Hyponatremia is a frequent cause of seizures with unsuspected cause in infants younger than 6 months of age. Infants with hyponatremic seizures have poorer outcomes than normonatremic infants, underscoring the need for prompt diagnosis and treatment. In infants with seizures of unknown cause and hypothermia (core body temperature of 36.5°C or lower), the possibility of hyponatremia should be investigated and empirical treatment with 2–6 mL of 3% saline solution per kg considered.

▶ All of us are aware that hyponatremia can be a serious cause of seizures. Were you aware, however, that hyponatremia causes as many as 70% of such seizures in infants younger than 6 months who have no fever and have had a generalized seizure. Hyponatremia is being increasingly recognized as a cause of seizures in infants, particularly those less than 6 months old. Such infants generally have tonic-clonic seizures, hypothermia, and depressed respirations. Their seizures are prolonged and respond poorly to standard anticonvulsant medications. This report shows us the extraordinarily high incidence of hyponatremia as a cause of seizures in this young age group and demonstrates the severity of such seizures and the utility of certain specific clinical findings in identifying patients with hyponatremic seizures.

The next time you see an infant with a generalized convulsion and a decreased core body temperature, think hyponatremia. The chance of a low serum sodium level is so high that you may want to try an empirical dose of 3% saline, 2–6 mL/kg. The latter can do relatively little harm and could be lifesaving. Of course, there is no substitute for a serum sodium determination, but these do take time.

In Utero Exposure to Phenobarbital and Intelligence Deficits in Adult Men

Reinisch JM, Sanders SA, Mortensen EL, et al (Indiana Univ, Bloomington; Inst of Preventive Medicine, Copenhagen; Harvard Univ, Cambridge, Mass)
JAMA 274:1518–1525, 1995
6–13

Background.—Behavior problems, learning disabilities, and deficits in intelligence may be more common among individuals exposed to barbiturates prenatally. The association between phenobarbital exposure in utero and intelligence score deficits in men was investigated. Whether exposure variables and/or postnatal environmental factors mediate the magnitude of the postnatal effect was also studied.

Methods.—Two double-blind studies were conducted. Participants were men born at the largest hospital in Copenhagen between 1959 and 1961. Exposed and unexposed members of this birth cohort were matched on a variety of maternal variables. The former group was exposed to phenobarbital during gestation through maternal medical therapy. Their mothers had no history of a CNS disorder and no other psychopharmacologic treatment during pregnancy. The first study included 33 exposed men and 52 control subjects, and study 2 included 81 exposed men and 101 control subjects.

Findings.—Verbal intelligence scores were significantly lower than predicted among men exposed prenatally to phenobarbital. The magnitude of these negative effects was increased by lower socioeconomic status and being the product of an unwanted pregnancy. Exposure in the last trimester of pregnancy was most harmful.

Conclusions.—Exposure to phenobarbital during prenatal development can adversely affect long-term cognitive performance. Poor outcomes are magnified by detrimental environmental conditions that interact with the prenatal biological insult. The timing of drug use appears to play an important role in the seriousness of the consequences.

► One last comment on anticonvulsants and intelligence. Did you know that adult men who were exposed to phenobarbital during gestation because of maternal medical treatment have a lower intelligence quotient (IQ) than their peers? Apparently they do, and the IQ difference is approximately 0.5 SD below the mean. This effectively means that men so exposed have about a 5-point lower IQ. Phenobarbital is a great drug but clearly must be used only when unequivocally indicated.

Transient Dystonia of Infancy, a Result of Intrauterine Cocaine Exposure?

Beltran RS, Coker SB (Loyola Univ Med Ctr, Maywood, Ill)
Pediatr Neurol 12:354–356, 1995

6–14

Introduction.—Intrauterine exposure to cocaine may lead to a broad range of neurologic sequelae (Table 1). An exposed newborn infant was encountered with generalized dystonic movements, and 3 other exposed infants had transient torticollis, a form of focal dystonia.

Case Report.—A male, 3,300-g infant was delivered by cesarean section at 38 weeks' gestation to a woman who had abused cocaine prenatally. She had inhaled crack cocaine about 3 times per week in the past trimester but denied other forms of abuse. When seen 3 hours after birth, the infant deviated his head to the right and had a right incurvature of the neck and spine. The tonic, apparently involuntary movements lasted longer than 30 seconds but did not occur during sleep. The spine episodically flexed dorsally with the infant prone. Computed tomography, MR, and electroencephalographic studies all were normal. The infant did well, and posturing became gradually less frequent during the first 4 months of life.

Discussion.—Prolonged dystonia is seen in some adult cocaine users, along with vocal and motor tics. Although the marked postural abnormalities seen in the present infant have not previously been described,

TABLE 1.—Reported Neurologic Sequelae of Intrauterine
Cocaine Exposure

Intrauterine infarction
Neonatal seizures
Electroencephalographic abnormalities
Microcephaly
Intracranial hemorrhage
Abnormal neurobehavioral development (per NBAS)
Abnormal acoustical cry characteristics
Mobius syndrome
Electroclinical sleep discordance
Delayed visual maturation, optic nerve abnormalities

Abbreviation: NBAS, neonatal behavioral assessment score.
(Reprinted by permission of the publisher from Beltran RS, Coker SB: Transient dystonia of infancy, a result of intrauterine cocaine exposure? *Pediatr Neurol* 12:354–356, Copyright 1995 by Elsevier Science Inc.)

torticollis is very common. The possibility of cocaine exposure should be considered whenever a newborn infant exhibits abnormal posturing.

▶ A dystonia is a sustained simultaneous contraction of agonist and antagonist muscles resulting in unusual postures. Dystonias are rarely manifested clinically in the newborn period, and as a clinical sign, dystonias do not appear until months or years of age. Early-onset dystonia has a very limited differential diagnosis and includes benign infantile dystonia, benign paroxysmal torticollis, and Sandifer syndrome (a dystonia associated with gastroesophageal reflux). Benign infantile dystonia is not seen until after 4 months of age and usually involves abnormal limb posturing only. Benign paroxysmal torticollis of infancy is characterized by cyclical regular dystonic attacks (parents are often able to predict the next episode). Sandifer syndrome may produce contortions of the neck resembling focal dystonia in infancy, but attacks are clearly related to feeding and are caused by gastroesophageal reflux. Because of the extremely limited differential diagnosis, it seems reasonable to assume that the etiology in the infants described was related to maternal cocaine use, because other causes of dystonia would be unheard of in the nursery. Dystonia, as one manifestation of the neurologic complications of cocaine abuse, has been described in older children and adults.[1]

Based on the cases abstracted, you should conclude that any newborn with abnormal posturing must be evaluated for cocaine exposure. Only time will tell whether there are permanent sequelae for these infants.

Reference

1. Casas-Parera I, et al: *Medicina (Buenos Aires)* 54:35, 1994.

Predictors of Persistence and Remission of ADHD Into Adolescence: Results From a Four-year Prospective Follow-up Study
Biederman J, Faraone S, Milberger S, et al (Massachusetts Gen Hosp, Boston)
J Am Acad Child Adolesc Psychiatry 35:343–351, 1996   6–15

Background.—Follow-up studies have consistently shown that attention-deficit hyperactivity disorder (ADHD) persists into adolescence and young adulthood in many individuals. However, there is little information on the predictors of persistence and remission.

Methods.—Follow-up data were available on 128 boys with ADHD. At study enrollment, all were between the ages of 6 and 17 years. A group of boys without ADHD was studied for comparison. At 4 years, the subjects were assessed by Diagnostic and Statistical Manual (DSM)-III-R structured diagnostic interviews. Blind raters evaluated psychiatric diagnoses, cognitive achievement, and social, school, and family functioning.

Findings.—Eighty-five percent of the boys with ADHD still had the disorder at 4 years and were classified as having persistent ADHD. Fifteen percent were termed remitters. Half the boys who remitted did so in childhood and the other half in adolescence. Factors predicting persistent ADHD were family history of the disorder, psychosocial adversity, and comorbidity with conduct, mood, and anxiety disorders.

Conclusions.—Most boys with ADHD continue to have the disorder for at least 4 years. In a minority of boys, ADHD remits early in its development. Persistent ADHD may be predicted by familiality, adversity, and psychiatric comorbidity.

▶ This report comes from a group that previously showed that ADHD is familial in some children and can be a highly persistent disorder. Taken with all other similar studies in this area, these findings stress the importance of family factors, either genetic or psychosocial, as risks for persistence of ADHD. Children with a higher comorbid disruptive behavior, mood disorders (major depression or bipolar disorders), and anxiety disorders are more likely to have persistent ADHD.

For the family, and for those who provide care to a family, the question of whether a given child with ADHD will have a persistent illness is of great clinical importance. Although the results of this study are not definitive, they do provide some guidelines. First, although there are some differences in the profile of ADHD symptoms between persistent and nonpersistent cases, such differences are not tremendously dramatic. In contrast, familiality, adversity, and comorbidity are predictive of persistence or late remission. Children who have none of these risk factors may have a relatively good prognosis.

The average person who cares for children will see a lot of ADHD. About 3% of school-aged youngsters and adolescents qualify for such a diagnosis, and approximately 750,000 kids in the United States currently receive psychostimulants to treat ADHD. Unfortunately, about 25% do not respond adequately to treatment. Even those who do respond do so at some risk; studies of tricyclic antidepressants (such as desipramine) have shown an untoward incidence of sudden death, which has made some care providers a bit squirrely about this class of drug.[1] For nonresponders, treatment with clonidine may provide a viable alternative.[2] Preliminary evidence is emerging that an additional class of drugs, represented by carbamazepine, may also be an effective alternate treatment in children with features of ADHD.[3]

Attention-deficit hyperactivity disorder is a good news/bad news story. The good news is that there are quite effective treatments. The bad news, to some extent, is that some with ADHD can expect to have it probably for the rest of their lives. Most of us know adults who probably have ADHD. Properly focused, the energies of such individuals frequently allow them to excel in ways that the non-ADHD adult cannot. Thus, it's not all gloom and doom for those who grow up to be a little more active than the rest of us.

References

1. Riddle MA, et al: *J Am Acad Child Adolesc Psychiatry* 30:104, 1991.

2. Hunt R, et al: *J Am Acad Child Adolesc Psychiatry* 24:618, 1985.
3. Silva RR, et al: *J Am Acad Child Adolesc Psychiatry* 35: 352, 1996.

Sexual Abuse in Childhood and Deliberate Self-harm

Romans SE, Martin JL, Anderson JC, et al (Otago Med School, Dunedin, New Zealand)
Am J Psychiatry 152:1336–1342, 1995   6–16

Background.—A relationship between being sexually abused as a child and engaging in self-damaging or suicidal behavior later in life often has been posited. Childhood abuse also may relate to borderline personality disorder, which may feature recurrent suicidal or self-mutilating behavior. High rates of deliberate self-harm have been correlated with childhood sexual abuse in a wide range of settings, including social agency clients, female inpatients, walk-in emergency clinic patients, and adolescents at a mental health center.

Objective.—This association was examined in a random community sample of 252 women younger than 65 years who reported having been sexually abused in childhood and 255 others who gave no such history.

Findings.—Women reporting sexual abuse in childhood were married less often than the control subjects and had lower socioeconomic status. They had relatively high rates of depression, anxiety, and eating and substance-use disorders. They also evinced more social, sexual, and interpersonal problems. All but 1 of 23 women who described deliberately harming themselves had been sexually abused as children. The most common form of self-harm was an overdose. Suicidal ideation correlated significantly with a history of childhood sexual abuse. Women who later harmed themselves were especially likely to have been abused many times; to have been abused by a father or stepfather; and to have been subjected to force. The same women were especially likely to come from psychosocially disadvantaged families.

Implications.—Childhood sexual abuse should always be thought of when a woman is being evaluated for self-destructive behavior or suicidal ideation. Every effort should be made to help those women who were abused as children to avoid sexually exploitative relationships.

▶ There is an important and straightforward lesson to be learned from this report. Any time you are evaluating a teenager, particularly a teenage girl, who has attempted suicide, carefully explore the possibility of that youngster having been sexually abused earlier in childhood. An etiologic link has long been postulated between sexual abuse at an early age and borderline personality disorders that can lead to suicide, suicide threats, or self-mutilating behaviors. Even eating disorders have also on occasion been suspected to be linked to sexual abuse in childhood. The linkage becomes most apparent during the college years. The problem is exacerbated if the individual enters a sexually exploitative relationship during high school or college. From such a relationship the teenager consciously or subconsciously recalls the abuse that was suffered earlier.

Remember, although only a minority of sexually abused children grow up to be adults who report deliberate self-harm, a fairly high proportion of all self-harming women report a history of sexual abuse in childhood. It's worth looking for.

Case Study: Electroconvulsive Therapy in Adolescents

Moise FN, Petrides G (Sagamore Children's Psychiatric Ctr, Dix Hills, NY; State Univ of New York, Stony Brook)

J Am Acad Child Adolesc Psychiatry 35:312–318, 1996   6–17

Background.—Although electroconvulsive therapy (ECT) has been used widely in the treatment of adults with many forms of mental illness, it is rarely used in adolescents. Lack of experience, fears that seizures may damage a developing brain, and families' reaction to such treatment are among the factors limiting the use of ECT in adolescents. The case literature that is available on ECT in this patient population has yielded ambiguous conclusions regarding its efficacy. One experience was reviewed to better define the indications for and efficacy of ECT in adolescents.

Methods.—The records of patients undergoing ECT at 1 center between 1983 and 1993 were reviewed. Thirteen patients were aged 16–18 years. Therapy was performed according to the institution's standard protocol in these cases (Table 1).

Findings.—Ten patients were classified as responders and 3 as nonresponders. Electroconvulsive therapy was most useful for patients with a diagnosis of affective illness, unspecified psychosis, or catatonia. Schizophrenic patients also showed some improvement. Eight patients were followed up through telephone interviews. Five patients continue to be asymptomatic 3 years after treatment. The remaining 3 relapsed within 12 months, despite maintenance pharmacotherapy.

Conclusion.—Within the limitations of this study, ECT appears to be as effective and safe in 16- to 18-year-olds with severe psychiatric illness as it is in adults. This treatment may be most appropriate in adolescents with disorders that, had they occurred in adulthood, would have been considered for and treated by ECT.

▶ Electroconvulsive therapy has been, for most of us, a treatment modality clothed in mysticism, yet it has survived more than 60 years of scrutiny in the psychiatric arena. Its primary indications remain depressive and manic disorders, especially those with excitement, suicidality, and catatonia. Even as we end this century, more than 30,000–40,000 patients receive ECT each year. A small percentage of these numbers represent children and adolescents. The ECT in adolescents is limited largely by lack of experience, fears that the resultant seizures may "damage" a developing brain, and the strong bias against the procedure by child and adolescent psychiatrists. A number

TABLE 1.—Demographic and Treatment Data

Case	Age	Sex	Admission Diagnosis	Discharge Diagnosis	No. of ECT	Electrode Placement	Catatonia	Outcome	Disposition
1	16	M	MDD with psychosis	MDD with psychosis	6	RUL	Staring, posturing	Responder	Home with follow-up
2	17	M	MDD	Bipolar disorder	16	Bil	No catatonia	Responder	Home with follow-up
3	16	M	Psychosis NOS	Psychosis NOS	8	Bil	No catatonia	Responder	Home with follow-up
4	16	M	MDD	Catatonia	3	RUL	Mutism, staring, posturing	Responder	Home with follow-up
5	18	F	Bipolar disorder	Bipolar disorder	1 (incomplete)	Bil	Posturing, rigidity, waxy flexibility	Nonresponder	Home with follow-up
6	18	M	Psychosis NOS	Schizophreniform disorder	(8 + 10) = 18	RUL + Bil	No catatonia	Nonresponder	Day hospital
7	17	M	Bipolar disorder	Schizophrenia	17	RUL	No catatonia	Responder	Day hospital
8	16	M	Catatonia	Catatonia	17	Bil	Mutism, staring	Responder	Home with follow-up
9	17	M	Psychosis NOS	Psychosis NOS	5	Bil	No catatonia	Responder	Day hospital
10	17	M	Psychosis NOS	Schizophreniform disorder	10	RUL	No catatonia	Responder	Drug rehabilitation program
11	17	M	Psychosis NOS	Schizophreniform disorder	20	Bil	No catatonia	Nonresponder	Group home
12	17	F	Catatonia	Bipolar disorder	15	Bil	Elective mutism, posturing, staring	Responder	Home with follow-up
13	16	M	Catatonia	Bipolar disorder	16	Bil	Staring, mutism, waxy flexibility	Responder	Day hospital

Abbreviations: ECT, electroconvulsive therapy; *MDD*, major depressive disorder; *NOS*, not otherwise specified; *RUL*, right unilateral; *Bil*, bilateral.
(Courtesy of Moise FN, Petrides G: Case study: Electroconvulsive therapy in adolescents. *J Am Acad Child Adolesc Psychiatry* 35:312–318, 1996.)

of states (Texas, California, Colorado, and Tennessee) strictly preclude the use of ECT below certain ages, which include early and late adolescence. In a recent issue of the *Lancet,* there was a plea for a ban on the use of ECT in adolescents.[1] The argument was that adolescents cannot give informed consent.

These warnings aside, ECT is still used in youngsters. Take, for example, the recent case report of an 8½-year-old girl.[2] This youngster had major depression with catatonic symptoms. While taking oral antidepressants, her symptoms worsened markedly. Significant morbidity appeared imminent. Electroconvulsive therapy was used and was reported to have been successful in treating both the catatonic and mood symptoms. No observable deleterious effects occurred. It should be noted that a review of the English language literature reveals no younger patient having been treated with ECT.

The report abstracted here did find ECT to be useful in the treatment of adolescents with severe psychiatric disorders. This finding is consistent with recent recommendations from the American Psychiatric Association. In some respect, this is a maverick report because present attitudes in adolescent psychiatry do not favor the use of ECT. It's not clear that the report abstracted will go too terribly far in reversing this negative attitude. Where this leaves the rest of us is clear. Caution in the use of ECT seems to exist and for good reason. When our planet is visited by extraterrestrials in the next millennium, will the period in the history of psychiatry that includes ECT be viewed as a period of enlightenment or one cast in the image of the Dark Ages? Given that "modern" psychiatry is in the process of burying Freud, one wonders, post Freud and ECT, where we are headed next.[3] Hopefully the "next" will be soundly based on new understanding of molecular neurobiology.

References

1. Baker T: *Lancet* 345:65, 1995.
2. Cizadlo BC, et al: *J Am Acad Child Adolesc Psychiatry* 34:322, 1995.
3. Tallis RC: *Lancet* 347:669, 1996.

Long-term Impact of Exposure to Suicide: A Three-year Controlled Follow-up

Brent DA, Moritz G, Bridge J, et al (Univ of Pittsburgh, Pa; Broward County Med Examiner, Fort Lauderdale, Fla; Pittsburgh Adolescent Alcohol Research Ctr, Pa; et al)
J Am Acad Child Adolesc Psychiatry 35:646–653, 1996   6–18

Background.—In a previous study of the effects of adolescent suicide on friends and acquaintances, the authors reported that exposed youths were at risk for recurrent depression. This finding was further explored in a 3-year, controlled follow-up of the friends of adolescents who committed suicide.

Methods.—The study included 166 friends and acquaintances of suicide victims and unexposed community control subjects. Periodic follow-up

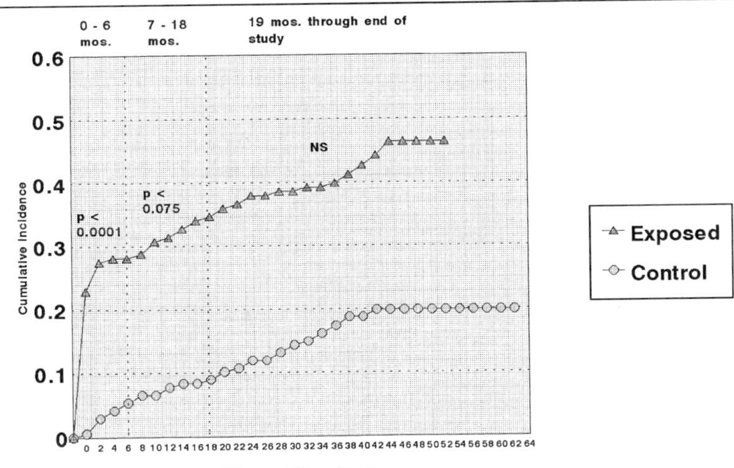

FIGURE 1.—Cumulative incidence of major depressive disorder in exposed vs. control subjects (initial acceptors and refusers). *Abbreviation: NS,* not significant. (Courtesy of Brent DA, Moritz G, Bridge J, et al: Long-term impact of exposure to suicide: A three-year controlled follow-up. *J Am Acad Child Adolesc Psychiatry* 35:646–653, 1996.)

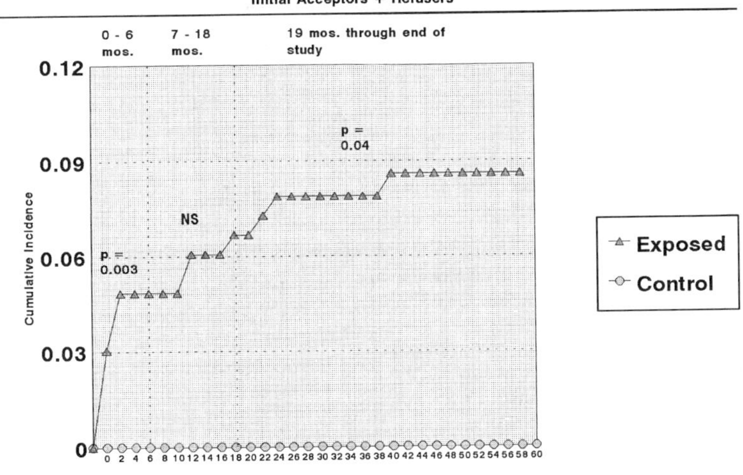

FIGURE 2.—Cumulative incidence of posttraumatic stress disorder in exposed vs. control subjects (initial acceptors and refusers). *Abbreviation: NS,* not significant. (Courtesy of Brent DA, Moritz G, Bridge J, et al: Long-term impact of exposure to suicide: A three-year controlled follow-up. *J Am Acad Child Adolesc Psychiatry* 35:646–653, 1996.)

was done using the Schedule for Affective Disorders and Schizophrenia for School-Age Children, Epidemiologic and Present Episode versions.

Findings.—The exposed and unexposed groups had a comparable incidence of suicide attempts during follow-up. However, rates of baseline and incident psychotherapy were greater in the exposed group. The exposed individuals had an increased incidence of depression and anxiety that was most pronounced in the 6 months after the friend's suicide. The exposed group also had an increased incidence of posttraumatic stress disorder (PTSD) throughout the follow-up period. Youths who knew about their friend's suicide plans were at the highest risk for incident depression and PTSD during the 3 years of follow-up (Figs 1 and 2).

Conclusions.—Exposure to suicide among youths has a relatively long effect. The friends of suicide victims had an increased incidence of depression, anxiety, and PTSD throughout the follow-up period. However, an adolescent's suicide does not appear to increase the risk of suicidal behavior among friends and acquaintances.

▶ This past summer, *Good Morning America* aired a series on raising children. For whatever reason, the producers of this show chose as their kickoff topic the question of whether our schools are teaching too much self-esteem. Apparently, the concern is that teaching kids to feel good about themselves in the absence of having something to feel good about produces a youngster who becomes an adult without substance behind the self-esteem, without true grit.

What does all this have to do with suicide? Suicide is the ultimate antithesis of self-esteem. If there is an ultimate antithesis to self esteem, there is a penultimate as well. That penultimate is the feeling held by the closest friend of someone who commits suicide. Such youngsters may have actually witnessed their friend's suicide. Others may simply have learned of the suicide when it was done. How the survivors fare is what this report is all about.

This report tells us much. It is a 3-year follow-up of not quite 200 teenagers whose best friends committed suicide. These kids continue, even after 3 years, to show high rates of depression and anxiety. Posttraumatic stress disorders were common. Fortunately, even though the incidence of PTSD didn't seem to wane over a 3-year period, depression and anxiety did. Most importantly, however, exposure to suicide among friends of suicide victims does not have the effect of provoking an increased incidence of suicide attempts via an imitation or contagion mechanism. In fact, the opposite phenomenon may occur. Peers exposed to suicide frequently confide that the experience of their friend's suicide had an inhibitory effect on their own future suicidal behavior, because they had seen the terrible devastation experienced by friends and family alike.

These findings have direct clinical implications for the psychological management of youths exposed to an adolescent suicide. Because the occurrence of imitative suicidal behavior in close friends of suicide victims is rare, the emphasis on intervention for these peers really needs to look well beyond the short-run prevention of imitation. The long-term problems that need to be dealt with to prevent lasting disability include depression, anxiety, and PTSD. Many of these kids, independent of their exposure, are vulnerable to the development of psychological disorders solely on the basis of high rates of personal and family history of psychiatric disorders.

This commentary opened with the observation that *Good Morning America* had taken an interest in the "feel-good-about-yourself" method of teaching that goes on within our schools today. Although *Good Morning America* did attempt to strike a balance in terms of the debate about such teaching methodologies, one was clearly left with the sense that we've gone overboard with making kids feel good about themselves. This may be right, even when it comes to kids who commit suicide. Obviously, such youngsters do not feel good about themselves, but psychiatrists tell us that the impulse for suicide often occurs in individuals who previously had no problems with their self-esteem, but for whatever reason, now find no basis for feeling good about themselves. It is critical for us to teach self-esteem, but only when we are certain that we have created a solid foundation upon which that esteem is based.

Without a better understanding of depression in childhood, we will continue to see children and teenagers doing harm to themselves. The consequences of even a failed suicide attempt are not minor. Granboulan et al. tell us what happens to such children in the long haul.[1] In a study of 265 adolescents who were hospitalized between 1971 and 1980 in a psychiatry unit after a suicide attempt, 39% of these individuals showed signs of improvement, 22% appeared to be unchanged, and 33% were worse. Unfortunately, only 32% of patients had received continuing and ongoing follow-up care. Fifteen subjects had died, only 1 of a natural cause. Of the remaining 14, 5 had committed suicide and 9 had died from unnatural or violent causes other than suicide, the cause of death appearing in all cases to be closely linked to the individual's previous adolescent disorder.

Reference

1. Granboulan V, et al: *Acta Psychiatr Scand* 91:265, 1995.

Psychological Effects of Hurricane Andrew on an Elementary School Population

Shaw JA, Applegate B, Tanner S, et al (Univ of Miami, Fla)
J Am Acad Child Adolesc Psychiatry 34:1185–1192, 1995   6–19

Introduction.—A spectrum of posttraumatic psychological sequelae has been reported in children after a natural disaster. To study the evolution of the psychological sequelae after disaster, posttraumatic symptomatology and the emotional and behavioral indices of psychopathology were studied in elementary school-age children in 2 communities after Hurricane Andrew struck.

Methods.—A total of 106 children were studied, including 62 who had lived directly in the path of the hurricane (HI-IMPACT school) and 44 in a comparable elementary school north of Miami (LO-IMPACT school). The Posttraumatic Stress Disorder Reaction Index (PTSDRI) was administered and the Teacher's Report Form (TRF) was completed 8 and 32 weeks after the hurricane. In addition, data were obtained from the schools' regional database of all discipline reports to analyze 21 measures of disruptive behavior during the school year.

Results.—Posttraumatic symptoms were present in 87% of the children at the HI-IMPACT school and 80% of the children at the LO-IMPACT school. At 8 weeks, there were no statistically significant differences between the 2 groups in the overall prevalence of posttraumatic symptomatology, but the HI-IMPACT school had twice as many students with severe symptoms. At 32 weeks, there was significant reduction in posttraumatic symptomatology, but moderate and severe distress was still present in many students in the HI-IMPACT school. The TRF showed a marginal reduction only in anxiety and depression among the boys at the HI-IMPACT school, whereas the HI-IMPACT girls had significantly lower scores for internalizing, externalizing, anxiety/depression, social problems, delinquent behavior, and aggressive behavior, whereas there was a trend toward more psychopathology in the LO-IMPACT school at 8 weeks. There were no statistically significant changes in the TRF scores at 32 weeks, although there was a trend toward higher scores for both sexes at the LO-IMPACT school. At the HI-IMPACT school, disruptive behavior decreased significantly for 2 marking periods, had a mild rebound in the third marking period, then returned to the previous year's level. At the LO-IMPACT school, disruptive behavior was significantly increased until the last marking period, when it returned to the previous year's level.

Conclusions.—The severity of psychological distress correlated with proximity to the impacted area. However, the comparable prevalence of mild and moderate posttraumatic symptomatology suggests a role for anticipatory anxiety. The persistence of posttraumatic symptomatology is likely related to the secondary effects of the destruction. The reduced indices of psychopathology and disruptive behavior in the HI-IMPACT school may reflect dampened behavioral responses related to shock immediately after the disaster. The increased indices of psychopathology and disruptive behavior in the LO-IMPACT school may be related to the disruption associated with increases in the school population after the hurricane and to the relatively decreased mental health resources in areas not directly affected by the hurricane. This suggests that there is an evolution of psychological distress symptoms after a natural disaster, both in the impacted areas and in the peripheral areas, which may require mental health intervention.

▶ One individual's stressor is another's stimulus. What this report fails to do is tell us which school-aged youngster is more likely to experience posttraumatic stress disorder and which is not, given the same environmental stressors. It's obvious, however, that for those who do experience the problem, it can be quite significant. What happened on August 24, 1992, was indeed a devastating event. Hurricane Andrew blew through south Miami with a vengeance. Winds of 164 miles/hr damaged more than 100,000 homes, apartments, and trailers, leaving 85,000 individuals unemployed and causing 35 deaths. More than 10,000 children in south Dade county (about 25% of the overall school population) were not able to return to their schools because of the devastation that had occurred. A year later, the school districts around the devastated area had a 13% increase in enrollment because of damage to where these affected children had previously attended school. As many as half of the young children 2 months after the event showed symptomatology consistent with the standard definition of posttraumatic stress disorder.

The younger child was not alone with this problem. Adolescents showed similar problems, albeit at a lower frequency. Approximately 3% of adolescent males and 9% of adolescent females had evidence of posttraumatic stress disorder.[1] Obviously the older we get, the better we handle stress. As we put years behind us, either we've seen or experienced it all or we just don't have that much to lose anymore. It's the young among us that we need to worry about.

As we learn more about the psychological impact of stress, such as exposures to serious natural disorders, we also learn that psychological stress is capable of producing a wide variety of physiologic responses. Were you aware, for example, of the effect of psychological stress on wound healing? Investigators at Ohio State University have evaluated the latter and have drawn some interesting conclusions. They evaluated 13 women caring for demented relatives and 13 matched for age and family income. Needless to say, those caring for seriously demented relatives were under an unusual amount of psychological stress. All participants agreed to undergo a 3.5-mm punch biopsy of the skin. Time to complete wound healing was then assessed by photography of the wound and response to bubbling of the skin when hydrogen peroxide was applied (healing was defined as no foaming). It took those who were under stress a full 9 days longer for their wound to heal (48.7 vs. 39.3 days).[2] Actually, if you look back through the literature, somewhat analogous findings were described by Holms many years ago.[3] Some time ago it was shown that stressful situations such as divorce, death of a spouse, or loss of a job were much more likely to cause an individual to have tuberculosis develop and to be less likely to recover from it. The link between stress and susceptibility to disease appears to be pinpointed to corticotropin-releasing hormone.[4]

Impaired physiologic responses and delayed wound healing in response to stress have some very significant implications. If you need elective coronary bypass surgery, or even something as simple as a hair transplant, schedule its timing carefully and make sure that your head is on straight well in advance of going under the knife.

References

1. Garrison CZ, et al: *J Am Acad Child Adolesc Psychiatry* 34:1193, 1995.
2. Kiecolt-Glaser JK, et al: *Lancet* 346:1194, 1995.
3. Lerner BH: *Ann Intern Med* 124:673, 1996.
4. Licinio J, et al: *Lancet* 346:104, 1995.

7   Child Development

Melatonin Treatment of a Non-24-hour Sleep–wake Cycle in a Blind Retarded Child
Lapierre O, Dumont M (Université de Montréal)
Biol Psychiatry 38:119–122, 1995   7–1

Background.—The light-dark cycle is the strongest known synchronizer of the endogenous circadian pacemaker on the 24-hour cycle. This may explain the high incidence of circadian rhythm abnormalities that occurs in blind persons. If other time indicators such as social cues are also absent, which happens with severe mental deficits, the sleep-wake cycle will probably free-run on a non–24-hour cycle in accordance with the individual's endogenous circadian pacemaker. Melatonin has been given experimentally to blind persons with sleep and vigilance problems associated with delayed or free-running sleep-wake cycles. The experimental melatonin treatment of a blind, retarded child was described.

Case Report.—Girl, 5 years, was referred to a sleep clinic because of a free-running sleep-wake cycle. The girl had severe mental and psychomotor retardation, had not developed language, and could not walk by herself. Her parents reported that she had never slept through the night for more than a few days in a row and that she tended to fall asleep about 1 hour later every day. Sleep diary data showed that her sleep-wake cycle free-ran on a regular 25.2-hour period (Fig 1). All other attempts to regulate the child's sleep pattern had failed. After the child's spontaneous sleep-wake cycle was close to the desired schedule—from 8 PM to 6 AM—melatonin treatment was begun. After a 4-day trial period, the administration of the oral melatonin suspension, 0.5 mg in aqueous solution with 2% ethanol, was fixed at half an hour before the desired bedtime. The treatment immediately synchronized the child's sleep-wake cycle. She slept well, with less than 30 minutes of wakefulness in the night. Sleep duration was also extended by 1.5 hours. As a result, the girl was no longer irritable, cried less, and reacted more to the presence of her parents. Six weeks after treatment was begun, she was able to go to a day-care center for the first time. At a 20-month assessment, the girl's sleep-wake cycle and total sleep time remained stable, and there were no adverse effects.

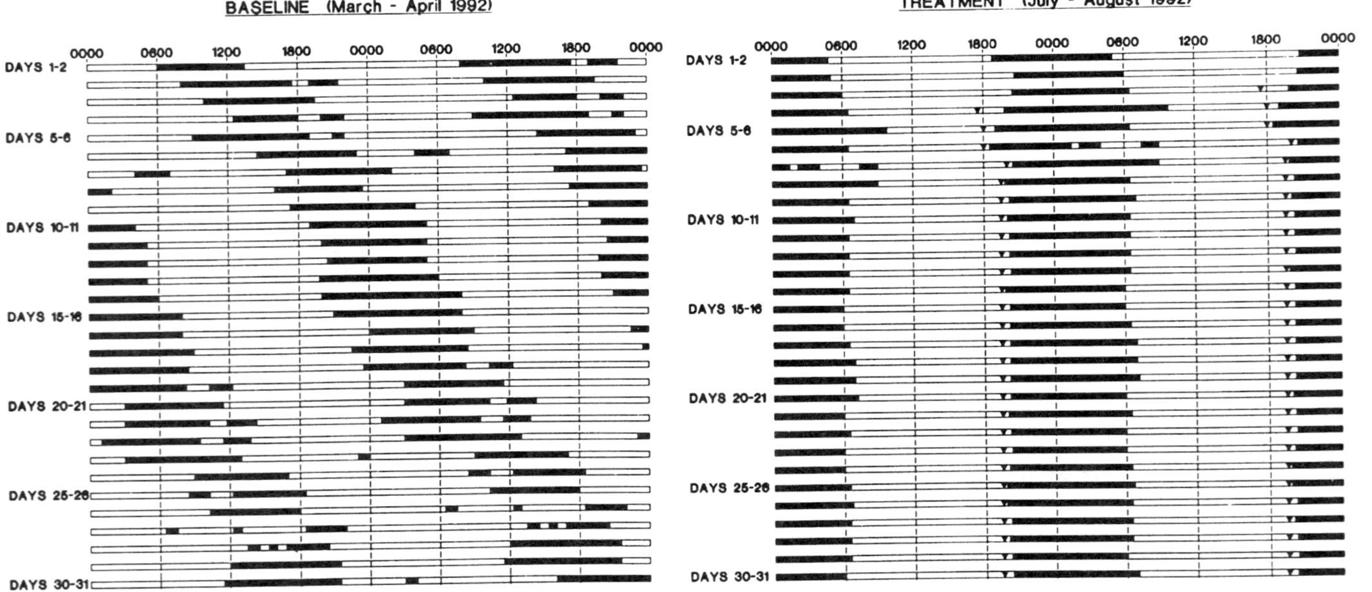

FIGURE 1.—Sleep diary data, double-plotted for 30 days. *Black bars* represent times when the child was asleep, as reported by the parents. The **left panel** presents baseline data, collected in March–April, 1992. The **right panel** presents the first 27 days of melatonin treatment (July–August, 1992). Treatment was initiated on day 4. *Triangles* represent the time of melatonin administration (Reprinted by permission of Elsevier Science Inc. from Lapierre O, Dumont M: Melatonin treatment of a non-24-hour sleep–wake cycle in a blind retarded child. *Biol Psychiatry* 38:119–122, Copyright 1995 by the Society of Biological Psychiatry.)

Conclusions.—With a normalized sleep schedule, this patient was able to get more sleep, which markedly improved her mood and learning capabilities. The treatment also greatly relieved her parents' exhaustion.

▶ Many factors trigger the timing of sleep onset in each of us. The light-dark cycle is the most powerful synchronizer known to pattern our circadian pacemaker on a 24-hour cycle. This accounts for the high incidence of circadian rhythm abnormalities found in blind people. This does not mean that all blind children and adults do not sleep well. In the presence of other time indicators, such as social cues, the absence of a circadian rhythm does not always prevent a blind person from adapting to a 24-hour schedule, although many do complain of sleep difficulties. However, if such time indicators and social cues are weak, as would be potentially true of a child with a severe mental handicap in association with blindness, the sleep-wake cycle runs free on a non–24-hour period. That's exactly what went wrong with this 5-year-old blind and mentally retarded child whose clinical problem was detailed in the above abstract. She was born with severe microophthalmia and had no light perception since birth. She had a partial trisomy 22. She literally had no sleep pattern whatsoever, but almost immediately after the institution of melatonin therapy, given at 7:50 PM each day, she normalized and actually was able to go to a day-care center for the first time in her life.

If you haven't heard much about melatonin and its use for sleep disorders, chances are that you've been on a sabbatical somewhere, perhaps on Mars. It's had extensive coverage on "60 Minutes" and "Prime Time Live." There are more than 2 dozen articles in the past couple of years on its usefulness for certain conditions found in childhood. Blind children who are not retarded and are having sleep difficulties are ideal candidates for trying this therapy. There are many studies that support its use for this purpose.[1] It can even help some children with epilepsy.[2] If you were on sabbatical and want to be brought up to speed about melatonin, read the article that describes the relevance of the pineal gland to the pediatric age population. It's an article by Cavallo et al., which appeared a couple years back in the *Journal of Pediatrics.*[3] For a summary of the usefulness of melatonin for jet lag, shift work, and seasonal affective disorders, see the review by Bonn.[4]

To date, melatonin has proved to be a safe therapeutic agent, but this statement must stand the test of time. It is certainly safer than almost all "hypnotics." The only problem you might have is difficulty finding it. Health food stores can't stock it fast enough.

P.S.: Melanatonin is also emerging as an alternative therapy for chronic refractory sarcoidosis.[5] Will there be an end to the purported benefits of this mystical agent?

References

1. Tzischinsky O, et al: *Chronobiol Int* 8:168–175, 1991.
2. Miyamoto A, et al: *Jpn J Psychiatry Neurol* 44:432, 1990.
3. Cavallo A, et al: *J Pediatr* 123:843, 1993.

4. Bonn D: *Lancet* 347:184, 1996.
5. Cognoni ML: *Lancet* 346:116, 1995.

Rates of Seasonal Affective Disorder in Children and Adolescents
Swedo SE, Pleeter JD, Richter DM, et al (Natl Inst of Mental Health, Bethesda, Md)
Am J Psychiatry 152:1016–1019, 1995   7–2

Background.—Seasonal affective disorder, a form of recurrent major depression, begins during childhood in one third of adult patients. However, there has been relatively little research on this disorder in children and adolescents.

Methods.—A total of 2,267 students at a middle school and high school in a Washington, D.C., suburb were given a modified version of the Seasonal Pattern Assessment Questionnaire. The response rate was 82.5%. The diagnosis of seasonal affective disorder was made when scores exceeded 18 and when the change of seasons was reported to be at least a "pretty bad" problem.

Findings.—There were 60 probable cases of seasonal affective disorder among the 1,835 surveys analyzed, for a frequency of 3.3%. Age and the frequency of the disorder were directly associated. The rate of the disorder was higher among postpubertal girls. Differences between those with and without the probable diagnosis were noted in the symptom patterns, especially for "feel worst," "least energy," "most irritable," and "socialize least."

Conclusions.—Seasonal affective disorder may occur in 1.7% to 5.5% of children and adolescents aged 9–19 years. Puberty appears to be associated with a greater rate of the disorder, especially among girls. Future research should more fully investigate this possible relationship.

▶ Another article dealing with the consequences of light, or not enough light. As much as we've tended to think of seasonal affective disorder as being a disease of adults, it is also a problem for children and adolescents. Until this report appeared, we didn't know how much of a problem seasonal affective disorder was in children and adolescents. It is a problem. If the results of this pilot study are generalizable, 3.3% of the 31 million children aged 10–18 years in the United States may have this mood-affecting entity. Thus, more than 1 million children may have winter blues, and these blues have nothing to do with school blues.

Biochemists and physiologists tell us that seasonal affective disorder is probably a nondisease, meaning that it is a normal biophysical response to the absence of light. In other words, winter depression is a naturally occurring rhythm of blues. It increases in prevalence in northern areas and in regions with a high proportion of overcast fall and winter days. It remits in the spring. It is characterized by sadness, anxiety, decreased involvement in work and social activities, increased appetite, carbohydrate craving, weight gain, hypersomnia, and psychomotor involution. To date, the most effective therapy seems to be the use of full-spectrum bright artificial light, but some drug therapies, including treatment with monoamine oxidase inhibitors, may be effective. To learn more about the use of phototherapy for seasonal affective disorder, read the report by Lafer et al.[1] Melatonin may also help. As a last-ditch effort, if light therapy and monoamine oxidase inhibitors don't work, you might try short-acting β-blockers. Propranolol, 60 mg or less, given in the very early morning hours at dawn, can induce a remission of depression in three quarters of adolescents.[2] If all these treatments fail, try lavender oil. The latter helps with the insomnia associated with seasonal affective sleep disorders.[3]

One last pearl. Because the management of seasonal affective disorder can be complex and lengthy, to get a handle on who might respond best to light therapy, take a very careful history to determine whether your patient craves sweets in the afternoon. A high intake of sweets in the second half of the day in teenagers who have seasonal affective disorder turns out to be the best predictor of a rapid and persistent response to light therapy.[4] Presumably, the intake of sweets acts either on similar neurochemical substrates to those affected by light or provides a behavioral marker for individuals susceptible to light response.

Clearly there is a lot we don't know about seasonal affective disorder and winter blues. We need a lot more research to shed "light" on this interesting entity.

References

1. Lafer B, et al: *Am J Psychiatry* 15:1081, 1994.
2. Schlager DS: *Am J Psychiatry* 151:1383, 1994.
3. Hardy M, et al: *Lancet* 346:701, 1995.
4. Crauchi K, et al: *Psychiatry Res* 46:107, 1993.

Distorting Reality for Children: Body Size Proportions of Barbie and Ken Dolls
Brownell KD, Napolitano MA (Yale Univ, New Haven, Conn)
Int J Eat Disord 18:295–298, 1995   7–3

Objective.—The increasing prevalence of eating disorders has raised interest in what determines ideals of body image, but most work in this area has involved adults. For this reason, bodily proportions in popular dolls of each sex and the degree to which they deviate from those of healthy young adults was determined.

Methods.—Measurements of the hips, waist, chest, and neck were taken from 2 young adults, a 22-year-old woman whose height was 5 ft 2 in. and weight 125 lb, and a man aged 32 years whose height was 6 ft and weight 185 lb. The same measurements were made on Barbie and Ken dolls.

Findings.—For the woman to attain the proportions of the Barbie doll, she would have to increase 40% in height, 14% in the chest, and 11% in neck length, and at the same time have a 21% smaller waist and a 7% smaller neck circumference (Fig 1). The man would have to become 28% taller, with a 30% increase in the waist, and a 27.5% increase in the chest, and a 51% increase in neck circumference.

Implication.—Insofar as dolls represent ideals of body shape and weight for the children who play with them, these ideals are highly unrealistic.

▶ If an analysis of the first names of couples married in the past 25 years were to be done, it is likely that you would find a deficit of couples whose first names were Barbara and Kenneth. No one wants to be stigmatized by being a Barbie or a Ken.

Our society overemphasizes ideal body size. The report abstracted is not the first of its type. Other examples include the original report by Garfinkel and Garner and a later one by Wiseman et al. showing how Miss America contestants have fallen increasingly below the healthy weights of adult females.[1, 2] Because much less attention has been paid to the exposure of children to ideals for shape and weight, the study abstracted was designed to examine body proportions in the popular dolls, Barbie and Ken, to determine the extent to which they actually vary from the proportions of young, healthy adults. They do indeed vary.

Just how dysmorphic are Barbie and Ken? If normal women and men had the body proportions that Barbie and Ken have, a normal woman would have to have an increase in height of 24 in., would have to increase her chest size by 5 in., have a longer neck by 3.2 in., would have to decrease her waist size by 6 in., with shrinkage of her neck size (circumference) by 0.2 in. Men would be no better off. A true "Ken" adult male would have to be 20 in. taller than average, have a 10-in. increase in waist size, and an 11-in. increase in chest size. His neck size (circumference) would have to increase by almost 8 in. A live Barbie would be 7 ft 2 in. tall and her mate 7 ft 8 in.

Please do not write this article off as "fluff." Children do imprint, image-wise, what they see around them. There have been 10 times more Barbie dolls manufactured in this country than there are actual children living at this point (800 million dolls sold; annual revenues greater than $1 billion).

Yes, Ken and Barbie are atypical. The only real-life analogies to them are Wonder Woman and Captain Marvel.

References

1. Garfinkel PE, Garner DM: *Anorexia Nervosa: A Multidimensional Perspective.* New York: Brunner/Mazel, 1982.
2. Wiseman CV, et al: *Int J Eat Disord* 11:85, 1992.

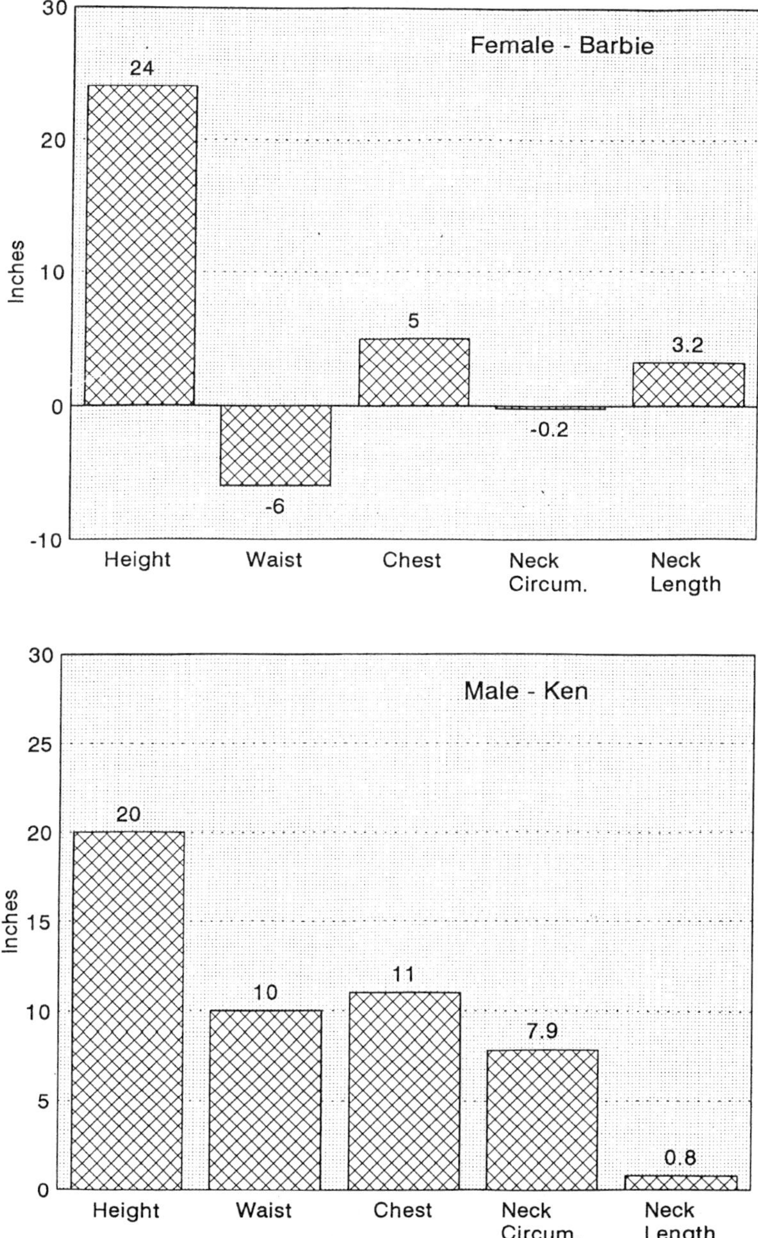

FIGURE 1.—Number of inches body parts would have to change for a young, healthy adult woman and man to achieve the proportions of Barbie and Ken, respectively. (Courtesy of Brownell KD, Napolitano MA: Distorting reality for children: Body size proportions of Barbie and Ken dolls. *Int J Eat Disord* 18:295–298, Copyright 1995. Reprinted by permission of John Wiley & Sons, Inc.)

Time Use and Mathematics Achievement Among American, Chinese, and Japanese High School Students

Fuligni AJ, Stevenson HW (Univ of Michigan, Ann Arbor)
Child Dev 66:830–842, 1995

Background.—There has been little formal study of how children from different cultures spend their time, despite the potential importance of such knowledge for understanding child and adolescent development. The few formal studies that have been done on time use among children and adolescents have almost always focused on only 1 or 2 activities. Time use and mathematics achievement among United States, Chinese, and Japanese high school students were studied.

Methods.—Representative samples of 578 students in grade 11 in Minneapolis, Taipei, and Sendai were surveyed. The individuals were 16 and 17 years of age. The amount of time spent on a wide variety of activities was elicited.

Findings.—In all 3 groups, studying, interacting with peers, and watching television were the most common activities. However, the relative importance of each activity was different among groups. Chinese students spent significantly more time than United States students on academic pursuits, such as going to school and after-school classes and studying.

TABLE 2.—Hours per Week Spent in Selected Activities Out of School

Activities	United States M	SD	Taiwan M	SD	Japan M	SD	F	Scheffé Contrasts
Academic:								
Studying (general)	10.1	7.4	16.4	10.5	11.4	8.8	30.15**	T > J, U**
Weekday	1.6	1.3	2.3	1.5	1.5	1.2	22.31**	T > U, J**
Saturday	.6	1.0	1.7	1.9	1.7	1.5	34.98**	T,J > U**
Sunday	1.5	1.1	3.2	2.7	2.0	1.7	42.76**	T > J, U**
Studying (math)	3.4	3.4	4.4	4.5	2.4	3.0	13.05**	T > J**
Lessons	.5	1.4	2.6	3.7	.8	1.6	41.77**	T > J, U**
Reading	4.8	6.0	6.5	5.0	5.0	5.2	6.89**	T > U*
Work:								
Employment	12.0	9.6	4.0	11.4	1.5	5.6	60.10**	U > T, J**
Chores	3.1	3.2	2.0	2.9	2.8	5.2	6.33*	U > T*
Leisure:								
Extracurricular	14.0	10.4	9.5	9.1	11.0	8.7	13.02**	U > T**
Watching TV	12.0	9.5	15.1	9.4	16.7	8.7	12.15**	T > U*; J > U**
With friends	18.4	12.3	8.8	9.1	12.4	12.0	38.79**	U > T, J**
Dating	4.7	4.5	.9	2.7	1.1	2.7	75.33**	U > T, J**
Alone	11.5	8.6	11.7	9.7	12.5	8.8	.68	...

Note: $n = 179$–204 (U, United States); $n = 213$–220 (T, Taiwan); $n = 138$–152 (J, Japan).
Studying (general) is sum of $5 \times$ weekday hours plus Saturday and Sunday hours.
* $P < 0.01$.
** $P < 0.001$.
(Courtesy of Fuligni AJ, Stevenson HW: Time use and mathematics achievement among American, Chinese, and Japanese high school students. *Child Dev* 66:830–842, 1995.)

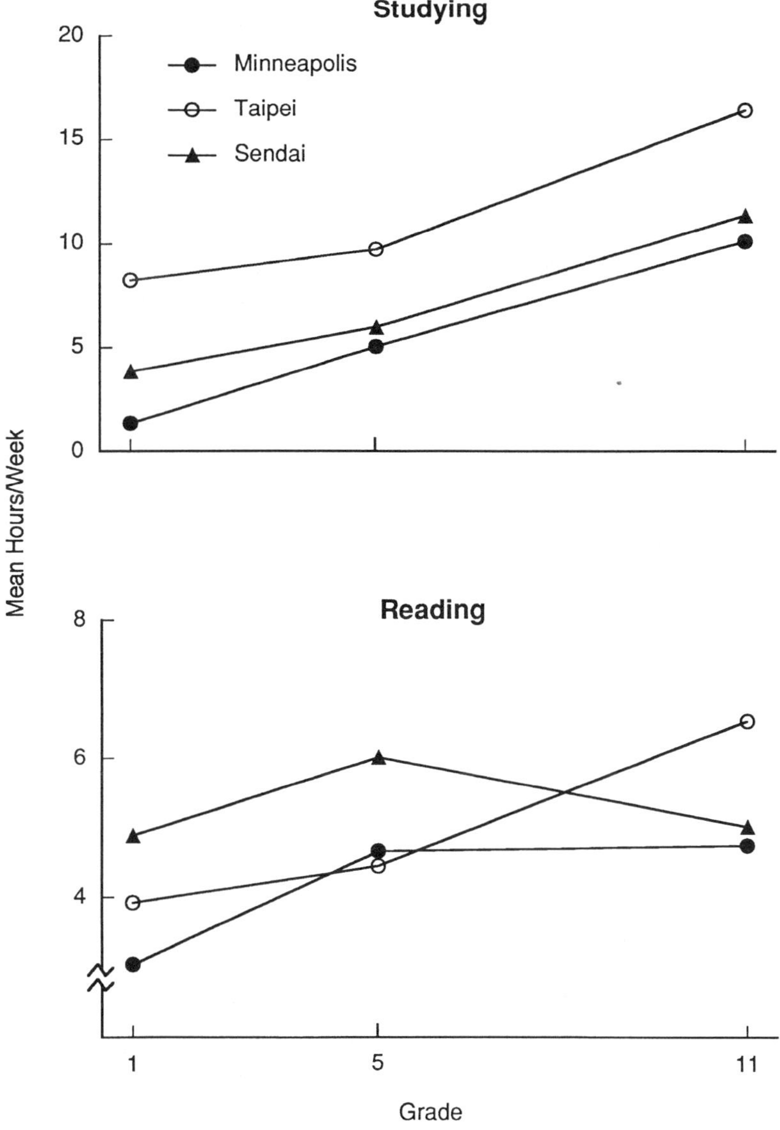

FIGURE 1.—Age trends in time spent studying and doing homework and time spent reading for pleasure, according to location. (Courtesy of Fuligni AJ, Stevenson HW: Time use and mathematics achievement among American, Chinese, and Japanese high school students. *Child Dev* 66:830-842, 1995.)

Although Japanese students did not spend significantly more time studying or going to after-school classes than United States students, the Japanese students did spend more time in school. Students in the United States spent more time working and socializing (Table 2; Figs 1 and 2). Differences in time use among groups were associated with cross-cultural and individual differences in math achievement.

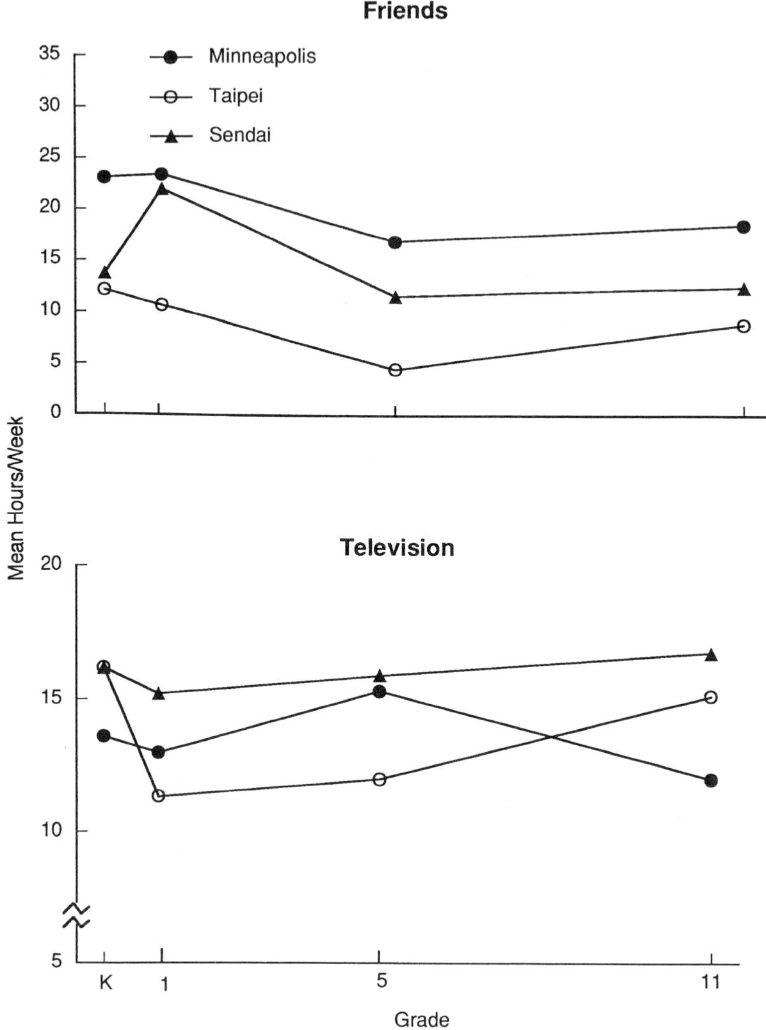

FIGURE 2.—Age trends in time spent playing with friends and time spent watching television, according to location. (Courtesy of Fuligni AJ, Stevenson HW: Time use and mathematics achievement among American, Chinese, and Japanese high school students. *Child Dev* 66:830–842, 1995.)

Conclusions.—The most striking aspect of students' lives in the United States was the amount of time spent working and dating. The students generally reported that both these activities interfered with their schoolwork. Employment among teenagers is relatively rare in Japan and Taiwan and ubiquitous in the United States, consuming as much time as studying. Similarly, teens in the United States spent much more time socializing with friends and were far more involved in dating than teens in the other 2 cultures.

▶ There are data, good data, documenting that students in East Asian countries consistently outperform their American peers in academic achievement, particularly in mathematics and science. To explain these differences, the American media have portrayed East Asian high school students as spending most of their waking time going to school, attending after-school classes, and studying. American students, in contrast, are depicted as academic couch potatoes for whom schoolwork is only one of many areas that occupy their interest. Sports, jobs, social life, dates, and television are often viewed as consuming a significant proportion of time that otherwise would be available for studying. If students from Minneapolis, Taipei (Taiwan), and Sendai (Japan) are representative of their respective countries, we now have the answer to why American students possibly do less well.

Japanese students are more similar in their use of time to American students than to Chinese students. The most assiduous of the Chinese students are the ones who were best described by the typical stereotype regarding Asian students. Nevertheless, even Chinese students participate in sports and extracurricular activities, spend time with their friends, and engage in various types of social and artistic activity. Thus, although the amount of time spent on academic activities in instruction, practice, and review is positively related to academic success, this success does not seem to require adolescents to give exclusive emphasis to academic work. On the other hand, the most striking aspect of American students' lives is the amount of time spent working and dating, activities they agree interfere with schoolwork. Relatively rare in Japan and China, youth employment is ubiquitous in the United States, occupying as much time as does studying. Additionally, adolescents in Minneapolis report substantially more time socializing with friends and a far greater involvement in dating than do their peers in Japan or China.

It's fairly clear that employment, watching television, and excessive socialization with friends are the archrivals of academic achievement. Students in Japan and China who participate in these activities, to a greater extent than those who do not, do not achieve the same level of academic accomplishment. It is therefore believable that the problem in the United States relates to these 3 elements.

Sissiness, Tomboyism, Sex-role, Sex Identity and Orientation
McConaghy N, Zamir R (Prince of Wales Hosp, Randwick, New South Wales, Australia)
Aust N Z J Psychiatry 29:278–283, 1995   7–5

Introduction.—Two types of self-rating studies have been used to study masculinity and femininity. Either personality traits considered to be masculine (M) and feminine (F) are examined, or those behaviors that appear to be statistically more frequent in one sex than in the other (so-called sex-linked behaviors) are studied. Consistent associations are observed between sex-liked behaviors and the ratio of homosexual to heterosexual feelings (Ho/Het) in men, but there is little if any indication of a relationship between self-reported M-F sex roles and Ho/Het in either sex.

Objective and Methods.—These 2 research approaches were compared in a study of 66 male and 51 female second-year medical students attending a class in human behavior. Without knowing about the study, the students completed a series of instruments including the Bem Sex-Role Inventory (BSRI) and the Sex-Linked Behaviors Questionnaire.

Findings.—Fifty-three men and 37 women were currently aware only of heterosexual feelings. One man described exclusively homosexual feelings. In neither men nor women did the Ho/Het ratio correlate significantly with the BSRI M and F scores. High M scores in women correlated closely with a number of "tomboyish" behaviors. In men but not women, opposite sex–linked behaviors characterized as "sissy" or "tomboyish" correlated significantly with self-reported Ho/Het.

Implication.—If Ho/Het and the ratio of same to opposite sex–linked behaviors develop on a biological basis, it may be that the critical intrauterine periods when these ratios are established overlap much more in males than in females.

▶ This report is a good example of well-intended psychology gone amuck. In part it attempts to show whether boys who manifest "sissy" behavior and girls who act like "tomboys" grow up to be adults with tendencies toward homosexuality and lesbianism. The study says that boys who are shy about participating in outdoor sports, particularly of the contact variety, and who keep a tidy room, according to these authors, are at risk of mixed homosexual and heterosexual feelings. The same is said to be true of girls in the opposite way. If either plugs in classical music CDs instead of pop rock, watch out!

In an era of greater acceptance and tolerance of diversity, one wonders why we continue to see reports such as this. Yes, there are truly extremes that kids and adults can manifest (one would be worried about a boy who continuously dresses in female clothes, uses cosmetics, jewelry, and carries a handbag). More commonly, however, youngsters who are a bit out of the mainstream probably are just fine, and we shouldn't call a great deal of attention to their non–totally conforming behavior. Besides, there are no data whatsoever to suggest that modification of such behaviors, in the long run, really makes any difference.

To say all this differently, boys will be boys and girls will be girls. Let's let it go at that.

Effects of Children With Down Syndrome on Parents' Activities
Barnett WS, Boyce GC (Rutgers—State Univ of New Jersey; Utah State Univ, Salt Lake City)
Am J Ment Retard 100:115–127, 1995   7–6

Background.—Researchers have long studied the effects of mentally retarded children on their families. Early investigators tended to conclude that such children were a source of significant psychological stress and adversity for parents and siblings. However, other research raises the possibility that these investigators may have misjudged the relative importance of various problems. More recent research has assessed family life more broadly. How the presence of a mentally retarded child may affect the daily activities of families was studied.

Methods and Findings.—Data on the time spent on various daily activities were obtained from diaries kept by 2 samples of parents with at least 1 child younger than 17 years. Parents in the first sample had a child with Down's syndrome, and parents in the other sample did not. Patterns of time use differed substantially between groups. Compared with mothers of healthy children, the mothers of a child with Down's syndrome spent about 7 hours per week less doing paid work and about 9 hours a week more caring for the child. Time involved in social activities was reduced by about 3 hours. Compared with fathers of healthy children, the fathers of children with Down's syndrome increased the amount of time caring for the child by 4 hours a week and reduced the amount of time in social activities by 2 hours a week. These changes were small compared with the estimated effects on mothers' time use but large compared with the time use of fathers of healthy children.

Conclusions.—Mothers and fathers of a child with Down's syndrome spent more time on child care and less time in social activities compared with the mothers and fathers of healthy children. The mothers of children with Down's syndrome also reduced their time in paid employment.

▶ Never attempt to understand the issues confronting another person until you've walked a mile in his or her shoes. This report does walk us through the daily lives of those who care for children with mental retardation. In this report, the mental retardation was caused by Down's syndrome. It's easy for someone who has not cared for a retarded child in his or her own family to suggest that this report must be flawed in its conclusions. The study tells us that children with mental retardation may be a source of significant psychological stress and adversity for parents. Other studies have suggested that siblings may also be affected.[1] If there is a flaw in this study, the flaw is that we do not learn whether there may be significant positive effects of caring for and having a child with Down's syndrome in one's family. Sure, mothers are not able to work as much (7 hours a week less) and have less free time for social activities. Dads too, albeit to a lesser degree, experience the same consequences. Surely, these "adversities" are offset in some families by the satisfaction and love that these parents derive from their relationship with their child.

If there is anything that we do learn from this report, it is that all of us must be sensitive to the fact that parents of handicapped children have fewer degrees of freedom than other parents and can, at times, experience stresses that most of us cannot begin to fully understand.

Reference

1. Farber B: Family and crisis: Maintenance of integration in families with a severely mentally retarded child. *Monogr Soc Res Child Dev* 25 (serial No. 11), 1960.

The Effect of Sugar on Behavior or Cognition in Children: A Meta-analysis
Wolraich ML, Wilson DB, White JW (Vanderbilt Univ, Nashville, Tenn; US Naval Hosp, Yokosuka, Japan)
JAMA 274:1617–1621, 1995   7–7

Background.—Shannon, in 1922, proposed that sugar-containing foods might adversely affect behavior. Half a century later, the lay literature began implicating sugar as causing "functional reactive hypoglycemia." Today the presumed relationship between sugar and behavior is used as a self-defense in court cases. Two possibilities are cited: an allergic response to refined sugar, and a reactive hypoglycemic state similar to that seen in adults.

Objective.—A meta-analysis was carried out on 23 studies featuring a within-subject design in which the individuals consumed a known amount of sugar, and there was a placebo condition consisting of an artificial sweetener. Study participants, parents, and research staff all were blinded. The studies were conducted from 1982 to 1994.

Results.—There was no evidence from these studies that sugar (chiefly sucrose) influenced either behavior or cognitive performance. In all instances the confidence interval included zero, despite considerable variation in the types of children studied, their ages, and preexisting dietary conditions. A small effect was not ruled out.

▶ There hasn't been a moment in the history of refined sugar that hasn't been troubled by controversy. If you weren't aware, refined sugar first became a nutritional concern in this country after the Civil War, when it was thought that this form of sugar had poor nutritional value. By 1922, the first flags were being raised about refined sugar causing hyperactivity. To this day we still see reports of kids who "bounce off the wall" after a spoonful of sugar. The whole problem became even more perturbing in the 1970s when table sugar was suspected to cause "functional reactive hypoglycemia." The latter is the basis of the classic "Twinkie" defense still used in the courtroom to write off bad behavior.

This report follows by 1 year an earlier study by the same investigators that examined the effects of diets high in sucrose or aspartame on the behavior and cognitive performance of children.[1] Even with megadose refined sugar or aspartame, no behavioral or cognitive problems were detected, not even in children previously described as being sugar sensitive.

It is not likely that we've heard the last word on potential side effects of sweeteners: the real stuff—sugar—or aspartame or saccharine. For what it's worth, there is one bit of encouraging news with respect to one of these products, aspartame. Were you aware that aspartame has now been documented to inhibit hunger and food intake? Indeed it does. In a double-blind study in which individuals were asked to swallow capsules containing aspartame (234–470 mg), a marked negative effect on appetite was seen.[2] Before you assign this phenomenon to *Ripley's Believe It Or Not*, recognize that it is well known that phenylalanine (a constituent of aspartame) releases cholecystokinin. The latter substance takes the edge off an appetite very quickly.

Anyone who has studied biology in high school knows that our tongue contains specific taste buds to allow us delight in perceiving sweet taste. What a waste it would be if we were denied one of life's small pleasures, refined sugar (or even an artificial sweetener). This study by Wolraich et al. should be considered definitive. No more on this topic. Jackie Gleason was right ..."how sweet it is."

P.S. Quiz question: Do you know how much refined sugar (in pounds) the average American eats during the course of a year? The answer is 120 pounds, according to a commercial for EQUAL starring Jamie Lee Curtis.

References

1. Wolraich ML, et al: *N Engl J Med* 330:301, 1994.
2. Rogers PJ, et al: *Physiol Behav* 47:1239, 1990.

What Do Children Worry About? Worries and Their Relation to Anxiety
Silverman WK, La Greca AM, Wasserstein S (Florida Internatl Univ, Miami; Univ of Miami, Fla)
Child Dev 66:671–686, 1995   7–8

Introduction.—Too little attention has been given to the worries that preoccupy young children and how they may relate to anxiety. From the clinical viewpoint, worry may be viewed as a central element in several *Diagnostic and Statistical Manual of Mental Disorders, edition 4*, anxiety disorders of children.

Methods.—A group of 141 boys and 132 girls in grades 2 through 6 at public school in a large metropolitan area were given a number of self-report measures and subsequently were individually interviewed about their worries. The measures used included the Social Anxiety Scale for Children–Revised, the Revised Children's Manifest Anxiety Scale, the Test Anxiety Scale for Children, and the Childhood Anxiety Sensitivity Index.

Findings.—Children described approximately 8 distinct worries on average. These most commonly had to do with health, school, and personal harm. Girls reported more worries than boys, and black children more than white or Hispanic children. Health concerns included those relating to the health of another, such as a parent, as well as surgery, specific bodily symptoms, and becoming ill. Contracting AIDS was a distinct area of concern. Most school worries revolved around tests and grades, being called on, and teachers. The chief worry concerning personal harm referred to physical attack or harm from others, such as robbery, stabbing, and mugging. Children rated as highly anxious reported significantly more worries—and more areas of worry—than did those with a comparatively low level of anxiety.

Summary.—Worries about physical harm and being attacked were the most prominent concerns expressed by study children. Health also is a frequent cause of worry by young children. Worry and anxiety are related but distinct constructs.

▶ This report tells us what our children worry and don't worry about. Children's worries are clearly a barometer of what is contemporary within our society. In the 1950s, those growing up had as their top worry a fear of being done in by a hydrogen bomb. There wasn't a kid in the country who thought that crawling under a desk was going to save him or her. Today, the top concerns are health issues. Nuclear warfare is far down the list, along with fears of aliens and animal attacks.

Worry is part of life. It is not to be avoided, but it is to be reckoned with. Our kids should not be so presumptuous as to think they might have no worries whatsoever; the trick is to minimize anxiety and to avoid becoming a worrywart.

Childhood Social Circumstances and Psychosocial and Behavioural Factors as Determinants of Plasma Fibrinogen
Brunner E, Smith GD, Marmot M, et al (Univ College London; Bristol Univ, England; St Mary's Hosp, Portsmouth, England)
Lancet 347:1008–1013, 1996   7–9

Introduction.—Adults with high plasma fibrinogen concentrations are at elevated risk of coronary heart disease. For unknown reasons, fibrinogen concentration is inversely associated with socioeconomic status. Three groups of factors were studied as possible determinants of plasma fibrinogen concentration—early life circumstances, current social and psychological circumstances, and health behaviors.

Methods.—The analysis used data from a cross-sectional study of British civil servants performed from 1985 to 1988. The analysis included 2,095 men and 1,202 women between 45 and 55 years of age. All patients provided blood samples for measurement of fibrinogen. They also completed a questionnaire covering their demographic characteristics, education, employment grade, parents' occupation, health behaviors, and work characteristics.

Results.—In both men and women, adult plasma fibrinogen concentration was inversely associated with certain indicators of childhood environment, namely adult height, father's social class, and subject's education. Fibrinogen concentrations were higher for subjects of lower socioeconomic status, the difference between the top and bottom employment grade was 0.22 g/L in women. The influence of employment grade was not explained by childhood circumstances. As assessed by personal managers, the subjects' control over their work was inversely related to fibrinogen concentration. The same was true for self-rated control over work for men but not for women. For men, being in the bottom third of the distribution of control over work, self-rated and externally assessed, was associated with a 0.16 g/L higher fibrinogen level than in men in the top third. Fibrinogen concentrations were higher in current cigarette smokers and lower in moderate alcohol users.

Conclusion.—Many different factors, starting in childhood, influence the fibrinogen concentration in adulthood. Fibrinogen may be a useful indicator of the biological processes responsible for the higher rates of coronary disease in the lower socioeconomic strata. Childhood, and even in utero, factors appear to have a lifelong influence on coronary risk.

▶ This report is proof positive that the tree grows not far from where the acorn has fallen, or something like that. To say this differently, the seeds of adult coronary artery disease find their origins in what happens to us as youngsters. This does not refer solely to our early experiences with cholesterol. It refers to those "stressors" that children experience in terms of poverty, social deprivation, and similar factors that set the thermostat for our blood fibrinogen levels. Although adversity builds character, it also builds fibrinogen. As important as fibrinogen is in stopping bleeding, it has other implications as well. A single fibrinogen measurement can now be used, to some extent, to predict fatal and nonfatal cardiovascular events which will occur as much as a decade or 2 later in life. Together with other hemostatic factors, fibrinogen may promote atherosclerotic changes and thrombosis by its effects on platelet aggregation, blood viscosity, and foam cell formation. Some believe that the relationship between fibrinogen and coronary artery disease is not causal, but rather the result of some confounding factor—a consequence, rather than a cause, of a disease process. Whatever the true basis is for the relationship between fibrinogen levels and heart attacks, the relationship does exist.

The message is pretty clear: Children and adults need to chill out, keep their cool in spite of adversity, and thereby learn to live longer and healthier lives.

Bone Lead Levels and Delinquent Behavior

Needleman HL, Riess JA, Tobin MJ, et al (Univ of Pittsburgh, Pa; Carnegie Mellon Univ, Pittsburgh, Pa)
JAMA 275:363–369, 1996

7–10

Background.—In children who have had lead poisoning, aggressive behavior has often been observed after an acute toxic episode. However, there has been only 1 published study of the relation of lead exposure to discipline problems, juvenile delinquency, and adult criminality. The role of lead exposure, at levels experienced by schoolchildren, as a risk factor in the genesis of antisocial behavior was investigated.

Methods.—Five hundred three first-grade boys were initially selected, based on a risk scale for antisocial behavior, from 850 at public schools. All 850 boys had scored in the upper 30th percentile of the distribution on a self-reported antisocial behavior scale. A control group included 301 students scoring in the lower 70% of the distribution. Bone lead measures were obtained.

Findings.—Borderline associations were found between teachers' scores of aggression, delinquency, and externalizing, and the boys' lead concentrations at 7 years of age, after adjustment for covariates. When the boys were 11 years of age, parent reports (Fig 2) showed significant associations between lead and several Child Behavior Checklist (CBCL) cluster scores,

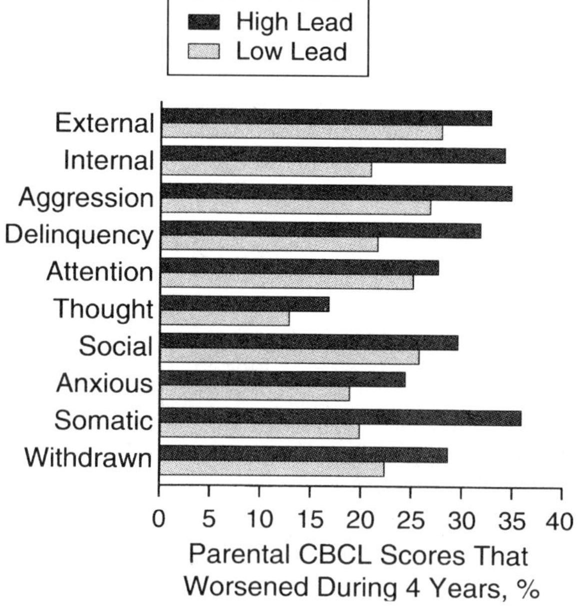

FIGURE 2.—The change in parental Child Behavior Checklist *(CBCL)* scores during 4 years in relation to bone lead concentrations. Subjects are classified as "high lead" (above the median) and "low lead" (below the median). (Courtesy of Needleman HL, Riess JA, Tobin MJ, et al: Bone lead levels and delinquent behavior. *JAMA* 275:363–369, Copyright 1996, American Medical Association.)

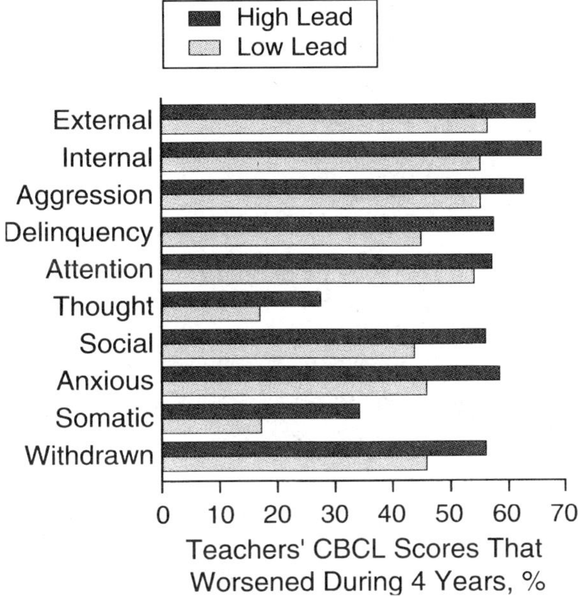

FIGURE 3.—The change in teachers' Child Behavior Checklist *(CBCL)* scores during 4 years in relation to bone lead concentrations. Subjects are classified as "high lead" (above the median) and "low lead" (below the median). (Courtesy of Needleman HL, Riess JA, Tobin MJ, et al: Bone lead levels and delinquent behavior. *JAMA* 275:363–369, Copyright 1996, American Medical Association.)

including somatic complaints and delinquent, aggressive, internalizing, and externalizing behavior. Teachers' reports (Fig 3) showed significant relationships between lead and somatic complaints: anxious/depressed behavior; social problems; attention problems; and delinquent, aggressive internalizing, and externalizing behavior. Boys with high lead concentrations had higher scores on delinquency self-reports at 11 years of age and were also more likely to get lower scores on all CBCL items during the 4 years of observation. High levels of bone lead were correlated with an increased risk of exceeding the clinical score for attention, aggression, and delinquency (Fig 4). A positive correlation was found between lead level and both verbal and full scale intelligence quotient (Table 6).

Conclusions.—Lead exposure in boys is correlated with an increased risk for antisocial and delinquent behavior. The effects of lead exposure seem to follow a developmental course.

▶ If these investigators are correct and if the findings reported can be extended to the population of the country as a whole, the contribution of lead to delinquent behavior would be very substantial. Even though mean blood levels in children have decreased 77% (from 13.7 μg/dL to 3.2 μg/dL) between 1976 and 1991, still many thousands of children continue to have toxic lead exposures, especially in minority communities. For example, the prevalence of blood lead concentrations more than 10 μg/dL in non-Hispanic blacks is 21%.[1]

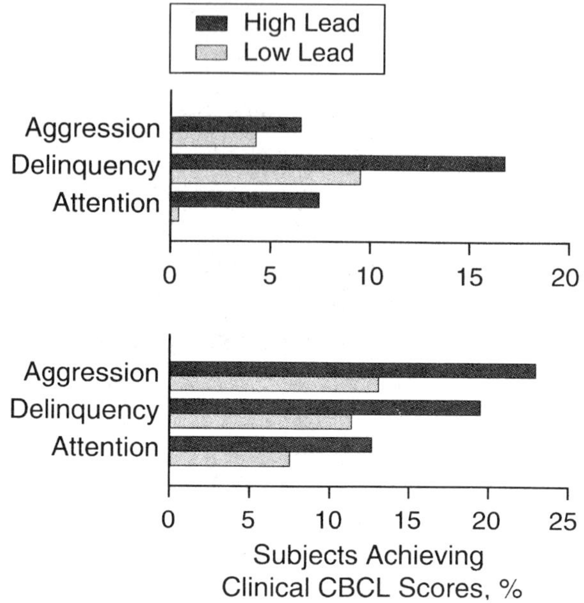

FIGURE 4.—The association between bone lead concentration and clinical Child Behavioral Checklist *(CBCL)* (T >70) scores for aggressions, delinquency, and attention. Subjects are classified as "high lead" (above the median) and "low lead" (below the median). Both parents' CBCL scores (**top**) and teachers' scores (**bottom**) are displayed. (Courtesy of Needleman HL, Riess JA, Tobin MJ, et al: Bone lead levels and delinquent behavior. *JAMA* 275:363–369, Copyright 1996, American Medical Association.)

There is one other aspect of the data presented that is extremely worrisome. Will these youngsters grow up to be antisocial adults? To say this differently, how predictive are the measurements which Needleman et al. have taken? Because it is generally accepted that antisocial behaviors are among the most stable of human attributes, showing continuities from childhood to adulthood that match those of measures of intelligence, it seems likely that there is a reasonable possibility that many adults who are ill mannered, ill tempered, and perhaps in jail may have experienced lead poisoning as children.

If there is any good news in all of this, it is that because blood lead concentrations have been steadily decreasing, perhaps we will be seeing a whole new generation of youngsters growing up to be normally socially adapted adults, free of aggressive, and possibly criminal, behavior. If you believe this theory, there is a bridge in New York City that you should look into buying.

Reference

1. Pirkle JL, et al: *JAMA* 272:284, 1994.

TABLE 6.—Bone Lead Concentrations and Intelligence Quotient (IQ), Attention, and Neurobehavioral Evaluation System Scores*

Test	Mean Low-Lead Level	Mean High-Lead Level	P
Wechsler Intelligence Scale for Children-Revised			
Verbal IQ	96.54	101.08	0.006
Performance IQ	102.18	103.14	.68
Full-scale IQ	99.14	102.15	.07
Attention Battery			
Factor 1			
Focus/execute	−.043	−.017	.71
Factor 2			
Reaction time/vigilance	.112	−.143	.09
Factor 3			
Continuous Performance Test errors	−.018	.068	.62
Factor 4			
Shift	.002	.079	.55
Neurobehavioral Evaluation System			
Finger tapping, No. of taps	122.96	122.79	.96
Reaction time, mean ms†	351.73	356.54	.68
Reaction Time SD, ms†	138.87	139.56	.94
Serial digit learning†	3.11	2.68	.26
Pattern recognition, mean latency, on correct trials	5.27	5.08	.30
Associate learning across three trials, No. correct per trial	3.41	3.29	.46
Associate recall, No. correct	3.44	3.30	.55

* Covariate-adjusted mean scores are given. Covariates in the model are the same as in Tables 2, 3, and 4. IQ score analyses are not adjusted for age.

† Lower scores indicate better performance.

(Courtesy of Needleman HL, Riess JA, Tobin MJ, et al: Bone lead levels and delinquent behavior. *JAMA* 275:363–369, Copyright 1996, American Medical Association.)

8 Adolescent Medicine

Which Teen Mothers Choose Norplant?
Stevens-Simon C, Wallis J, Allen-Davis J (Univ of Colorado Health Science Ctr, Denver)
J Adolesc Health 16:350–353, 1995

8–1

Objective.—Because repeat teenage pregnancies present risks to both mother and child, prevention of additional pregnancies is very important. Whether there are differences between teen mothers who choose Norplant and those who do not was studied.

Methods.—A total of 187 poor, multiracial girls, aged 13–18 years, at risk for repeat pregnancies were studied. Risk factors included youth, poverty, marriage, school failure, no career plans, numerous siblings, not living with parents, poor social support, no day care, depression, new boyfriend, older boyfriend, dissatisfied with previous pregnancy, dissatisfied with sex of baby, problem pregnancy or delivery, desire for more children, encouraged to have more children, and no birth control.

Results.—Norplant was inserted into 100 of the patients (Table 1). Norplant users were more likely to have poor grades, more than 1 child, less desire for more children, and problems with other contraceptive methods or remembering to use contraceptives.

TABLE 1.—Sociodemographic Factors

Factor	Norplant User	Norplant Refuser
Number	100	87
Chronologic age (mean w SD:years)	16.9 w 1.2	17.0 w 1.3
Race: N (%)		
White	53 (53)	43 (49)
Black	24 (24)	27 (31)
Hispanic	23 (23)	15 (17)
Other	0 (0)	2 (2)
Medicaid dependent: N (%)	98 (98)	81 (93)
Primigravida: N (%)	73 (73)	67 (77)
Primiparous: N (%)	79 (79)*	78 (90)
Married: N (%)	11 (11)	7 (8)

* $P = 0.04$.

(Reprinted by permission of Elsevier Science Inc. from Stevens-Simon C, Wallis J, Allen-Davis J: Which teen mothers choose Norplant? *J Adolesc Health* 16:350–353, Copyright 1995 by the Society for Adolescent Medicine.)

Conclusion.—Teen mothers at highest risk of repeat pregnancy are more likely to select Norplant as a postpartum contraceptive. Additional studies are needed to examine the part depression and social support play in the selection of postpartum contraceptives.

▶ The prevention of a repeat adolescent pregnancy should be a laudable goal, because the incidence of low birth weight and prematurity increases with each additional adolescent pregnancy, and the likelihood of completing high school, having a job, and being self-supporting decreases. There are substantial data to show that in the absence of intensive postpartum follow-up, the incidence of repeat adolescent pregnancy averages 30% in the first year after the first delivery and is 25% to 50% during the second year.[1] The results of this study are encouraging because they do not support the hypothesis that those adolescent mothers who are at highest risk for repeat adolescent pregnancy are least likely to select Norplant as a postpartum contraceptive. Rather, many investigators have reported that adolescent mothers who do poorly in school are more likely to drop out of school and have more children than their academically successful peers. Litt has reported that past compliance behavior is a good predictor of future compliance behavior.[2]

Although neither Norplant nor Depo-Provera are new agents, the recent approval for their use as contraceptives by the Food and Drug Administration (FDA) has extended their availability to many teenagers. Most individuals involved in the care of children are concerned about these 2 agents. Some of these concerns include a worry that the incidence of sexually transmitted diseases will increase when contraception becomes technically uncoupled from disease prevention. Others are concerned that Norplant has been looked to to solve some of society's basic ills. Within days of FDA approval, the availability of Norplant mobilized those looking for a "quick fix" to many of contemporary society's pressing social problems by embracing this new contraceptive as a potential panacea. An editorial in the *Philadelphia Inquirer* encouraged readers to think about Norplant as a tool in the fight against poverty in the black community.[3] Not long afterward, legislators in Louisiana and Kansas proposed legislation to offer financial reimbursements to women receiving public assistance who agreed to have implants done with Norplant.[4]

It is obvious that agents such as Depo-Provera and Norplant do produce solutions, but they also raise issues that demand to be addressed. Iris Litt,[5] editor of the *Journal of Adolescent Health,* recently commented on this topic with the following words: "Is it not too early to plan to prospectively follow our adolescent patients who elect these contraceptive methods, gather uniform information, both biological and psychological, at standard intervals and to pool the result in data? Are we ready for a national registry?" What Dr. Litt is referring to is the need to address all the unanswered questions surrounding 1-stop contraception. If we care about our adolescents, perhaps we should take Dr. Litt's suggestions seriously. Are we ready for a national registry?

References

1. Stevens-Simon C, et al: *Pediatr Ann* 20:322, 1991.
2. Litt IF: *Pediatrics* 75:693, 1985.
3. Editorial, "Poverty and Norplant: Can Contraception Reduce the Under Class," *Philadelphia Inquirer,* 12 Dec 1991.
4. Lewin T: "A Plan to Pay Welfare Mothers for Birth Control," *New York Times,* 9 Feb 1991, p 18.
5. Litt IF: *J Adolesc Health* 16:337, 1995.

Experience With Side Effects and Health Risks Associated With Norplant Implant Use in Adolescents
Rosenthal SL, Biro FM, Kollar LM, et al (Univ of Cincinnati, Ohio; Children's Hosp Med Ctr, Cincinnati, Ohio)
Contraception 52:283–285, 1995

8–2

Background.—Although levonorgestrel implants are thought to be especially advantageous for adolescents, this contraceptive method may be associated with adverse effects and increased negative health risks. The medical records of adolescents with Norplant implants placed as part of their care in a hospital-based clinic for teenagers were reviewed to determine possible side effects and health risks.

Methods.—The 72 patients studied had had their implants placed at least 1 year previous to the chart review and attended at least 1 follow-up visit after insertion. The mean age of the patients was 15.5 years. Sixty-eight percent of the young women were black, and 29% were white. Norplant implants were in place for a median of 18 months, with a range of 12–29 months.

Findings.—Norplant implants were removed from 24 patients 8–34 months after insertion. A modest increase in mean and median weight was recorded. Bleeding irregularities also occurred. Norplant implantation did not appear to affect condom use or the acquisition of sexually transmitted diseases (STDs).

Conclusions.—The adolescents had an excellent rate of Norplant continuation, an overall modest weight gain, and no change in the risk of STD acquisition. One common side effect was irregular bleeding. Preimplantation counseling should include a discussion of menstrual irregularities and the avoidance of STD acquisition.

▶ Rosenthal and associates present another report about Norplant, one showing us its therapeutic pros and cons. The benefit of Norplant (basically its effectiveness) is balanced by the knowledge that side effects do exist with its use. This has led many to accept its therapeutic benefits with mixed emotions (...remember the definition of mixed emotions: the feeling you have when your mother-in-law drives over a cliff in your new Porsche). What this report does is to shift the risk-benefit ratio more in favor of recommending Norplant to a selected population of teenagers who are at reasonably high risk of getting pregnant.

What are the concerns with Norplant implants? These concerns include irregular uterine bleeding, weight gain, and the potential that there will be a disincentive to use condoms, resulting in an increased risk of STDs. In this report, after a year of Norplant use, the average teenager gained about 6 lbs. The majority also had bleeding that was either irregular in length or interval or both. Neither of these 2 problems, weight gain or bleeding, offset the desire to continue Norplant, however. The other good news was that Norplant use did not diminish the use of condoms. There was no increase in the prevalence of STDs with Norplant use.

To say all the above differently, with proper counseling and appropriate selection of those to use it, Norplant works. Benefits can be achieved with minimal risks.

Our apologies to mothers-in-law.

Pregnancy, Abortion, and Birth Rates Among US Adolescents: 1980, 1985, and 1990

Spitz AM, Velebil P, Koonin LM, et al (Natl Ctr for Chronic Disease Prevention and Health Promotion, Atlanta, Ga; Natl Ctr for Health Statistics, Hyattsville, Md)
JAMA 275:989–994, 1996   8–3

Background.—The United States has higher rates of pregnancy and birth among adolescents than other developed countries. Adolescent pregnancy has a substantial public health impact and high costs for society and individuals. The rates of pregnancy, abortion, and birth to adolescents in the United States for the years 1980, 1985, and 1990 were analyzed.

Methods.—Data for the retrospective analysis were drawn from a number of sources, including the Centers for Disease Control and Prevention, the National Center for Health Statistics, and the National Survey of Family Growth. Rates of pregnancy, abortion, and birth were calculated for girls aged 15–19 years and for those younger than 15 years of age. Trends were analyzed with and without adjustment for sexual experience.

Results.—Pregnancy rates for girls aged 15–19 years remained stable from 1980 to 1985. However, the last half of the 1980s saw a 9% increase, for a 1990 rate of 96 pregnancies per 1,000 teenaged girls. At the same time, rates of sexual experience increased even faster, to the point where the pregnancy rate among sexually experienced teens actually decreased by about 8% during the 1980s. The abortion rate in this age group remained stable, at about 36 abortions/1,000 throughout the period studied. There was a 4% decrease in birth rate from 1980 to 1985. However, this was followed by an 18% increase, for a 1990 birth rate of 60/1,000. A similar pattern was noted for sexually experienced girls in this age group.

About 3% of pregnancies and abortions in 1990 were in girls less than 15 years of age. However, the 1980s saw a 15% increase in the number of births to these younger adolescents, whose trends in pregnancy, abortion, and birth rates were similar to those of the older group. A declining

TABLE 5.—Birth Rates and Number of Births Among All Adolescent Girls and Sexually Experienced Adolescent Girls, by Race/Ethnicity and Age Group

Race/Ethnicity	Age Group, y	No. of Births 1980	1985	1990
All adolescent girls				
All races*	<15	2.8	2.9	3.6
	15–19	53.0	51.0	59.9
	15–17	32.5	31.0	37.5
	18–19	82.1	79.6	88.6
White	<15	1.4	1.4	1.9
	15–19	45.4	43.3	50.9
	15–17	25.5	24.4	29.5
	18–19	73.2	70.4	78.0
Black	<15	10.4	10.7	12.7
	15–19	97.9	95.4	112.8
	15–17	72.5	69.4	82.3
	18–19	134.9	132.4	153.0
Hispanic†	<15	...	...	6.2
	15–19	...	...	99.9
	15–17	...	...	65.7
	18–19	...	...	147.2
Sexually experienced adolescent girls				
All races*	<15	33.0	34.1	43.1
	15–19	113.0	102.1	109.1
	15–17	100.9	88.1	91.5
	18–19	128.1	115.4	119.1
White	15–19	101.0	89.2	95.9
	15–17	84.4	74.0	76.0
	18–19	119.1	103.8	105.9
Black	15–19	166.0	160.3	162.1
	15–17	164.5	146.9	145.8
	18–19	169.7	170.6	183.9
Births		No. 1980	1985	1990
Sexually experienced adolescents	<15	10 169	10 220	11 657
	15–19	552 161	467 485	521 826

Note: Rates are per 1,000 teenaged girls, except rates for girls under 15 years of age, which are per 1,000 girls 13 and 14 years of age. All rates are based on unrounded numbers.

* Includes races other than white or black.

† Data are available for Hispanic births for all states and the District of Columbia for all adolescent girls only for 1990. Hispanics can be of any race.

(Courtesy of Spitz AM, Velebil P, Koonin LM, et al: Pregnancy, abortion, and birth rates among US adolescents: 1980, 1985, and 1990. *JAMA* 275:989–994, Copyright 1996, American Medical Association.)

abortion rate and stable pregnancy rate in the late 1980s led to a 26% increase in the birth rate (Table 5).

Conclusion.—Adolescent pregnancy and birth rates continue to be high in the United States, even in the face of efforts to address the problem. Nearly all of these pregnancies are unintended, so intensified initiatives to reduce the adolescent pregnancy rate are needed. Problems to be overcome include the ongoing controversy regarding sex education, lack of access to contraception, and irresponsible presentations of sexual behavior in the media.

▶ Pregnancy rates among United States teenagers go up and they go down and they go up again. In the 1970s, birth rates among adolescents actually declined sharply, probably because of the legalization and availability of abortion; for reasons that are not clear, these rates then leveled off until 1988, when they rose to a new peak for 10- to 17-year-olds. Over the course of the 1980s, there was a decline in legal abortions among sexually active adolescent girls. Changing attitudes toward out-of-wedlock parenthood and decreasing access to physicians who provide abortions may explain this.

At the same time, there has been an enormous increase in births to unmarried adolescents, from less than 15% of all births in this age group in 1960 to nearly 65% by 1988. Again, changing social attitudes toward out-of-wedlock births, improvement in support in schools for pregnant teenagers, and the increasing difficulty adolescent fathers have in finding jobs to support families may explain much of this phenomenon. While all this has been happening, a parallel trend in the rates of sexually transmitted diseases among adolescents during the 1980s suggests that sexually active teenagers are not using effective birth control methods, including condoms.

A superb commentary on the Spitz article tells us that intervention in this cycle of increasing pregnancy among adolescents is needed. It tells us that the goal of postponing initiation of sexual experimentation until psychosocial maturity is not as difficult a goal as it may appear, nor is preparation for first and subsequent intercourse by counseling regarding appropriate methods that protect against both pregnancy and sexually transmitted diseases. Put these approaches together with school-based clinics, the provision of universal health insurance, and the improvement in training of health care providers in the area of adolescent health, and perhaps during the next decade we will see pregnancy rates in adolescents waning rather than waxing.

This commentary on pregnancy ends with a quiz. Who said: "Marriage be set for girls 18, for men at 37 or somewhat less"? The answer to this is Aristotle. He noted that women performed best at child-bearing when they were young, just as they do in gymnastics and marathon running. In the days when life expectancy was low, it was clearly prudent to begin a family while still young. In some countries, however, the trend is going the other way. Were you aware that for the first time in recorded history, in Great Britain the number of births for every 1,000 British women in their early 30s now exceeds that in women in their early 20s. This is not quite true yet here in the United States.[1]

Reference

1. Gosden R, et al: *BMJ* 311:1585, 1995.

Medical Complications in Male Adolescents With Anorexia Nervosa
Siegel JH, Hardoff D, Golden NH, et al (Long Island Jewish Med Ctr, New Hyde Park, NY; B'nai Zion Med Ctr, Haifa, Israel)
J Adolesc Health 16:448–453, 1995   8–4

Background.—Because only 5% to 10% of patients with anorexia nervosa (AN) are male, there are few reports describing medical complications in male patients with AN. Data on 10 male patients with AN treated at 1 medical center between 1978 and 1990 were presented.

Methods and Patients.—The charts of these patients were reviewed retrospectively. The patients' ages ranged from 9.5 years to 22 years, with 7 of 10 patients in their teens. Eight patients were white, 1 was Hispanic, and 1 was Asian.

Findings.—All were malnourished, weighing 80% or less of their ideal body weight. Their mean body mass index was 13.5. Eight patients were below the 50th percentile in height, with 3 being below the 10th percentile. Seven of 9 patients had structural brain changes on CT scans. More than half had mild anemia relative to their Tanner stage. Initial mean heart rates were 68.3 beats/min. Three of 4 patients with heart rates of 80 or more had serious medical problems and severe malnutrition. Cardiac complications were discovered in 2 patients, and a life-threatening electrolyte disturbance was documented in another (Table 1).

Conclusions.—The proportion of male adolescent anorectics with medical problems appears to be high. This may result from difficulty in establishing the diagnosis and delays in seeking medical help. A higher index of suspicion for congestive heart failure and closer medical monitoring are warranted for malnourished adolescents with AN and relatively increased heart rates.

▶ If you are like this editor, you tend not to think about a boy having AN. Unfortunately, it would seem that boys are not immune. For every 20 girls with this eating disorder, there will be 1 or 2 boys with it as well, and these boys tend to be very sick. Why they tend to be relatively more ill is not answered by this report. Perhaps AN is not diagnosed promptly in boys, resulting in delayed medical treatment. The admonishment of the authors seems correct when they recommend a higher index of suspicion for congestive heart failure in boys with AN.

The treatment of teenagers with eating disorders presents some interesting problems to care providers. Therapy can be time-consuming, prolonged, and extremely costly. Lack of care or insufficient treatment can result in chronic disease, social or psychiatric morbidity, and even death. Barriers to care include lack of eligibility for insurance, inadequate insurance, low reimbursement rates, and lack of access to appropriate interdisciplinary teams. In most insurance plans, the scope of benefits for treatment of eating disorders is insufficient. The use of Diagnostic Related Groupings (DRGs) typically allows too short a time for adequate inpatient treatment. The labeling of the disorder as a purely psychiatric illness by some insurance companies limits the number of hospitalizations permitted per year, restricts the number of outpatient visits, and establishes lifetime caps on coverage that precludes payment of medical practitioners. In addition, some institutions have age-limit policies that negatively affect treatment and limit access to care. Many plans limit the number of nutrition visits to 1 per year and the number of mental health visits to 6 or fewer.

TABLE 1.—Patient Profiles

Patient	Age	HX	BMI	IBW %	HT %	Tanner Stage	Initial Heart Rate	Medical Complications				
								Cardiac	Other	Short Stature < 10%	Anemia	Structural Brain Changes
J.M.	12 yrs 3 mths	Hispanic with illness duration of 8 months	11.9	68	30	2	80		Hypernatremic dehydration (serum sodium = 172 meq/l)	−	−	ND
C.K.	9 yrs 5 mths	Caucasian preadolescent with a 3-month history of restrictive eating behavior, extreme fear of being fat, and a 13-lb. weight loss	12.9	65	95	1	64			−	+	−
E.S.	22 yrs 8 mths	Caucasian athletic young adult who had restrictive eating behavior and weight loss over two years duration	16.9	76	50	5	56			−	+	+
T.F.	16 yrs 5 mths	Caucasian with a 15-lb. weight loss over five months, and one year of restrictive eating behavior	13.7	70	15	4	80			−	+	+
K.H.	14 yrs 9 mths	Caucasian with restrictive eating behavior resulting in a 10-lb. weight loss over the preceding eight months	11.5	67	7	2	86	SVT	Delayed puberty	+	+	−
S.M.	19 yrs 6 mths	Caucasian who presented to another hospital for cardiopulmonary resuscitation. At our facility he had multiple episodes of tachycardia which resolved with nutritional rehabilitation	10.9	43	8	5	92	Cardiopulmonary arrest, tachycardic episodes		+	+	+

R.F.	15 yrs 11 mths	Caucasian who initially began to lose weight to enhance his athletic abilities with restrictive eating behavior leading to a 50-lb. weight loss over 12 months. He was seen as an outpatient and was lost to follow-up	15.9	80	28	5	42		−	−	+
L.P.	17 yrs 10 mths	Caucasian with a 154-lb. weight loss over 2 years and peripheral muscular weakness on presentation. His symptoms improved with nutritional rehabilitation and a diagnosis of neuropathy secondary to nutritional deficit was made	12.4	59	27	4	45	Neuropathy, neutropenia, anemia, thrombocytopenia	−	+	+
J.P.	15 yrs 1 mth	Caucasian of Greek ancestry with a 20-lb. weight loss in 3 months and a 40-lb. total loss over 10 months. He had restrictive eating behavior, extreme body image distortion and was an excessive exerciser. He had an initial elevated erythrocyte sedimentation rate of 27 and a negative medical work-up for other causes of cachexia	14.9	71	65	4	74		−	+	+
S.S.	16 yrs 9 mths	Asian of Indian descent who initially began to lose weight to enhance his athletic abilities. His vegetarian restrictive food intake resulted in a 20-lb. weight loss over 8 months	14.0	74	5	4	64		+	−	+

Abbreviations: *BMI,* body mass index; *IBW,* ideal body weight; *ND,* not done.
(Courtesy of Siegel JH, Hardoff D, Golden NH, et al: *J Adolesc Health* 16:448–453, 1995.)

Unless these basic problems are solved, no adolescent, male or female, stands an even chance at getting better. Finally, to read one of the best reviews ever written on eating disorders in adolescents, see the excellent article by Fisher et al.[1]

Reference

1. Fisher M, et al: *J Adolesc Health* 16:420, 1995.

The Cost of Comprehensive Preventive Medical Services for Adolescents

Gans JE, Alexander B, Chu RC, et al (American Med Assoc, Chicago; Michigan State Univ, Lansing; Actuarial Research Corp, Annandale, Va)
Arch Pediatr Adolesc Med 149:1226–1234, 1995   8–5

Background.—A focus on preventive measures is especially appropriate for adolescents, for whom the most serious health problems—including unplanned pregnancy, sexually transmitted diseases, and substance abuse—are more behavioral than biomedical. The American Medical Association has published a set of clinical practice suggestions, the *Guidelines for Adolescent Preventive Services* (GAPS), that address the needs of adolescents 11–21 years of age in the areas of immunization, health promotion, and health screening. Plans to include such services in basic health care coverage mandates inquiry into their costs and benefits.

Methods.—Prevalence rates of various morbidities common in adolescents were derived from national surveys. Costs were estimated from published data and adjusted for 1992 dollars. Costs of preventive services were taken from a 1993 survey of insurance coverage plans. The conditions considered included pregnancy, sexually transmitted diseases, AIDS/HIV infection, alcohol and drug use, vehicular injuries, unintentional injuries, and mental disorders.

Findings.—Estimated physician payments made by insurance companies for preventive services under a fee-for-service payment system approximated $130 per adolescent per year. This amounts to a total of just over $5 billion if all those aged 11–21 years in the United States received GAPS-recommended services. An administrative markup of 12.5% was taken into account. Approximately 80% of the total expenditures would be for routine services such as physician fees, vaccines, and cholesterol screening for those not at risk. The remaining 20% represents payment for services given to those at high risk for sexually transmitted diseases.

Discussion.—It remains to be demonstrated that primary care providers are able to actually alter adolescent behaviors. It appears that to break even fiscally, preventive measures would have to eliminate 15% of all adolescent morbidity.

▶ In December 1992, the American Medical Association released a set of clinical practice recommendations known as the *Guidelines for Adolescent*

Preventive Services (GAPS).[1, 2] The GAPS recommendations address the content and delivery of clinical preventive services for adolescents aged 11–21 years, including immunizations, health promotion, and screening for a range of health problems. The model for GAPS is the existing series of routine, well-child visits from birth through 5 years of age. The estimated payments to physicians by insurance companies for adolescent preventive services under an indemnity-type fee-for-service payment system would be approximately $130 per adolescent per year, on average, in 1992 dollars. This would be approximately $5.1 billion in 1992 dollars if every 11- to 21-year-old adolescent in the United States received these services recommended by GAPS. Specifically, all adolescents would receive screening and health guidance, all 11-year-old adolescents would receive the immunizations recommended by GAPS, and half of all adolescents would undergo serum cholesterol screening. All sexually active adolescents would undergo testing for chlamydia and gonorrhea, and high-risk sexually active adolescents would undergo testing for HIV and syphilis.

To say all this differently, if all 11- to 21-year-old adolescents received a preventive services visit, with an administrative markup of 12.5%, the cost to insurers of paying providers for clinical preventive services would be approximately $5.1 billion at a 100% participation rate.

When summarizing any article dealing with preventive services and cost-effective medicine, one must cut to the chase. Do the types of preventive services for adolescents discussed here break even or save money? The data are fairly clear. To break even and "save" the $5.1 billion required for preventive services, GAPS would have to reduce adolescent morbidities by about 15% across the board. Can we as clinicians produce this level of prevention and cost savings? Can we get health insurers to buy into the concept of preventive medicine? Indemnity payers primarily pay for catastrophic events and profit when no claim for services is made; preventive care would increase cost for the short haul. Furthermore, profit is driven primarily on a year-to-year basis, so long-term gains from prevention hold little financial interest. Physicians in an indemnity system have incentive to provide preventive service only when they are adequately reimbursed.

In a capitated system, risks and benefits reside more directly with the payer, because the payer incurs the cost of both prevention and catastrophic events. Therefore, it is in the payer's interest to ensure that routine care is provided and that such care helps to avoid catastrophic events.

If there is a benefit associated with managed care, it should be a benefit associated with preventive medical services for all ages, including adolescents. The data from this report show that if adolescents receive preventive care that reduces their rate of illness by just 15%, preventive care has more than paid for itself. Given the nature of adolescent illnesses, preventive services should be able to easily reduce rates of illness by that amount. If we can convince insurers to go for the long-haul benefit of preventive care, they, we, and the children we care for will all profit.

References

1. American Medical Association: *Guidelines for Adolescent Preventive Services.* Chicago, American Medical Association, 1992.
2. Elster AE, et al: *AMA Guidelines for Adolescent Preventive Services: Recommendations and Rationale.* Baltimore, Md, Williams and Wilkins, 1994.

Adolescents' Perceptions of Factors Affecting Their Decisions to Seek Health Care

Ginsburg KR, Slap GB, Cnaan A, et al (Univ of Pennsylvania, Philadelphia; Children's Hosp of Philadelphia; School District of Philadelphia)
JAMA 273:1913–1918, 1995
8–6

Introduction.—Increasing efforts are under way to improve access to health care for adolescents, but most work in this area has been conducted from the adult perspective. Little effort has been made to learn directly about the needs and expectations of adolescents and what might deter their seeking care. Adolescents are not merely passive recipients of care but instead actively evaluate services and interactions.

Objective and Methods.—The barriers that adolescents believe exist in obtaining health care were studied in 6,821 ninth-grade students at 39 of 42 public high schools in Philadelphia. A series of group techniques and surveys were used to ensure that ideas were generated and prioritized by the adolescents themselves. Initially focus groups were held to frame study questions, and the nominal group approach used to generate responses by students. Three surveys then were conducted to determine the importance of responses, and another one to relate the chief responses to care-seeking decisions. Finally, focus groups were held to clarify which variables correlated with the decision to seek care.

Observations.—The final survey used Likert scale ratings to order 31 items according to how strongly they influenced the decision to seek health care (Table 2). The most influential factors were hand washing by providers, the use of clean instruments, an honest and respectful attitude toward patients, and a high level of knowledge. Other prominent factors were equal treatment of all patients, maintenance of confidentiality, and the provider being seronegative for HIV. The preferred characteristics remained constant regardless of gender, race, and socioeconomic status. Factor analysis demonstrated that competent providers and infection control are very important elements in the decision to seek health care.

Implication.—In deciding whether to obtain health care, adolescents are more concerned about issues of cleanliness and control of infection–especially HIV infection—than about specifics of site and service or outreach characteristics.

▶ This study is unique, but what makes it unique is almost ironic. It is one of very few studies that have attempted to explore how health care providers, health care sites, and outreach strategies affect an adolescent's deci-

TABLE 2.—Final Ranking and Distribution of Ratings for the Top 31 Items Influencing the Decision to Seek Health Care*

Item†	Final Ranking‡	% of Students Assigning Likert Rating	
		Rating=4	Rating=5
Providers wash hands	1	14	73
Providers use clean instruments	1	12	74
Providers are honest with patients	1	15	72
Providers and staff are respectful	2	18	68
Providers and sites are clean	2	16	69
Providers are knowledgeable	2	15	69
Providers are careful not to mix things up	2	17	67
Providers are experienced	2	18	65
Providers are HIV-negative	2	15	68
Providers and staff treat all patients equally	2	17	66
Providers emphasize confidentiality	3	20	63
Providers are up-to-date	4	23	58
Out-of-pocket costs are low	4	21	59
Providers and staff relate well to teens	4	25	56
Provider is the same for all visits	4	28	52
Contraception is available	4	23	55
Staff is happy and friendly	4	27	52
Waiting room time is short	4	26	52
Appointments are made easily	5	27	49
Teens can go on their own	6	25	51
Providers prepare teens for procedures	7	28	46
Visits and testing can be anonymous	7	25	49
24-hr crisis centers are available	7	25	47
Teens have their own medical card	8	25	45
Sites are near home	8	30	41
Teen-only sites are available	8	27	43
Counseling is available	8	30	40
Teens help design the health care system	8	30	40
Sites provide job counseling	9	29	39
Sites offer incentives for health care	9	21	41
Sites provide entertainment while waiting	9	23	37

* Students ($n = 6,821$) were asked to rate each item on a scale of 1 ("Definitely would not make me more likely to come for care") to 5 ("Definitely would make me more likely to come for care").

† Items are listed by order of their mean Likert ratings.

‡ A Bonferroni calculation was done to determine the proper significance level for the total sample. Items that did not differ by $P < 0.002$ by the sign test were assigned the same final ranking.

(Courtesy of Ginsburg KR, Slap GB, Cnaan A, et al: Adolescents' perceptions of factors affecting their decisions to seek health care. *JAMA* 273:1913–1918, Copyright 1995, American Medical Association.)

sion to seek care. It does this by actually asking the adolescent all the appropriately relevant questions. This report from the City of Brotherly Love comes none too soon. Although most adolescents are healthy, adolescence is the age group in which mortality rates have increased most dramatically. Unintentional injury, homicide, and suicide are the leading causes of death among teens. All of these are preventable, assuming teenagers access health services, including mental health and substance abuse services.

We learn from this report that teenagers are not a very trusting lot. They well recognize that it has only been in recent times that the uniqueness of adolescence has been appreciated. The adolescents in this report articulate fairly clearly what they want from care providers: honesty, sensitivity, respect toward young people, and the ability to relate to teens.

We can't expect teenagers to take an active role in their own health; that just doesn't happen. Therefore it is increasingly important that we, as care providers, be proactive when it comes to health and prevention of disease among our adolescent patients. To learn more about adolescent health research, particularly as related to legal perspectives, see the excellent commentary on this subject by Abigail English.[1]

Reference

1. English A: *J Adolesc Health* 17:277, 1995.

Fluoxetine in the Treatment of Premenstrual Dysphoria
Steiner M, for the Canadian Fluoxetine/Premenstrual Dysphoria Collaborative Study Group (McMaster Univ, Hamilton, Ontario; McGill Univ, Montreal; Univ of Toronto; et al)
N Engl J Med 332:1529–1534, 1995   8–7

Background.—Premenstrual syndrome, characterized by a cluster of symptoms (most commonly, tension, irritability, and dysphoria) occurring in the late luteal phase, is reported to affect 3% to 8% of North American women during their reproductive years. No cause has been identified, and no treatment has been consistently effective. Similar to depression and anxiety states, serotonin dysregulation has been implicated in the pathogenesis of premenstrual dysphoria. Because fluoxetine therapy inhibits the reuptake of serotonin, it was hypothesized that it would be effective in treating premenstrual dysphoria. This hypothesis was tested in a multicenter, randomized, double-blind, placebo-controlled trial.

Methods.—A total of 313 women, aged 18–45 years, with a diagnosis of late-luteal-phase dysphoric disorder participated in the study, and 180 completed it. The women were given placebo for 2 menstrual cycles for a washout period, then were randomly assigned to treatment with placebo or either a 20-mg or 60-mg dose of fluoxetine per day. Symptoms of tension, irritability, and dysphoria were measured with visual analogue scales at baseline, during the follicular and late luteal phases of each cycle, and at the end of the study. The frequency of side effects was noted.

Results.—Either dose of fluoxetine was significantly more effective than placebo in reducing tension, irritability, and dysphoria as early as the first cycle of treatment. Visual analogue scores were reduced by 50% during the luteal phase of the first treated cycle in 46 of the 96 women given 20 mg of fluoxetine, in 49 of the 86 women given 60 mg of fluoxetine, and in only 21 of the 95 women given placebo. The rates of response remained consistent during the 6 cycles of the trial in the 180 women who completed the protocol (Fig 1). The most common side effects were insomnia, nausea, tremor, fatigue, dizziness, anorexia, somnolence, sweating, visual disturbance, dry mouth, minor cardiovascular symptoms, and yawning. Their frequency was dose related.

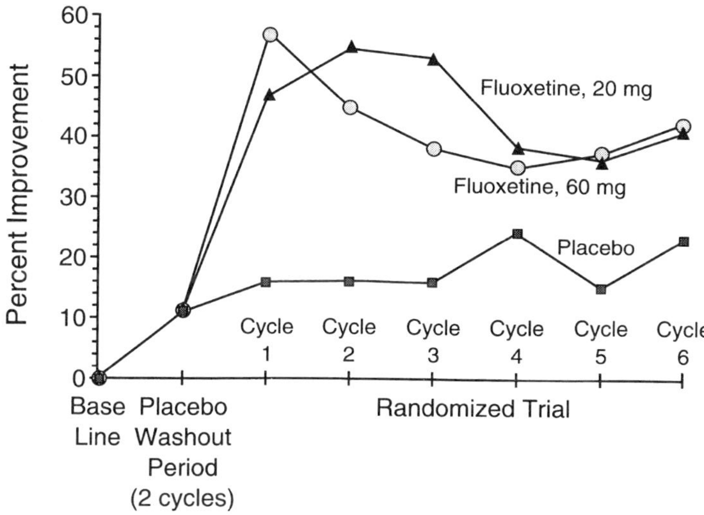

FIGURE 1.—Percent improvement in total luteal-phase scores of visual analogue scale for the 180 women who completed the protocol ($P < 0.001$). The degree of improvement recorded during the placebo washout period did not differ between groups (mean improvement, 11.2%) (Reprinted by permission of *The New England of Medicine* from Steiner M, for the Canadian Fluoxetine/Premenstrual Dysphoria Collaborative Study Group: Fluoxetine in the treatment of premenstrual dysphoria. *N Engl J Med* 332:1529-1534, Copyright 1995, Massachusetts Medical Society.)

Conclusions.—Fluoxetine, taken at doses of 20 mg or 60 mg per day, was significantly more effective than placebo in relieving symptoms associated with premenstrual syndrome. The 2 doses were equally effective, but significantly more adverse side effects were experienced by women taking the larger dose.

▶ Three cheers for these authors. Not only have they devised a new method to treat an old problem, but they also changed the name of that old problem, a name that was saddled with denotations and connotations that were often inappropriate. The previous name was "premenstrual syndrome (PMS)." The new name is "premenstrual dysphoric disorder (PMDD)." Those loathing PMS now have PMDD, which is a totally treatable entity.

By way of background, the technical term for PMS and PMDD is LLPDD, late-luteal-phase dysphoric disorder, which fortunately is attenuated to PMDD. Premenstrual dysphoric disorder is characterized by a cluster of symptoms appearing regularly during the week before and disappearing within a few days after the onset of menstrual bleeding. Tension, irritability, and dysphoria are among the prominent symptoms. Surveys indicate that PMDD affects up to 3% to 8% of North American women during adolescent and adult years, with a substantial negative impact on functional health. Because the cause of this disorder is unknown, it's not surprising that during the past half century, more than 50 different treatment options have been suggested, based on the popular hypothesis du jour. To date, however, although some treatments, such as medical or surgical ovariectomy and anxiolytic drugs, have been found to be superior to placebos, no treatment has been uniformly effective.

So, what is the treatment for PMDD à la *The New England Journal of Medicine?* It is a treatment based on the fact that PMDD shares many of the features of depression and anxiety states that have been linked to a serotonergic dysregulation. Indeed, there is a body of evidence showing that serotonin may be important in the pathogenesis of PMDD. Because fluoxetine (Prozac) selectively inhibits serotonin reuptake, it should come as no surprise that it is the latest in treatment fads for the management of PMDD. The report abstracted shows how useful it can be.

Should such heavy hitters as fluoxetine be used in teenagers with PMDD? Depending on the dosage used, it can cause significant side effects that make PMDD pale by comparison. Fortunately, a low dosage (20 mg/day) usually works if the drug is preordained to work in a particular patient. Also, don't forget the reports of the occurrence of a preoccupation with suicide during fluoxetine treatment.[1] Although the association between suicidal ideation and fluoxetine therapy has now been refuted, there is still litigation about this issue in the courts.[2]

Of all the health problems in society, PMDD cumulatively affects more individuals than virtually anything else. Whether medical historians will look back on the mid-1990s as the time when fluoxetine conquered PMDD is something for those individuals to decide. For right now, it would be best to view a complex drug, such as a serotonin reuptake inhibitor, as something to be called in at the eleventh hour, only after time has expired on more traditional treatment options. To learn more about PMDD, read the excellent review of the topic by Rubinow et al.[3]

Dysphoria isn't the only complication related to menstrual cycles. Are you aware of an entity called catamenial pneumothorax? Catamenial pneumothorax is a condition characterized by recurrent spontaneous pneumothoraces associated with the onset of menstruation. The majority of women who experience this disorder are women in their late 30s and early 40s. The pneumothoraces are right-sided and occur within 72 hours of the onset of menstruation. Congenital diaphragmatic fenestrations allow air to enter the chest from the peritoneal cavity. Such fenestrations are more common on the right side and explain the occasional development of right-sided pneumothoraces after pneumoperitoneum. The diaphragmatic openings may be caused by endometrial implants, which slough during menstruation and eventually form small holes. Most affected adolescents and women have evidence of pelvic endometriosis.

Air probably enters the chest from the peritoneal cavity during menstruation when the cervix dilates, the mucous plug is lost, and uterine contractions squeeze air into the peritoneum. Treatment of this unusual condition is ovulation suppression with gonadotropin-releasing hormone analogue, which prevents catamenial pneumothoraces caused by endometriosis. The only alternative is tubal ligation, which may be fine for a woman who has had all the children she desires but is not a great alternative for a teenager.

Catamenial pneumothorax is proof positive that there is more than one way to get air into one's chest.[4]

References

1. Teicher MD: *Am J Psychiatry* 147:207, 1990.
2. Mann JJ, et al: *Arch Gen Psychiatry* 48:1027, 1991.
3. Rubinow DR, et al: *N Engl J Med* 332:1574, 1995.
4. Ekford SD, et al: *Lancet* 347:734, 1996.

Anabolic-steroid Use, Strength Training, and Multiple Drug Use Among Adolescents in the United States

DuRant RH, Escobedo LG, Heath GW (Children's Hosp, Boston; Harvard Med School, Boston; Ctrs for Disease Control and Prevention, Atlanta, Ga)
Pediatrics 96:23–28, 1995   8–8

Introduction.—Some claim that adolescents who use anabolic steroids to make their muscles larger and stronger and to enhance their athletic performance will at the same time avoid alcohol and marijuana. There is some evidence, however, that the opposite may be the case.

Objective.—The relationship between anabolic steroid use and the use of other drugs was explored in data from a randomized survey of children enrolled in public and private schools in all states, the 1991 Centers for Disease Control and Prevention Youth Risk Behavior Survey. The study population included 12,272 students in the ninth through twelfth grades.

Findings.—Males were more likely than females to have used anabolic steroids, but no significant age trend was apparent (Table 2). Steroid use was more prevalent in students reporting the use of alcohol and other drugs and those who had used cocaine at any time. Anabolic steroid use correlated with the frequency of cigarette smoking, drinking alcohol, and using marijuana as well as other drugs. On multiple regression analysis, use of injected drugs was the closest correlate of anabolic steroid use (Table 5). This relationship was strongest in the Western states. Steroid use was least frequent in the northeastern part of the country.

Implication.—Adolescents who use anabolic steroids are also likelier than others to use multiple drugs and to inject drugs.

▶ This report is important because it demystifies the individual who abuses anabolic steroids. A myth has developed that adolescents who use anabolic steroids to increase muscle size for cosmetic reasons and to improve strength and endurance do not use other drugs such as alcohol, marijuana, and cocaine because these substances would harm their health. If you look back through the literature, you will find that there are reports showing that the frequency of anabolic steroid use by ninth graders is associated with the use of cocaine, injected drugs, alcohol, marijuana, cigarettes, and smokeless tobacco.[1, 2] The report abstracted shows that anabolic steroid users drink,

smoke pot, and sometimes do hard drugs. If you're treating a teenager who lives in the South, put an exclamation point after the preceding sentence.

Why these data are important is fairly obvious. Despite sanctions against the illicit use of anabolic steroids in the United States, thousands of adolescents continue to use them. Steroid use is a marker for an even more serious problem of substance abuse. Anabolic steroid use prevention efforts must go far beyond the athlete on the playing field. In fact, coaches have long recognized this. They worry most about the athlete who looks muscle-bound but is performing poorly. Now we know why. The abuse of other substances is the culprit.

No commentary regarding athletic endeavors during the teenage years would be complete without some mention of what's new in girls' competitive sports. The latest is a study that recently appeared and that examined a large number of women athletes to determine whether phase of menstrual cycle affected athletic performance.[3] The teenagers studied were tested during early follicular and midluteal phases of the menstrual cycle. Cycle phases were confirmed by serum estradiol and progesterone assays. No significant differences were observed throughout the menstrual cycle in weight, performance body weight, sum of skin folds, hemoglobin concentrations, hematocrit, maximum heart rate, maximum minute ventilation, maximum respiratory exchange ratio, anaerobic performance, endurance to time of fatigue, or isokinetic strength. That's the good news. The bad news is that both absolute and relative oxygen ventilation were low during the midluteal phase of the menstrual cycle.

Thus, coaches might want to be aware that menstrual cycle phases do affect aerobic exercise capacity, with potential implications for individual athletes. Overall, however, one would be hard-pressed to base tactical decisions on this type of information. No cross-country race or track event is worth a coach's invasion of a teenager's privacy.

References

1. DuRant RH, et al: *N Engl J Med* 328:922, 1993.
2. DuRant RH, et al: *N Engl J Med* 329:889, 1993.
3. Lebrun CM, et al: *Med Sci Sports Exerc* 27:437, 1995.

Sports Participation in an Urban High School: Academic and Psychologic Correlates
Fisher M, Juszczak L, Friedman SB (Cornell Univ, Manhasset, NY; Albert Einstein College, Bronx, NY)
J Adolesc Health 18:329–334, 1996   8–9

Background.—Although physical activity is acknowledged to be important in adolescent health care, surprisingly little attention has been paid to adolescents' level of participation in athletic activities and to the relationship between these activities and physical and emotional well-being. No study has comprehensively assessed the positive and negative effects of sports participation on adolescents' lives. The positive and negative correlates of sports participation among inner-city youths were investigated.

Methods.—An anonymous questionnaire was distributed to 838 students in gym classes at a New York City high school. Sixty-five percent were in grades 9 and 10 and 36% were in grades 11 and 12. Sixty-three percent of the students were black; 27%, Hispanic; and 10%, other. Thirty percent of the students had grade point averages of A or B; 38% had a C average; and 32% had a D or F average.

Findings.—All students reported some sports participation. Thirty-seven percent played 1 or 2 sports; 29%, 3 or 4; and 24%, 5 or more. Twenty percent played on local teams. Twelve percent participated in junior or senior varsity sports. Thirty percent said they did not play sports during the week, 34% reported playing 1 or 2 hours per day, and 36% played for 3 or more hours a day during the week. On the weekends, 34% reported no participation; 26%, 1 or 2 hours a day; and 40%, 3 or more hours. Most commonly played were basketball, volleyball, baseball, and weight lifting. Reasons reported for participation were enjoyment, recreation, and competition. Eighty-six percent of the students considered school to be extremely or very important, and 35% felt that sports were extremely or very important. Many students believed they would definitely or probably get an athletic scholarship. Boys spent more time participating in sports, played more team sports, and had greater expectations about having a future in sports. Involvement in sports was unrelated to academic performance or scores on the Rosenberg Self-Esteem Scale or Depression Self-Rating Scale. Eleven percent of the boys and 4% of the girls had used steroids at least once. Twenty-one percent of the boys and 6% of the girls tried to gain weight for sports, and 20% of both sexes tried to lose weight for sports. Fifteen percent of the students had been injured during sports in the previous year.

Conclusions.—Most of the students were involved in athletics. Many had unrealistic expectations for a future in sports, and some reported unhealthy practices in an attempt to enhance performance. Sports involvement was unassociated with academic performance, self-esteem, or depression.

▶ To paraphrase a law of physics, for every swing of a pendulum, there is an equal and opposite swing the other way given enough time. There has been much touting with respect to the benefits of participation in high school athletic programs. Clearly such programs can improve one's physical health. Some have even suggested that they prevent juvenile delinquency. Others have said that such activity is a motivating factor to exercise later in life. There are even a small number who believe that data exist to show a positive effect of sports participation by adults on self-esteem, depression, and other healthy lifestyles.[1] However, the swing of the pendulum the opposite way is demonstrated in several recent reports in adolescents that question the advantages of competitive sports, including the possibility that sports participation may mislead some adolescents into believing they have the potential to become professional athletes.[2, 3]

What do students expect when they participate in gym classes or play on junior or senior varsity teams? This report tells us that many do it for enjoyment and fun, but more than half of boys think that it will lead to a college athletic scholarship (girls are more realistic about this). When you realize that the chances of a high school athlete playing in the National Basketball Association or the National Football League are truly one in a million (or less), those who engage in competition for such reasons would be better off spending a comparable amount of time at McDonald's and using the $4.50 an hour to get someone to buy lottery tickets for them.

One thing that sports certainly appear good for is weight control. About equal numbers of boys and girls either intentionally lost weight or tried to gain a little bit of weight to get within the "competitive" range. As much as this editor disdains exercise, he does believe that there is benefit to participating in high school competitive sports. The benefits, in general, are obvious, despite a 15% incidence of injury. Sporting activities are for the young. It is better to get it out of your system early.

References

1. Morgan WP, et al: *Med Sci Sports Exerc* 17:94, 1985.
2. Fejgin N: *Soc Sport J* 11:211, 1994.
3. Harris L, et al: High school students' attitudes on human rights, community activity and steps that might be taken to ease racial, ethnic, and religious prejudice. The Reebok Foundation and Northeastern University Center for the Study of Sport in Society, October 1990.

The Patterns and Predictors of Smokeless Tobacco Onset Among Urban Public School Teenagers
Hu FB, Sussman S, Hedeker D, et al (Univ of Illinois, Chicago; Univ of Southern California, Los Angeles; Univ of Memphis, Tenn)
Am J Prev Med 12:22–28, 1996   8–10

Background.—Although cigarette smoking has declined recently, the use of smokeless tobacco has increased. Smokeless tobacco, like cigarette smoking, is associated with significant harmful effects, including cancer of the mouth, larynx, throat, and esophagus. The determinants of smokeless tobacco use were investigated in a large, urban, ethnically diverse sample of adolescents.

Methods.—A total of 6,695 students in 7th grade attending 47 urban public schools completed questionnaires. The students again completed questionnaires in 8th grade, with 73.4% of the students responding both times. The questionnaires had questions about lifetime and current use of smokeless tobacco and other substances. Information on psychosocial predictors was also sought, with questions on family, peer, and intrapersonal variables. The predictive significance of the variables was analyzed with logistic regression analyses.

Results.—The prevalence of smokeless tobacco use was significantly higher among boys than among girls and among whites than among blacks, Hispanics, and other ethnicities. Overall, trying smokeless tobacco at least once was reported by 19.5% of the boys and 4.5% of the girls in 7th grade and 21.6% of the boys and 5.3% of the girls in 8th grade. Smokeless tobacco use was significantly associated with cigarette smoking and alcohol and marijuana use. Of the family variables, family structure, family conflict score, and parental alcohol use were significantly associated with adolescent smokeless tobacco use. Of the peer variables, the number of peers smoking, parties with friends during the preceding month, and sports activities during the preceding week were all significant predictors. Smokeless tobacco use was also significantly predicted by the following intrapersonal variables: low grades in school, high risk-taking and stress scores, and valuing excitement or fun over physical health, but not religiosity.

Conclusions.—The use of smokeless tobacco among adolescents can be predicted by many of the same psychosocial factors that predict cigarette smoking, suggesting a problem-prone behavior model for predicting both. Therefore, similar prevention and intervention strategies may be effective in reducing both cigarette smoking and smokeless tobacco use in urban adolescents.

▶ The things kids, and sometimes parents, put in their mouths never fails to amaze. Would you believe that 1 in 5 boys and 1 in 20 girls have chewed smokeless tobacco? A problem that was once unique to rural areas, and originally to the Wild West, is now an urban cowboy dilemma. Virtually every convenience store now sells Skol or another leading brand of smokeless tobacco.

Smokeless tobacco is a form of addiction, no worse than the cigarette habit, but no better. We have been extremely aggressive, more or less, about tobacco smoking; we need to be equally aggressive in our campaigns against smokeless tobacco. Maybe we need some catchy phrases. Here's one, smokeless tobacco addicts are "dumb skols"—nothing like a little negative advertising.

Tobacco is indeed a dirty weed. It has no real benefits for the average teenager. Possibly, the only indication for chewing or other forms of tobacco might be for the adolescent who has Tourette's syndrome. Did you know that substantial acute improvement of tics has been reported after the application of transdermal nicotine patches?[1] It is just possible that high-dose nicotine will desensitize brain nicotinic receptors, which are involved with the pathophysiology of Gilles de la Tourette's syndrome. When all else fails, reach for the Skol, if and only if, you run into a patient with Tourette's syndrome.

Reference

1. Dursun SN, et al: *Lancet* 344:1577, 1994.

The Residual Cognitive Effects of Heavy Marijuana Use in College Students

Pope HG Jr, Yurgelun-Todd D (Harvard Med School, Boston)
JAMA 275:521–527, 1996   8–11

Background.—Although more than 40 studies have been published in the past 30 years on the residual effects of cannabis on neuropsychological performance, methodological problems make the findings of this research difficult to interpret. A single-blind comparison of regular and infrequent marijuana users was reported.

Methods.—Two groups of college undergraduates were studied. The first consisted of 65 heavy users, who reported smoking marijuana a median of 29 of the past 30 days and who also had cannabinoids in their urine. The second group consisted of 64 light users, who reported smoking a median of 1 of the last 30 days and had no cannabinoids in their urine. Testing was done after a minimum of 19 hours of supervised abstinence.

Findings.—The heavy users had significantly greater impairments in attentional/executive functions, which was especially evident on their greater perseverations on card sorting and reduced word-list learning. Between-group differences persisted after controlling for potential confounding variables, such as estimated levels of premorbid cognitive functioning and use of alcohol and other substances.

Conclusions.—Residual neuropsychological effects are associated with heavy marijuana use, even after a day of supervised abstinence. However, it is still unknown whether this impairment is caused by drug residue in the brain, a withdrawal effect, or a frank neurotoxic effect.

▶ If these data are validated, it would seem that pot is more of a mind-numbing than mind-expanding substance of abuse, a finding that is particularly relevant in the 90s. After well over a decade or two of declining use, marijuana's popularity has increased markedly among adolescents in this country in the past 3 or 4 years. This having been said, the findings of this report must be properly placed in context. Most of the cognitive impairments noted are not large relative to normal cognitive variability among individuals. The degree of intellectual impairments seen would not make a heavy marijuana user stand out in a crowd. On the other hand, such deficits aren't going to go a long way toward improving one's Scholastic Aptitude Test or Graduate Record Examination scores, much less one's grade point average.

Marijuana has gotten a lot of attention lately. You can see that in the press. When the latter covers the arraignment of Woody Harrelson on a charge of growing marijuana for personal use and does so on evening prime time news, there is still a lot of mileage left in this weed. Maybe Woody had been using too much of his own stuff and the resultant impairment is what got him caught. In any event, no longer can we give 3 "cheers" (pardon the pun) for those who have become a little bit dumber by having their brains scrambled a bit by a touch of cannabis.

One final comment about smoking, marijuana and otherwise. For a long time it had been thought that women who smoke might have a lower risk of breast cancer. Not so. Although smoking does have an antiestrogen effect that theoretically might decrease an individual's risk of cancer, the fact that cigarette smoking is such a strong carcinogen overrides this effect, at least as shown in a recent report.[1] Women who smoke have a 1.6-fold increased risk of breast cancer. Furthermore, they have breast cancer develop 8 years earlier, on average, than do nonsmokers (59 years of age vs. 67 years of age). How many more fatal consequences of smoking are needed before cigarettes are labeled as drugs?

Reference

1. Bennick EK, et al: *BMJ* 310:1431, 1995.

Law Officers' Views on Enforcement of the Minimum Drinking Age: A Four-state Study

Wolfson M, Wagenaar AC, Hornseth GW (Univ of Minnesota, Bloomington; HealthPartners Inc, Bloomington, Minn)
Public Health Rep 110:428–438, 1995   8–12

Introduction.—Passage of laws declaring the minimum legal drinking age to be 21 years in all states in the United States has been shown to reduce the rates of underage drinking and of youth involvement in alcohol-related traffic accidents. However, the mechanisms explaining this effect are not known. The role of law enforcement has not been elucidated. Through interviews with law enforcement personnel, the social and political context of drinking age enforcement, constraints to enforcement, and recommendations on improving enforcement efforts were investigated.

Methods.—Semistructured interviews were conducted with police supervisors and line officers in 15 law enforcement agencies (8 city police agencies and 7 county sheriff agencies) selected to represent areas of both high and low arrest rates for liquor law violations involving those younger and older than 21 years.

Results.—Whereas the incidence of underage alcohol-impaired driving has decreased, it was reported that the incidence and severity of underage drinking has remained the same or worse. Underage drinkers most commonly get alcohol from legal-age purchasers and relatively rarely from the use of false identification. The officers reported that minimum age enforcement was a relatively low priority in the community and that parents often considered underage drinking a rather benign offense. There has been generally satisfactory compliance with the law from the owners and managers of alcoholic beverage establishments. Reported constraints to enforcement included personnel shortages, a lack of juvenile detention facilities, the difficulty of identifying the source of confiscated alcohol, a perceived lack of effective penalties imposed by the courts, the excessive processing and paperwork, the lack of public status, and the unreasonable burden of proof required for arrest. Recommendations focused largely on merchants and other adults and included increasing penalties for merchants who provide liquor to minors, labeling individual beer kegs to enable tracing to the purchaser, and penalties for parents. Recommendations regarding the youth included imposing more effective sentences, including denying driver's license privileges and community-service penalties connected to alcohol abuse, such as working in a detoxification center.

Conclusions.—There are significant obstacles to enforcement of the minimum drinking age. Enforcement efforts aimed at suppliers, rather than youth, appear to be more promising. Research is needed on the sources of supply.

▶ All states now have age 21 drinking laws. Despite the passage of "21," we seem to have failed to put a significant dent in the incidence of underage drinking. It has been estimated that 2 of every 1,000 occasions of illegal drinking by youth younger than 21 years will actually result in an arrest. When law enforcement actions are taken, they are typically focused on individual young drinkers rather than on commercial outlets or private individuals who may be supplying alcoholic beverages to youth. There is only 1 chance in 10 when a 16- to 20-year-old individual is arrested for drinking that someone will go after the source of the alcohol provided to that teenager.

The report abstracted shows the lethargy with which some law officers approach the minimum drinking age. The police aren't solely to blame for this. They perceive an acceptance of youth drinking by many segments of their communities and do not receive significant encouragement from community members to increase enforcement efforts. Complicating enforcement efforts is that many states allow underaged individuals to obtain and possess alcohol in certain circumstances, as long as they don't drink it. Five states allow underaged youth to possess alcohol if they do not intend to consume it, and 6 states have no laws against minors attempting to or actually purchasing alcohol. Many states allow individuals younger than 21 years to possess and consume alcohol in private residences, private establishments, or when accompanied by a legal guardian 21 years or older. Twenty-one states have no specific statutory language that prohibits the consumption of alcohol by minors, although possession of the same alcohol may be prohibited. Sixteen states have no statutory language explicitly prohibiting the deliberate misrepresentation of age by youth to obtain alcohol, and 19 states do not explicitly prohibit youth from using false identification to obtain alcohol.

Don't think that state Alcoholic Beverage Control (ABC) agencies do very much, either. In 1 study, 27% of counties in a state with fairly clear-cut underaged drinking laws had no ABC actions against any outlet during a 3-year period for violations of sale of alcohol to minors. In Texas, 41% of counties had made no arrests in a recent 3-year period for adults furnishing alcohol to minors.[1]

So what is the point of all this? The point is pretty straightforward. If we can't get serious about underage drinking as parents, as members of a community, as those who provide the tax dollars that pay the salaries of our police officers, why should our young get serious?

Reference

1. Wagenaar AC, et al: *Public Health Rep* 110:419, 1995.

Severe Ethanol Intoxication in an Adolescent

Morgan DL, Durso MH, Rich BK, et al (Univ of Texas, Dallas; Parkland Mem Hosp, Dallas; North Texas Poison Ctr, Dallas)
Am J Emerg Med 13:416–418, 1995

8–13

Background.—Death of severe ethanol intoxication can result from respiratory depression, hypoglycemia, or hypothermia. Most reports of patients with very high blood ethanol levels have been about adults. A MEDLINE search revealed only 3 reports of young children and none of adolescents with blood ethanol levels exceeding 500 mg/dL. An adolescent with severe ethanol intoxication was described.

Case Report.—Boy, 15 years, was brought to an emergency department (ED) with status epilepticus. He had no significant medical history. Three hours before presentation, he began drinking beer and vodka with his friends. After consuming an unknown amount of alcohol, he fell to the ground in a generalized tonic-clonic seizure. Intermittent seizures continued with no return of consciousness, while his friends took him to the ED. Initial tests obtained minutes after his arrival showed an ethanol level of 757 mg/dL, with a serum osmolality of 482 mOsm/kg. He required mechanical ventilation and substantial amounts of benzodiazepines. Aspiration pneumonia complicated his hospital course, but no episodes of hypoglycemia occurred. He was placed on hemodialysis for 2.8 hours, which accelerated ethanol elimination but did not appear to improve his clinical outcome. The patient was discharged on day 11 with no neurologic deficits. At a 2-month follow-up examination, he was doing well with no obvious sequelae.

Conclusions.—Optimal treatment for severe ethanol intoxication includes aggressive supportive care with attention to ventilation, adequate perfusion, hypothermia avoidance, monitoring of serum electrolytes, and frequent determinations of blood glucose with rapid hypoglycemia treatment. Dialysis increases the rate of ethanol elimination from the blood, although it has not been proven to improve the clinical outcomes of patients with severe ethanol intoxication and high concentrations of blood ethanol.

▶ Some articles are important because they change the way we think about disease processes. Some are important because they tell us about dramatic new therapies. Some are important merely because they show us the unusual, the 1-in-a-million case. This report falls into the latter category. Would you believe that a 15-year-old could achieve a blood alcohol level of almost 760 mg/dL and still survive! In fact, this youngster beats by 15 mg/dL any other nonadult in terms of highest blood ethanol level. His serum osmolality reached 482 mOsm/kg, which is probably also a record or near a record level. At these levels of osmolality, the human body can't even freeze, at least not easily.

It's not likely that you'll see a child as intoxicated as this teenager was. To achieve these extraordinary blood alcohol levels, he had to consume three fifths of vodka, a 12-pack of beer, and several margaritas over the course of a day. Most teenagers can't afford this much booze.

Everyone knows that alcohol and driving can cause accidents, but this commentary closes with an interesting twist on accident rates and teenagers. If your teenager has the option of taking driver's education and getting his or her driver's permit during either the fall or spring semester, choose fall. The reason for this choice is pretty complex. It has to do with daylight savings time. More than 25 countries shift to daylight savings time each spring and return to standard time in the fall. The spring shift results in the loss of 1 hour of sleep (the equivalent of traveling one time zone to the east), whereas fall shift permits an additional hour of sleep (the equivalent of traveling one time zone to the west). Although a 1-hour change may seem like a minor disruption in the cycle of sleep and wakefulness, most studies have shown that sleep pattern is disturbed in the average individual for as many as 5 days after each time shift. This theoretically would lead to the prediction that the spring shift, involving the loss of an hour of sleep, might lead to an increased number of lapses of attention during daily activities, such lapses increasing the probability of accidents. In fact, this has been documented in Canada. The loss of 1 hour of sleep associated with the spring shift to daylight savings time increases the risk of automobile accidents by approximately 8% in the first few days after clocks move ahead. The fall shift backward results in a decrease in accidents of approximately the same magnitude.[1] The likelihood of accidents is far less when one falls back rather than springs ahead.

Reference

1. Coren S, et al: *N Engl J Med* 334:92, 1996.

9 Therapeutics and Toxicology

Recommendations for Off-label Use of Intravenously Administered Immunoglobulin Preparations
Ratko TA, Burnett DA, Foulke GE, and the University Hospital Consortium Expert Panel for Off-Label Use of Polyvalent Intravenously Administered Immunoglobulin Preparations (Univ Hosp Consortium, Oak Brook, Ill; Univ of California, Davis; Georgetown Univ Med Ctr, Washington, DC)
JAMA 273:1865–1870, 1995

9–1

Background.—All formulations of polyvalent IV immunoglobulin (IVIG) licensed for use in the United States are labeled as replacement therapy for patients with particular forms of primary immunodeficiency. These products also are commonly used for off-label purposes not mentioned in the product labeling approved by the Food and Drug Administration (FDA) for marketing. The high cost of such usage makes it important for providers to have objective information with which to guide their use of IVIG.

Objective.—A University Hospital Consortium–sponsored expert panel was convened to search databases for English-language reports and review articles dealing with clinical use of IVIG.

Methods.—Eight board-certified physicians working in various areas including immunology participated in the process, as did 2 hospital pharmacists. Both MEDLINE and EMBASE were searched, yielding 201 review articles and 1,904 original reports published in the years 1982–1994. A set of recommendations was formulated that reflected total agreement based on the published evidence. The major issues were whether available IVIG preparations are therapeutically and pharmacologically equivalent, and which off-label uses are justified by the available evidence.

Recommendations.—The expert panel made specific recommendations for 53 off-label indications (table). In general, IVIG is considered to be indicated only if conventional measures are contraindicated, have failed, or cause intolerable side effects. Intravenous immunoglobulin products may be viewed as therapeutically equivalent and therefore interchangeable. Pharmaceutical differences between various products should be taken into account, along with the patient's clinical and functional status,

TABLE.—University Hospital Consortium (UHC) Expert Panel Consensus Recommendations for Off-Label Use of IV Immunoglobulin (IVIG)

Clinical Category	No. of Reports	Total No. of IVIG Recipients	Combined IVIG Response, No. (%)*	Evidence Grade† (No. of IVIG) Recipients	UHC Expert Panel Consensus
Hematology					
Anemia, aplastic	2	2	2 (100)	III (2)/IV	Evidence does not support IVIG use.
Anemia, autoimmune hemolytic (AIHA)	16	75	38 (51)	II-3 (46)/III (29)	Evidence does not support routine use of IVIG, IVIG may have a role in patients with warm-type AIHA that does not respond to corticosteroids.
Anemia, Diamond-Blackfan	2	5	0	III (5)/IV	Evidence does not support IVIG use.
Aplasia, pure red cell	6	16	13 (81)	II-3 (10)/III (6)	Evidence does not support routine use of IVIG. IVIG may be used in patients with documented parvovirus B19 infection and severe anemia.
Factor VIII inhibitors, acquired	7	12	7 (58)	III (12)	Evidence does not support IVIG use.
Hemolytic disease, neonatal	4	30 (Prenatal)	28 (83) Live births	II-3(24)/III (6)/IV	Evidence does not support IVIG use.
	2	12 (Postnatal)	10 (83)	II-3 (9)/III (3)/IV	
Hemophagocytic syndrome	2	4	4 (100)	III (4)	Evidence does not support IVIG use.
Leukemia, acute lymphoblastic	1	30	No individual data	I	Evidence does not support IVIG use.
Myeloma, multiple	1	42	No individual data	I	Evidence does not support routine use of IVIG. It may have a role in patients with stable (plateau phase) disease and high risk of recurrent infections.
Neutropenia, immune-mediated	12	25	19 (76)	II-3 (12)/III (13)	Evidence does not support routine use of IVIG. IVIG may have a role in severe illness that does not respond to other modalities or when the latter are contraindicated.
Purpura, posttransfusion	5	10	7 (70)	II-3 (4)/III (6)	IVIG may be considered as first-line therapy in severely affected patients.
Thrombocytopenia, neonatal alloimmune	4	10 (Prenatal)	9 (90)	II-3 (7)/III (3)	Evdience does not support routine use of IVIG. IVIG may be used in neonates with severe immune thrombocytopenia if other interventions are unsuccessful or contraindicated. Maternal antenatal infusion may be considered.
	13	42 (Postnatal)	32 (76)	II-3 (17)/III (25)	
Thrombocytopenia, nonimmune	6	8	8 (100)	III (8)	Evidence does not support IVIG use.
Thrombocytopenia, refractoriness to platelet transfusions	11	70	36 (51)	1 (7)/II-3 (47)/III (16)	Evidence does not support routine use of IVIG. IVIG may have a role in patients with severe thrombocytopenia of documented immune basis for whom other modalities are unsuccessful or contraindicated.
TTP/HUS	13	33	16 (48)	II-1 (20)/III (13)/IV	Evidence does not support IVIG use.

Condition					
Transfusion reaction, hemolytic	1	1	1 (100)	III	Evidence does not support IVIG use.
von Willebrand's syndrome, acquired	7	8	8 (100)	III (8)	Evidence does not support IVIG use.
Infectious diseases (prophylaxis: infections)					
Neonates, high-risk hypogammaglobulinemic	13	2154	17% RR reduction	I (2154)	Evidence does not support routine use of IVIG. IVIG prophylaxis may have a role in LBW infants (< 1500 g) or in setting with high baseline infection rate or morbidity.
HIV infection, adults	…	…	Not determined	IV	Evidence does not support IVIG use.
Surgery of trauma	6	313	31% RR reduction	I (313)	Evidence does not support IVIG use.
Transplantation, solid organ	7	153	29% RR reduction	I (72)/II-2 (81)	Evidence does not support routine use of IVIG. IVIG may be used in CMV-seronegative recipients of CMV-seropositive organs.
Infectious diseases (treatment: mortality)					
Neonates, high-risk hypogammaglobulinemic	2	44	63% RR reduction	I (44)/IV	Evidence does not support IVIG use.
Surgery or trauma, adults	1	12	23% RR reduction	I (12)/IV	Evidence does not support IVIG use.
Neurology					
Epilepsy, pediatric intractable	11	162	87 (54)	II-1 (10)/II-3 (147)/III (5)	Evidence does not support routine use of IVIG. IVIG may have a role in certain syndromes (eg, West, Lennox-Gastaut) as a last resort, especially in patients who may be candidates for surgical resection.
Guillain-Barré syndrome	11	128	75 (59)	I (74)/II-3 (44)/III (10)	IVIG is recommended as an equivalent alternative to plasma exchange in children and adults.
Motor neuron syndromes	2	17	9 (53)	I (12)/II-3 (5)	Evidence does not support IVIG use.
Multiple sclerosis	1	10	No individual data	II-2	Evidence does not support IVIG use.
Myasthenia gravis (MG)	9	102	75 (74)	II-3 (102)	Evidence does not support routine use of IVIG. IVIG may be considered in patients with severe MG to treat acute severe decompensation when other treatments have been unsuccessful or are contraindicated.
Myelopathy, HTLV-I associated	1	14	10 (71)	II-3	Evidence does not support IVIG use.
Neuropathy, paraproteinemic	1	2	2 (100)	III	Evidence does not support IVIG use.
Plexopathy, progressive lumbrosacral	1	2	2 (100)	III	Evidence does not support IVIG use.
Polyneuropathy, chronic inflammatory demyelinating	7	111	67 (60)	I (22)/II-3 (89)	IVIG is recommended as an equivalent alternative to plasma exchange in children and adults.
Obstetrics, spontaneous abortion (recurrent)	8	52	35 (67) Live births	II-3 (44)/III (8)	Evidence does not support IVIG use.
Pulmonology, asthma and inflammatory chest disease	5	60	13 (72) of 18 with individual data	II-1 (23)/II-3 (36)/III (1)	Evidence does not support IVIG use.
Rheumatology					
Arthritis, rheumatoid (adult and juvenile)	5	42	22 (52)	II-3 (39)/III (3)	Evidence does not support IVIG use.

(Continued)

TABLE (cont.)

Dermatomyositis	4	28	21 (75)	I (15)/II-3 (11)/III (2)	Evidence does not support routine use of IVIG. IVIG may be used in patients with severe active illness for whom other interventions have been unsuccessful or intolerable.
Myositis, inclusion body	2	13	3 (23)	II-3 (13)	Evidence does not support IVIG use.
Polymyositis	3	17	13 (76)	II-3 (14)/III (3)	Evidence does not support routine use of IVIG. IVIG may be used in patients with severe active illness for whom other interventions have been unsuccessful or intolerable.
Systemic lupus erythematosus (SLE)	13	42	25 (60)	II-3 (28)/III (14)	Evidence does not support routine use of IVIG. IVIG may be used in patients with severe active SLE for whom other interventions have been unsuccessful or intolerable.
Vasculitic syndromes, systemic	4	25	21 (84)	II-3 (23)/III (2)	Evidence does not support routine use of IVIG. IVIG may be used in patients with severe active illness for whom other interventions have been unsuccessful or intolerable.
Miscellaneous					
Adrenoleukodystrophy	1	1	1 (100)	III	Evidence does not support IVIG use.
Behçet's syndrome	1	1	1 (100)	III	Evidence does not support IVIG use.
Chronic fatigue syndrome	2	37	10 (27)	1 (37)	Evidence does not support IVIG use.
Cystic fibrosis	1	8	No individual data	I	Evidence does not support IVIG use.
Diabetes mellitus	2	18	No individual data	I (8)/11-2(10)	Evidence does not support IVIG use.
Endotoxemia	1	10	10 (100)	II-2 (10)	Evidence does not support IVIG use.
Heart block, congenital	1	1	1 (100)	III	Evidence does not support IVIG use.
Nephropathy, membranous	1	9	8 (89)	II-3	Evidence does not support IVIG use.
Nephrotic syndrome	1	10	0	I	Evidence does not support IVIG use.
Ophthalmopathy, euthyroid	2	8	8 (100)	I (7)/III (1)	Evidence does not support IVIG use.
Otitis media, recurrent	3	38	16 (42)	II-2 (22)/II-3 (16)	Evidence does not support IVIG use.
Renal failure, acute	1	17	73% RR reduction	I	Evidence does not support IVIG use.
Uveitis	1	1	1 (100)	III	Evidence does not support IVIG use.

*Combined response is presented for comparative discussion purposes only; it does not imply any statistical significance.

†Study quality: I, evidence obtained from at least 1 properly designed randomized, controlled trial; II-1, evidence obtained from well-designed controlled trials without randomization; II-2, evidence obtained from well-designed cohort or case-control analytic studies, preferably from more than 1 center or research group; II-3, evidence obtained from multiple time series with or without the intervention, or dramatic results in uncontrolled experiments; III, opinions of respected authorities, based on clinical experience, descriptive studies (case reports), or reports or expert committees; and IV, insufficient evidence to ascertain role (UHC Expert Panel).

Abbreviations: TTP/HUS, thrombotic thrombocytopenic purpural hemolytic uremic syndrome; *RR*, relative risk; *LBW*, low birth weight; *CMV*, cytomegalovirus; *HTLV-I*, human T-cell lymphotropic virus type I.

(Courtesy of Ratko TA, Burnett DA, Foulke GE, et al: Recommendations for off-label use of intravenously administered immunoglobulin preparations. *JAMA* 273:1865–1870, Copyright 1995, American Medical Association.)

when choosing a product. It is not possible, at present, for manufacturers to ensure that their IVIG preparations are free of viral contamination.

▶ You would think that with a product as expensive as IVIG, someone would call a time-out on the distribution of these products for off-label uses. In the United States, the land of the free, we are not likely to see this happen, perhaps with good reason. This report tells us that there are more than 50 different disease indications for the administration of IVIG. With few exceptions, these indications are based on data that are derived almost exclusively from uncontrolled case reports and open series, rather than from randomized, controlled trials.

For some diseases, particularly many of the debilitating or fatal conditions for which IVIG has been suggested, it is highly improbable that we will ever see randomized comparative trials to evaluate IVIG therapy. This is primarily because of ethical concerns about randomization of seriously ill patients to either placebo treatment or unproven intervention with IVIG, but it is also because of the high cost of multicenter trial designs necessary to achieve adequate study power. Even some largely nonfatal common disorders fall into this latter category. Take, for example, idiopathic thrombocytopenic purpura (ITP) in children. We all know that IVIG raises platelet counts quickly in children with ITP. What we don't know is whether IVIG (vs. steroids vs. nothing) actually reduces the mortality rate of this disease. The reason is that the mortality rate is sufficiently low that a randomized control trial would require more than 14,000 children in each treatment arm to demonstrate effectiveness. Lacking such demonstrative studies, chances are we'll continue to use IVIG in ITP and other disorders until someone pulls the plug on us.

It is not likely, however, that anyone's going to pull the plug on IVIG therapy. Off-label use means the application of a particular drug for a disease that has not been sufficiently studied to permit FDA approval for a specific use. Nonetheless, the FDA does not push anyone's button with respect to off-label IVIG use. Off-label IVIG therapy is, in general, consistent with the FDA's nonconstraint of physicians in the art and practice of medicine. The FDA's stance on this issue is that a pharmaceutical agent that has received marketing approval for at least 1 indication may be prescribed for any use based on rational scientific theory, expert medical opinion, or controlled clinical studies.[1] An approved label is not intended to set a standard of medical practice. Rather, a drug should be used in a manner that is consistent with good medical practice and in the best interest of a patient. It is doubtful that off-label use of IVIG in this context presents any greater liability risk than would off-label use of any other pharmaceutical product.

Read this report in detail. It tells a great deal. It suggests that IVIG is indicated only if standard approaches have failed, become intolerable, or are contraindicated. There are relatively few conditions in which IVIG is clearly the therapy of choice. In fact, if you look at the entire list of uses for IVIG that was generated by the expert panel that has established consensus recommendations on its use, you will see that the only clear-cut indications for IVIG, above all other alternative therapies, are the Guillain-Barré syndrome and chronic inflammatory demyelinating polyneuropathy. Again, this does not mean that it cannot be used for other purposes.

Lastly, recognize that with current IVIG manufacturing processes, there is no absolute guarantee of freedom from viral contamination in the finished product. We need to remind ourselves of this and be wary of the potential risk of viral transmission, albeit perhaps vanishingly small.

Reference

1. Use of approved drugs for unlabeled indications. *FDA Drug Bull* 12:4, 1982.

A Comparison of Cathartics in Pediatric Ingestions

James LP, Nichols MH, King WD (Univ of Alabama, Birmingham)
Pediatrics 96:235–238, 1995

9–2

Background.—In the setting of toxic ingestion, cathartics are often used in conjunction with activated charcoal to shorten the passage of the charcoal-toxin complex through the gastrointestinal tract. However, there have been no studies comparing the effectiveness of cathartic agents used in pediatric patients. Therefore, the time to first stool and number of stools within 24 hours were compared among 3 cathartic agents used with activated charcoal in pediatric patients after toxic ingestions.

Methods.—During an 11-month period, 116 children, aged 1–5 years, with suspected acute ingestions were treated with activated charcoal. In addition, the patients were randomly assigned to receive either sorbitol, magnesium citrate, magnesium sulfate, or water. The parents or nurses were then interviewed by telephone at 1, 4, 8, and 24 hours after cathartic administration to obtain information about the time of first stool, the number of stools, and side effects. The physicians, nurses, parents, and interviewers were all unaware of the cathartic used.

Results.—The mean time to first stool was 8.48 hours in the sorbitol group, 12.84 hours in the magnesium citrate group, 22.65 hours in the magnesium sulfate group, and 14 hours in the water group (Table 2).

TABLE 2.—Cathartic Mean Times to First Stool With Cathartic Comparisons*

Cathartic	Mean Time to First Stool (h)	Cathartic Comparison†	Difference Between the Means With 90% CI
Sorbitol	8.4	Sorbitol vs MgCit	4.4 (0.3, 8.4)
MgCit	12.84	Sorbitol vs MgSO$_4$	14.2 (9.7, 18.7)
MgSO$_4$	22.65	Sorbitol vs water	5.5 (1.3, 9.8)
Water	14.0	Water vs MgSO$_4$	8.6 (4.0, 13.3)
		MgCit vs MgSO$_4$	9.8 (5.3, 14.3)

Abbreviations: MgCit, magnesium citrate; MgSO$_4$, magnesium sulfate.
* Significant differences in mean time to first stool were detected among cathartic agents by analysis of variance with least-significant difference multiple-comparison procedure (F = 9.29; P = 0.01).
† All agent comparisons are significant at the 0.10 level.
(Courtesy of James LP, Nichols MH, King WD: A comparison of cathartics in pediatric ingestions. Reproduced by permission of *Pediatrics*, Vol 96, pp 235–238, Copyright 1995.)

TABLE 3.—Cathartic Mean Number of Stools With Cathartic Comparisons*

Cathartic	Mean Number of Stools in 24 h	Cathartic Comparison†	Difference Between the Means With 90% CI
Sorbitol	2.97	Sorbitol vs MgCit	1.1 (0.4, 1.8)
MgCit	1.79	Sorbitol vs water	1.1 (0.4, 1.9)
MgSO$_4$	1.65	Sorbitol vs MgSO$_4$	1.2 (0.5, 2.0)
Water	1.75		

Abbreviations: MgCit, magnesium citrate; MgSO$_4$, magnesium sulfate.
 * Significant differences in number of stools produced were detected among cathartic agents by analysis of variance with a least-significant difference multiple-comparison procedure (F = 3.49; P = 0.018).
 † All agent comparisons are significant at the 0.10 level.
 (Courtesy of James LP, Nichols MH, King WD: A comparison of cathartics in pediatric ingestions. Reproduced by permission of *Pediatrics*, Vol 96, pp 235–238, Copyright 1995.)

Sorbitol also induced a significantly higher number of stools within 24 hours than the other cathartics, which were comparable (Table 3). There were no side effects in 80% of the patients. Emesis was the most common side effect and occurred significantly more frequently in patients treated with sorbitol than with the other agents. Other side effects, including diarrhea, cramping, and constipation, were evenly distributed among the treatment groups.

Conclusions.—Because sorbitol administration is associated with a shorter mean time to the first stool and more stools than magnesium-containing cathartics, it is recommended along with activated charcoal for management of pediatric toxic ingestions. All of the studied cathartics were well tolerated in single doses.

▶ In the stooly race to the john, sorbitol beats out magnesium citrate and magnesium sulfate. In fact, sorbitol wins hands down, coming in 50% faster in terms of time to the first stool after administration of a cathartic. A report like this doesn't seem like it's based on rocket science, but realize that although cathartics have been used since ancient times, until this report appeared, we really did not know how well cathartics worked, nor how quickly, when used in patients after exposures to poisons.

It does seem logical that a cathartic should be used after a toxic ingestion. Indeed, the Poisindex recommends the administration of either a saline cathartic or sorbitol with activated charcoal.[1] However, remember the following:

- If sorbitol is given in excess or in multiple doses, it can cause hypernatremic dehydration and even death.[2]
- Cathartics should be withheld in caustic ingestions.
- Cathartics should be withheld in the absence of bowel sounds.
- Cathartics should be withheld in patients with histories of recent bowel surgery.
- Magnesium-containing cathartics should not be administered to patients with renal disease.
- Because of the potential for fluid and electrolyte disturbances, sorbitol should not be used in children younger than 12 months.

If you follow the above do's and don'ts, chances are a sorbitol cathartic may be of potential benefit. Remember: if it's a rush to the can you seek, think 50% sorbitol.

References

1. Rumack BH (ed): *Poisindex Information Systems.* Denver, Micromedex, 1994, p 79.
2. Farley TA: *J Pediatr* 109:719, 1986.

Prostaglandin-induced Cortical Hyperostosis: Case Report and Review of the Literature

Gardiner JS, Zauk AM, Donchey SS, et al (Seton Hall Univ, South Orange, NJ; St Joseph's Hosp and Med Ctr, Paterson, NJ)
J Bone Joint Surg (Am) 77–A:932–936, 1995   9–3

Background.—Prostaglandin E has been proven effective in the treatment of newborns with congenital cardiac defects who are dependent on the patency of the ductus arteriosus for pulmonary blood flow. However, this treatment has been associated with cortical hyperostosis in the diaphyses of the long tubular bones and in the ribs, scapulae, and clavicles. The skeletal changes and long-term effects after prostaglandin therapy in 1 patient were presented, along with a literature review.

Case Report.—Boy, born at 32 weeks' gestation and weighing 1,200 g, had respiratory distress syndrome and needed continuous positive pressure of the nasal airway. Systemic arterial oxygen saturation began to decrease when he was 28 days old. An echocardiogram showed tetralogy of Fallot. Intravenous prostaglandin E_1, 0.05 µg/kg/min, was administered, evoking a sudden increase in oxygen saturation. At 133 days of age, the patient was found to have hard swellings and reduced range of motion in the joints in all extremities. Cortical hyperostosis was documented radiographically in the bones of the upper and lower extremities and in the ribs, scapulae, and clavicles. The patient's serum alkaline phosphatase level was 550 IU/L. At 147 days of age, a Blalock-Taussig shunt was performed successfully, and IV prostaglandin was stopped. At 18 months of age, the patient showed no signs of cortical hyperostosis. His range of motion in all joints in all extremities was normal.

Discussion.—Eighteen additional cases of prostaglandin-induced cortical hyperostosis were identified in the literature (Table 1). There appears to be no association between the dosage of prostaglandin and cortical hyperostosis onset. In the 18 previously described patients and in the current patient, the long bones showed cortical hyperostosis. The ribs were in-

TABLE 1.—Summary of Reported Data on Patients Who Had Prostaglandin-induced Cortical Hyperostosis

Study	Case	Sex	Birth Weight (g)	Duration of Treatment (Days)	Peak Alkaline-Phosphatase Level (IU/L)	Dosage of Prostaglandin E (µg/kg/Min.)	Duration between Start of Prostaglandin-E Therapy and Diagnosis (Days)	Duration between End of Prostaglandin-E Therapy and Resolution of Hyperostosis (Days)	Bones and Soft Tissues Affected
Ueda et al. (1980)	1	M	2650	109	348	0.04–0.01	61	43	Long bones, ribs
	2	F	2750	48	Normal	0.05–0.01	134	Not reported	Long bones
Abe et al. (1982)	3	Not reported	3220	49	2081	0.02–0.08	30	90	Long bones, ribs
	4	Not reported	1910	37	2010	0.04–0.02	30	Not reported	Long bones, ribs
Ringel et al. (1982)	5	M	3600	53	Normal	0.1	50	Not reported	Long bones, ribs, scapulae
Alpert et al. (1984)	6	Not reported	3350	46	Not reported	0.045–0.040	64	2 yrs.	Long bones
Hoevels-Guerich et al. (1984)	7	Not reported	Not reported	97	Normal	0.05–0.025	49–56	150	Long bones, cranial sutures, eyelids
	8	Not reported	Not reported	95	Normal	0.05–0.025	49–56	90	Long bones, cranial sutures
Poznanski et al. (1985)	9	M	2000	49	Not reported	Not reported	20	Not reported	Long bones, ribs, clavicles
	10	M	Not reported	56	Not reported	Not reported	16	Not reported	Long bones, ribs clavicles
	11	M	Not reported	42	Not reported	Not reported	20	Not reported	Long bones, ribs, clavicles
Williams (1986)	12	F	2300	39	Not reported	0.05	17	77	Long bones, ribs clavicles
Jureidini et al. (1986)	13	M	2300	96	Normal	0.05	73	Died at 96 days	Long bones, hands
	14	M	1880	33	Normal	0.05	36	Not reported	Long bones
Host et al. (1988)	15	M	3100	59	Slightly elevated	0.04–0.025	50	270	Long bones
	16	F	3800	78	Not reported	0.09–0.008	46	62	Long bones
Jorgensen et al. (1988)	17	F	Not reported	79	Not reported	0.09–0.008	46	Died at 144 days	Long bones
Drvaric et al. (1989)	18	F	1460	76	567	0.1	36	21 (mild regression of bone changes)	Long bones, ribs
Present study (1995)	19	M	1200	119	550	0.05	105	18 mos.	Long bones, ribs, clavicles, scapulae, eyelids

(Courtesy of Gardiner JS, Zauk AM, Donchey SS, et al: Prostaglandin-induced cortical hyperostosis: Case report and review of the literature. *J Bone Joint Surg [Am]* 77-A:932–936, 1995.)

volved in 10 infants, the clavicles in 5, and the scapulae in 2. Cranial suture widening was noted in 2 patients. Another 2 had swollen, thickened eyelids. In 6 infants, serum alkaline phosphatase levels were increased. Characteristic hyperostotic changes occur 16–134 days after prostaglandin treatment is begun and disappear 6 weeks to 2 years after treatment is stopped.

▶ Imagine the following scenario. You're seeing a 1-year-old infant in the emergency department who appears to have a fairly run-of-the-mill case of bronchiolitis. You obtain a chest radiograph and see evidence of periosteal irregularities, including new bone formation and hyperostosis. These findings are seen in the ribs and clavicles. You're tempted to report the parents of this child to your hospital abuse team. Fortunately, before doing so, you stumble across the article abstracted above, which shows you that if this infant is a neonatal nursery graduate who received prostaglandins, you already have a reason for the boney abnormalities without calling into play the potential for child battering.

In the 20 years or so since prostaglandin E has been used to treat newborns who have congenital cardiac defects and who require that their ductus arteriosus remains open, literally thousands of such infants have been exposed to this pharmaceutical agent, which is capable of inducing a number of complications. Side effects include apnea, congestive heart failure, flushing, convulsions, jitteriness, diarrhea, fever, hypertrophy of the eyelids, widening of the cranial sutures, swelling of the fingers and toes, and cortical hyperostosis. Obstruction of the gastric outlet has also been reported, supposedly caused by mucosal hyperplasia.[1] As far as the bones are concerned, hyperostotic changes are seen, with new bone formation that can involve ribs, clavicles, scapulae, and long bones. Because prostaglandins are rapidly inactivated when they pass through the lungs, you would think that administering this class of drugs would not have any systemic effects. Unfortunately, in an infant who has congenital heart defects with right-to-left shunting of blood, pulmonary blood flow is decreased and the clearance of prostaglandins is markedly reduced. Add to this the effect of furosemide treatment, which stimulates the renal production of prostaglandin E, and you have a lot of this substance floating around in sick newborns.

If there is any value to this report, it is the listing of the differential diagnosis of the type of bone lesions seen in these children. There are many metabolic, traumatic, neoplastic, inflammatory, and idiopathic disorders of the skeleton that can cause diffuse periosteal formation of bone in an infant. This can result from intrauterine fractures, osteogenesis imperfecta, battered-baby syndrome, Wiskott-Aldrich syndrome, a neoplasm, osteomyelitis, trauma associated with chest physiotherapy, infantile cortical hyperostosis (Caffey disease), maternal syphilis, or congenital cytomegalovirus infection. Before jumping to the wrong conclusion about what might result in such serious looking bone abnormalities, stop and think about this list. Please note that prostaglandin-induced cortical hyperostosis, although self-limited, may be very painful for infants and will restrict joint motion. It does go away, but it can take as long as 2 years to do so.

Reference

1. Ritter M, et al: *J Arthroplasty* 3:185, 1988.

Pediatric Arsenic Ingestion
Cullen NM, Wolf LR, St Clair D (Wright State Univ, Dayton, Ohio; Egland Air
Force Base, Niceville, Fla)
Am J Emerg Med 13:432–435, 1995   9–4

Background.—Dimercaptosuccinic acid (DMSA) has been proven effective in the treatment of arsenic toxicity in animals. However, because of the rarity of acute arsenic intoxication in human beings, there is little information on its use in patients.

Case Report.—Girl, 22 months, ingested about 1 oz of 2.27% sodium arsenate, an ingredient in ant killer that had been stored in the basement. Within 30 minutes, the child had profuse vomiting and diarrhea, and became lethargic. Her vital signs at the emergency department (ED) were blood pressure, 96/72 mm Hg; pulse, 160 beats/min; respiratory rate, 22 breaths/min; and temperature, 96.5°F. Ipecac was administered, and gastric lavage was done. No radiopaque material was seen on an abdominal radiograph. During transfer to a children's hospital ED, she continued to vomit and remained tachycardic. Her blood pressure was 103/39 mm Hg; pulse, 69 beats/min; and respirations, 43 breaths/min on arrival at the ED. One IM dose of British antilewisite (BAL), 3 mg/kg, was given about 9 hours after ingestion. Twelve hours after ingestion, the patient was asymptomatic except for reduced urine output and periods of sinus tachycardia. The patient was given 250 mg of D-penicillamine (DP) every 6 hours for a total of 9 doses. On day 6, she was discharged. Three days later, however, she was readmitted because of a high urine arsenic level. A diffuse erythematous rash was also observed. Treatment with DMSA was begun. The patient remained asymptomatic and was discharged on DMSA treatment at a dosage of 10 mg/kg every 8 hours. Laboratory values, including renal and hepatic function and a complete blood cell count, remained normal. There were no long-term sequelae, although the patient was lost to follow-up.

Conclusions.—The symptoms of arsenic ingestion usually appear in 30–60 minutes. If the arsenic is taken with food, the symptoms may be delayed. Toxicity severity depends on the amount and form of the arsenic ingested. There are 2 distinct clinical presentations of acute arsenic toxicity: acute paralytic syndrome and acute gastrointestinal syndrome. Acute massive arsenic intake can result in the acute paralytic syndrome, characterized by cardiovascular collapse, CNS depression, and death within hours. The most common presentation of arsenic poisoning is acute gastrointestinal syndrome. Patients with this syndrome may initially have a metallic or garlic-like taste associated with dry mouth, burning lips, and/or dysphagia. Violent vomiting begins, sometimes progressing to frank hematemesis. Diarrhea is often profuse. Stools range from "rice water" to hematochezia. The gastrointestinal symptoms result from the intestinal injury caused by dilatation of splanchnic vessels, resulting in mucosal vesiculation. Rupture of the vesicles causes bleeding, diarrhea, and protein-wasting enteropathy. Severe gastrointestinal symptoms often lead to dehydration and electrolyte imbalance and, in some cases, the development of hypotension and hypoxia. Although the patient described had tachycardia and reduced urine output, she remained normotensive.

▶ Arsenic is quite a noble substance. Did you know the word is derived from the Greek word "arsenikon," meaning potent? As early as 2,000 BC, the word became synonymous with the term poison. It was considered "the perfect poison" for many reasons, including its physical qualities (odorless and nearly tasteless, with a sugarlike appearance), its ability to cause a slow, painful death, and the inability to detect it in the human body unless actually looked for. Arsenic poisoning is thought to be responsible for the deaths of such luminaries as Britanicus (by Nero in 55 A.D.—the first documented case), Popes Pius III and Clemente XIV (the latter by Pope Alexander VI and Caesar Borgia's son), Charles Frances Hall (by his mutinous crew), and Napoléon Bonaparte[1] ... no wonder Agatha Christie found arsenic sufficiently interesting that it was her poison of choice for her novels.

Most of us don't think much about arsenic these days, but it is all around us. In fact it's quite ubiquitous. Most of us ingest 0.5–1.0 mg a day in the form of food (particularly fish and crustaceans). It was in heavy production throughout the 1950s and 1960s for use in insecticides and rodenticides, but beginning in the 1970s, arsenic was largely replaced by less toxic products. Unfortunately, lots of the old stuff is still around, as the case history in the report abstracted proves.

You may want to read this report in some detail because it catalogues the often mysterious clinical presentation of signs and symptoms related to arsenic poisoning. If you do suspect arsenic poisoning, seek help unless you are thoroughly familiar with its management. Various supportive measures and chelation therapy are not for those who are unseasoned with respect to medical toxicology. This is not a minor league entity. The potential complications of therapy alone should be enough to scare off the weak-hearted.

Reference

1. Keynes M: *Lancet* 344:276, 1994.

The Relationship Between Idiopathic Mental Retardation and Maternal Smoking During Pregnancy

Drews CD, Murphy CC, Yeargin-Allsopp M, et al (Emory Univ, Atlanta, Ga; US Public Health Service, Atlanta, Ga; Batelle Ctrs for Public Health Practice and Education, Atlanta, Ga)
Pediatrics 97:547–553, 1996   9–5

Introduction.—Several effects on fetal and infant development can be attributed to maternal smoking during pregnancy, including low birth weight and increased risk of sudden infant death syndrome and perinatal mortality. Although some studies have reported cognitive and achievement deficits in the children of smokers, these findings have not been consistent. There has been little study of an association between maternal smoking and serious intellectual disabilities. The potential relationship between maternal smoking during pregnancy and idiopathic mental retardation was examined in a case-control study of 10-year-old children.

Methods.—A total of 221 children with idiopathic mental retardation and 400 randomly selected control children without MR or conditions associated with mental retardation were studied. All of the children were aged 10 years in 1985–1986. The mothers of the study children were interviewed to obtain information about their use of cigarettes and alcohol during pregnancy, reproductive history, and maternal age at delivery. The family's socioeconomic status was classified using the median income of the families living in the same census block group as the residence listed on the child's birth certificate during the year of the child's birth. Birth certificates provided additional data on maternal education, birth weight, race, and sex. The relationship between smoking and mental retardation was analyzed with logistic regression models.

Results.—Compared with children of women who did not smoke during pregnancy, there was a 75% increase in the prevalence of mental retarda-

---

TABLE 4.—Relationship Between Maternal Cigarette Smoking Into the Second Trimester of Pregnancy and the Prevalence of Idiopathic Mental Retardation Among 10-year-old Children, Metropolitan Atlanta, 1985 and 1986

Model	Smoking Any Time Into the Second Trimester of Pregnancy			Amount of Smoking in the Second Trimester of Pregnancy					
	No	Yes	(95% CI)	None	<1 pack/day	(95% CI)	≥1 pack/day	(95% CI)
OR	1.0	1.75	(1.20–2.55)	1.0	1.76	(1.12–2.76)	1.80	(1.02–3.17)
OR$_{adj}$*	1.0	1.65	(1.05–2.60)	1.0	1.55	(0.91–2.65)	1.92	(0.98–3.77)
OR$_{adj}$†	1.0	1.53	(0.95–2.45)	1.0	1.40	(0.80–2.46)	1.87	(0.92–3.79)

*Adjusted OR, controlling for sex, maternal age, race, economic status, parity, maternal education, and alcohol use during pregnancy.

†Adjusted OR, controlling for all of the above variables plus low birth weight (very low birth weight, low birth weight, and normal birth weight).

Abbreviations: OR, odds ratio; *CI,* confidence interval.

(Courtesy of Drews CD, Murphy CC, Yeargin-Allsopp M, et al: The relationship between idiopathic mental retardation and maternal smoking during pregnancy. Reproduced by permission of *Pediatrics* Vol 97, pp 547–553, Copyright 1996.)

tion in the children of women who did smoke during pregnancy. The rates of idiopathic mental retardation increased with increasing frequency of smoking during pregnancy, even after controlling for low birth weight. Compared to the children of women who stopped smoking during the last 2 trimesters of pregnancy, the children of women who smoked through the first 2 trimesters had a 60% greater prevalence of mental retardation (Table 4). The dose-response relationship was also seen in these children, even after controlling for low birth weight.

Conclusions.—Maternal smoking during pregnancy significantly and independently increases the risk of idiopathic mental retardation in the child. There is a linear dose-response relationship between the amount of smoking and the prevalence of idiopathic mental retardation. Therefore, smoking interventions represent a method of substantially preventing idiopathic mental retardation.

▶ If the data from this report are correct, we now have 858 reasons why no one should smoke, much less smoke when pregnant. The data seem very believable despite the complexity of what must be taken into account when attempting to tease out smoking as one of multiple potential causes of mental retardation. The very fact that there is a linear relationship between the number of cigarettes smoked per day and the prevalence of mental retardation in the offspring of such smokers, adds an enormous degree of validity and believability to the conclusions that were reached. These data aside, the most chilling conclusion from this report is that if these findings represent a causal relationship, the attributable risk among exposed women is very high. Thirty-five percent of cases of idiopathic mental retardation occurring among children of women who smoke directly relate to the mothers' smoking habit. What a guilt trip these mothers face if they ever fully understand the impact of their smoking.

Exactly why maternal smoking might cause an IQ deficit in an individual's offspring is speculative at best. It's possible that smoking may have a direct, toxic effect on the fetus. It could alter maternal ability to supply nutrients during pregnancy. Smoking is known to cause an increase in maternal complications of pregnancy and to produce some degree of fetal hypoxemia. It is unlikely, however, that the effect of maternal smoking on mental retardation occurs through the same mechanism as the effect of smoking on birth weight because, as has been found in other studies, controlling for birth weight neither eliminates nor substantially reduces the observed association between smoking and mental retardation. One should be aware that the children of smokers are more likely to display aggressive behaviors and be less attentive than children of nonsmokers.[1] Such behaviors could increase the likelihood that a child will not perform well on an IQ test of the type given in this report.

If you need more convincing (unlikely) about the morbidity seen in children as a result of the use of tobacco products by other people, see the article by Di Franza.[2] Each year among American children, tobacco is associated with an estimated 284–300 deaths from lower respiratory tract illnesses and fires initiated by smoking materials, 354,000–2.2 million episodes of otitis media,

5,200–165,000 tympanotomies, 14,000–21,000 tonsillectomies and/or adenoidectomies, 529,000 physician visits for asthma, 1.3–2 million visits for coughs, and, in children younger than 5 years of age, 260,000–436,000 episodes of bronchitis and 115,000–190,000 episodes of pneumonia. These data are another 8 reasons why adults should stop smoking. Have you lost count?

References

1. Weitzman M, et al: *Pediatrics* 90:342, 1992.
2. Di Franza JR, et al: *Pediatrics* 97:560, 1996.

Randomized, Double Blind Comparison of Brand and Generic Antibiotic Suspensions: II. A Study of Taste and Compliance in Children
El-Chaar GM, Mardy G, Wehlou K, et al (St John's Univ, Jamaica, NY; Schneider Children's Hosp of Long Island Jewish Med Ctr, New Hyde Park, NY)
Pediatr Infect Dis J 15:18–22, 1996   9–6

Background.—Children are more likely to comply with oral liquid medications if those medications taste good. Generic preparations commonly prescribed to save cost may taste worse than brand name products, thus negatively affecting compliance. The taste of, and compliance with, brand name and generic formulations of common antibiotic suspensions were compared.

Methods.—Fifty-three antibiotic suspensions were distributed at pediatricians' offices between August and December 1994. Because of attrition, additional preparations of trimethoprim-sulfamethoxazole were also distributed. Children aged 3–14 years were eligible for the study. Taste was evaluated using verbal and visual assessment methods. Compliance was determined by measuring the amount of drug returned after use. Medications and evaluation sheets were returned by 10 of 15 patients given cephalexin, 10 of 14 given erythromycin-sulfisoxazole, and 16 of 24 given trimethoprim-sulfamethoxazole.

Findings.—The 10 children in the cephalexin and erythromycin-sulfisoxazole groups reported that the brand and generic medications tasted the same. Fifteen of the 16 children in the trimethoprim-sulfamethoxazole group said the brand product tasted better than the generic preparation. The percentage of returned/expected amount of medication was, respectively, 114.3% and 102% for the brand name and generic cephalexin formulations; 100% and 80% for the brand name and generic erythromycin-sulfisoxazole suspensions; and 96% and 86% for the brand name and generic trimethoprim-sulfamethoxazole formulations.

Conclusions.—Not all brand name oral liquid antibiotics taste better than the generic formulations. All children complied with both brand name and generic medications, although most preferred the taste of brand name trimethoprim-sulfamethoxazole to that of the generic formulation.

▶ In an era of cost containment, there is a great push to write prescriptions for generic pharmaceuticals. When making a decision to use a generic drug, one must always entertain 2 considerations: is the generic brand as therapeutically effective as a brand name product?; and is the generic drug as likely to be taken? The likelihood with which the recipient of a prescription will complete a course of treatment, more often than not, is based on how well a medicine "goes down." As far as kids are concerned, antibiotic suspensions that taste better have a greater likelihood of being used in their entirety.

So how would you determine whether one liquid antibiotic preparation is more palatable than another? Theoretically, you could have the equivalent of a wine tasting party, but because antibiotic tasting is not entirely risk-free, this approach is probably less than ideal. What these investigators did was to take children aged 3–14 years who were receiving antibiotic suspensions for treatment of infections and did verbal and visual assessments as to whether 1 drug or another seemed to be better received. The predictable conclusion would be that no differences would be found. Overall, that is exactly what was seen. Brand name liquid antibiotics do not necessarily taste better than their cheaper generic counterparts.

All in all, this is a great study. Its only flaw is the assumption that medicines are supposed to taste good. A generation or more ago, the saying "take your medicine" meant something, i.e., something less than pleasant. Now we're creating a coddled generation of offspring who not only willingly take their medicine but perhaps even enjoy doing so. Someone once said that the only thing that separates us from the apes is our willingness to take drugs. This report only further reinforces this distinguishing characteristic.

Carbohydrate and Alcohol Content of 200 Oral Liquid Medications for Use in Patients Receiving Ketogenic Diets
Feldstein TJ (Children's Health Care-Minneapolis)
Pediatrics 97:506–511, 1996   9–7

Background.—To help maintain a ketotic state, patients with intractable seizure disorders are given a ketogenic diet, in which they must follow a strict low-carbohydrate intake. However, many of these patients require medication, and some pharmaceutical products—especially oral liquid formulations—contain significant amounts of carbohydrate. Therefore each medication taken by the patient following a ketogenic diet must be evaluated. Oral liquid drug products were assessed for their carbohydrate content.

Methods and Findings.—A list of 200 oral liquid drug products was compiled, and the manufacturers were asked to provide the carbohydrate and alcohol content of those products. The information is presented in tabular form. Many of the medications on the list included significant amounts of carbohydrate in the form of sucrose, fructose, sorbitol, and glycerin.

Discussion.—A table providing information on the carbohydrate and alcohol content of various oral liquid medications is presented. Although medications in tablet or capsule form may also contain carbohydrate excipients, the total number of carbohydrate per dose is usually much lower. The information provided in the table should be useful in designing a low-carbohydrate drug regimen for the patient on a ketogenic diet. The quantities listed are subject to change and should be confirmed again with the manufacturers.

▶ Most of us don't tend to think too much about the sugar content of the medications we use. What makes liquid medications palatable, in most instances, is the carbohydrate content, which can cause problems on occasion. Children with specific forms of carbohydrate intolerance may require a thought or 2 before a prescription is written. In the article abstracted, we see that those who are on ketogenic diets, who of necessity should have diets with very little in the way of carbohydrates, frequently taken over-the-counter or prescription medications containing carbohydrates. Such medications obviate any theoretical advantage of a ketogenic diet. One doesn't need to worry about diabetic children and the sugar content of medications, because it isn't enough to produce poor control of diabetes. There is some sugar, however, enough that if you are stuck in a situation where a child with diabetes becomes hypoglycemic and you have no access to orange juice, you could give a dose of amoxicillin to get rid of the jitters.

There is recent information about the dental complications of carbohydrates in liquid medications. In a study of almost 100 children ages 2–17 years, those taking liquid medications for conditions such as epilepsy, cystic fibrosis, chronic renal failure, asthma, recurrent urinary tract infections, and chronic constipation are at a markedly increased risk of dental caries, particularly of the anterior teeth.[1] As for any child, the risk of caries can be reduced by the use of fluoride-containing toothpaste. In fact, 1 recent study has shown that regular fluoride toothpaste use reduces caries by as much as one third.[2] Lastly, we probably should be taking a clue from the Finns about what they are doing to reduce the number of cavities, especially in adolescents. In Finland, the chewing of xylitol gum is quite common. The anticariogenic effects of xylitol were first shown in studies in the 1970s.[3] Not long after, chewing gum was then suggested as a practical vehicle for xylitol-related caries prevention, inasmuch as gum would allow the xylitol to remain in the mouth long enough to have some effectiveness. Xylitol is also a nice sweetener for chewing gum.

The use of chewing gum has been considered a health-damaging behavior because of the cariogenic effect of sucrose and the fact that many perceive chewing gum as an improper social habit. Knowing that most teenagers eschew good manners at least on occasion, one might capitalize on their proclivity to chew gum (xylitol-laced) to do something good. Just don't emphasize the benefits. If nothing else, it is better than chewing tobacco.[4]

References

1. Maguire A, et al: *Caries Res* 30:16, 1996.
2. Mathiesen AT, et al: *Caries Res* 30:29, 1996.
3. Scheinin A, et al: *Acta Odontol Scand* 33(suppl 70):307, 1995.
4. Honka LA, et al: *Caries Res* 30:34, 1996.

Identification of Children at Risk for Lead Poisoning: An Evaluation of Routine Pediatric Blood Lead Screening in an HMO-insured Population
Haan MN, Gerson M, Zishka BA (Univ of California, Davis; Kaiser Permanente Med Ctr, Vallejo, Calif)
Pediatrics 97:79–83, 1996   9–8

Objective.—The Centers for Disease Control and Prevention (CDC) have suggested that routine screening for lead poisoning need not be continued in low-risk children. The prevalence of lead poisoning in children receiving regular checkups was determined, as well as the sensitivity, specificity, and negative predicative value of selected CDC questions in identifying an exposed population.

Methods.—Survey data and blood samples were collected during regular checkups of 636 children, aged 12–60 months, cared for in 4 Kaiser Permanente Medical Care Program locations. Parents were asked whether their child (1) lived in or visited a house with peeling paint built before 1960; (2) lived in or visited a house built before 1960 that was being or had been recently remodeled; (3) had a sibling or playmate treated for lead poisoning; (4) lived with an adult with a job or hobby involving lead exposure; and (5) lived near industry involved with lead products.

Results.—A total of 220 children were white, 197 black, 98 Hispanic, 94 Asian, and 27 other or mixed. Blood lead levels were less than 10 µg/mL for 94% of children. Blood levels decreased with age and were 25% higher in blacks than in non-Hispanic whites. Age of housing was significantly related to blood lead levels, with mean levels 19% higher in children living in housing 10–20 years old and 29% higher in children living in housing older than 20 years as compared with levels in children living in housing less than 10 years old. From 25.7% to 33.1% of respondents said that a household member was employed in a job having lead exposure, and 87.5% of households reported practicing a lead-related hobby. After multivariate linear regression analysis, however, no association was found between screening criteria and blood lead levels.

Conclusion.—Although the study confirms that minority and low-income children are at higher risk of lead poisoning, the CDC questionnaire did not appear to be useful as a screening tool to identify at-risk children but does have a high negative predictive value.

▶ This report was the final stake in the heart of the 1991 CDC recommendations for universal blood lead screening.[1] If CDC recommendations for universal screening were implemented in the Northern California Kaiser Permanente Medical Care Program pediatric population, and if each child were screened at 1 year and at 2 years of age as per the early recommendations, the total cost for blood lead analysis (currently $13.50 per test) would exceed $4 million in a 5-year period with relatively little yield. This estimate does not include the cost of retesting, staff time spent in follow-up, or member time spent attending appointments. Less tangible costs, such as the emotional and financial impact of a diagnosis of elevated lead values on the child and family, are not calculable.

This report teaches us that well-intended recommendations do not always prove to be effective. Specifically, the CDC booklet *"Preventing Lead Poisoning in Young Children"* has recommended that all physicians evaluate children for lead poisoning by asking parents 5 questions: Does your child live in or regularly visit a house with peeling or chipping paint built before 1960? Does your child live in or regularly visit a house built before 1960 with recent, ongoing, or planned renovation or remodeling? Does your child have a brother or sister, housemate, or playmate being followed or treated for lead poisoning? Does your child live with an adult whose job or hobby involves exposure to lead? Does your child live near an active lead smelter, battery recycling plant, or other industry likely to release lead? If Northern California holds true for the rest of the country, only the question related to job or hobby activity seems to have predictive value. As we gradually withdraw from these early CDC recommendations, it still may be worthwhile to ask whether these job or hobby risk factors exist. The most common potentially lead-related occupations are construction, steel welding and cutting, police work, plumbing, painting and paint manufacturing, and auto repair. The most common lead-using hobby activities include making stained-leaded glass; making fishing sinkers or bullets; working with cars, car parts, or car batteries; soldering; shooting guns at a firing range; painting pictures; painting a house or furniture; working with model cars or boats; and making pottery.

Nationwide, mean blood lead levels have fallen by two thirds according to the third National Health and Nutrition Examination Survey findings.[2] This decrease in average blood lead levels only further increases the feasibility of approaches emphasizing targeted rather than universal blood lead screening among children. The use of risk assessment instruments that are effective will be vital. Clearly the types of questionnaires proposed by the CDC in the early part of this decade are no longer effective for many urban and suburban children. Clearly they do not work for children in rural settings.[3]

References

1. US Department of Health and Human Services. Centers for Disease Control: Preventing lead poisoning in young children: A statement by the Centers for Disease Control. October 1991. Atlanta, Ga: USDHHS, 1991.
2. Pirkle JL, et al: *JAMA* 272:284, 1994.
3. Schaffer SJ, et al: *Pediatrics* 97:84, 1996.

The Relationship of Bone and Blood Lead to Hypertension: The Normative Aging Study

Hu H, Aro A, Payton M, et al (Harvard Med School, Boston; Harvard School of Public Health, Boston; Dept of Veterans Affairs, Boston)
JAMA 275:1171–1176, 1996   9–9

Background.—Although low-level lead exposure is known to be neurotoxic in children, its toxicity in adults is unclear. Previous studies have shown mixed and/or weak associations between lead exposure and blood pressure. Measuring long-term lead accumulation in bone rather than recent exposure in blood may be a better biological marker for investigating the possible link between lead exposure and hypertension. This relationship was analyzed as part of the Veterans Administration Normative Aging Study.

Methods.—The analysis included 590 men who were seen for regular follow-up visits in the larger study and for whom there were data on all variables of interest. All underwent in vivo measurement of lead levels in cortical and trabecular bone—the tibia and patella, respectively—by K x-ray fluorescence. Blood lead levels were measured as well by graphite furnace atomic absorption spectroscopy. The subjects were considered hypertensive if they were taking daily antihypertensive medication or if their blood pressure at examination was 160/96 mm Hg or higher.

Results.—The mean blood lead level was only 0.30 µmol/L, suggesting little recent lead exposure. Bone lead levels were consistent with those reported in other populations, with means of 22 µg/g of bone mineral in the tibia and 32 µg/g in the patella. The 146 hypertensive men had significantly higher blood and bone lead levels than the 444 nonhypertensive men; means in the hypertensive group were 0.33 µmol/L in the blood, 24 µg/g of bone mineral in the tibia, and 35 µg/g of bone mineral in the patella. Logistic regression analysis was performed to assess the contribution of age, race, body mass index, family history of hypertension, history of ethanol use, pack-years of smoking, dietary sodium intake, dietary calcium intake, and blood and bone lead levels to hypertensive status. The significant variables in this model were body mass index, family history of hypertension, and tibia lead level. As the tibia lead level increased from the midpoint of the lowest quintile to the midpoint of the highest quintile— from 8 to 37 µg/g of bone mineral—the odds ratio for hypertension increased to 1.5.

Conclusion.—Long-term accumulation of lead in the body, as reflected by cortical bone lead levels, appears to be an independent risk factor for hypertension in adults. The mechanism of this relationship is unknown. Prospective epidemiologic studies of the link between bone lead and cardiovascular health and basic scientific studies of the long-term toxicity of lead are needed.

▶ This report made it into the YEAR BOOK OF PEDIATRICS even though it deals exclusively with adults. The data are pretty clear. Adults exposed over long periods to even low concentrations of lead have a much greater risk of hypertension than expected. The importance of these data to children are fairly obvious. Children grow up to be adults.

Why low levels of lead exposure cause hypertension is not known. One thing that is known, however, is that low-level exposure to lead impairs renal function in middle-aged and older men.[1] Even if blood lead levels never exceed 10 µg/dL in adults, there is an inverse correlation between blood lead levels and renal function. Fortunately, the reduction in lead levels in the average United States population, attained through rigorous environmental controls during the past 2 decades, may have a benefit in reducing renal damage and death to a degree far greater than was ever expected merely on the basis of a reduction in short-term toxicity related to lead poisoning.

One final comment having to do with lead: With so many states these days allowing private citizens to pack a side arm, the risk of lead poisoning is increasing. The risk relates to exposure to volatilized lead in the air at indoor shooting ranges.[2] It appears that pistols emit various particles, including lead from their barrels, when they are fired. About 50% of the lead is in inhalable particles. The particles also contain other toxic elements such as antimony, copper, arsenic, and barium. Most gun clubs that have these ranges rarely clean the dust that is generated, and few provide external ventilation. Given the fact that it is not at all unusual for individual gun club members to shoot between 2,000 and 3,000 rounds a week, you can see that a lot of gun slingers these days may be harming their kidneys and also causing hypertension. Also, given the fact that some such individuals often have a disdain for authority and friendly advice, including health warnings, it is likely that we will continue to see them at home on the range and with lead in their bones.

For a superb overview on the treatment guidelines for lead exposure in children, see the American Academy of Pediatrics Committee on Drugs report.[3]

References

1. Kim R, et al: *JAMA* 275:1177, 1996.
2. McDonald P: *Lancet* 343:856, 1994.
3. American Academy of Pediatrics Committee on Drugs: *Pediatrics* 96:155, 1995.

Methylene Blue–induced Phototoxicity: An Unrecognized Complication
Porat R, Gilbert S, Magilner D (Albert Einstein Med Ctr, Philadelphia)
Pediatrics 97:717–721, 1996   9–10

Objective.—Several different complications of exposure to methylene blue in newborns have been reported, most involving prenatal exposure to the dye, used either to detect amniotic fluid leaks or differentiate sacs of twins. Few studies have reported hemolytic anemia and hyperbilirubinemia occurring after postnatal use of methylene blue, and there have been no reports of complications of phototherapy for hyperbilirubinemia. Photosensitization is reported as a complication of prenatal exposure to a very large dose of methylene blue.

Case Report.—Girl was born at 27 weeks' gestation with a birth weight of 1,090 g to an African-American mother. The mother had been admitted to the hospital with contractions and probable rupture of the membranes. Amniocentesis with injection of 10 mL of 1% methylene blue confirmed rupture of the membranes. The infant, delivered by cesarean section, required ventilator support for respiratory distress syndrome. Her skin was stained deep blue, except for small areas under the chin and the inguinal folds, which gradually became blue over the next day. The patient received 2 exchange transfusions for methemoglobinemia, hemolytic anemia, and hyperbilirubinemia, as well as phototherapy for hyperbilirubinemia. A few hours after exposure to phototherapy, the exposed areas turned from dark blue to red and maroon (Fig 2). This was followed by formation of bullae, which showed signs of a phototoxic reaction on pathologic examination. Desquamation developed, continuing even after phototherapy was stopped and eventually affecting an estimated 35% of the total body surface. Skin sloughing continued for a few days, followed by re-epithelializa-

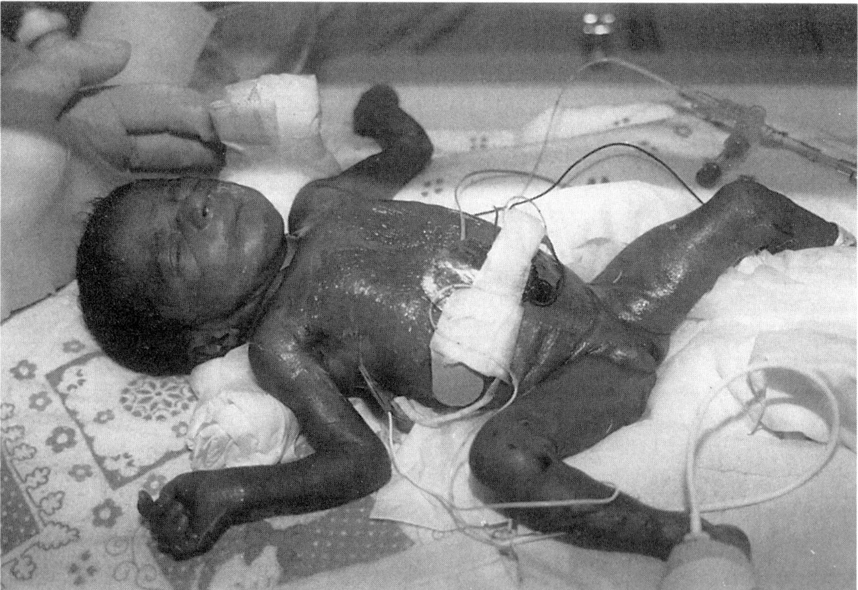

FIGURE 2.—Photograph of the infant at 5 days of age. Extensive redness, bullae, and excoriation of the skin in the areas exposed to phototherapy are shown. Note that areas in the inguinal folds and under the chin gradually became blue. (Courtesy of Porat R, Gilbert S, Magilner D: Methylene blue–induced phototoxicity: An unrecognized complication. Reproduced by permission of *Pediatrics*, Vol 97, pp 717–721, Copyright 1996.)

TABLE 2.—Clinical Characteristics and Hospital Course of Neonates With Methylene Blue Toxicity

Author, Year	Birth Weight, kg	Gestational Age, wk	Amount Given	Route	Exposure Time	Hospital Course
Plunkett, 1973	4 cases	UN	3.5 mL 1% (35 mg)	IA	1 d–5 wk	Hemolysis, ↑ bili (1 died)
Cowett et al, 1976	2.8	35	1 mL 1% (10 mg)	IA	3 h	RD, hemolysis, ↑ bili, EX ×2, Photo
Serota et al, 1979	3.4	41	20 mL 1% 200mg	IA	24 h	RD, hemolysis, ↑ bili, Photo
Spahr et al, 1980	3.12	37	1 mL 1% (10 mg)	IA	3 d	RD, 20% Met Hg, hemolysis, ↑ bili, Photo
Kirsch and Cohen, 1980	1.22	31	2–3 mL 0.1%	OG	At age	Hemolysis, ↑ bili,
	1.18	31	×2 (4–6 mg)	OG	1 wk	3 blood transfusions
	(1 case)	UN	UN	IA	UN	Hemolysis, ↑ bili, died at 8 d of age
Crooks, 1982	3.15	38	7 mL 1% (70 mg)	IA	3 d	RD, hemolysis, ↑ bili, EX ×2, Photo
McEnerney and McEnerney, 1983	2	34	2 mL 1% (20 mg)	IA	14 h	RD, Met Hg 4.1, hemolysis, ↑ bili, EX ×2, Photo
Troche, 1989	0.92	26	1 mL 1% (10 mg)	IA	18 h	↑ bili, Photo, inaccurate pulse oxymetry
Fish and Chazen, 1992	2.61	35	10 mL 1% (100 mg)	IA	12 h	Hemolysis (Hct 18), Met Hg, ↑ bili, Photo, blood transfusion
Sills and Zinkham, 1994	2.4	37	UN (several boluses)	OG	2 d	Severe hemolysis, ↑ bili, Photo, multiple gastrointestinal perforation, died, red skin on chest → denuded
	2.58 Type II butyric aciduna	37	50 mg	IV	4 d	↑ bili, Photo, died, bullae and desquamation of hands (autopsy: bluish discoloration of hands, vitreous, thalamus)
Present case	1.09	27	10 mL 1% (100 mg)	IA	9 h	↑ Met Hg, (7.8%) hemolysis, ↑ bili, EX ×2, Photo, severe phototoxic reaction (redness → desquamation of 35% of body surface)

Note: Perpendicular arrow indicates "elevated"; *parallel arrow* indicates "became."
Abbreviations: UN, unknown; *IA*, intra-amniotic; *OG*, orogastric; *bili*, bilirubin; *RD*, respiratory distress; *EX*, exchange transfusion; *photo*, phototherapy; *Met Hg*, methemoglobin.
(Courtesy of Porat R, Gilbert S, Magilner D: Methylene blue–induced phototoxicity: An unrecognized complication. Reproduced by permission of *Pediatrics*, Vol 97, pp 717–721, Copyright 1996.)

tion, which was complete by 3 weeks of age. The patient was left with several areas of depigmentation on her abdomen and extremities.

Discussion.—Methylene blue–induced phototoxicity is a newly reported complication in infants with high prenatal exposure to methylene blue and subsequent treatment with phototherapy. The occurrence of methylene blue phototoxicity in this case may have resulted from the high dose of dye relative to the small size of the patient and the young gestational age (Table 2). Obstetricians and pediatricians should be aware of the proper dosing and potential toxic effects of methylene blue.

▶ It's strange that in this era of modern newborn medicine, we still resort to old techniques, such as injecting methylene blue into amniotic fluid to determine whether membranes are ruptured (if so, blue dye can readily be seen in the vagina). Methylene blue is a good agent, except when it is not. When it is not, it is an absolutely no-good agent. In the newborn, it can cause Heinz body hemolytic anemia; hyperbilirubinemia; methemoglobinemia; respiratory distress; skin staining and, because of skin staining, interference with pulse oximetry. The infant reported here was exposed to methylene blue when obstetricians injected it into the mother's amniotic fluid. There was concern regarding premature rupture of membranes and chorioamnionitis. A lot of methylene blue must have been used because the infant came out purple and voided blue urine for 6 days.

Why this child got into trouble with shedding of the skin is a bit speculative, but there is probably a good explanation. In small doses, methylene blue can be used to treat methemoglobinemia by hastening the conversion of methemoglobin to hemoglobin. In a large dose, however, it has the opposite effect and oxidizes hemoglobin, resulting in methemoglobin formation. It also results in a brisk hemolytic anemia because of the oxidative damage it causes. It is also a photosensitizing compound with a peak absorption at 665 nM, which is within the wavelength of light emitted by phototherapy units. Photo-activated methylene blue causes structural damage to cell membranes. Once inside cells, it destroys lysosomes and also binds to DNA within the nucleus of cells. There, superoxide ions damage DNA and interfere with cell functions. The net result of this is pretty straightforward: The skin will blister after what first appears to be a sunburn.

It is not known whether methylene blue–induced phototoxic skin damage results in any permanent sequelae, such as a long-term risk of melanoma. Time will have to tell us the answer to this. In the meantime, use methylene blue only in low doses. There are better and truly safer ways to tell whether amniotic fluid is leaking.

Respiratory Failure From Corn Starch Aspiration: A Hazard of Diaper Changing

Silver P, Sagy M, Rubin L (Schneider Children's Hosp, New Hyde Park, NY; Albert Einstein College of Medicine, New Hyde Park, NY)
Pediatr Emerg Care 12:108–110, 1996   9–11

Introduction.—There are numerous reports of the health hazards of aspiration of talcum-based baby powders used in diaper changing. Many pediatricians have therefore recommended cornstarch instead of talcum powder for routine skin care. An infant was seen with acute severe pneumonitis and respiratory failure resulting from cornstarch powder aspiration during diaper changing.

Case Report.—Boy, 1 month, was brought to the emergency department with respiratory distress, which had lasted several hours. The infant had been in good health until that day. He was pale and lethargic and had intercostal retractions with grunting. He had coarse, bilaterally diminished breath sounds. On 50% of inspired oxygen, his arterial blood gas revealed a pH of 7.13, PCO_2 of 53 mm Hg, and a PO_2 of 46 mm Hg. The patient was admitted to the pediatric ICU, treated with IV ampicillin and cefotaxime, intubated, and placed on mechanical ventilation with 100% of inspired oxygen. The ventilator settings were as follows: a peak inspiratory pressure of 43 cm H_2O, positive end-expiratory pressure of 7 cm H_2O, and intermittent mandatory ventilation rate of 45 breaths/min. A large number of crystal-like structures were found in his tracheal aspirate, which proved to be cornstarch on further study. The infant was treated with a 7-day course of methylprednisolone. His health status began improving on his second day of hospitalization, and daily chest radiographs revealed gradually clearing infiltrates. He was slowly weaned from the ventilator, enabling extubation on hospital day 5 and hospital discharge after 6 additional days.

Discussion.—The use of cornstarch during diapering is potentially extremely hazardous for the infant's respiratory health. Parents should be informed of this hazard and advised that no powder is necessary for routine infant skin care. If powder is used, it should be carefully kept away from the infant's face. For any infant with acute respiratory failure and pneumonitis who has a history of powder use during diapering, cornstarch pneumonitis should be included in the differential diagnosis.

▶ Aspiration of talcum-based baby powder during diaper changes is well known. According to the Long Island Regional Poison Control Center located at the Nassau County Medical Center in New York, there are approximately 200 reports per year nationally of talcum powder aspiration and ingestion by infants.[1] In some of these cases, the child was reported to have placed the baby powder container in his or her mouth, possibly mistaking the powder container for a milk bottle. Although the majority of babies who aspirate talcum powder don't have any problem, some patients do have severe lung disease. Mortality rates as high as 20%[2] have been reported. The risks associated with talcum powder use have led a fair number of pediatricians to recommend the use of cornstarch powder for routine infant skin care.

So, is cornstarch a safe substitute for talcum powder? No, if you believe this report. Before this report appeared, there had been no reports of cornstarch powder aspiration resulting in pneumonitis. This report, however, describes an infant with a severe bilateral pneumonitis from the aspiration of cornstarch. The data are pretty convincing because cornstarch crystals were found deep within the child's airway at the time of intubation.

Should we be instructing parents about the potential dangers of cornstarch as we have reminded them about those of talcum powder? Perhaps yes; perhaps no. One case such as this does not a series make. Chances are that cornstarch is safer than talcum powder. It's certainly safer than other lubricants like WD 40.

References

1. Caraccio T: Long Island Regional Poison Control Center. Nassau County Medical Center, East Meadow, New York. Direct Communication.
2. Brouillette F, Weber M: *Can Med Assoc J* 119:354, 1978.

Adverse Reactions in Children During Long Term Antimicrobial Therapy
Uhari M, Nuutinen M, Turtinen J (Univ of Oulu, Finland)
Pediatr Infect Dis J 15:404–408, 1996   9–12

Background.—Long-term antimicrobial therapy can be effective in immunologically healthy children with recurrent urinary tract infections or recurrent otitis media. Methodological difficulties and the expense of prospective trials restrict the availability of reliable data on adverse reactions of antibiotics in general use. However, the importance of obtaining reliable data on adverse reactions to long-term antimicrobial therapy prompted a retrospective study of adverse reactions to long-term antimicrobial therapy for recurrent urinary tract infections in immunologically healthy children.

Methods.—The hospital records of 1,825 randomly selected children (including 1,607 girls and 218 boys) receiving long-term antimicrobial therapy for the treatment of recurrent urinary tract infections between 1976 and 1985 were reviewed. Overall, the female patients received 5,066 courses of treatments, and the male patients received 607 courses. Nitrofurantoin was used most commonly, followed by sulfonamide.

Results.—There were adverse reactions in 10.4% of the courses of treatment, which resulted in drug discontinuation in 8.2%. Abdominal discomfort was the most common adverse reaction to nitrofurantoin treat-

TABLE 2.—Numbers of Adverse Reaction Events and Rates With 95% Confidence Intervals Relative to Antimicrobial Therapy Given to Girls Less Than 2 Years of Age

Adverse Reaction	Nitrofurantoin (1)			Sulfonamides (2)			Trimethoprim (3)			1 + 2		
	N	R	95% CI	N	R	95% CI	N	R	95% CI	N	R	95% CI
Nausea, vomiting	23	12.5	7.9–18.8	2	1.7	0.2–6.0	1	3.0	1.9–26.7	20	21.0	12.7–32.1
Refusal	11	6.0	3.0–10.7	1	0.8	0.02–4.6	0	0.0		12	13.0	6.4–21.8
Urticaria	6	3.3	1.2–7.1	9	7.4	3.4–14.1	0	0.0		7	7.3	2.9–15.0
Drug fever	1	0.5	0.01–3.0	0	0.0		0	0.0		0	0.0	
Blood dyscrasia	0	0.0		1	0.8	0.02–4.6	0	0.0		1	1.0	0.03–5.8
Diarrhea	1	0.5	0.01–3.0	0	0.0		1	3.0	1.9–26.7	0	0.0	
Other adverse reactions	0	0.0		1	0.8	0.02–4.6	0	0.0		1	1.0	0.03–5.8
All	42	23.0	17.4–29.6	14	11.0	6.3–19.4	2	6.0	0.74–22.0	41	43.0	32.3–60.2

Abbreviations: R, events per 100 years at risk; *CI*, confidence interval.
(Courtesy of Uhari M, Nuutinen M, Turtinen J: Adverse reactions in children during long term antimicrobial therapy. *Pediatr Infect Dis J* 15(5):404–408, 1996.)

TABLE 3.—Numbers of Adverse Reaction Events and Rates With 95% Confidence Intervals Relative to Antimicrobial Therapy Given to Girls Aged 2–15 Years

Adverse Reaction	Nitrofurantoin (1)			Sulfonamides (2)			Trimethoprim (3)			1 + 2			2 + 3		
	N	R	95% CI	N	R	95% CI	N	R	95% CI	N	R	95% CI	N	R	95% CI
Nausea, vomiting	55	3.8	2.8–4.9	18	3.4	2.0–5.4	7	2.3	0.9–4.7	64	7.1	5.4–9.0	2	2.8	0.3–10.0
Refusal of the drug	34	2.3	1.6–3.3	8	1.5	0.6–3.0	2	0.7	0.1–2.4	39	4.3	3.1–5.9	1	1.4	0.0–7.7
Urticaria	22	1.5	0.9–2.3	26	5.0	3.2–7.2	6	2.0	0.7–4.3	18	2.0	1.2–3.1	1	1.4	0.0–7.7
Drug fever	2	0.1	0.0–0.5	0	0.0		0	0		3	0.3	0.1–1.0	0	0	
Blood dyscrasia	1	0.1	0.0–0.4	1	0.2	0.0–1.1	2	0.7	0.1–2.4	1	0.1	0.0–0.6	0	0	
Diarrhea	0	0.0		5	0.9	0.3–2.2	1	0.4	0.0–1.8	0	0.0		1	1.4	0.0–7.7
Other reactions	22	1.5	0.9–2.3	16	3.0	1.7–4.9	3	1.0	0.2–2.9	23	2.5	1.6–3.8	3	4.2	0.9–12.2
All	136	9.3	7.8–11.0	74	14.0	11.0–17.6	21	6.9	4.2–10.5	148	16.4	13.8–19.2	8	11.1	4.8–21.9

Abbreviations: R, events per 100 years at risk; *CI*, confidence interval.
(Courtesy of Uhari M, Nuutinen M, Turtinen J: Adverse reactions in children during long term antimicrobial therapy. *Pediatr Infect Dis J* 15(5):404–408, 1996.)

TABLE 4.—Numbers and Rates of the Recurrences per 100 Person-years at Risk With 95% Confidence Intervals of the Rate During Preventive Antimicrobial Therapy According to the Drug Used

Antimicrobial	Girls <2 yr			Girls 2–15 yr			Boys <2 yr		
	N	Rate	95% CI	N	Rate	95% CI	N	Rate	95% CI
Nitrofurantoin	13	7.1	3.8–12.1	141	9.7	8.1–11.4	14	18.6	10.1–31.3
Sulfonamides	36	29.7	20.6–41.1	143	27.1	22.9–32.0	22	29.9	18.6–45.2
Trimethoprim	8	24.3	10.5–48.0	84	27.4	21.9–33.9	2	22.0	2.7–79.4
Nitrofurantoin + sulfonamide	18	18.7	11.1–29.6	91	10.1	8.1–12.3	6	8.9	3.3–19.3
All	75	17.3	13.6–21.7	459	14.4	13.1–15.7	44	19.5	14.2–26.2

Abbreviation: CI, confidence interval.
(Courtesy of Uhari M, Nuutinen M, Turtinen J: Adverse reactions in children during long term antimicrobial therapy. *Pediatr Infect Dis J* 15(5):404–408, 1996.)

ment, whereas allergic skin reactions were the most common adverse reactions to sulfonamide treatment. Adverse events were more frequent in association with nitrofurantoin treatment in patients younger than 2 years of age (Table 2), whereas patients aged 2–15 years had more frequent adverse events in association with sulfonamide treatment (Table 3). A protocol involving the alternation of drugs increased the rate of adverse reactions and did not reduce recurrences. There was a recurrence rate of 9.4 episodes/100 person-years at risk with nitrofurantoin treatment and of 26.7 episodes/100 person-years at risk with sulfonamide treatment, which was not affected by age or sex (Table 4).

Conclusions.—Long-term treatment with nitrofurantoin or sulfonamides is safe in the prevention of recurrent urinary tract infection, causing no serious adverse reactions. Resistance to nitrofurantoin treatment develops slowly among the bacteria causing urinary tract infections, making this agent a particularly advantageous choice.

▶ How comforting. By and large, antibiotics rarely cause significant adverse reactions. Those that do tend to be in the nitrofurantoin or sulfonamide category. Even then, don't expect to see too much of an adverse reaction rate, as this series showed only 11 adverse events per 100 person-years at risk among children younger than 2 years of age. Not bad. When you recognize, however, how many millions of children are treated with antibiotics each year, you must never lose sight of the fact that agents such as trimethoprim-sulfamethoxazole can cause fever, liver damage, renal injury, and bone marrow suppression. Anaphylaxis that is mediated by IgE can occur, particularly in children with AIDS receiving this agent as part of the prevention or treatment of *Pneumocystis carinii* infection. Thank goodness a simple method for oral desensitization to this antibiotic has recently been described.[1]

Reference

1. Palusci VJ, et al: *Pediatr Infect Dis J* 15:456, 1996.

Hypertrophy of the Tongue Associated With Inhaled Corticosteroid Therapy in Premature Infants

Linder N, Kuint J, German B, et al (Tel Aviv Univ, Israel)
J Pediatr 127:651–653, 1995   9–13

Introduction.—Hypertrophy of the tongue developed in 3 infants who received inhalational therapy with beclomethasone for respiratory distress.

Clinical Features.—All 3 infants were born prematurely at 26–29 weeks' gestation; 2 weighed less than 1,000 g at birth. The infants were initially treated for bronchopulmonary dysplasia, severe respiratory distress, and severe hyaline membrane disease, respectively. All the infants received dexamethasone systemically shortly after birth, and subsequently were

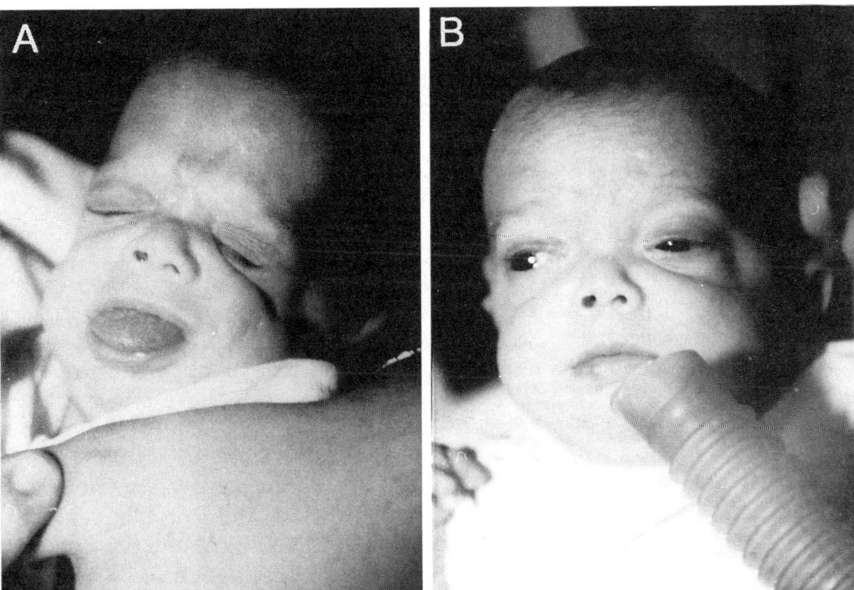

FIGURE 1.—Patient 1. **A**, severe tongue hypertrophy and oral candidiasis after corticosteroid inhalations. **B**, face of same infant at 7 months of age, showing disappearance of glossomegaly. (Courtesy of Linder N, Kuint J, German B, et al: Hypertrophy of the tongue associated with inhaled corticosteroid therapy in premature infants. *J Pediatr* 127:651–653, 1995.)

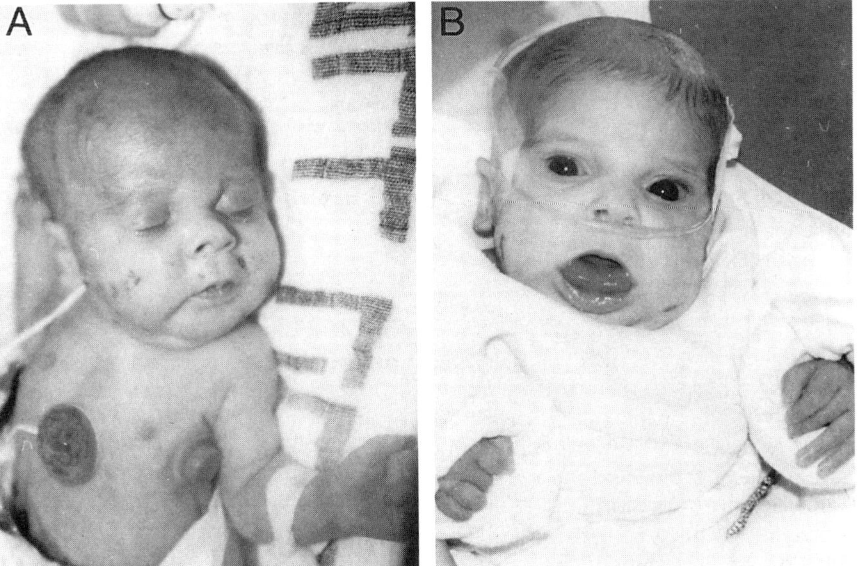

FIGURE 2.—Patient 2. **A**, face after extubation, before corticosteroid inhalations were started. **B**, severe hypertrophy of the tongue 1 month after initiation of corticosteroid inhalations. (Courtesy of Linder N, Kuint J, German B, et al: Hypertrophy of the tongue associated with inhaled corticosteroid therapy in premature infants. *J Pediatr* 127:651–653, 1995.)

given aerosolized beclomethasone. Two of the infants received inhaled salbutamol as well. Marked hypertrophy of the tongue (Figs 1 and 2) was observed after 2–4 weeks of inhalational steroid treatment. The macroglossia subsided gradually after inhalational treatment was replaced by systemic steroid.

Discussion.—Hypertrophy of the tongue may develop in premature infants given inhaled beclomethasone. It may lead to dysphagia, respiratory obstruction, apnea, or cyanosis. Treatment may continue unless obstruction develops or there are feeding problems.

▶ This report will prove to be one of the clinical pearls of the year. Were you aware that aerosolized steroids would make the tongue bigger? This editor was not. One can only conclude from this report that tongue hypertrophy is a possible side effect in premature infants receiving inhalations of beclomethasone. It takes 2–4 weeks for the tongue to increase in size. Fortunately, the hypertrophy disappears gradually after discontinuation of therapy.

Why big tongues develop in infants exposed to topical steroids is not clear. Steroids can reduce thyroxine secretion, but this was not a problem in these infants. Tongue hypertrophy could also have been caused by localized edema from steroids. There did not appear to be evidence of infection or glossitis as a cause of tongue enlargement. Steroids given systemically can increase the heart muscle size. Is it possible that when inhaled they do the same thing to the tongue?

Whatever the cause of tongue hypertrophy in infants receiving inhaled steroids, one must be certain that there are no other conditions present that also cause macroglossia. These conditions include cystic hygroma, Down's syndrome, Beckwith-Wiedeman syndrome, glycogenosis type II, and ectopic thyroid. Of this lengthy list, macroglossia is reversible only in those kids who have it on the basis of steroid exposure.

Tricyclic Medication in Children and the QT Interval: Case Report and Discussion
Alderton HR (Univ of Toronto)
Can J Psychiatry 40:325–329, 1995   9–14

Introduction.—Tricyclic drugs are commonly used to treat major depressive disorders, separation anxiety disorder, and attention deficit hyperactivity disorder in children. Although serious side effects are rare, there is evidence that tricyclic therapy may have adverse cardiac effects. Three unexpected deaths in children treated with desipramine have raised concerns about prolonged QT interval as a possible mechanism for cardiac effects. A child with prolonged QT syndrome diagnosed during tricyclic therapy was described.

Case Report.—Girl, 12 years, with a history of learning difficulty and conflict with her parents had symptoms of inattentive-ness, forgetfulness, and impulsiveness. Attention deficit hyperactivity disorder, predominantly inattentive type, along with learning disorder, motor skills disorder, and adjustment disorder with mixed anxiety and depressed mood were diagnosed. Recommendations included individual psychotherapy, family therapy, and psycho-stimulant medication. Psychostimulant therapy brought improved attention and concentration, but with side effects of anorexia, delayed sleep initiation, and irritability. Therefore, after a baseline ECG was obtained, she was started on nortriptyline. An ECG was obtained before each dose increment. Although nortriptyline, 0.51 mg/kg per day, brought clinical improvement, her QT interval corrected for heart rate (QTc) was higher than 0.45 seconds. Trials of desipramine, which caused adverse side effects and only partial clinical response, and amitriptyline, which was well tolerated but also increased the QTc unacceptably, followed. She underwent a treadmill exercise test, which showed that her QT interval did not shorten during and after exercise, and Holter monitoring, which showed a borderline QTc value at rest. Idiopathic long QT syndrome was diagnosed, and avoidance of drugs prolonging the QT interval, including tricyclics, was recommended.

Discussion.—Long QT syndrome should be strongly suspected if there are possible symptoms or family history, even if the baseline resting ECG is normal. These patients should undergo exercise testing and Holter monitoring before tricyclic therapy is initiated. Tricyclic therapy is contraindicated in patients with a baseline QTc greater than 0.425 seconds or if the QTc exceeds 0.45 seconds during treatment.

▶ If you are a user of tricyclic drugs, this report should be on your reading list because it shows how much trouble you can get into on rare occasions in terms of serious, life-threatening side effects in some children for whom you may prescribe these agents for the treatment of major depressive disorders, attention deficit hyperactivity disorders, and enuresis. What this article does is show us the kinds of circumstances in which serious consequences of tricyclic use can occur. After the death of a 6-year-old child with school phobia who was treated with a high bedtime dose of 14 mg of imipramine per kg was reported by Saraf in 1974, guidelines were developed for maximum permitted dose and increases in pulse rate, blood pressure, and PR and QRS intervals on ECG.[1] Cardiovascular guidelines now include a PR interval less than 0.21 seconds, QRS lengthening to a maximum of 30% over baseline, a resting pulse rate to a maximum of 130 beats/min, and a maximum systolic blood pressure of 130 mm Hg and a maximum diastolic pressure of 85 mm Hg.[2] After 3 unexpected deaths in boys aged 6–9 years treated with desipramine, attention has additionally focused on prolongation of the QT interval as a possible mechanism of sudden death in children receiving tricyclic medications. As readers of the YEAR BOOK OF PEDIATRICS know, the QT interval represents the time taken for ventricular depolarization during systole and repolarization before the next beat. It has long been recognized that excessive QT prolongation is associated with potentially fatal dysrhythmias, including torsades de pointes and ventricular tachycardia and fibrillation. A recommended limit for the QTc is 0.45 when using tricyclics in children.

The long QT syndrome in the case reported as part of this abstract was idiopathic. There are acquired causes of long QT syndrome including metabolic disorders, diffuse myocardial disease, and drugs, including tricyclics, phenothiazines, and quinidine. This report teaches us that children who have idiopathic long QT syndrome probably should not receive any pharmacologic agent that would make their problem worse. This includes tricyclics. Further, to identify increased susceptibility to tricyclics in children from these or other causes, it is strongly recommended that a baseline ECG be obtained before tricyclic use and after each dose increase. Inclusion of an upper limit for baseline QTc of 0.425 is strongly recommended. The author of this report suggests that until more is known about the significance of the QT interval and sudden death, it is not advisable to exceed the 0.45 QTc limit without cardiac consultation. Immediate cardiac consultation is advised if the baseline QTc exceeds 0.425 seconds. If very low doses of tricyclics result in a prolonged QT interval, this may suggest that the child has underlying idiopathic prolonged QT syndrome, which should be evaluated.

Cardiac arrhythmias resulting in death from the use of psychopharmacologic agents are a rare circumstance, one that is totally preventable with appropriate care and monitoring.

References

1. Saraf K, et al: *Psychopharmacologia* 37:265, 1974.
2. Ryan ND: *J Child Adolesc Psychopharmacol* 1:21, 1990.

10 The Genitourinary Tract

Analysis of Meatal Location in 500 Men: Wide Variation Questions Need for Meatal Advancement in All Pediatric Anterior Hypospadias Cases
Fichtner J, Filipas D, Mottrie AM, et al (Mainz Univ, Germany)
J Urol 154:833–834, 1995   10–1

Objective.—Correcting hypospadias involves straightening the penis and repositioning the meatus to what is believed to be the normal site at the tip of the glans. Because the tip of the glans might not be the normal site, the location of the meatus was studied in 500 men in an attempt to avoid complications and preserve function.

Methods.—The distance from the corona to the tip of the glans was measured in 500 men, aged 38–75 years, and classified as A (anterior third/tip of the glans), B (middle third), or C (posterior third near the corona) (Figure).

Results.—Meatal location was located at A in 275 men, at B in 160 men, and C (anterior hypospadias) in 65, including 49 glanular, 15 coronal, and 1 subcoronal. Ten of the latter 16 patients and their partners were unaware of any deformity, and all except 1 homosexual patient had fathered children. None had problems with sexual intercourse or voiding in a standing position. Only the patient with subcoronal hypospadias had penile curvature.

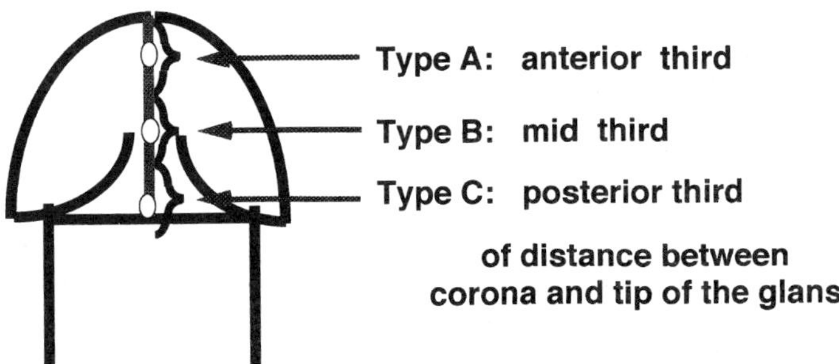

FIGURE.—Classification of meatal location in relation to tip of glans and corona. (Courtesy of Fichtner J, Filipas D, Mottrie AM, et al: Analysis of meatal location in 500 men: Wide variation questions need for meatal advancement in all pediatric anterior hypospadias cases. *J Urol* 154:833–834, 1995.)

Conclusion.—Only 55% of normal men had the meatus located at the tip of the glans. Because even the 13% with anterior hypospadias had no functional complaints, the need for reconstructive surgery to correct the condition in the absence of penile curvature is questioned.

▶ You may complain that this report of where the penile meatus is located in 500 men, with a mean age of 57 years, is stretching the boundaries of material for inclusion in the YEAR BOOK OF PEDIATRICS. Well, think again. Because it is unlikely that the penis has a built-in transport mechanism to move its meatus with age, adult men and the location of their penile meatus are the same as boys in this regard. That having been said, this report tells us an important truth. Some 45% of men, and by inference boys, are not "normal" if normal means having your urethral opening at the tip of your penis. Thirteen percent of otherwise normal adult men (and presumably boys) have hypospadias without knowing it, and some 32% have their meatus halfway between the "normal" position and the point defining true hypospadias.

None of this would be very important except for 2 facts. No one has ever reported the actual frequency of the position of the penile meatus in otherwise normal boys and men. Secondly, because none of these individuals with "abnormal" position of their meatus had any functional difficulties, one wonders whether urologists, at the time of a repair of a hypospadias in a youngster, ought to be too aggressive in getting the meatal opening exactly where it is theoretically supposed to be. Making the meatus open at the tip of the glans during a surgical procedure for repair of hypospadias can involve extensive dissection and a risk that may have little benefit if the alternative is simply to move the meatus close to the tip, but not quite there, a much less complex procedure for the surgeon.

By this point in reading this commentary, every male reader of the YEAR BOOK has checked to see whether he is in the 55% group or the 45% group. If you're in the latter, you're still a stand-up guy because no one in this series had any difficulty in voiding in the upright position, as these persons' shoe-makers will attest to.

Testicular Autotransplantation: A 17-year Review of an Effective Approach to the Management of the Intra-abdominal Testis
Bukowski TP, Wacksman J, Billmire DA, et al (Univ of Cincinnati, Ohio)
J Urol 154:558–561, 1995
10–2

Objective.—The outcomes were reported for 23 patients who underwent 27 testicular autotransplantations during a 17-year period. All patients had at least 1 intra-abdominal testis, a finding that accounts for approximately 5% of all undescended testes.

Patients and Methods.—Patients ranged in age from 1.4 to 20 years at the time of operation (median, 4.5 years). In each case, the intra-abdominal testis was initially determined to be too high to permit conventional

TABLE 1.—Results of Testicular Autotransplantation in 27 Cases of Intraabdominal Testes

Operation Yr.	Pt. Age at Operation (yrs.)	How Identified	Hospital Stay (days)	Operative Time (hrs.)	Side Operation	Size at Followup
1993	17	Prune-belly syndrome	6.0	4.5	Rt.	Good
1992	1.4	Laparoscopy	4.0	5.0	Lt., previous failed rt. Fowler-Stephens procedure	Good
1992	2.0	Abdominal exploration	3.0	4.0	Rt.	Good
1992	4.5	Inguinal exploration	2.0	4.0	Lt.	Good
1992	3.2	Laparoscopy	Not available	Not available	Lt.	Good
1991	7.3	Laparoscopy	2.0	4.5	Solitary lt. testis	No follow-up
1991	7.3	MRI	4.0	4.0	Rt.	No follow-up
1991	2.0	Inguinal exploration	4.0	4.0	Rt.	Good
1991	2.8	Inguinal exploration, human chorionic gonadotropin	Not available	4.5	Rt.	Good
1990	2.2	Inguinal exploration, human chorionic gonadotropin	4.0	5.0	Lt.	Good
1990	6.3	Inguinal exploration	3.0	4.0	Rt.	Good
1987	2.6	Inguinal exploration	Not available	Not available	Lt.	Good
1990	3.3	Inguinal exploration	3.0	3.5	Lt.	Good
1989	4.5	Inguinal exploration	2.0	3.5	Rt.	Good
1989	2.2	Inguinal exploration	Not available	Not available	Lt.	Good
1988	5.3	Inguinal exploration, human chorionic gonadotropin	Not available	Not available	Lt. autotransplantation, rt. Fowler-Stephens procedure	Good/lt. greater than rt.
1988	18	Prune-belly syndrome, MRI	6.0	7.0	Lt.	Lt. greater than rt.
1987	17	Not available	Not available	9.5	Rt.	No follow-up
1985	Not available	Not available	Not available	Not available	Rt.	Good
1981	Not available	Not available	Not available	Not available	Rt.	Good
1981	Not available	Not available	Not available	Not available	Lt.	Good
1981	9.0	Not available	Not available	Not available	Rt.	Good
1979	3.0	Not available	Not available	Not available	Rt.	Good
1980	15	Not available	Not available	Not available	Lt.	Good
1980	9.0	Not available	Not available	Not available	Lt.	Poor
1978	1.9	Not available	Not available	Not available	Rt.	Good
1977	20	Not available	Not available	Not available	Lt.	Good

TABLE 2.—Comparison of Present and Previous Autotransplantation Series

Reference	No. Testes	No. Pts.	Age	% Success	Follow-up	Method Identified
Romas et al	4	3	5–8	100	6–15 mos.	Retroperitoneal exploration
Silber	4	4	5–24	100	6–8 mos.	Not available
Upton et al	10	7	2–18	60	6 mos.–4 yrs.	Inguinal exploration
O'Brien et al	13	11	4–24	55	1–6 yrs.	Inguinal exploration
Garibyan et al	9	9	4–13	100	9–18 mos.	Retroperitoneal and inguinal exploration
Bianchi	12	10	3–15	83	1–2 yrs.	Retroperitoneal and inguinal exploration
Shioshvili	6	5	20–42	100	2–12 mos.	Not available
Harrison et al	12	10	Less than 1–14	100	6–30 mos.	Laparoscopy
Boddy et al	8	Not available	Not available	88	6 mos.–4.25 yrs.	Not available
Present study	27	23	1–20	96	2 mos.–14 yrs.	Retroperitoneal and inguinal exploration

(Courtesy of Bukowski TP, Wacksman J, Billmire DA, et al: Testicular autotransplantation: A 17-year review of an effective approach to the management of the intra-abdominal testis. *J Urol* 154:558–561, 1995.)

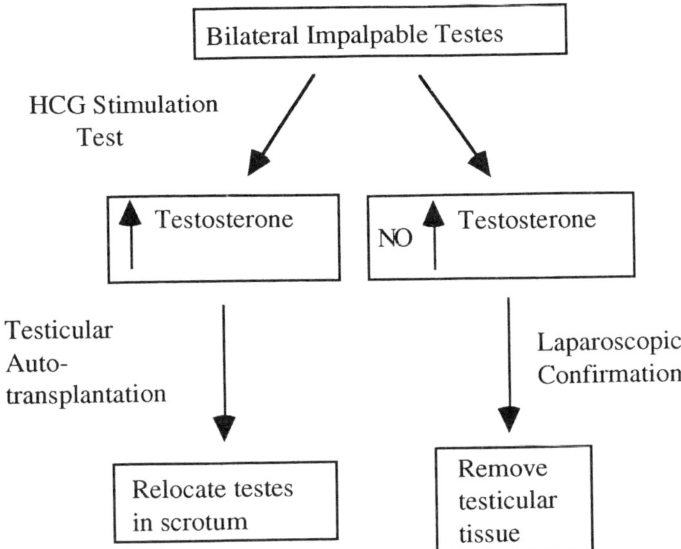

FIGURE.— Algorithm for treatment of intra-abdominal testes. *Abbreviation: HCG,* human chorionic gonadotropin. (Courtesy of Bukowski TP, Wacksman J, Billmire DA, et al: Testicular autotransplantation: A 17-year review of an effective approach to the management of the intra-abdominal testis. *J Urol* 154:558-561, 1995.)

orchiopexy, because successful positioning in the scrotum would require transection of the spermatic vessels. The surgical technique involved mobilization of the testicle, with a wide strip of peritoneum taken with the vas deferens. The testicle was brought out through a scrotal incision and secured in the dartos pouch. Microvascular anastomosis was used to maximize testicular blood supply, using the inferior epigastric vessels.

Results.—All patients had a minimum follow-up of 1 year. The median operative time was 4.25 hours, with 40–90 minutes required for vascular anastomoses. A palpable intrascrotal testicle was achieved in all but 1 of the 24 testicular autotransplantations evaluated at follow-up. Venous engorgement resulted in atrophy in 1 case, but the testicle was stable in size, shape, and consistency in the remaining cases (Table 1). In 3 cases, a previous contralateral Fowler-Stephens procedure had failed. Puberty has been or is being completed successfully in those patients who are old enough.

Discussion.—These results, together with those of other series, suggest that testicular autotransplantation is the most successful orchiopexy technique for the management of a high undescended testicle (Table 2). With improvements in instrumentation, the procedure can be performed in patients as young as 1 year. The authors recommend that all patients with bilateral undescended testes have at least 1 testis treated by microvascular transfer to optimize future gonadal function (Figure).

▶ These investigators obviously believe that the hormonal value of a viable testicle far outweighs the risk of malignancy. They also believe that efforts directed at saving potentially healthy tissue are well worthwhile. This report is an impressive summary of a long-term experience with a technically challenging surgical undertaking. Testicular autotransplantation, particularly in the young child, is a technical tour de force. In the 20 years since the first successful autotransplantation of an intra-abdominal testicle to the scrotum by microvascular techniques, few physicians have had the opportunity to gain a great deal of experience.[1] Even in a large center such as Cincinnati, the site of this report, only 1 child a year, on average, was operated on with this technique. It must be tough to maintain one's operative skills under such conditions.

This report still leaves a number of unanswered questions, not the least of which is whether it is worthwhile to undertake such heroic surgery for the intra-abdominal testis. The fertility potential of an intra-abdominal testis is much worse than that of a testis that has achieved a lower point of descent. In a recent commentary,[2] Snyder comments that "if there is a good contralateral testis in the scrotum, the intra-abdominal testis may be unworthy of orchiopexy and could be removed. In patients with bilateral descended testes, I think that it is important to recognize that infertility is likely to be a problem even after successful orchiopexy."

What to do with an intra-abdominal testis or even a high one that has not descended remains as controversial today as 2 decades ago when the potential option of microvascular surgery first became available. Sure, one would like to preserve hormonal function and possibly even fertility...but at what cost? Currently the cost minimally is a quite rigorous surgical procedure and a lifelong risk of malignancy, even in the surgically corrected testis. Is it worth it? It will probably take another 2 decades to find out.

References

1. Silber SJ, et al: *J Urol* 115:452, 1976.
2. Snyder HM: *J Urol* 154:562, 1995.

Breast-feeding and Inguinal Hernia
Pisacane A, de Luca U, Vaccaro F, et al (Università di Napoli, Italy; Ospedale Santobono, Naples, Italy)
J Pediatr 127:109–111, 1995   10–3

Introduction.—Inguinal hernias occur in about 15 per 1,000 live births and are characterized by the layers of the processus vaginalis failing to fuse normally during the last few weeks of gestation. Reduced secretion of human chorionic gonadotropin and changes in fetal testicular function have been associated with inguinal hernia. A gonadotropin-releasing hormone, contained in human milk, could play a role in the developmental physiology of the neonate. The association between infant feeding and inguinal hernia was investigated.

Methods.—One hundred children up to 12 months of age who were hospitalized because of inguinal hernia and 399 infant controls were included in the study, which evaluated whether they were breast-fed, the duration of breast-feeding, and whether they were exclusively breast-fed. Other information gathered included sex, type of birth, maternal education, number of other children in the household, and birth weight.

Results.—The group of children with inguinal hernias was breast-fed significantly less often than were the children who served as controls: 31% of patients were never breast-fed compared with 18% of controls. A significant dose-response risk reduction was associated with exclusive breast-feeding. Patients were exclusively breast-fed for a mean of 48.7 days, whereas controls were exclusively breast-fed for 94.8 days. Factors such as birth weight, type of birth, sex, number of children in the family, or maternal education did not affect the association.

Discussion.—A reduced risk of inguinal hernia in infants may be associated with breast-feeding. To support the hypothesis that human milk can promote closure of the inguinal canal, more data are needed.

▶ It's easy to accept the conclusions of a report that reinforces one's prejudices. The prejudice here is a strong bias toward the merits of breast-feeding. Recognizing that this editor is biased in this manner, let it be said that the prevention of inguinal hernias is the 163rd reason to breast-feed.

Having read this abstract, you're probably concerned that although the report sounds good, it has no scientific basis in theory. Not so. In most term infants, the inguinal canal is still open, closing only during the first few months after birth. The factors that favor its closure are not entirely known. Human milk contains several hormones, some of which might stimulate neonatal testicular function and accelerate the descent of the testes and the closure of the inguinal canal.[1] One of these hormones could be gonadotropin-releasing hormone.[2]

There isn't a parent in the world who would not want to prevent the onset of diabetes in his or her child. Very few parents would want their child to have a hernia if it could be avoided. Both conditions occur with higher frequency in bottle-fed babies. Discuss these points with new parents so that they don't discount the value of breast-feeding at a time when there is a flurry of direct advertising of formulas to the public.

References

1. Koldobsky O, et al: *J Pediatr Gastroenterol Nutr* 6:172, 1987.
2. Palmon A, et al: *Proc Natl Acad Sci U S A* 91:4994, 1994.

Acute Scrotal Symptoms Due to Perforated Appendix in Children: Case Report and Review of Literature

Friedman SC, Sheynkin YR (Maimonides Med Ctr, Brooklyn, NY)
Pediatr Emerg Care 11:181–182, 1995   10–4

Introduction.—Acute scrotal swelling and pain in a child with no previous urologic history is assumed to be torsion unless another cause is proven. Acute appendicitis is rarely considered in the differential diagnosis. However, a case is reported in which the patient had acute left scrotal swelling, which was secondary to a perforated appendix.

> *Case Report.*—Boy, 7 years, had a 2-day history of nausea, vomiting, and anorexia. Painful left scrotal swelling developed 5–6 hours before admission. His physical examination revealed no fever, normal bowel sounds, no hernia, a soft abdomen with mild tenderness in the left lower quadrant, and an absent cremasteric reflex. A presumptive diagnosis of left testicular torsion was made, and he was taken to the operating room where a herniated spermatic cord with pus in the processus vaginalis was discovered. Further investigation with laparotomy revealed a perforated appendix in the retrocecal and retroileal position, which was removed. The patient was given ampicillin, gentamicin, and metronidazole and discharged without complications on day 5.

Discussion.—It is likely to be difficult to differentiate between testicular torsion and the more rare scrotal swelling secondary to acute appendicitis in the emergency department. However, a patent processus vaginalis or pus found within a patent processus vaginalis, hernia sac, or tunica vaginalis should prompt laparotomy to identify the source of the inflammatory process, which may be intra-abdominal.

▶ The differential diagnosis of acute scrotal swelling in children rarely includes acute appendicitis. That is what makes this report important.

Scrotal swelling isn't the only urologic sign of acute appendicitis. Irritative and obstructive voiding problems, hematuria, pyuria, obstruction of the ureters, urinary retention, and fistulas between the appendix and the bladder have all been reported as complications of appendicitis.

Why the scrotum swells in some boys who have appendicitis isn't entirely clear, but it is most likely related to the presence of a patent processus vaginalis. Surgeons are well aware that if they find pus within a patent processus vaginalis at the time of exploration of a scrotum, they must perform an exploratory laparotomy.

The presence of perforated appendix and acute scrotal symptoms represent an unusual phenomenon, but it is not one to be forgotten.

Validity of G1-cells in the Differentiation Between Glomerular and Non-glomerular Haematuria in Children
Lettgen B, Wohlmuth A (Univ of Essen, Germany)
Pediatr Nephrol 9:435–437, 1995   10–5

Objective.—Microhematuria is a common finding in school-age children. The distinction between glomerular and nonglomerular hematuria is essential in avoiding unnecessary diagnostic procedures. The proportion of dysmorphic erythrocytes seen in the urine sediment by phase-contrast microscopy has been used to differentiate glomerular from other causes of hematuria. However, this interpretation is highly subjective and difficult to standardize. Whether counting G1-cells—a particular type of dysmorphic erythrocyte that appears to be specific for glomerular hematuria—is a reliable method of distinguishing between glomerular and nonglomerular hematuria was determined.

Methods.—Urine specimens from 100 children and adolescents with microhematuria or macrohematuria were studied by phase-contrast microscopy to determine the percentage of G1-cells. The clinical diagnosis of glomerular hematuria was made according to renal biopsy results, physical examination findings, laboratory test values, and family history.

Results.—The clinical diagnosis was glomerular hematuria in 51 patients (group 1) and nonglomerular hematuria in 49 patients (group 2). Patients in group 2 had various causes of hematuria including urinary tract infection, urolithiasis, hypercalciuria, and hematuria caused by urologic surgery or diagnostic procedures. The percentage of dysmorphic erythrocytes in this group was only 6%, compared with 42% in group 1. The percentage of G1-cells was 19% in group 1 vs. 0.6% in group 2. When the criterion of 30% or greater dysmorphic erythrocytes was used as the definition of glomerular hematuria, sensitivity was 71%, specificity 100%, and diagnostic efficiency 85%. When the criterion of 5% or more G1-cells was used, sensitivity, specificity, and efficiency all improved to 100%.

Conclusions.—Counting G1-cells by phase-contrast microscopy appears to be a valuable technique of differentiating between glomerular and nonglomerular hematuria in children and is more sensitive and efficient than determining the percentage of dysmorphic erythrocytes. The diagnostic rate is unaffected by the use of fresh urine samples without acidification and concentration. A 5% cutoff level of G1-cells is proposed for the differentiation of glomerular and nonglomerular hematuria.

▶ The search for the perfect tool to differentiate between glomerular and nonglomerular hematuria has been under way for years. The more we learn about ways to differentiate causes of blood in the urine, the more we learn that a simple look at the shape of urine red blood cells is as valuable a technique as any other.

Children who have blood in the urine are not a rarity. It has been estimated that between 0.5% and 4% of school-aged children will at one time or another have dipstick-positive urine for blood.[1] The causes of such hematuria range from totally benign entities to more serious ones such as stones, tumors, trauma, and importantly, serious glomerular diseases. Early differentiation between glomerular and nonglomerular hematuria is important to avoid unnecessary and invasive diagnostic procedures such as cystoscopy and radiologic evaluation of the urinary tract. It was Birch and Fairley who first differentiated glomerular hematuria from other causes of hematuria by determining the number of misshapen red blood cells in spun urine using a phase-contrast microscope.[2] Red blood cells that originate in damaged glomeruli exhibit a wide range of morphologic appearance. With nonglomerular hematuria, red cells are much more uniform in size. The problem with looking at these red blood cells is that the technique is somewhat subjective.

This report attempts to remove subjectivity by counting what are known as G1-cells, cells characterized by a donut shape with 1 or more blebs. The investigators found that when you define glomerular hematuria on the basis of greater than 5% G1-cells, the sensitivity and specificity of this simple technique are both 100%.

The only thing more eloquent than the technique described by Lettgen and Wohlmuth is the technique of actually sizing urine red blood cells the same way you size red blood cells in a routine complete blood cell count. With electronic counting equipment, you can actually get the equivalent of a red cell distribution width (RDW) of red blood cells in urine. Soon we will be seeing standards that will help us to easily distinguish between glomerular and nonglomerular red blood cells. A high RDW of urine red cells will indicate a glomerular origin of the hematuria, and a low RDW, a nonglomerular cause of the hematuria. How much simpler could it be?

While on the topic of red blood cells in the urine, please be aware of the problem characterized by the following fictitious case scenario: Your first patient of the day is a 5-year-old whom you treat for bilateral otitis media. He is sent home with a prescription of amoxicillin (250 mg/5mL, a 150-mL bottle dispensed). Late that afternoon, the mother calls you with the following story. She is concerned because she sees blood in the child's urine. She also confesses that the child downed half of the bottle of amoxicillin. There is no history of urinary frequency, pain, fever, edema, or trauma. The mother brings in the child and the bottle of amoxicillin. The latter has 75 mL left. The ingested amoxicillin dose is estimated at 120 mg/kg. The urine is bright red with a specific gravity of 1.020. The urine is dipstick positive for hemoglobin and protein. Microscopy shows many red blood cells. What is going on here? The child in this fictitious case scenario is very close in description to a real child described by Belko and colleagues.[3] Several children actually have been reported to have hematuria and renal failure after amoxicillin overdose. Any penicillin in high concentration can cause acute tubulointerstitial nephritis. Some children even have papillary necrosis develop. Death can result. The child in question did have mild renal failure but recovered fully.

References

1. Vehaskari VM, et al: *J Pediatr* 95:676, 1979.
2. Birch DF, et al: *Lancet* 2:845, 1979.
3. Belko J, et al: *Pediatr Infect Dis J* 14:917, 1995.

IgA Nephropathy: Long-term Prognosis for Pediatric Patients
Wyatt RJ, Kritchevsky SB, Woodford SY, et al (Univ of Tennessee, Memphis; LeBonheur Children's Med Ctr, Memphis, Tenn; Crippled Children's Found Research Ctr, Memphis, Tenn; et al)
J Pediatr 127:913–919, 1995
10–6

Introduction.—Immunoglobulin A nephropathy is the most common form of chronic glomerulonephritis seen in individuals of European or Asian descent. Few studies have followed affected children into the adult years.

Objective.—Clinical and renal histologic data were available for 103 patients in whom IgA nephropathy was diagnosed before 18 years of age, 40 of whom were followed for 10 years or longer after renal biopsy. The overall average follow-up interval was 8½ years.

Initial Status.—About three fourths of patients had macroscopic hematuria at the time symptoms began. Renal function was reduced at the outset in 13 patients. Sixteen percent of patients initially had microscopic hematuria and proteinuria.

Course.—Fourteen of the 103 patients have had end-stage renal disease (ESRD) develop, and 3 others have a glomerular filtration rate (GFR) less than 50 mL/min/1.73 m². Two of the 24 steroid-treated patients subsequently had ESRD. Progressive renal insufficiency and ESRD were asso-

TABLE 2.—Clinical Pattern at Onset of Symptoms for Patients Having 10 Years of Follow-up and Apparent Stable Renal Function as Compared to Those With Progressive Disease

	Stable function (n = 34) (%)	ESRD or progressive CRI (n = 17) (%)
Patients		
Male	74	71
Female	26	29
Race		
White	97	76
Black*	3	18
Native American	0	6
Hypertension	0	24
Biopsy grade†		
1	26	0
2	35	12
3	35	88
Proteinuria‡		
<1 gm 1.73 m²/24 hr	59	18
>1 gm <3 gm/1.73 m²/24 hr	38	47
>3 gm 1.73 m²/24 hr	3	35

* White vs. black race: *P* = 0.0371.
†*P* = 0.0013; 1 patient did not have biopsy-grade determination.
‡*P* = 0.0014.
Abbreviations: ESRD, end-stage renal disease; *CRI*, chronic renal insufficiency.
(Courtesy of Wyatt RJ, Kritchevsky SB, Woodford SY, et al: IgA nephropathy: Long-term prognosis for pediatric patients. *J Pediatr* 127:913–919, 1995.)

ciated with the severity of renal pathology and the degree of proteinuria (Table 2). No patient with stable renal function had transient reductions in GFR. The overall predicted kidney survival rate from the apparent onset of illness was 94% at 5 years, 87% at 10 years, and 70% at 20 years. The outcome could not be related to the age at clinical onset of disease or to gender, but black patients had a poorer outcome than whites.

Conclusion.—In general, the outcome of IgA nephropathy in children is similar to that in adults. Those with persistent clinical abnormalities should continue to be followed nephrologically in adult life.

▶ IgA nephropathy is not a good-news diagnosis, as we can see from this report. Although the majority of children who have this form of renal disease will do well, about 15% will progress to ESRD. Because IgA nephropathy is the most commonly occurring form of chronic nephritis in children of European or Asian descent and is the nephropathy associated with Henoch-Schönlein purpura, a fairly frequent problem in the pediatric population, this topic quickly becomes one of some importance.

There isn't much in the way of well-designed studies to tell us the best way to manage IgA nephropathy. Many pediatric nephrologists use steroids.[1] In adults with this problem, fish oil and high doses of intravenous immune globulin (IVIG) have been shown to have some efficacy.[2] Because no rigorously controlled pediatric trials have been done, no standard form of therapy can be recommended. Fortunately, the National Institutes of Health (NIH) is funding a collaborative study that may solve this problem soon.

For more on the topic of the long-term follow-up of renal function in IgA nephropathy, see the report of Berg.[3] He also shows that many children with IgA nephropathy do not have a benign clinical course. Boys with persistent proteinuria, in particular, manifest a significant decrease in renal function over time.

References

1. Waldo FB: *Am J Kidney Dis* 13:55, 1989.
2. Rostocker G, et al: *Ann Intern Med* 120:476, 1994.
3. Berg UD: *Arch Dis Child* 66:588, 1991.

Recombinant Human Growth Hormone in Infants and Young Children With Chronic Renal Insufficiency

Fine RN, for the Genentech Collaborative Study Group (State Univ of New York, Stony Brook; Genentech Inc, South San Francisco; Univ of Alabama, Birmingham)
Pediatr Nephrol 9:451–457, 1995   10–7

Objective.—Children with structural renal abnormalities resulting in chronic renal insufficiency (CRI) often are significantly growth retarded by age 2 years. A multicenter trial of recombinant human growth hormone (rhGH) enrolled 125 children with CRI, 30 of whom were less than 2½ years of age. A randomized, placebo-controlled design was used in which one third of patients were assigned to receive placebo and two thirds received rhGH.

Study Plan.—All children studied had irreversible renal insufficiency with a creatinine clearance between 5 and 75 mL/min per 1.73 m² of body surface. In addition, all participants had a height below the 3rd percentile for their chronological age and a bone age of less than 10 (girls) or 11 (boys) years. In the first 2 study years, 19 patients received rhGH subcutaneously in a daily dose of 0.05 mg/kg and 11 received placebo injections.

Results.—In all age groups, children given rhGH grew significantly more rapidly than placebo recipients. Both height and body weight gains were greater in actively treated patients. Muscle circumference measurements also indicated better growth in these children. The serum creatinine level increased by 0.9 mg/dL on average over 2 years in placebo recipients and by 0.5 mg/dL in children given rhGH. Adverse events were similarly frequent in the 2 groups of children.

Conclusion.—Young children with CRI may safely receive daily rhGH treatment, and can expect to grow significantly more rapidly as a result. Starting GH treatment before growth is severely limited will optimally stimulate growth before renal transplantation.

▶ Although there has been a surfeit of publications dealing with the use of GH in older children, this is the first study of any size that has examined its potential benefits in infants and very young children with renal failure. If you are caring for such a child, this report, in full length, should be on your reading list because it shows how important as well as possible it is to maintain adequate growth in affected children.

The impact of growth retardation caused by CRI is dramatic in infants and young children. In the first 2 years of life, the average normal child will grow 37 cm. Thus, it's understandable how CRI during infancy can impact one's final height later in life. Growth hormone–treated children with CRI were 5 cm longer at the end of the first year of treatment and an additional 2 cm longer after 2 years of treatment.

Should every infant and toddler with CRI receive GH? This query is not answered by this report. Clearly there are multiple factors that contribute to growth retardation in infants with renal failure, the most common of which is inadequate nutritional intake. Don't start GH therapy unless you are feeding adequate amounts of calories. Calories alone, however, will not do it.

There are potential negative consequences of GH treatment that should be thought about. Theoretically, GH treatment could have adverse effects on renal function because it increases the glomerular filtration rate; therefore, hyperfiltration might be produced, leading to glomerulosclerosis and a more rapid decrease in renal function. Fortunately, none of the children in this series had this problem, probably because their kidneys were "gone" to begin with. Other consequences of GH therapy did not occur. For example, none of the infants and toddlers had significant glucose intolerance or had osseous consequences, such as slipped capital femoral epiphysis or avascular necrosis of the femoral head.

Growth hormone therapy is expensive, but recognize that you are dealing with such small individuals that the amounts required are not exactly the same as would be required in a 10-year-old child. More importantly, you have only 1 shot at addressing short stature in these children. Strike while the iron is hot. To learn more about pediatric end-stage renal disease, its cause, and its management, see the superb review article from the United States Renal Disease Society.[1]

Reference

1. United States Renal Disease Society: *Am J Kidney Dis* 26:S112, 1995.

A Comparison of Amitriptyline, Vasopressin and Amitriptyline With Vasopressin in Nocturnal Enuresis

Burke JR, Mizusawa Y, Chan A, et al (Mater Misericordiae Children's Hosp, South Brisbane, Australia; Royal Children's Hosp, Queensland, Australia)
Pediatr Nephrol 9:438–440, 1995   10–8

Introduction.—Nocturnal enuresis can be managed nonpharmacologically, with motivated counseling, bladder stretching, self-hypnosis, or a conditioning alarm, or pharmacologically, with tricyclic antidepressants or desmopressin. The potential benefit of treating primary nocturnal enuresis with a combination of desmopressin and amitriptyline was compared with the benefit of treatment with each agent alone.

Methods.—A total of 45 patients, aged 6–17 years with primary nocturnal enuresis who had not been treated for enuresis during the preceding 6 months, were randomly assigned to treatment with either desmopressin, amitriptyline, or both in standardized doses. The frequency of wet nights was recorded during a 2-week run-in period with no medication, a 16-week treatment period, and a 12-week follow-up without medication. Fourteen consecutive dry nights were designated a cure, and more than 2 wet nights in 2 weeks were designated a relapse.

Results.—The mean wet nights per week decreased from 5.8 to 3.3 in the amitriptyline group, from 6 to 4.7 in the desmopressin group, and from 6.3 to 3.3 in the amitriptyline and desmopressin group. There were cures in 3 children in the amitriptyline group, 1 child in the desmopressin group, and 4 children in the amitriptyline and desmopressin group, but 7 of these 8 children relapsed during the follow-up. The efficacy of amitriptyline alone and of the combination of amitriptyline and desmopressin did not differ significantly. Treatment with amitriptyline alone or with amitriptyline and desmopressin was statistically superior to treatment with desmopressin alone at weeks 6, 8, and 10. There were no significant side effects to any of the treatment options.

Conclusions.—In the treatment of primary nocturnal enuresis, amitriptyline was more effective than desmopressin and there was no additional treatment benefit with combining amitriptyline and desmopressin.

▶ The reason for selecting this article was not to make a strong case for the use of pharmacologic agents over other treatments as part of the management of enuresis, but rather to show that sometimes more (in this case, a combination of treatments) is not better than less. Also, inclusion of this article should not lead one to believe that amitriptyline is the treatment of choice for enuresis. Treatment must be tailored. In most instances, the best treatment, and the one that will serve the patient well, is the use of a conditioning alarm. Conditioning alarms do have high initial cure rates (approaching 80%). The rub with conditioning alarms is a fairly high relapse rate after an initial response. What have been lacking in the literature are reports combining therapies such as desmopressin with a tricyclic drug or an enuretic alarm. The purpose of this report was to investigate the benefit of a combination of desmopressin and amitriptyline. The outcome was pretty straightforward. Amitriptyline alone is as effective as a combination of 2 pharmacologic approaches.

Enuresis would not be much of a problem were it not for its stigmatizing nature and that, even at 20 years of age, 1% of adults wet the bed. What is sorely needed is a basic understanding of why the Maker decided to equip humans with a voiding mechanism that doesn't fully mature in everyone. There must be a cause that we don't know about yet.

One last comment having to do with enuresis. Were you aware that children who are pyromaniacs have a much higher incidence of enuresis? They do![1] Psychologists are having a field day trying to figure out the link between fire setting and enuresis, particularly in boys, who have the equipment to put out brush fires.

Reference

1. Schleider K, et al: *Monatsschr Kinderheilkd* 140:277, 1992.

Fever Can Cause Pyuria in Children
Turner GM, Coulthard MG (Royal Victoria Infirmary, Newcastle upon Tyne, England)
BMJ 311:924, 1995   10–9

Introduction.—Pyuria often is considered a key factor in diagnosing urinary tract infection in children. It is not considered likely that pyuria will be found in febrile children who do not have urinary tract infection.

Objective.—The possibility that fever itself can promote pyuria in the absence of infection was examined in 157 children with a mean age of 2.7 years who were seen in a pediatric day unit. Seventy of them had a temperature of 38°C or higher. Moderate pyuria was defined as $10–100 \times 10^6$ leukocytes per liter of uncentrifuged midstream or bag-collected urine.

Findings.—Thirty of the 70 febrile children (43%) but only 6% of those without fever had moderate pyuria, a significant difference. Obvious pyuria of at least 100×10^6 leukocytes per liter occurred in 6 febrile children (9%) but in no afebrile child. A higher leukocyte excretion rate, not an increased concentration of urine, was responsible.

Implication.—True pyuria is not infrequent in febrile children even in the absence of urinary tract infection. Awareness of this possibility will avoid unneeded investigation and inappropriate antibiotic treatment.

▶ This editor was taught years ago that fever was capable of producing white blood cells in the urine. Unfortunately, this observation seemed to be based on anecdotes alone. Observations without foundations are often described as old wives' tales. Well, apparently tales can come true as this report provides testimony to. Moderate pyuria (10–100 white blood cells per L) occurs in 43% of febrile children. Obvious pyuria (more than 100 white blood cells per L) occurs in 9% of febrile children.

Why children with fever have white blood cells in their urine isn't clear from this report. Pyuria in such circumstances is not caused by the presence of a highly concentrated urine. This was ruled out. The suggestion is that pyuria results from a nonspecific feature of fever in acute childhood illnesses and reflects a generalized increase in white cell migration, perhaps mediated by changes in membrane permeability or white cell motility. Whatever the cause, the next time you see a child with a high fever and some white cells in the urine, don't automatically assume that the culprit is a urinary tract infection.

While on the topic of medical folklore, is cranberry juice useful in the management of urinary tract infections? Every medical student since 1914 has been taught that cranberry juice is useful in the management of patients with urinary tract infections.[1] Nonetheless, it wasn't until somewhat recently that it was unequivocally documented that elderly individuals who drank cranberry juice were 42% as likely to have organisms in the urine as were similar aged individuals who did not ingest this liquid.[2] As importantly, if an individual had a urinary tract infection in the previous month, the risk of having persistence of a urinary tract infection was reduced by 75% if one drank cranberry juice. Yes, cranberry juice does work. The assumption is that cranberry juice interferes with bacterial adhesion to the lining of the urinary tract because it is now documented that cranberry juice as an acidifier to prevent urinary tract infection really isn't much of an acidifier. One can slug down as much as 2 liters of the stuff a day, and it is still not likely that one will experience a decrease in urine pH. Overall, however, one must clearly say: "Ocean Spray, Über Alles."

References

1. Blatherwick NR: *Arch Intern Med* 14:409, 1914.
2. Arvon J, et al: *JAMA* 271:751, 1994.

Uroradiologic Evaluation of Children With Urinary Tract Infection: Are Both Ultrasonography and Renal Cortical Scintigraphy Necessary?
Sreenarasimhaiah V, Alon US (Univ of Missouri, Kansas City)
J Pediatr 127:373–377, 1995

10–10

Objective.—The results of 3 investigative methods were compared in a prospective masked study of children with a clinical diagnosis of acute pyelonephritis. Fifty children 2 months to 15 years of age were studied.

Methods.—All patients underwent renal scanning with technetium-99m–labeled glucoheptonate (GHS). All but 2 of them also underwent renal ultrasonography (RUS). Both studies were done within 2–4 days after admission to the hospital. Two patients had intravenous pyelography, and 49 patients had voiding cystourethrography (VCUG).

Findings.—The findings of GHS were abnormal in 79% of the 48 patients who also had RUS, and the latter study was abnormal in 42%. The 2 studies agreed on the status of 57 of 96 renal units, 21 of which were abnormal. The VCUG demonstrated vesicoureteral reflux (VUR) in 4 renal units that had normal findings on both GHS and RUS. Fifteen children in all had VUR. In 7 kidneys, only RUS was abnormal, usually demonstrating mild-to-moderate pelvic dilatation secondary to VUR. The combination of GHS and VCUG demonstrated abnormalities in all but 2 of 64 affected renal units.

Recommendation.—Renal ultrasonography has a number of advantages over renal scintigraphy, including its much lower cost, ready availability, and noninvasiveness. If GHS is to be part of the initial workup, it can be combined with VCUG and RUS left for use in a few selected patients.

▶ The day that ^{99m}Tc-labeled GHS renal scans (at $750 per study) become part of the routine evaluation of the kidneys of a child with a urinary tract infection, this editor's shingle is coming down in protest. It should be only on rare occasions that one would need to resort to this technology. Rare occasions mean rare. It is a great test, but it is one that can be spared from overuse by good clinical judgment and common sense.

To learn more about the pros and cons of renal scanning, see the commentary: "To DMSA or Not, That Is the Question."[1]

Reference

1. Sloves TL: *Pediatr Radiol* 25:546, 1995.

Urinary Tract Infections in Cocaine-exposed Infants

Gottbrath-Flaherty EK, Agrawal R, Thaker V, et al (Columbus–Cabrini Med Ctr, Chicago; Loyola Univ, Chicago; Univ of Chicago)
J Perinatol 15:203–207, 1995
10–11

Background.—Infants exposed to cocaine prenatally reportedly have an increased incidence of genitourinary tract abnormalities. Children with genitourinary tract anomalies have a greater incidence of urinary tract infections (UTIs). Thus the incidence of UTIs in cocaine-exposed infants was investigated.

Methods.—One hundred ten infants were prospectively studied. Urine was collected from infants ranging in age from birth to 40 weeks or at a mean age of 5 weeks. Ultrasonography was performed in 89 of these infants. Ninety-eight infants not exposed to cocaine who underwent urine culture for suspected sepsis served as a control group.

Findings.—Sixteen percent of the ultrasound examinations were abnormal. Of this group, 14% had positive urine culture results that met the criteria for UTI (Table 2). Only 4% of control infants had infections. This between-group difference was significant. Seventy-nine percent of the patients with abnormal ultrasound findings had negative urine cultures. In 85% of those with UTIs, ultrasound findings were normal (Table 3).

Conclusions.—Infants exposed prenatally to cocaine have a high incidence of UTI. Thus urine culture screening is indicated for these patients. Infants with positive urine culture findings should undergo further assessment, including renal ultrasonography, voiding cystourethrogram, and possibly a 2,3-dimercaptosuccinic acid renal scan.

▶ No one ever said cocaine was good for you. As far as infants are concerned, not only is it not good, but the "not good" can last a lifetime. As a result of cocaine use during pregnancy, women have a number of complications when they are pregnant, including poor weight gain, abruptio placentae, premature labor and delivery, and precipitous delivery. The infants can have intrauterine growth retardation, microcephaly, neurobehavioral and neurophysiologic abnormalities, and CNS hemorrhage. Cocaine-exposed infants have an increased risk of thrombosis. Their organs may be malformed. They may have prune-belly syndrome, pseudohermaphroditism, hydronephrosis, and ambiguous genitalia. The report abstracted confirms earlier stud-

TABLE 2.—Incidence of UTI in 110 Cocaine-exposed Infants

	Number with UTI*	%
Total	15/110	14
Male	8/15	53
Female	7/15	47

* Male/female ratio, 1.1:1.
Abbreviation: UTI, urinary tract infection.
(Courtesy of Gottbrath-Flaherty EK, Agrawal R, Thaker V, et al: Urinary tract infections in cocaine-exposed infants. *J Perinatol* 15:203–207, 1995.)

	TABLE 3.—Incidence of Abnormal Renal Ultrasounds in 110 Cocaine-exposed Infants		
Urinary tract infections		15/110	14%
Abnormal renal ultrasounds		14/89	16%
Urinary tract infections with abnormal ultrasound		1/13*	15%
Urinary tract infections with normal ultrasound		11/13*	85%
Abnormal ultrasound without urinary tract infections		11/14	79%

* Two infants with urinary tract infections did not have ultrasonography.
(Courtesy of Gottbrath-Flaherty EK, Agrawal R, Thaker V, et al: Urinary tract infections in cocaine-exposed infants. *J Perinatol* 15:203–207, 1995.)

ies, which suggest that mothers who use cocaine during pregnancy have a fivefold higher risk of having an infant with a urinary tract abnormality.[1] In addition, we now learn that cocaine-exposed infants have a higher risk of UTIs, regardless of whether they have urinary tract anomalies. Where will all this end?

Why infants of cocaine-abusing mothers have UTIs is not known. The suspicion is that cocaine interferes with normal peristalsis, causing poor urinary tract emptying; this leads to urinary stasis, resulting in UTIs. Because there is little correlation between the frequency of UTI and anatomical abnormalities, this concept of poor clearance function leading to UTI seems to make sense.

Does every infant whose mother is an addict require abdominal ultrasonography? Probably not, even though a high frequency of anomalies will be found. What does seem reasonable, however, is to screen such infants at some point in early life for a UTI. One infant in 7 will be found to have a treatable problem. This is a frequency high enough to merit concern, screening, and treatment.

Infants with UTIs demonstrate once again how the ills of our society roll downhill to our youth. How do we get our children properly aligned in the food chain?

Reference

1. Chasnoff IJ, et al: *Teratology* 37:201, 1988.

Urinary Tract Infections and Cholelithiasis in Early Childhood

Hes FJ, de Jong TPVM, Bax NMA, et al (Wilhelmina Children's Hosp, Utrecht, The Netherlands)
J Pediatr Gastroenterol Nutr 21:319–321, 1995   10–12

Introduction.—The incidence of cholelithiasis in childhood is increasing, usually associated with hemolysis, ileal resection, total parenteral nutrition, or hereditary susceptibility. Seven cases have been reported in which cholelithiasis was associated with urinary tract infections (UTIs). Three more infants with recurrent UTIs in whom gallstones developed were described.

Case 1.—Boy, 1 month, had right-sided reflux nephropathy after a UTI. At the age of 1.5 years, he was evaluated for recurrent UTIs. Abdominal ultrasonography revealed a gallstone, which had not been evident on an ultrasonogram at the age of 1 year. At 2 years, he was again evaluated for monthly abdominal pain. His biochemistry values were normal except for slightly increased serum cholesterol, triglyceride, and bile salt levels. He had no family history of gallstones. Cholecystectomy confirmed the presence of a small stone in the cystic duct and a larger stone in the gallbladder.

Case 2.—Boy, 1 month, with pyelonephritis, severe dehydration, electrolyte abnormalities, and a tender abdomen had right-sided obstructive uropathy, which was surgically corrected at the age of 4 months. At 6 months, a follow-up IV pyelogram revealed some shadows, which were identified as gallstones with ultrasonography. These had not been visible on a previous ultrasonogram. He had no family history of gallstones, normal serum bilirubin and liver enzyme levels, and no parameters indicating hemolysis. Because he remained asymptomatic and had no further recurrent UTIs, no treatment was planned.

Case 3.—Girl, 9 months, received a diagnosis of UTI, complicated by left-sided pyelonephritis and urethral stenosis. She had refractory recurrent UTIs. At 4 years, abdominal ultrasonography revealed 2 mobile gallstones not detected at 9 months. When she was 5 years of age, she had pain after eating and occasional white stools. She had no family history of cholelithiasis and normal serum bilirubin, liver enzymes, and γ-glutamyltransferase levels. Two gallstones were found at cholecystectomy.

Conclusions.—These patients provide added evidence of the association between childhood cholelithiasis and recurrent UTIs. Therefore, children with recurrent UTIs should be monitored for the development of cholelithiasis, and children with gallstones should be examined for accompanying UTIs.

▶ Chances are, if you have cared for a child with gallstones, you immediately jumped to the conclusion that there was a high likelihood that that child had some sort of hemolytic process. Not necessarily so. Only about 20% of cases of cholelithiasis in children are secondary to hemolytic anemias.[1] Other things to search for include congenital anomalies of the biliary tree, the use of parenteral nutrition, prior ileal resection, significant dehydration, and a hereditary susceptibility. To this list must now be added UTIs. The 3 infants described in this study, when combined with previously reported cases, bring to a total of 10 the number of cases of combined cholelithiasis and UTIs.

You will have to judge whether 10 cases truly make a series as opposed to coincidence. A little math, however, shows that these cases must represent more than coincidence. If cholelithiasis and UTIs were independent phenomena, the frequency of the combination on a purely mathematical basis should be no more than one case in a million. The demographics of the population base that formed these 10 cases show that the incidence of cholelithiasis and UTI is 1 case in 30,000.

Why gallstones develop in children with UTIs is speculative at best. Two possible mechanisms could be considered. First, infection, as seen in gram-negative sepsis, could have a lithogenic effect on bile by decreasing the bile salt–independent flow.[2] Second, dehydration resulting from UTIs, a common development in infants, could cause the bile to become lithogenic.

The lesson to be learned from these case reports is straightforward. Unexplained abdominal pain in a child with a UTI should trigger a consideration of the possibility of gallstones. Secondly, if you happen to be performing an ultrasound of the kidney as part of the evaluation of a UTI, ask the ultrasonographer to look at the gallbladder as well. Assuming there is no extra charge, it's possible that every now and then you will make an interesting secondary diagnosis of gallstones. If the ultrasonographer is surprised at the finding, tell him or her that this is now the 11th case of a well-described association.

References

1. Friesen CA, et al: *Clin Pediatr* 28:294, 1989.
2. Zimmerman HJ, et al: *Gastroenterology* 77:362, 1979.

Effect of Circumcision on Incidence of Urinary Tract Infection in Preschool Boys

Craig JC, Knight JF, Sureshkumar P, et al (Royal Alexandra Hosp for Children, Sydney, Australia)
J Pediatr 128:23–27, 1996   10–13

Background.—Several different types of studies have suggested that the uncircumcised state is associated with an increased incidence of urinary tract infection (UTI). However, it is still not generally accepted that circumcision prevents UTI. The relationship between circumcision and UTI was examined in a case-control study of boys younger than 5 years of age.

Methods.—The study took place at a large, ambulatory pediatric service, from which both case and control subjects were drawn. The cases were 144 preschool-aged boys (median age, 6 months) with microbiologically proven and symptomatic UTI. They were compared with 742 control boys (median age, 21 months) without UTI. The proportion of circumcised boys was compared in the 2 groups, and the strength of the association between circumcision and UTI was expressed as an odds ratio. The potential confounding or modifying effects of age were examined as well.

Results.—Just 1% of the boys with UTI were circumcised, compared with 6% of the control boys. The calculated odds ratio was 0.21, with 95% confidence intervals of 0.06 to 0.76. Age had no apparent influence on circumcision's protective effect against UTI. Seventy-nine percent of UTI risk in the study sample was attributable to circumcision status.

Conclusions.—Preschool-aged boys who are circumcised are less likely to have symptomatic UTI than their circumcised peers. This is true at all ages from birth to 5 years.

▶ As time passes, the more we learn about the relationship between UTI and circumcision status, the clearer the relationship is—being uncircumcised puts you at risk for infection. Before this report, the added risk was felt to be mostly, if not exclusively, in boys younger than 1 year of age.[1] We learn from this study that infant boys are not the only boys at risk.

Australia is an ideal country in which to examine the pros and cons of the circumcised vs. uncircumcised state. In the land down under, only 1 boy in 5 is circumcised. That's enough, however, to look at risk ratios of things such as infection. Up to the age of 5, boys who are circumcised have one fifth the chance of developing a UTI, compared with their "intact" friends. In fact, 80% of the risk of a UTI in boys younger than age 5 in that country can be attributed to circumcision status.

Data such as these must be put into perspective. The data are not so dramatic as to make circumcision a public health cause célèbre. Although every study that has examined the relationship between circumcision status and UTI has found an increased risk of UTI in those who are uncircumcised, if you examine the data closely, you'll see that in order to prevent a single urinary tract infection in a boy, you have to circumcise 99 youngsters. To say this differently, no matter what your circumcision status, UTI is fairly uncommon in young boys. Given the fact that the complication rate of circumcision is reported to range from 0.2% to 5%, one can calculate that in a cohort of 100 boys circumcised to prevent 1 urinary tract infection, 0.2–5 boys will have complications of their circumcision, hopefully of a minor nature. Given the delicacy of the organ involved, minor, of course, is in the eye (or hand) of the beholder.

In the immortal words of Roseanne Roseanna Danna, "If it isn't one thing, it's another." If you get circumcised, you might have some complications. If you don't get circumcised, you run a risk of UTI. Given the lack of science in all of this, it's reasonable that decisions about circumcision probably will continue to be based on cultural perceptions rather than medical dogma.

For more on the topic of neonatal circumcision and the controversy that still surrounds it, see the review by Roberts.[2] Also, in the past year, we learned that all healthy males who are circumcised without any complications can be expected to void, and it is unnecessary to delay hospital discharge merely to make this observation.[3] The average time to first void after circumcision is a mean of 5.3 hours. There's a pearl.

References

1. Wiswell TE, et al: *Pediatrics* 83:1011, 1989.
2. Roberts JA: *South Med J* 89:167, 1996.
3. Perlmutter DF: *Pediatrics* 96:1111, 1995.

11 The Respiratory Tract

Infant Sleep Position Following New AAP Guidelines
Gibson E, Cullen JA, Spinner S, et al (Thomas Jefferson Univ, Philadelphia)
Pediatrics 96:69–72, 1995
11–1

Background.—Because the prone sleep position has been implicated as a risk factor for sudden infant death syndrome (SIDS), in 1992 the American Academy of Pediatrics (AAP) recommended that healthy term infants sleep on the side or back rather than in the prone position. The recommendation has not yet received support from integrated marketing and educational initiatives.

Objective.—How well pediatricians and the public are following the AAP recommendation was assessed by interviewing 737 parents of infants 1–6 months of age. They represented 97% of parents seen at 2 pediatric clinics and 2 private practices who were invited to participate.

Findings.—Initially, 25% of infants in the clinic group and 41% of practice infants were put to bed in the supine position or lying on the side. In the second 4-month period, the figures increased to 58.5% and 63%, respectively (Table 1). Parents often cited health professionals as having influenced the decision, but other family members and family tradition also were seen as influential in some cases. A majority of infants of all ages awoke in the same position in which they had been put to sleep (Figure).

Implications.—Health professionals should take a more active role in advocating that parents avoid placing their infants in the prone position to sleep. As more parents adopt this practice, it will be of interest to determine its effect on the rate of SIDS.

TABLE 1.—Percent of Infants Sleeping Supine or on Side

	Clinic	Practice	Total	*P* value
September-December 1993	29/115 (25.2%)	35/86 (40.7%)	64/301 (31.8%)	<.02
January-April 1994	268/458 (58.5%)	49/78 (62.8%)	317/536 (59.1%)	NS
P value	<.001	<.005	<.001	

Abbreviation: NS, not significant.
(Courtesy of Gibson E, Cullen JA, Spinner S, et al: Infant sleep position following new AAP guidelines. Reproduced by permission of *Pediatrics*, Vol 96, pp 69–72, Copyright 1995.)

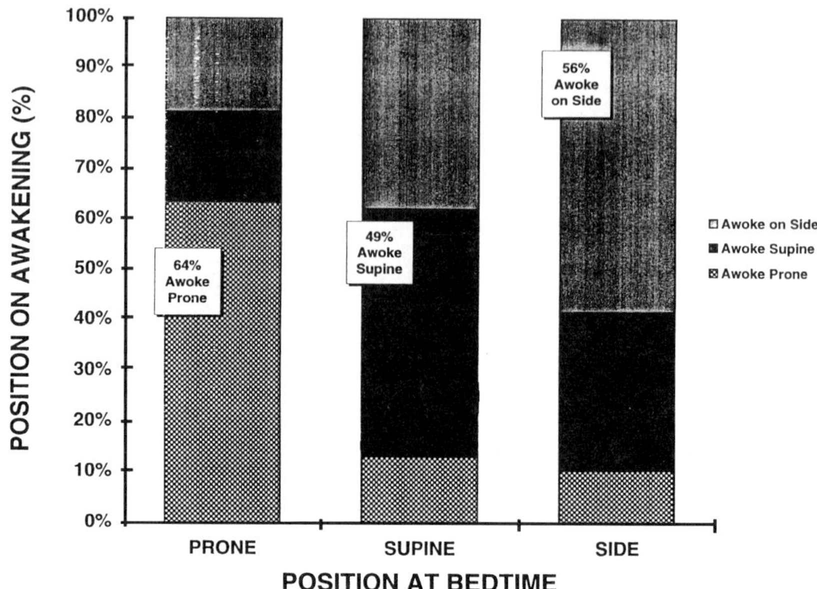

FIGURE.—Position at bedtime compared with position on awakening. (Courtesy of Gibson E, Cullen JA, Spinner S, et al: Infant sleep position following AAP guidelines. Reproduced by permission of *Pediatrics*, Vol 96, pp 69–72, Copyright 1995.)

▶ It was in 1992, after review of the international evidence by the National Institute of Child Health and Development, that the AAP recommended that healthy term infants be put to sleep on their side or back. This recommendation unleashed a firestorm of opinion about the relative merits of infant sleep positioning. Differences of opinion do exist about the applicability of international studies to the United States population and the physiology of prone vs. supine positioning. Questions have also been raised about the potential effect on the SIDS rate should the change to supine position become widespread. Although the Academy has recommended a change to supine position for infants' sleep, this recommendation has not yet been supported by integrated marketing or widespread educational efforts.

What we see from this report is that the percentage of infants sleeping on their side or supine has increased in the United States, but it has not reached the levels of 75% to 90% reported in other countries. By mid-1994, this percentage in the United States was about 60%.

The National Institute of Child Health and Development, with the support of the Surgeon General's office, has recently announced a "back to sleep" campaign aimed at changing infant sleep practices in the United States. Chances are that this campaign will be effective given the experience of other countries. This editor has had reservations about sleep positioning recommendations, as have others. These types of reservations can easily be changed if careful data are obtained, in a controlled fashion, to document what does what in terms of reducing the SIDS rate. Sometimes it's easy to focus on one thing, such as infant sleep position, when in fact many other variables are changing that might positively influence death rates from SIDS.

Skull Morphology Affected by Different Sleep Positions in Infancy

Huang C-S, Cheng H-C, Lin W-Y, et al (Natl Taiwan Univ, Taipei; Chang Gung Mem Hosp, Taipei, Taiwan)
Cleft Palate Craniofac J 32:413–419, 1995   11–2

Objective.—Although some observations have suggested that sleep positions can affect the shape of the head, there have been no studies documenting this relationship. Whether the skull can be deformed by sleep position was studied in infants with cleft lip and palate.

Methods.—Sleep position was determined for 81 infants aged 1 month with cleft lip and/or palate. Height, weight, head circumference, head width and length, and cephalic index were recorded at 1, 3, and 6 months. Growth changes between periods were compared between the supine and prone sleep groups and between the sexes.

Results.—A total of 27 infants were in the supine sleep group, 23 in the prone sleep group, and 19 in the mixed sleep group. There were 64 infants in the first observation, 70 in the second, and 66 in the third. No significant difference was noted between the heights at different ages. Body weight of the mixed sleep group was higher than the other 2 groups after 3 months and significantly higher than that of the supine group by 6 months. Head circumference increased similarly in all groups. Head width was wider, head length shorter, and cephalic index larger for the supine group. Head width was narrower, head length longer, and cephalic index smaller for the prone sleep group. The mixed sleep group fell in the middle of all measurements. All measurements for boys were significantly higher than for girls at 6 months.

Conclusion.—Regardless of sleeping position, the infant's head circumference will grow normally. The shape, however, will differ depending on sleeping position.

▶ An alarming story, actually an exposé on unnecessary neurosurgical procedures perfomed for craniosynostosis in infants who were put to sleep in the supine position, appeared in *USA Today* in February 1996. The mistake in diagnosis was an honest one in most cases. Consider such infants innocent bystanders in the rush to the supine sleep position. The explanation for this is provided by Huang et al., who have shown that infants placed in the supine position are more likely to develop brachycephaly, characterized by a short, broad cranium.

Please note that whether an infant is placed supine or prone, the head circumference will grow normally, although the shape will not be the same. One might think that as soon as an infant starts rolling over during sleep (at about 4 months of age), the skull would finally assume whatever shape it would otherwise have, regardless of early sleep positioning. Apparently not so, because data exist to show that older infants become accustomed to early sleep position.

All of these data are empowering to parents. Parents can now choose the shape of their infant's calvaria. Remember: prone equals a shape like a boat; supine equals a shape like a bowling ball.

Sleeping Position and Sudden Infant Death Syndrome in Norway 1967–91

Irgens LM, Markestad T, Baste V, et al (Univ of Bergen, Norway)
Arch Dis Child 72:478–482, 1995

11–3

Objective.—A population-based national study was undertaken in Norway covering the years 1967–1991 in an attempt to relate infant sleeping position to the rate of sudden infant death syndrome (SIDS). Since the early 1980s, SIDS has been routinely monitored in Norway.

Methods.—A single-page questionnaire regarding sleep position was sent to a random sample of 34,799 mothers who had given birth in one of the 20 largest maternity institutions in the country. Samples were collected

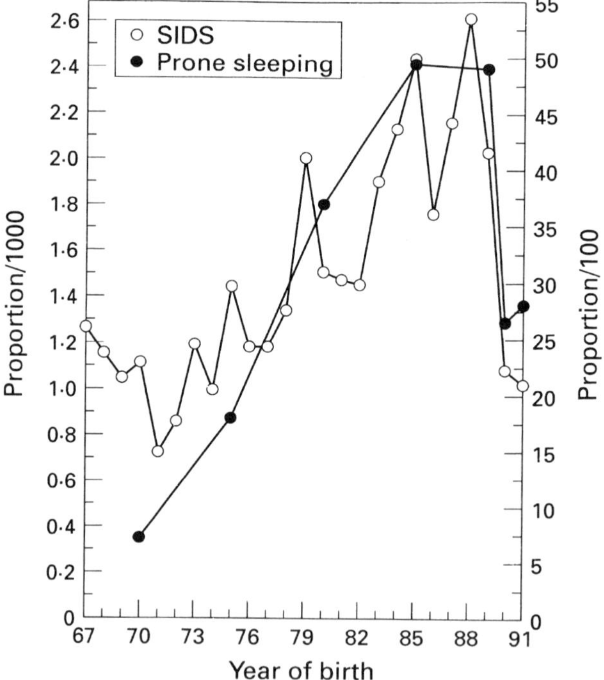

FIGURE 1.—Occurrence (proportion/100 infants) of sleeping in prone position at the age of 3 months and occurrence of sudden infant death syndrome (*SIDS*) (proportion/1,000 survivors of the perinatal period) by year of birth. Data obtained from the 20 largest maternity institutions in Norway, 1967–1991). (Courtesy of Irgens LM, Markestad T, Baste V, et al: Sleeping position and sudden infant death syndrome in Norway 1967–91. *Arch Dis Child* 72:478–482, 1995.)

at 5-year intervals starting in 1970. The response rate was 70%, and 92.5% of respondents claimed to be certain about their infant's sleep position at age 3 months.

Findings.—The proportion of infants who slept prone increased regularly from 1970 to 1989, peaking at 49%, and subsequently decreased to 28% in 1991 (Fig 1). The rate of SIDS increased from 1.1 cases per 1,000 infants in 1970 to 2.6 in 1988, and decreased to 1.1 per 1,000 in both 1990 and 1991. After adjusting for breast-feeding, maternal smoking during pregnancy, birth order, maternal age, and birth weight, the proportion of prone sleeping remained the only significant variable associated with SIDS.

Conclusion.—This and other studies are establishing sleeping in the prone position as a prominent risk factor for SIDS, but the mechanisms responsible remain to be clarified.

▶ The authors present another report on the relationship between SIDS and sleeping position. This study confirms the association between prone sleeping and SIDS, at least in Norway. Importantly, the authors are careful to state that an association does not necessarily represent a causal relationship. For example, one could speculate, as the authors do, that the association might be the effect of a brain stem lesion that causes both SIDS and, before death, a preference for prone sleeping. If this were the case, a reduction in the prone sleeping proportion of all infants would not necessarily reduce the SIDS rate in the population. However, it did appear that an abrupt reduction of prone sleeping in Norway was followed by an equally abrupt drop in the SIDS rate. The observations do suggest that the association represents a causal relationship of considerable interest from a preventive viewpoint.

Accumulating evidence from the United States and other parts of the world forces us to accept a relationship between prone sleeping and SIDS, even though common sense makes you wonder why this is so. The mechanisms involved are far from clarified, and many challenges exist to explain why a position that has been the preferred position of sleep by mothers for their infants from time immemorial is risky to certain infants. Although a fair percentage of pediatricians still ponder the issue of prone vs. supine, it does seem, at least for now, that supine is the way to go for term infants.

Vulnerability of Respiratory Control in Healthy Preterm Infants Placed Supine

Martin RJ, DiFiore JM, Korenke CB, et al (Case Western Reserve Univ, Cleveland, Ohio)
J Pediatr 127:609–614, 1995

11–4

A Dilemma.—In an effort to prevent sudden infant deaths, there is mounting pressure to avoid the prone sleeping position for all infants, even preterm infants without respiratory distress. Nevertheless, these infants are better oxygenated and less often apneic when maintained in the prone

TABLE.—Response of Ventilatory Measurements, End-Tidal P_{CO_2}, and O_2 Saturation to Hypercapnia

| | Active sleep | | | | Quiet sleep | | | |
| | Supine | | Prone | | Supine | | Prone | |
	Normo-capnia	Hyper-capnia	Normo-capnia	Hyper-capnia	Normo-capnia	Hyper-capnia	Normo-capnia	Hyper-capnia
Respiratory rate* (breaths/min)	64 ± 2	71 ± 3	56 ± 3	69 ± 2	56 ± 3	68 ± 3	53 ± 3	67 ± 3
Tidal volume ($ml \cdot kg^{-1}$)	6.9 ± 0.3	10.4 ± 0.6	7.0 ± 0.4	11.1 ± .06	6.0 ± 0.2	11.3 ± 0.6	6.2 ± 0.3	11.8 ± 0.7
Minute ventilation ($ml \cdot min^{-1} \cdot kg^{-1}$)	439 ± 29	745 ± 52	380 ± 26	767 ± 50	333 ± 21	781 ± 58	318 ± 16	790 ± 59
End-tidal P_{CO_2} (mm Hg)	40 ± 1	60 ± 1	41 ± 1	60 ± 1	41 ± 1	60 ± 1	41 ± 2	61 ± 1
O_2 saturation (%)†	96 ± 1	97 ± 1	97 ± 0	99 ± 0	97 ± 1	98 ± 1	98 ± 1	99 ± 0

*$P < 0.05$ for effect of position on respiratory rate across sleep states and levels of CO_2.
†$P < 0.01$ for effect of position on O_2 saturation across sleep states and levels of CO_2.
Abbreviations: P_{CO_2}, partial pressure of carbon dioxide; O_2, oxygen.
(Courtesy of Martin RJ, DiFiore JM, Korenke CB, et al: Vulnerability of respiratory control in healthy preterm infants placed supine. *J Pediatr* 127:609–614, 1995.)

position. Apnea in preterm infants has been ascribed to decreased central respiratory drive, which may be compounded by obstruction of the upper airway.

Objective and Methods.—Respiratory stability was assessed in 19 healthy premature infants by comparing the ventilatory response to hypercapnia in the supine and prone positions. The mean gestational age was 30 weeks, and the average postnatal age at the time of study was 5½ weeks. All infants were clinically stable at the time of the study. Nasal airflow was measured using a pneumotachygraph incorporated in a nasal mask. During sleep, infants were exposed to 5% carbon dioxide (CO_2) and 40% oxygen in nitrogen for at least 30 seconds.

Results.—Infants breathed faster while supine and had lower oxygen saturation values, regardless of the stage of sleep or the CO_2 level (Table). There was no significant positional difference in the response of minute ventilation to CO_2. Infants studied while supine exhibited more asynchrony of rib cage and abdominal motion independent of the sleep state or CO_2 level.

Implications.—Preterm infants who are placed supine may be at risk of respiratory instability. If still recovering from neonatal apnea, an impaired ventilatory response to CO_2 might aggravate the problem. It may therefore not be a good idea to always avoid prone positioning for healthy preterm infants.

▶ Confusion, confusion. Although we are seeing reductions in postneonatal mortality and sudden infant death rates in association with the change to sleeping in the supine position, now this report appears to suggest a disclaimer to this approach, at least for preterm infants. The recommendation for supine, as opposed to prone sleep position, does present a dilemma for neonatologists and pediatricians caring for healthy preterm infants, because preterm infants in the prone position have better oxygenation, less chest-wall asynchrony, and a lower incidence of apnea. Such apnea in preterm infants may persist for weeks, even delaying hospital discharge. The cause of the neonatal apnea is multifactorial, but apnea has been attributed to decreased central respiratory drive, often compounded by upper airway obstruction. Consistent with this hypothesis is the observation that preterm infants with apnea have attenuated ventilatory responses to carbon dioxide in comparison with age-matched preterm infants without apnea. An impaired ventilatory response to the increase in arterial partial pressure of carbon dioxide that invariably accompanies apneic episodes would delay resolution of apnea and increase its severity.

The American Academy of Pediatrics Task Force on Infant Sleeping Position and SIDS (sudden infant death syndrome) has stated that prone sleeping should not be recommended for premature infants with respiratory disease. Data are not yet available to indicate whether this recommendation for avoidance of sleeping position has affected the incidence of SIDS in former preterm infants.[1] The authors of the report abstracted caution us that respiratory control may be vulnerable in preterm infants placed in the supine position at a time when there is no longer clinical evidence of respiratory disease and they are being prepared for hospital discharge. Such infants are often still recovering from clinically significant neonatal apnea. An impaired ventilatory response to carbon dioxide would be expected to aggravate this problem. The authors recommend that widespread avoidance of the prone position may not be an appropriate recommendation for healthy preterm infants. Confusion, confusion.

Reference

1. American Academy of Pediatrics Task Force on Infant Sleeping Position and SIDS: *Pediatrics* 93:820, 1994.

A Reexamination of the Risk Factors for the Sudden Infant Death Syndrome

Taylor JA, Sanderson M (Univ of Washington, Seattle)
J Pediatr 126:887–891, 1995

11–5

Objective.—Although earlier studies linked sudden infant death syndrome (SIDS) with being born to young, poor mothers of minority races, later evidence refuted that link. From data in the 1988 National Maternal and Infant Health Survey, the prevalence of risk factors among infants who died of SIDS and infants who died of other causes was compared.

Methods.—The 1988 survey included 3 cohorts: 9,953 live births, 5,332 infants younger than 1 year who died, and 3,309 fetuses older than 28 weeks who died. Only the first 2 cohorts were included in this analysis. Risk factors for SIDS were defined as birth weight less than 2,500 g (low birth weight), birth weight less than 1,500 g (very low birth weight), black race, male sex, maternal smoking during pregnancy, gestational age less than 37 weeks, 5-minute Apgar score less than 7, maternal age younger than 20 years, more than 2 previous pregnancies, and maternal education of less than 12 years.

Results.—There were 649 deaths resulting from SIDS and 1,221 deaths from other causes out of a final sample size of 11,734 infants. The odds ratios were significantly greater than 1 for the SIDS cohort as compared with the live birth cohort for all risk factors other than a 5-minute Apgar score less than 7. The odds ratios were also significantly greater than 1 for infants dying of other causes as compared with the live birth cohort for all risk factors except male sex. When the 2 infant death cohorts were compared, infants who died of SIDS were significantly more likely to have mothers who smoked and who had less than 12 years of education (Table 2). After controlling for education level, only maternal smoking remained significantly more common in the SIDS cohort, giving a risk factor of 30%.

Conclusion.—After comparing the generally accepted risk factors for SIDS, only maternal smoking was significantly associated with an increased risk of SIDS as high as 30%.

TABLE 2.—Odds Ratios Comparing Sudden Infant Death Syndrome (SIDS) Deaths With Non-SIDS Postneonatal Deaths

Characteristic	OR	95% CI
Black race	0.98	0.81–1.19
VLBW	0.25	0.18–0.34
LBW	0.32	0.25–0.40
Prematurity	0.52	0.39–0.65
Perinatal asphyxia	0.10	0.06–0.18
Male gender	1.22	0.98–1.52
High parity	1.07	0.86–1.33
Young maternal age	1.23	0.96–1.59
Low maternal education level	1.30	1.05–1.61
Maternal smoking during pregnancy	2.03	1.64–2.52
Multiple births	0.98	0.61–1.57

Abbreviations: VLBW, very low birth weight; *LBW*, low birth weight.
(Courtesy of Taylor JA, Sanderson M: A reexamination of the risk factors for the sudden infant death syndrome. *J Pediatr* 126:887–891, 1995.)

▶ What a powerful study, assuming the results hold up. Data from this nationally representative sample indicate that if women refrain from smoking while pregnant, up to 30% of SIDS cases might be prevented. Elimination of maternal smoking would have a far greater impact than the presumed putative effects of sleep positioning (prone vs. supine). This report debunks the perception that the majority of SIDS deaths are the result of prenatal or perinatal events or are caused by problems associated with less than advantageous social situations.

This is not the first study to show a relationship between maternal cigarette smoking during pregnancy and SIDS. Bergman et al.[1] identified maternal tobacco use as a risk factor for SIDS 20 years ago. Other researchers have corroborated this finding. Because maternal smoking during pregnancy was the only characteristic significantly more prevalent in the SIDS group than in infants dying of other causes suggests that prenatal tobacco exposure has a more direct relationship than other risk factors to SIDS. This is intriguing because Kinny et al.[2] found that prenatal exposure to nicotine might diminish an infant's arousal mechanisms; this might also explain some of the increased risk of SIDS associated with the prone sleep position. Some smart investigator should try to tease out whether the prone position alone or the prone position in association with maternal smoking is the true culprit explaining a large percentage of infants with SIDS.

This report represents reason number 891 to stop smoking. Perhaps Congress will create reason number 892 by allowing the Food and Drug Administration to declare nicotine a drug.

References

1. Bergman AB, et al: *Pediatrics* 58:665, 1976.
2. Kinny HC, et al: *Neuroscience* 55:1127, 1993.

Infant Room-sharing and Prone Sleep Position in Sudden Infant Death Syndrome

Scragg RKR, for the New Zealand Cot Death Study Group (Univ of Auckland, New Zealand)
Lancet 347:7–12, 1996

11–6

Background.—Evidence suggests that infants of ethnic groups in which parents generally share a bedroom with the baby have a lower risk of sudden death. The hypothesis that the presence of other family members in the infant's sleeping room is related to the risk of sudden infant death syndrome (SIDS) was tested.

Methods.—Seventy-eight percent of all births between 1987 and 1990 in New Zealand were included in the case-control study. The parents of 393 infants dying of SIDS between 28 days and 1 year of age were interviewed, along with the parents of 1,592 healthy infants.

Findings.—Compared with infants not sharing a room with 1 or more adults in the previous 2 weeks, those who did share a room had a relative risk of SIDS of 0.19, after controlling for confounders (Table 3). The relative risk among those sharing a room in the last sleep was 0.27. The relative risk of SIDS was unaffected by sharing a room with 1 or more children. A significant interaction was noted between not sharing a room with an adult and prone sleep position in the last sleep. Compared with infants sharing a room with an adult and not prone, infants not sharing a room and prone had a multivariate relative risk of 16.99; those sharing a room and prone, 3.28; and those not sharing a room and not prone, 2.60.

Conclusion.—These findings need to be confirmed by others before public health recommendations can be made. Until such confirmation, physicians should advise parents to share their room with their infant at night for at least the first 6 months, the age of greatest risk of SIDS. The interaction between room-sharing and prone sleep position suggests a common mechanism for both factors.

▶ This is not the first report to suggest that solitary sleeping may be a contributory factor to SIDS. Solitary sleeping, after all, is a fairly recent innovation in the evolution of Western societies. For example, Bangladeshi infants have a low risk of SIDS, but they typically sleep in the same room as their parents and siblings, as has been true for centuries.

The report abstracted here seems to clearly show that infants who share their sleeping room at night with 1 or more adults have a lower risk of SIDS in comparison with infants who do not share their sleeping quarters. These results have public health implications for populations with a high proportion of infants who do not share a room with an adult during sleep. If these data are to be believed, more than one quarter of infant sudden deaths could be prevented by new sleeping arrangements, although this proportion may now be lower given the fact that the prone sleeping postition is much less common.

TABLE 3.—Relative Risk of Sudden Infant Death Associated With Sharing a Room While Sleeping With an Adult or Child for Last Sleep

Person(s) sharing room	Maori and Pacific Islander infants				European infants				All ethnic groups			
	Number of:		Odds ratio (95% CI)		Number of:		Odds ratio (95% CI)		Number of:		Odds ratio (95% CI)	
	Cases	Controls	Univariate*	Multivariate†	Cases	Controls	Univariate*	Multivariate†	Cases	Controls	Adjusted for ethnic group*	Multivariate†
Adult												
Yes	128	289	0·61 (0·41–0·90)	0·24 (0·13–0·44)	37	458	0·34 (0·24–0·50)	0·23 (0·13–0·38)	165	747	0·44 (0·34–0·58)	0·26 (0·18–0·37)
No	69	140	1	1	153	669	1	1	222	809	1	1
Child												
Yes	84	108	2·06 (1·43–2·97)	2·55 (1·49–4·39)	27	153	1·06 (0·68–1·64)	0·76 (0·41–1·40)	111	261	1·56 (1·18–2·06)	1·39 (0·96–2·01)
No	113	319	1	1	162	968	1	1	275	1287	1	1
Adult/Child												
Yes/Yes	66	93	1·22 (0·73–2·02)	0·64 (0·31–1·28)	13	101	0·57 (0·31–1·04)	0·23 (0·10–0·50)	79	194	0·87 (0·59–1·27)	0·41 (0·26–0·64)
Yes/No	62	193	0·57 (0·35–0·93)	0·21 (0·11–0·42)	24	353	0·29 (0·18–0·46)	0·19 (0·11–0·35)	86	546	0·39 (0·28–0·54)	0·21 (0·14–0·33)
No/Yes	18	14	2·67 (1·16–6·12)	1·83 (0·60–5·64)	14	52	1·20 (0·65–2·24)	0·52 (0·22–1·22)	32	66	1·60 (0·98–2·62)	0·84 (0·45–1·58)
No/No	50	125	1	1	138	615	1	1	188	740	1	1

*Adjusted for time of day of last sleep.

† Adjusted for variables listed in Methods section of original article, plus room-sharing with an adult or child as appropriate.

(Courtesy of Scragg RKR, for the New Zealand Cot Death Study Group: Infant room-sharing and prone sleep position in sudden infant death syndrome. *Lancet* 347:7–12, Copyright by The Lancet Ltd., 1996.)

It is difficult to tell how well accepted this report will be. Parents in developed countries are generally advised that an infant should sleep in a room alone from an early age. The authors of this report clearly suggest that parents should be advised to sleep in the same room with their infant at night, at least until the child is 6 months old and past the highest risk of sudden infant death. For more on the topic of SIDS and room-sharing, see the editorial on this subject by Pharoah.[1]

One last comment: These data also explain one other important observation: the fact that Eskimos have such a low rate of sudden infant death syndrome. Room-sharing is sort of a necessity when you live in an igloo.

Reference

1. Pharoah P: *Lancet* 347:2, 1996.

Toxic Gas Generation From Plastic Mattresses and Sudden Infant Death Syndrome

Warnock DW, Delves HT, Campell CK, et al (Public Health Lab, Bristol, England; Southampton Gen Hosp, England; Univ of Southampton, England)
Lancet 346:1516–1520, 1995
11–7

Background.—Microbial generation of toxic gases from chemicals used as fire retardants in plastic cot mattress covers has been suggested as a cause of sudden infant death syndrome (SIDS). Apparently, the gases arsine, stibine, and phosphine were detected when polyvinyl chloride mattress covers used by infants dying of SIDS were incubated with silver nitrate and mercuric bromide test papers in petri dishes. These mattress covers were found to be contaminated with the fungus *Scopulariopsis brevicaulis*. However, there has not been enough evidence to support this hypothesis.

Methods.—Samples from 23 polyvinyl chloride mattresses used by infants who had died of SIDS were analyzed. They were incubated on malt agar plates until good microbial growth was obtained, and silver nitrate and mercuric chloride test papers were inserted. Color reactions were documented.

Findings.—The main organism recovered from all mattresses tested was not *S. brevicaulis*. Instead, a mix of common environmental *Bacillus* species was identified. Changes in test paper color were observed when bacterial growth was present. However, these reactions also occurred in control tests in which no mattress material was placed on the plates. In chemical and instrumental analyses of exposed test papers, the color reactions were not caused by deposits of antimony, arsenic, or phosphorus.

Conclusions.—Toxic gases from antimony, arsenic, and phosphorus do not appear to be a cause of SIDS. The plates containing bacterial growth showed more sulfur in test papers than those without such growth. Thus the test paper reactions were probably the result of sulfur-containing compound generation during bacterial growth on the agar medium.

▶ There are few more emotional topics than crib death. Currently, as many as 1 in 1,000 infants in this country die of SIDS. Parents of children who die of SIDS not only have to cope with grief, but also face guilt and recrimination when thinking that they might have been able to avoid the tragedy. Worse, they may face accusations from relatives and friends or even police investigation. The introduction of "back to sleep" campaigns for infants was followed by reductions in the incidence of SIDS in those countries that adopted the strategy of educating parents not to let their infants sleep prone. In some countries, the frequency of SIDS was cut in half.

Despite these types of improvements, the search continues for the underlying cause of SIDS. In 1989, rumblings began of a possible new cause of SIDS. A chemist, Barry Richardson, reported finding a fungus, *S. brevicaulis*, in the mattresses of SIDS cases.[1] The claim made was that incubation of infected materials generated toxic trihydride gases (stibine from antimony trioxide added as a fire retardant, phosphine from phosphate plasticizers, and arsine from the preservative 10,10'-oxybisphenoxyarsine or from arsenical impurities in antimony trioxide). In England, the Department of Health studied this problem, and in 1991 found no evidence that mattresses generated toxic gases. That might have been that except for some media coverage in 1994 by investigative reporters, which reopened the toxic-gas theory of SIDS. In Great Britain, this led to a panic over the relationship between SIDS and the mattresses infants were dying on. This also led to a fairly high-profile committee being set up in Great Britain that commissioned a study, the results of which are abstracted above. The study replaced hype with reality, demonstrating that there are no toxic gases emanating from infants' mattresses.

The British learned an expensive lesson that we have also learned in the United States: take an investigator with a pet theory and a crusading media and you have a bad pairing. The media does have a role in driving public opinion and reaction, but investigative reporters must be responsible and reasonable in their interpretations, especially in science reporting. Enthusiasm for a sensational story all too frequently overshadows cautious and careful reporting. Geraldo beware.

Reference

1. Richardson BA: *Lancet* 335:670, 1990.

Oxygen Desaturation of Selected Term Infants in Car Seats

Bass JL, Mehta KA (MetroWest Med Ctr, Framingham, Mass)
Pediatrics 96:288–290, 1995

Introduction.—Premature infants may be at risk of oxygen desaturation and/or apnea while positioned upright in car seats. This prompted the American Academy of Pediatrics to recommend a period of car seat monitoring before hospital discharge for infants born before 37 weeks' gestation. However, term infants with certain indications may also be at risk for oxygen desaturation or apnea. Car seat monitoring in selected term infants was evaluated.

Methods.—Twenty-eight term infants who were judged by their pediatrician to be at risk for oxygen desaturation or apnea were studied. The most common indication was low birth weight; others included genetic disorders or observed duskiness, apnea, or decreased transcutaneous oxygen desaturation in the nursery. Three infants had been discharged from the nursery and readmitted. All underwent 90 minutes of monitoring in an upright car seat, with observation for transcutaneous oxygen desaturation, apnea, or bradycardia.

Results.—A period of oxygen desaturation of less than 90% occurred in 8 (28.6%) of 28 monitored infants. Another 5 infants (18%) had borderline results, i.e., oxygen desaturation of 90% to 93% (Table 2). Monitoring yielded abnormal results in all 4 infants studied because of genetic syndromes. Two infants who were observed to be apneic by their parents after discharge from the nursery also had oxygen desaturation on monitoring. When 5 infants with borderline or abnormal results were retested in a supine-position car seat, 3 had normal results.

Conclusions.—Term infants with genetic syndromes, observed apnea, or other indications may be at risk for oxygen desaturation while in an upright car seat. Car seat monitoring before hospital discharge may be considered for such infants. Alternatively, supine-position car seats could be recommended for use during the early months of life unless medically contraindicated.

▶ It has been many years since the American Academy of Pediatrics recommended in 1974 that all infants riding in automobiles be placed in car

TABLE 2.—Car Seat Test Results: Full-term Infants

	N	Borderline tcSaO$_2$ (90-93%)		Abnormal tcSaO$_2$ (< 90%)	
		No.	%	No.	%
37 weeks	14	1	7.1	2	14.3%
> 37 weeks*	14	4	28.6	6	42.9%
Total ≥37 weeks	28	5	17.8	8	28.6%

Abbreviation: tcSaO$_2$, transcutaneous oxygen saturation.
*Includes 3 readmissions after discharge.
Source: MetroWest Medical Center, Framingham, Mass, March 1, 1992 to April 8, 1994.
(Courtesy of Bass JL, Mehta KA: Oxygen desaturation of selected term infants in car seats. Reproduced by permission from *Pediatrics*, Vol 96, pp 288–290, Copyright 1995.)

seats. The rub with this recommendation is that some infants are not saved, but rather are killed by their car seats. Preterm infants, in particular, are at such risk. This was first noted by Bull and Stroup in 1985 and a year later by Willet et al., who demonstrated that some premature infants are subject to periods of oxygen desaturation, occasionally associated with bradycardia, while upright in car seats.[1, 2] A study performed in 1992 by the same investigators of the report abstracted confirmed that 18% of preterm infants less than 37 weeks' gestation showed evidence of oxygen desaturation, bradycardia, or apnea when monitored in a car seat.[3]

The report abstracted extends these earlier findings to show that there may be a problem with some full-term infants when they are put into a car seat. Two groups in particular seem to be at risk: those with genetic disorders and those with a previously reported apneic event. Infants with genetic disorders would likely be at risk for car seat apnea because of hypotonia and other anatomical problems that might predispose to hypoventilation in the upright position. The Academy guidelines concerning transportation of children with special needs provide specific advice about proper positioning of children with disabilities.

If all the data about car seats are considered, some obvious conclusions can be drawn. Infants with genetic disorders, those with observed dusky or apneic spells and, less frequently, with respiratory symptoms, as well as all low-birth-weight infants should be considered at risk for oxygen desaturation in an upright car seat. Consideration should be given to monitoring these infants in their car seats before nursery discharge. Unfortunately, risk factors may not always be apparent at birth. Universal car seat screening of all full-term infants is impractical. The authors suggest that because supine-position car seats are readily available, perhaps all infants should be routinely transported in this position in the early months of life. This is a very controversial suggestion.

The bottom line is that no method of transportation is completely risk-free. Under no circumstances should parents be left with the impression that car seat use should be discouraged. The authors appropriately point out that despite reports of occasional oxygen desaturation in some infants, the car seat remains one of the most effective strategies available to protect infants from injury and death in the early years of life.

References

1. Bull MJ, Stroup KB: *Pediatrics* 75:336–339, 1985.
2. Willet LD, et al: *J Pediatr* 109:245–248, 1986.
3. Bass JL, et al: *Pediatrics* 91:1137–1141, 1993.

Sweat Chloride Concentrations in Infants Homozygous or Heterozygous for F_{508} Cystic Fibrosis

Farrell PM, Koscik RE (Univ of Wisconsin, Madison)
Pediatrics 97:524–528, 1996

11–9

Introduction.—Sweat testing for elevated chloride or sodium concentrations is a routine part of the diagnosis of cystic fibrosis (CF). However, there is little experience with sweat testing in infants younger than 2 months of age, and some studies have questioned whether sweat testing is a useful and reliable procedure in this age group. The ability to obtain an adequate sample of sweat and to evaluate sweat chloride levels in infants was examined in a 9-year experience.

Methods.—Pilocaparpine iontophoresis and measurement of sweat volume concentration were performed in 725 infants of known genotype. Most of the infants had screened positive for CF as newborns, based on immunoreactive trypsinogen testing. The subjects underwent DNA analysis for the 3 bp deletion at codon 508 of the CF transmembrane regulator gene (F508 mutation) whenever possible. Sweat tests were deemed successful if at least 50 mg of sweat was obtained.

Results.—Ninety-nine percent of infants had a successful sweat test, with no difference in the success rate for infants younger vs. older than 6 weeks. Normal subjects had a mean sweat chloride level of 10.6 ± 5.2 mEq/L. Patients with CF—whether they were F508 homozygotes, F508 compound heterozygotes, or had non-F508 mutations—had mean sweat chloride levels of about 100 mEq/L. Patients with cystic fibrosis who were F508 heterozygote carriers had a slight but significant elevation in sweat chloride concentrations compared with normals, with a mean value of 14.9 ± 8.4 mEq/L (Table 2).

Conclusion.—Sweat testing can be successfully performed in infants younger than 6 weeks who have positive newborn screening results for CF. However, the upper limit of normal for sweat chloride testing in infants

TABLE 2.—Infant Sweat Chloride Levels by Category of Infant Sweat Tested

Subjects (Genotype)	Age weeks	Sweat Chloride mEq/L	
	Mean (SD)	Mean (SD)	95% Confidence Interval
Normal (N/N) 184	9.3 (5.3)	10.6 (5.2)	9.9–11.3*
Normal (no gene data) 280	21.2 (13.1)	11.6 (5.3)	11.0–12.2
CF heterozygote carrier (N/F508) 128	8.8 (5.0)	14.9 (8.4)	13.4–16.4*
Infants with CF,(F508/F508) 61	10.5 (9.9)	100.0 (9.2)	97.6–102.4
Infants with CF, (cf/F508) 47	9.3 (9.3)	97.6 (15.3)	93.1–102.1
Infants with CF (cf/cf) 7	16.5 (17.3)	99.6 (14.1)	86.5–112.7

*Nonparametric 95% confidence intervals were 8.90–10.1 for the N/N group and 11.3–13.7 mEq/L for the N/F508 CF heterozygote carriers. The distributions of chloride values were skewed (not bimodal) in the 2 groups and were different ($P < 0.0001$) by the Wilcoxon rank sum text.

Abbreviations: N, normal DNA test revealing no F508 alleles; *CF*, cystic fibrosis; *F508*, 3-base pair deletion at codon 508 of the CF transmembrane regulator gene; *cf*, other CF transmembrane regulator mutation, i.e., mutant allele other than the F508 mutation.

(Courtesy of Farrell PM, Koscik RE: Sweat chloride concentrations in infants homozygous or heterozygous for F_{508} cystic fibrosis. Reprinted by permission of *Pediatrics*, Vol 97, pp 524–528, Copyright 1996.)

should be adjusted to 40 mEq/L, which is the mean value for CF heterozygotes plus 3 SD. Infants with sweat chloride levels of 40–60 mEq/L are likely to have CF and should be followed closely for the development of symptoms. Subclinical sweat chloride elevations, among other manifestations of CF, can be found in infants who are CF heterozygote carriers with 1 F508 mutant allele.

▶ This report is critically important for 3 reasons: It tells us that one can easily and readily do a sweat test on an infant less than 6 weeks of age; it shows us that carriers of CF do have quantitatively different sweat chlorides than truly normal individuals; and finally, it warns us that the upper limit of normal for sweat chloride should be revised downward from 60 mEq/L to 40 mEq/L. No longer can we accept the myth that sweat tests are unreliable in the very young infant.

What constitutes the upper limit of normal for sweat chloride has been a somewhat controversial issue over the years. Based on the data from this report, in infants who do not have CF and who are not carriers of CF, 30 mEq/L constitutes the mean + 2 SD and can be used as the upper limit of normal rather than the 60-mEq/L value traditionally used. The sticky wicket is the fact that a fair percentage of "normal" infants are CF carriers who may have chloride levels greater than 30 mEq/L. It was for this reason that the authors recommended that 40 mEq/L or greater be used to distinguish infants with CF, as this represents the mean + 3 SD–value for the group of CF carriers identified by DNA analysis.

For all practical purposes, during infancy, any sweat chloride value greater than 40 mEq/L has an extraordinarily low probability of being a true normal, assuming that the test was performed properly. Accordingly, if a young infant has a sweat chloride level between 40 and 60 mEq/L, a diagnosis of CF is quite likely and such infants should be followed as though they had CF. No one would question a sweat chloride level greater than 60 mEq/L, which is invariably diagnostic of CF. Using these parameters, one will not "overcall" a carrier as being a homozygous affected individual.

The old-fashioned sweat test has held up pretty well over the years. In case you have forgotten, it was in 1953 that di Sant'Agnese described sweat electrolyte disturbances associated with childhood pancreatic disease.[1] To learn more about carrier screening for CF, see the excellent review by Raeburn.[2] For a magnificent update on gene therapy for CF, see the review by Rosenfeld.[3]

References

1. di Sant'Agnese PA, et al: *Am J Med* 15:777, 1953.
2. Raeburn JA: *BMJ* 309:1428, 1994.
3. Rosenfeld MA, et al: *Chest* 109:241, 1996.

Correlation of Sweat Chloride Concentration With Classes of the Cystic Fibrosis Transmembrane Conductance Regulator Gene Mutations

Wilschanski M, Zielenski J, Markiewicz D, et al (Hosp for Sick Children, Toronto; Univ of Toronto)
J Pediatr 127:705–710, 1995

11–10

Introduction.—Mutations in the cystic fibrosis transmembrane conductance regulator (CFTR) gene have been shown to cause cystic fibrosis (CF). This gene encodes a protein that functions as a cyclic adenosine monophosphate (cAMP)–regulated chloride channel, which causes aberrant chloride conductance across the apical membrane of epithelial cells. The different types of mutations have been classified by the functional properties of the encoded gene product, which can prevent the formation of the intact CFTR protein product (class I), fail to reach the apical membrane (class II), reach the apical cell membrane but does not respond to stimulation by cAMP (class III), have changed channel properties that reduce the current (class IV), or reduce the synthesis or processing of normal CFTR (class V) (Figure). Possible differences in epithelial chloride conductance were investigated by studying chloride concentrations in the sweat of patients with the different classifications of mutations.

Methods.—Sweat chloride concentrations were measured in 455 patients with CF. The patients were grouped according to the molecular consequences of their CF mutations, and the sweat chloride data were compared among the functional classes.

Results.—The sweat chloride concentrations did not differ significantly in patients with functional class I, II, III, or V mutations (Table). However,

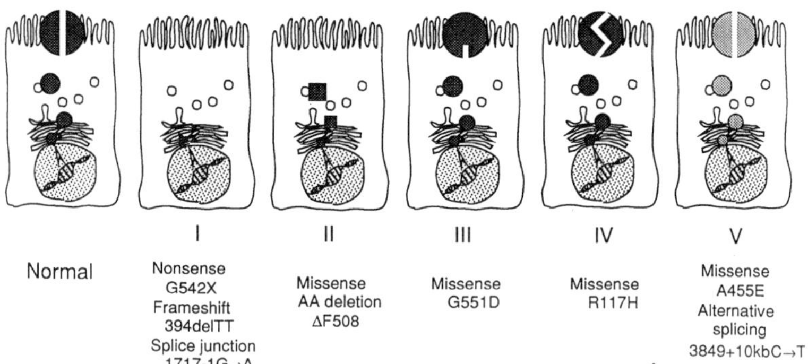

FIGURE—Molecular consequences of cystic fibrosis transmembrane conductance regulator (*CFTR*) mutations. **Normal,** CFTR correctly positioned at apical membrane of an epithelial cell, functioning as a chloride channel. **Class I,** no CFTR messenger RNA or no CFTR protein formed (e.g., nonsense, frameshift, or splice site mutation). **Class II,** trafficking defect. The CFTR mRNA formed, but protein fails to traffic to cell membrane. **Class III,** regulation defect. The CFTR reaches cell membrane but fails to respond to cyclic adenosine monophosphate stimulation. **Class IV,** channel defect. CFTR functions as altered chloride channel, **Class V,** synthesis defect. Reduced synthesis or defective processing of normal CFTR. Chloride channel properties are normal. (Courtesy of Wilschanski M, Zielenski J, Markiewicz D, et al: Correlation of sweat chloride concentration with classes of the cystic fibrosis transmembrane conductance regulator gene mutations. *J Pediatr* 127:705–710, 1995.)

TABLE.—Age and Sweat Chloride Values of 455 Patients With Cystic Fibrosis Classified by Genotypic Group and Function

Genotype group	Functional class	n	Age at diagnosis (yr)	Sweat chloride (mmol/L)
ΔF508/ΔF508	II	294	2.4 ± 4.5	104 ± 17
ΔF508/nonsense	I	41	3.6 ± 7.4	105 ± 17
ΔF508/frameshift	I	24	3.1 ± 5.3	111 ± 13
ΔF508/splice	I	20	3.6 ± 7.0	92 ± 16*
ΔF508/missense	III	48	3.7 ± 5.3	108 ± 22
ΔF508/missense	IV	17	6.2 ± 6.7*	95 ± 20*
ΔF508/reduced synthesis	V	11	9.8 ± 8.3*	101 ± 23

Note: Values for age at diagnosis and sweat chloride concentration are expressed as mean ± SD.
*Significant difference in comparison with ΔF508/ΔF508 ($P < 0.05$).
(Courtesy of Wilschanski M, Zielenski J, Markiewicz D, et al: Correlation of sweat chloride concentration with classes of the cystic fibrosis transmembrane conductance regulator gene mutations. *J Pediatr* 127:705–710, 1995.)

the patients with class IV mutations had a significantly lower mean sweat chloride level. However, among the patients with the class I mutations, those with the ΔF508/splice junction mutation had significantly lower sweat chloride values than did those with the ΔF508/stop or frameshift mutations.

Discussion.—Mutations that fail to produce a complete CFTR protein, produce a CFTR protein that does not reach the apical membrane, or produce a protein that does not respond to cAMP stimulation result in similar chloride conductance. However, if the mutated protein reaches the apical membrane, the chloride channel may be responsive to appropriate agonists. Therefore, determination of functional classes of CFTR mutations can illuminate the relationship between the genotype and phenotype.

▶ The list of gene defects that can present as CF continues to grow. Cystic fibrosis is caused by mutations in the CFTR gene, which encodes a protein of 1,480 amino acid residues. Approximately 70% of chromosomes affected in CF harbor a 3 base-pair deletion, resulting in the loss of a phenylalanine residue at position 508 (ΔF508).

It's been known for some time that there is a rough correlation between the type of gene mutation a child with CF has and whether that child is more or less likely to have pancreatic insufficiency. Also, there has been a rough correlation between sweat chloride values and the presence or absence of pancreatic insufficiency. Specifically, sweat chloride values are significantly lower for patients whose pancreas works as opposed to those with pancreatic insufficiency. The study abstracted helps pull some of this together. It appears that those with ΔF508 mutations are much more likely to have pancreatic insufficiency and higher sweat chloride values. There are other mutations that produce significantly lower, intermediate sweat chloride values. It is also possible to see normal sweat chloride values in certain genotypes of CF.

So what do we learn from all this? We learn that the most common CF mutation (ΔF508) remains a bad actor. Most patients with it will have pancreatic insufficiency and the highest sweat chloride values seen among patients with CF. Some children, however, are affected with milder variants, and it is important to know this because on the horizon there will be pharmacologic agents designed to stimulate chloride channel activity. Theoretically, these agents would work best in those patients who have the lowest values for sweat chlorides (the class IV mutations in this report).

Recent reports have clearly shown that normal sweat chloride values, even in those as low as 16 mmol/L, do not absolutely rule out the diagnosis of CF.[1, 2] In the case of a patient with a constellation of signs and symptoms suggestive of CF, but in whom the results of sweat testing are not clearly positive, no known CF mutations can be identified, and electrophysiologic testing is not practical, making a definitive diagnosis remains troublesome for us as clinicians. Such individuals may very well warrant mutation analysis despite their normal sweat chloride test.

It's important for all of us to keep track of the evolving saga that links the gene mutation of CF with its clinical expression. Clearly, CF is not 1 disease anymore; therefore, therapies tailored to specific subsets of the disorder may well be the wave of the future.

References

1. Highsmith WE, et al: *N Engl J Med* 331:974, 1994.
2. Stewart B, et al: *Am J Respir Crit Care Med* 151:899, 1995.

Neonatal Screening for Cystic Fibrosis: A Comparison of Two Strategies for Case Detection in 1.2 Million Babies
Wilcken B, Wiley V, Sherry G, et al (Royal Alexandra Hosp for Children, Sydney, Australia)
J Pediatr 127:965–970, 1995   11–11

Objective.—Two neonatal screening protocols for cystic fibrosis (CF) were used to assess more than 1.2 million infants in New South Wales, Australia, during a 13½-year period. Compliance with screening during this period exceeded 99%.

Methods.—Initially immunoreactive trypsin (IRT) was measured in dried blood spots, and a second sample was acquired from infants whose test results were positive. Since 1993, a positive IRT result was followed by direct gene analysis of the same sample to detect the common CF mutation ΔF508.

Results.—Of 1,015,000 infants tested by IRT alone, 389 had CF. A clinical diagnosis was made after negative screening (or an administrative error) in 30 instances. An early diagnosis was achieved in 92% of cases. All but 3 of 62 infants with CF were positive on IRT/DNA screening (Table 1). Forty-four of these infants were homozygous for ΔF508. Two of the 3 infants lacking a copy of the mutation received a diagnosis of CF early

TABLE 1.—Results of Neonatal Screening for CF, for Both Protocols

Protocol	IRT/IRT	IRT/DNA
Babies screened	1,015,000	189,000
Total CF cases known	389	62
Total high risk	117	9
Meconium ileus	80*	8
Sibling of known patients	47*	1
Unexpected cases	272	53
Detected by test	242	52
Not detected	30	1†
Babies receiving early diagnosis (%)	92	98
False-positive result		
First sample	6,984 (0.69%)	102‡ (0.054%)
Second sample	335‡ (0.033%)	NS

*Ten infants were in both high-risk categories.
†Three infants had a negative DNA test result: 2 of these were at high risk, with meconium ileus.
‡ Infants who required sweat tests but did not have CF.
Abbreviations: CF, cystic fibrosis; *IRT*, immunoreactive trypsin.
(Courtesy of Wilcken B, Wiley V, Sherry G, et al: Neonatal screening for cystic fibrosis: A comparison of two strategies for case detection in 1.2 million babies. *J Pediatr* 127:965–970, 1995.)

because they had meconium ileus. The false positive rate was 0.7% with IRT alone and 0.05% with IRT/DNA testing.

Implications.—Early experience with combined IRT/DNA screening for CF indicates that it is more efficient than IRT testing alone and that it provides equal or better early detection at minimal added cost. A small number of heterozygotes will be detected, but this is more than compensated for by fewer families being confronted with false positive test results.

▶ Another report dealing with screening for CF DNA mutations, this one combined with enzyme analysis. The search continues for the perfect screening and diagnostic newborn test for CF. It's been almost 20 years now since we heard about neonatal blood-spot screening with IRT assays. In case you've forgotten, a very high percentage of children with CF will have elevations in their IRT blood levels as a consequence of bile sludging. The problem with this way of approaching CF from a screening test point of view is that many kids without CF are detected (low specificity). What this report attempts to do is to combine neonatal enzyme screening together with DNA mutation analysis. More specifically, if the enzyme screen is positive, an immediate ΔF508 DNA assay is performed.

A word of warning. Not all children with CF have enough gastrointestinal involvement to raise their IRT levels. Also, as we all know by now, the ΔF508 mutation does not account for all patients with CF either. However, putting the two together does yield a reasonably sensitive and highly specific way to screen newborns for CF.

Cost Effectiveness of Antenatal Screening for Cystic Fibrosis

Cuckle HS, Richardson GA, Sheldon TA, et al (Univ of Leeds, England; Univ of York, England)
BMJ 311:1460–1464, 1995   11–12

Background.—Cystic fibrosis is the most common recessive condition in the United Kingdom. The carrier frequency appears to be as high as 1 in 25. The discovery of the principal genetic mutations involved in cystic fibrosis has made antenatal screening possible. An important consideration before such screening can be introduced into routine practice is its cost-effectiveness. The cost efficacy of different cystic fibrosis antenatal screening programs was compared.

Methods.—The screening process includes 4 components: information giving, DNA testing, genetic counseling, and prenatal diagnosis. Component costs were estimated using data from the literature and a pilot screening study. The cost of a screening program was then determined by summing up the components according to the specific screening strategy, the proportion of carriers detected by DNA testing, and the uptake of screening. It was assumed that 20% of the patients would have missing information on carrier status from previous pregnancies, that 20% would have changed partners between pregnancies, and that the rate of uptake of prenatal diagnosis would be 100%.

Findings.—Sequential screening was estimated to cost between £40,000 and £90,000 per affected pregnancy identified, depending on carrier detection rate and uptake. The cost of couple screening ranged from £46,000 to £104,000. A 10% change in the assumed proportion with missing information from a previous pregnancy resulted in a £4,000 change in cost. A 10% change in the proportion with new partners also had this effect, but only for couple screening. Screening costs would change directly in proportion to the uptake of prenatal diagnosis (Figure).

Conclusions.—The cost of cystic fibrosis screening is only somewhat higher than that of other established screenings, such as that for Down's syndrome. Thus there are no economic barriers to introducing cystic fibrosis screening into routine practice. However, there may be social, ethical, and political barriers to such screening.

▶ Another cost-effective analysis; in this case, one that is very well done. To understand what is going on here, one must accept the assumptions that were inherent in this type of study. In this report, only 1 cystic fibrosis gene mutation was screened (ΔF508). Another assumption was that 3 times out of 4, individuals will be willing to be screened. Also, the carrier detection rate using the single gene probe was estimated to be 80%. When one adds up the screening cost, the cost of genetic counseling for those couples found to be at risk, and then the cost for those who may want to undergo prenatal diagnosis, the total cost divided by the number of affected pregnancies shows that antenatal screening for cystic fibrosis runs up a bill per each affected pregnancy of between $65,000 and $160,000.

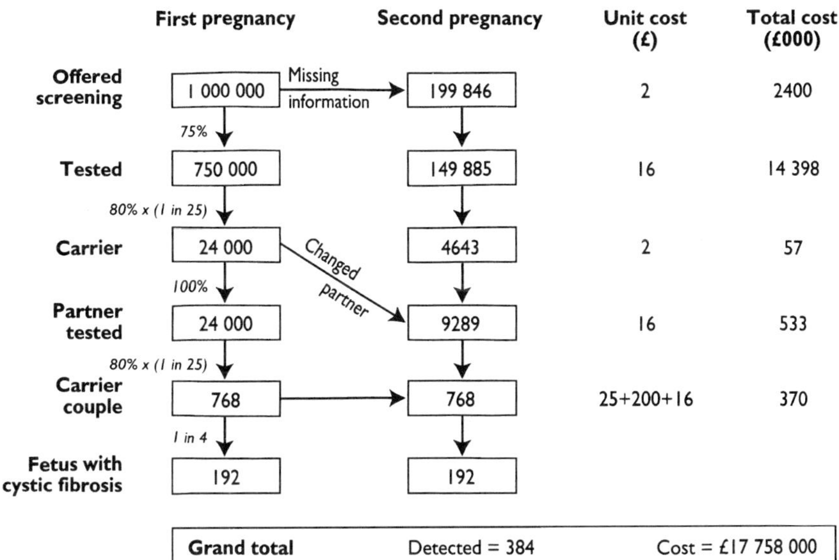

FIGURE.—Cost of a sequential antenatal screening program for cystic fibrosis. (Courtesy of Cuckle HS, Richardson GA, Sheldon TA, et al: Cost effectiveness of antenatal screening for cystic fibrosis. *BMJ* 311:1460–1464, 1995.)

As high as these numbers seem, they are actually lower than estimates from prior studies. Three previous studies have estimated the cost per affected birth avoided by antenatal screening to be $450,000 to $860,000, depending on the screening strategy.[1-3]

What do all these numbers mean? The numbers tell us that it is financially costly to screen for a pregnancy affected by cystic fibrosis. On the other hand, the cost of screening for this disease is probably considerably less than the estimated lifetime cost of currently available treatments. Also, the cost of screening for cystic fibrosis is somewhat higher than for established services such as screening maternal serum for Down's syndrome.

These authors conclude that there are no economic grounds for not introducing routine cystic fibrosis screening as part of all routine care and counseling. As you might suspect, the authors avoided any discussion of social, ethical, and political reasons for not doing so. Before anyone seriously considers routine antenatal screening, we must understand better the benefits we hope for and how they can be measured.

References

1. Asch DA, et al: *Am J Obstet Gynecol* 168:1, 1993.
2. Ginsburg G, et al: *Health Economics* 3:5, 1994.
3. Leu TA, et al: *Obstet Gynecol* 84:903, 1994.

A Cystic Fibrosis Mutation Associated With Mild Lung Disease

Gan K-H, Veeze HJ, van den Ouweland AMW, et al (Leyenburg Hosp, The Hague, The Netherlands; Sophia Children's Hosp, Rotterdam, The Netherlands; Dijkzigt Univ Hosp, Rotterdam, The Netherlands; et al)

N Engl J Med 333:95–99, 1995   11–13

Background.—In Dutch patients with cystic fibrosis (CF), the 2 most common mutations of the CF transmembrane conductance regulator gene on chromosome 7 are $\Delta F508$ and $A455E$. Preserved pancreatic function and residual secretion of chloride across membranes are associated with the A455E mutation. It is unknown whether this mutation is also correlated with less severe pulmonary disease in patients with CF.

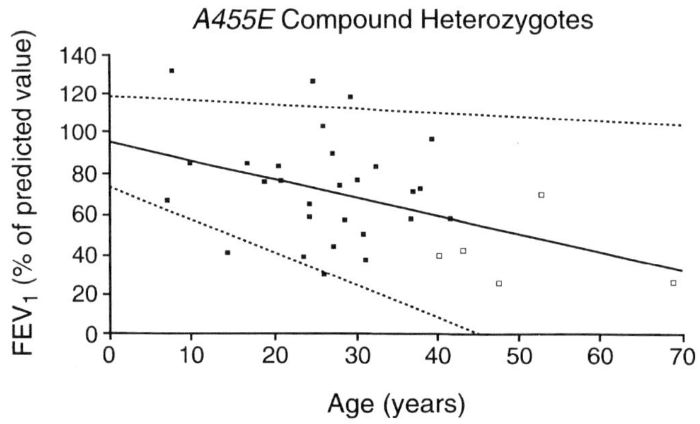

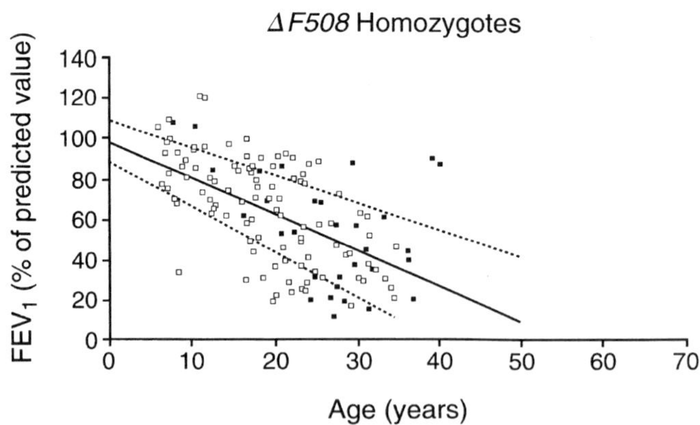

FIGURE 1.—Forced expiratory volume in 1 second (*FEV₁*) in 34 *A455E* compound heterozygotes and 130 *ΔF508* homozygotes, according to age. *Solid squares* represent patients included in the matched-pairs analysis; 4 *A455E* compound heterozygotes and 21 *ΔF508* homozygotes were not included because they were too young for pulmonary function testing. Regression lines (*solid lines*) and 95% confidence intervals (*dashed lines*) are indicated. The regression line had a slope of -0.0089 for *A455E* compound heterozygotes and -0.0178 for *ΔF508* homozygotes (*P* = 0.02). (Reprinted by permission of *The New England Journal of Medicine*, from Gan K-H, Veeze HJ, van den Ouweland AMW, et al: A cystic fibrosis mutation associated with mild lung disease. *N Engl J Med* 333:95–99, Copyright 1995, Massachusetts Medical Society.)

TABLE 1.—Characteristics of Pairs of ΔF508 Homozygotes and A455E Compound Heterozygotes Matched According to Sex and Age*

CHARACTERISTIC	No. OF PAIRS	ΔF508 HOMOZYGOTES	A455E COMPOUND HETEROZYGOTES†	P VALUE
Sex–no. (%)	33			
Male		16 (49)	16 (49)	NS
Female		17 (51)	17 (51)	
Age—yr	33			
Mean		22.9	23.0	NS
Range		0–40	1–41	
Age at diagnosis–yr	33	3.1 ± 3.9	15.0 ± 10.6	< 0.001‡
FEV$_1$—% of predicted value	29§	54.3 ± 28.4	73.9 ± 25.5	0.002‡
FVC—% of predicted value	29§	76.3 ± 24.4	88.7 ± 21.1	0.04‡
Pseudomonas colonization—no. (%)	33	20 (60.6)	11 (33.3)	0.02¶
Pancreatic insufficiency—no. (%)	33	31 (93.9)	7 (21.2)	< 0.001¶
Diabetes mellitus—no. (%)	33	9 (27.3)	0	0.004¶
Weight—(percentile)‖	33	61.0 ± 29.4	53.4 ± 30.3	NS
Height—(Percentile)				
Men	16	21.4 ± 25.0	42.0 ± 27.6	0.03‡
Women	17	38.1 ± 28.2	38.7 ± 29.4	NS

Abbreviation: NS, not significant; *FEV$_1$*, forced expiratory volume in 1 second; *FVC*, forced vital capacity.

*Plus-minus values are means ± SD.

†The following genotypes were identified: *A455E/ΔF508* (25 patients), *A455E/E60X* (4), *A455E/G542X* (2), *A455E/R553X* (1), and *A455E/1717-1G → A (1)*.

‡ By 2-tailed paired *t*-test.

§ Four patients were not old enough for pulmonary function testing.

¶ By 2-tailed exact binomial test.

‖ Weight was adjusted for height.

(Reprinted by permission of *The New England Journal of Medicine*, from Gan K-H, Veeze HJ, van den Ouweland AMW, et al: A cystic fibrosis mutation associated with mild lung disease. *N Engl J Med* 333:95–99, Copyright 1995, Massachusetts Medical Society.)

TABLE 2.—Frequency of ΔF508 and *A455E* Mutations in Various Countries

Study	Country/Region	No. of Chromosomes Screened	ΔF508	A455E
			%	
Present study	The Netherlands	556	73	7.0
Cystic Fibrosis Genetic Analysis Consortium	The Netherlands*	1043	77.1	3.0
Lindner et al.	Southwestern Germany	220	67	0
Cuppens et al.	Belgium	200	72.5	1.0
Super and Schwarz	Northwestern England	1008	82	0
Shrimpton et al.	Scotland	506	72.3	0.5
Claustres et al.	Southern France	262	63	0
Cutting et al.	Baltimore	163	76.1	0.6
Cutting et al., Zielenski et al.	Toronto	1030	68.4	0.2
Rozen et al.	Quebec	84	71	1
Rosen et al.	Saguenay-Lac St. Jean, Quebec	182	58	8
Cutting et al.	United States†	43	37	0
Cutting et al.	Israel‡	94	30	0

*Includes 31 *A455E* compound heterozygotes from the present study.

† Blacks were studied.

‡ Ashkenazi Jews were studied.

(Reprinted by permission of *The New England Journal of Medicine*, from Gan K-H, Veeze HJ, van den Ouweland AMW, et al: A cystic fibrosis mutation associated with mild lung disease. *N Engl J Med* 333:95–99, Copyright 1995, Massachusetts Medical Society.)

Methods and Findings.—Thirty-three patients with compound heterozygosity for the *A455E* mutation and age- and sex-matched patients homozygous for the *ΔF508* mutation were investigated. Group comparisons demonstrated that patients with the *A455E* mutation were older at diagnosis than *ΔF508* homozygotes. The mean patient ages in the 2 groups were 15 and 3.1 years, respectively. Twenty-one percent of the patients with the *A455E* mutation had pancreatic insufficiency, compared with 93.9% in the *ΔF508* group. None of the former group had diabetes, whereas 27.3% of the latter group did. Forced expiratory volume in 1 second (FEV₁) and forced vital capacity (FVC) were significantly greater in the *A455E* mutation group. *Pseudomonas aeruginosa* colonization was documented in 33.3% of the patients with the *A455E* and in 60.6% of those with the *ΔF508* mutation (Fig 1; Tables 1 and 2).

Conclusions.—The *A455E* mutation in these Dutch patients was significantly correlated with mild pulmonary disease. Because CF mortality depends mainly on the progression of pulmonary disease, patients with the *A455E* mutation have a better prognosis than those who are homozygous for the *ΔF508* mutation.

▶ Cystic fibrosis remains the most common lethal autosomal recessive disorder in the white population. One in 25 is an asymptomatic carrier. Since the cloning of the CF gene in 1989, there has been an explosion of information about the relationship between genotype and phenotype in affected patients. The most common mutation, *ΔF508,* is associated with pancreatic insufficiency and severe pulmonary disease. Until the report that is abstracted above appeared, no mutation associated with principally mild pulmonary disease had been found. Well, here it is, a mutation known as *A455E.* Affected patients have less severe pancreatic disease and very mild pulmonary disease, and CF is diagnosed when they are older. Their prognosis is obviously much better than that for the average patient, the latter having a median survival of just 27 years.

As an aside, whenever one discusses genetic mutations, one should be aware of the frequency of consanguinity in the populations being evaluated. Were you aware, for example, of how consanguinist the population is in Saudi Arabia? If you are not, you will be now. The overall rate of consanguinity in Saudi Arabia is 57.7% (as defined by first cousin, second cousin, and other close-relative marriages. The most frequent consanguinist marriages are between first cousins (28.4%). In the Samtah province, the rate of consanguinity is 80.6%. As high as these figures are, they don't begin to approach the rate of consanguinity in the Samaritans, a group of individuals numbering only 500 people, who have been genetically isolated for over 3,000 years. As you might suspect, the rate of consanguinity in this population is almost 100%. The lowest rate of consanguinist mating occurs here in the United States among Roman Catholics. In the majority of states, cousin marriages are illegal under statutes passed in the 19th and 20th centuries. All of this makes for some fairly interesting and complex family trees.[1] Abstract 11–15 shows the implications of ethnic intermarriage and its consequences for cystic fibrosis carrier screening.

Reference

1. El-Hazemi MAF, et al: *J Med Genet* 32:623, 1995.

Combined Lung and Liver Transplantation in Patients With Cystic Fibrosis: A 4½-year Experience

Couetil JPA, Houssin DP, Soubrane O, et al (Broussais Hosp, Paris; Cochin Hosp, Paris)
J Thorac Cardiovasc Surg 110:1415–1423, 1995   11–14

Background.—Patients with cystic fibrosis (CF), end-stage respiratory failure, and associated liver cirrhosis have been thought to be poor candidates for lung transplantation. After surgery, hepatic insufficiency results in high morbidity and mortality. The outcomes of combined lung and liver transplantation in 1 series of patients with CF and end-stage lung and liver disease were reviewed.

Methods.—Twenty-five patients were accepted to the program for combined transplantation. Between June 1990 and March 1995, 9 patients died awaiting organs, and 10 underwent transplant procedures. The procedures were heart-lung-liver transplantation in 5, en bloc double lung–liver transplantation in 1, sequential double lung–liver transplantation in 3, and bilateral lobar lung transplantation from a split left lung and reduced liver transplantation in 1. The transplant recipients were 5 females and 5 males, aged 10–24 years. The patients had a mean forced expiratory volume in 1 second of 29% and a mean forced vital capacity of 35% of predicted values. All patients had resistant *Pseudomonas* infections including 3 with *Pseudomonas cepaceia*. In addition, 2 patients had *Aspergillus* species. Cirrhosis was severe and associated with portal hypertension in all patients. Four patients had a history of esophageal variceal bleeding. Two had had previous portosystemic shunts. In the 2-stage operation, intrathoracic surgery was completed before the abdominal stage was begun. Because of the patients' poor clinical condition, cardiopulmonary bypass was done in all. Immunosuppression was achieved with azathioprine, cyclosporine, and prednisone.

Outcomes.—Two perioperative deaths occurred. One resulted from primary liver failure and the other from early lung dysfunction. Pulmonary infection was the most common cause of morbidity in the first 3 months after transplantation. Other complications, all treated successfully, were severe ascites in 3 patients, biliary stricture in 2, tracheal stenosis in 1, and bronchial stenosis in 1. In 3 patients, obliterative bronchiolitis developed, which was stabilized with FK 506 in 2 patients. The third underwent retransplantation at 38 months but eventually died of hemorrhage. One- and three-year actuarial survival was 70% (Fig 1). All survivors had significant functional improvement.

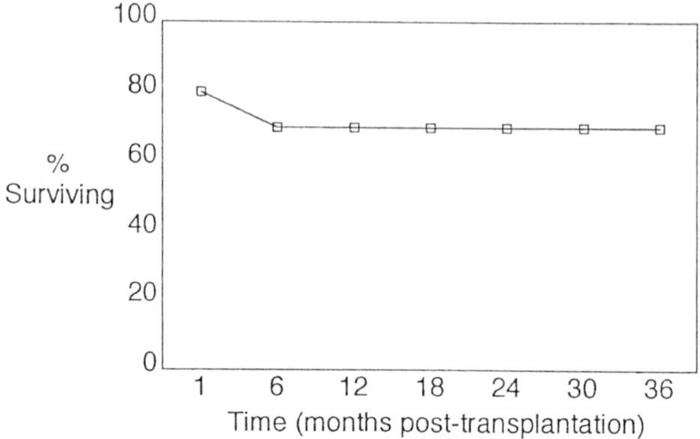

FIGURE 1.—Actuarial survival (Kaplan-Meier) of patients with cystic fibrosis having combined lung-liver transplantation. (Courtesy of Couetil JPA, Houssin DP, Soubrane O, et al: Combined lung and liver transplantation in patients with cystic fibrosis: A 4½-year experience. *J Thorac Cardiovasc Surg* 110:1415–1423, 1995.)

Conclusions.—Lung-liver transplantation can be done with a satisfactory outcome in patients with CF, chronic respiratory failure, and advanced cirrhosis. The morbidity and mortality was comparable to that of separate replacements.

▶ The very fact that of 25 patients with CF who were accepted for transplantation purposes, 9 died while waiting for a transplant, shows how desperately ill these children are and how a posttransplant survival at 3 years of 70% is so good by comparison. This is particularly true because the combination of lung and liver disease in these patients is particularly challenging for both surgical therapy and postoperative management. Such patients are often in poor nutritional condition caused by severe intestinal malabsorption and chronic infection with multiresistant organisms. In this series, all patients had problems with portal hypertension and life-threatening complications such as gastrointestinal bleeding. The 3-year follow-up data are virtually identical to those being reported for isolated unilateral or bilateral lung transplantation sans the liver.

As critically important as these data showing that combined organ transplantation can "salvage" some with CF who would otherwise die are at the same time, this report raises many other questions that demand answers. When is a patient sick enough to require such dramatic therapies? How useful are these therapies, overall, when there is such a shortage of donor organs? Is it possible to do a partial liver/lung transplant using living parent organs as is now being done with isolated lung transplant and isolated liver transplant? Lastly, although the genetic nature of CF is such that recurrence in transplant organs is highly unlikely, do we know this for sure, particularly with respect to the liver?

With all the unanswered questions still lurking about, it is clear to everyone that the holy grail of future management for CF remains the ongoing search for gene therapy. For an update on the topic of recent advances in the application of gene therapy to human diseases, and in particular to CF, see the excellent reviews of this topic by Hamania et al.[1] and Wilson et al.[2] It is not too early to anticipate the development of safe and efficient gene transfer technologies that will work to correct the basic pathophysiology of CF.

References

1. Hamania AG, et al: *Am J Med* 99:537, 1995.
2. Wilson JM: *J Clin Invest* 96:2547, 1995.

Ethnic Intermarriage and Its Consequences for Cystic Fibrosis Carrier Screening
Gilbert F, Arzimanoglou I, Schoelkopf J, et al (Cornell Univ, New York; MediGene Inc, Yonkers, NY)
Am J Prev Med 11:251–255, 1995   11–15

Background.—Cystic fibrosis (CF) is one of the most common recessively inherited diseases in the world. The frequencies of individual mutations can significantly vary among subgroups of different European ethnicities. For instance, 6 mutations account for more than 95% of total CF chromosomes in eastern European Jews, and less than 20 mutations account for more than 85% of total CF chromosomes in non-Jews from most of western and northern Europe. Among southern Europeans, however, panels including up to 62 mutations detect less than 75% of all CF chromosomes. As a result, the use of limited mutation panels for specific ethnic groups has been proposed. The authors recently introduced such a panel in their U.S. practice. The panel contained the CF mutations most commonly found in eastern European Jews.

Methods and Findings.—A total of 1,260 individuals participated in the screening program. About 6% overall and 7% of eastern European Jews had mixed ethnic parentage. In the next generation, the children of more than 25% of the couples participating in screening would be of mixed ethnic origin. Thirty-one percent of the couples in the next generation would include at least 1 eastern European Jewish partner. These findings are consistent with past analyses of intermarriage of Jews (Table 3). Thirty-five CF carriers were identified among the individuals tested. This result corresponded with an overall carrier detection rate of 81% of that predicted.

Conclusions.—In trying to determine who should be tested using the panel containing the CF mutations most commonly found in eastern European Jews, a high frequency of ethnic intermarriage was discovered among all patients—Jews and non-Jews. Clinicians in the United States must be careful about how they apply restricted mutation panels and calculate carrier risk. The significance of these findings extend beyond CF to other diseases, such as Tay-Sachs and Gaucher diseases.

TABLE 3.—Studies of Intermarriage Between Jews and Non-Jews

Study	Results
NJPS study (completed 1971 among Jewish couples, in marriages)	
Before 1925	< 2% involved a non-Jewish spouse
1940–1960	6% involved a non-Jewish spouse
1960–1964	12% involved a non-Jewish spouse
In 1971	8.1% of Jewish couples, overall, included a new-Jewish partner
NJPS study (completed 1990 among Jewish couples, in marriages)	
1975–1984	51% involved a non-Jewish spouse
1985–1990	57% involved a non-Jewish spouse
In 1990	31% of Jewish couples, overall, included a new-Jewish partner
UJA study (completed 1991, comparing Jewish couples in New York versus United States overall, those involving a non-Jewish spouse)	
Before 1965	5.5% of NY total versus 4.4% in US
1965–1974	15.4% of NY total versus 19.7% in US
1975–1984	26.1% of NY total versus 39.5% in US
1985–1991	26.3% of NY total versus 46.6% in US
In 1991	Of Jewish couples, overall, 20% in NY and 28% in US involved a non-Jewish partner
This study	
Of Jewish individuals from NY, most over 35, thus derived from couples married before 1985	7% report having one non-Jewish parent
Of Jewish couples from NY, most married since 1985	31% involved Jewish and non-Jewish partners

Abbreviations: NJPS, National Jewish Population Study; *UJA*, United Jewish Appeal.
(Courtesy of Gilbert F, Arzimanoglou I, Schoelkopf J, et al: *Am J Prev Med* 11:251–255, 1995, by permission of Oxford University Press.)

▶ This is a fascinating article. It attempts to show us how, with increasing ethnic intermarriage, difficulties arise with certain diseases vis-à-vis carrier screening. Take CF for example. Cystic fibrosis carrier frequencies among whites are between 1:25 and 1:30. In the 7 years since the gene abnormality was discovered, more than 400 CF mutations have been identified. Depending on what one's ethnicity is, however, the frequency of the specific mutations vary. For example, 6 mutations account for more than 95% of all CF chromosomes in Jews from eastern Europe. On the other hand, it takes about 20 mutations to account for about 85% of total CF chromosome abnormalities in non-Jews from most of western and northern Europe. When southern Europeans are considered (including Spaniards, Portuguese, Italians, and Greeks), CF screening panels have to include more than 60 mutations just to capture 75% of all CF carriers.

What does all this mean? It means, for example, that in eastern European Jews studied in Israel, the conditions that foster intermarriage in the United States do not apply; therefore the predominant CF mutation, W1282X, accounts for more than 50% of all CF chromosomes, and the deltaF-508 accounts for less than 30% of total CF chromosomes. On the other hand, among non-Jewish northern Europeans, W1282X constitutes less than 3%

and ΔF-508, some 75% of all CF chromosomes. In the series in the article abstracted, among people who were obligate carriers for CF who said they were of eastern European Jewish origin, the numbers did not match for gene abnormality frequency with studies of Jews in Israel. This presumably is a result of intermarriages.

All of these results would not mean much were it not for the important fact that unless there is a clear understanding about the background of populations being studied, appropriate panels of mutations to be screened for cannot be designed. It is not easily possible to screen for all 400 mutations that cause CF, so panels must be created that encompass the most frequent abnormalities. We see that you can't bet on stated ethnicity to set up such panels.

The significance of the findings of this report extends well beyond CF to other diseases, individual examples of which are more prevalent in particular ethnic or racial subgroups. These would include Tay-Sachs and Gaucher diseases in eastern European Jews, the β-thalassemias in populations from the Mediterranean basin, and phenylketonuria, which is much more common in whites than American blacks.

Ours is a country in which racial prejudice persists despite the fact that our society is truly a racial and ethnic melting pot. That having been said, bigots will soon have to start hating themselves, for we are truly more alike than we are different as molecular probes are proving.

Comparison of Nasal Prongs and Nasopharyngeal Catheter for the Delivery of Oxygen in Children With Hypoxemia Because of a Lower Respiratory Tract Infection

Weber MW, Palmer A, Oparaugo A, et al (Med Research Council Labs, Fajara, The Gambia; Children's Hosp, Hannover, Germany; Royal Victoria Hosp, Banjul, The Gambia)
J Pediatr 127:378–383, 1995   11–16

Rationale.—Maintaining hemoglobin oxygen saturation will limit deaths of children with pneumonia. The costliness of oxygen mandates the use of low flow rates, especially in developing countries. The World Health Organization has recommended both nasal prongs and the nasopharyngeal (NP) catheter; which of these methods is best remains uncertain.

Study Design.—These 2 methods of delivering oxygen were compared in children 1 week to 5 years of age who had acute lower respiratory tract infection and hypoxemia, defined as an arterial oxygen saturation (SaO_2) less than 90% as estimated by pulse oximetry. Using a crossover design, 62 children received oxygen by nasal prongs and 56 by NP catheter. Flow rates of 0.2–4 L/min were used to deliver humidified oxygen.

Effectiveness.—All but 6 of the 118 children were satisfactorily oxygenated at the peak flow rate of 4 L/min. Treatment time averaged 87.5 hours when treatment began with prongs and 95 hours when the NP catheter was used initially. Children consistently required less oxygen with the second delivery method. Twenty-six children reached an SaO$_2$ of 95% or higher at the lowest flow rate of 0.2 L/min regardless of which system was used. The 2 methods were equally well tolerated.

Complications.—Hypoxemic episodes were frequent in both groups. Nasal obstruction was more prevalent when the NP catheter was used. One child treated with prongs had nasal ulceration develop. One child in the catheter group had acute gastric distention and died.

Costs.—Oxygen therapy with nasal prongs cost $14.83 on average, compared with $15.73 for use of the NP catheter.

Conclusion.—Nasal prongs are as effective a means as the NP catheter for delivering oxygen to hypoxemic children, and in addition they are safer.

▶ Although this study was designed to be carried out in developing countries where one of the main causes of death in children is respiratory tract infection, the lessons to be learned can be applied equally well here at home. Two oxygen delivery systems are recommended by the World Health Organization: nasal prongs and NP catheters. There has been debate, however, over which method of delivery is preferable. Advocates of the nasal prongs claim that they are safer; advocates of the NP catheter contend that it is more effective in achieving adequate oxygenation. Expense is also an issue. How much should it cost to reduce morbidity and mortality rates for infants and young children? This is the query that the article by Weber et al. attempts to address. The authors conclude that nasal prongs are associated with less nasal obstruction than are nasal catheters and, in combination with good nursing care, successfully deliver oxygen to permit relative normalization of pulse oximetry values in most children with acute pneumonia. They also found that 24% of children younger than 2 months require a flow rate of more than 0.5 L/min to achieve adequate oxygenation. These observations are virtually identical to what has been found to be true in the respiratory care of adults.

There was a difference in cost associated with these 2 forms of oxygen delivery. This difference largely occurred because the manufacturer of NP catheters was located in Europe and the cost per catheter was just 20 cents (U.S. dollars), whereas nasal prongs imported from the United States cost between $2 and $5 each (a 10- to 25-fold difference). The actual difference in the cost of oxygen itself was negligible between the 2 methods of oxygen delivery.

Why we in the United States charge $5 for a piece of plastic when a somewhat more complicated NP catheter costs only 20 cents abroad is puzzling. Because nasal prongs have much less morbidity associated with them, hopefully somebody will figure out how to make a piece of plastic cheaply. Cost aside, nasal prongs are safer than NP catheters and deliver oxygen as effectively; therefore, they are a more appropriate method for oxygen delivery in developing countries, and in this country as well.

Grunting Respirations in Infants and Children

Poole SR, Chetham M, Anderson M (Univ of Colorado, Denver)
Pediatr Emerg Care 11:158–161, 1995   11–17

Objective.—Grunting respirations are known to be a symptom of serious illness—particularly pneumonia—in infants and young children. However, there is little information about the pathophysiology, differential diagnosis, or management of infants and children with grunting. Fifty-one pediatric patients with grunting were studied.

Methods.—The 51 patients were prospectively identified from among all patients between 1 month and 18 years of age who were seen in the emergency department of a children's hospital during a 5-month period. Their medical records were reviewed retrospectively.

Findings.—The children accounted for 0.3% of all patients seen in the emergency department during the study. The patients' mean age was 8 months. Three groups were identified according to mode of presentation. Fifty-five percent of the children were seen with mainly respiratory signs and symptoms, and each of them had a respiratory or cardiac condition. Twenty-five percent had a temperature greater than 38.5°C but no respiratory signs or symptoms. In all of these patients, the symptoms resulted from an infectious cause, with three fourths of patients having an invasive bacterial disease. The remaining 20% of patients did not have respiratory signs or fever; rather, they had any of a number of apparently painful conditions (Table 1). Seventy-eight percent of the study patients were admitted to the hospital.

Conclusions.—Three relatively distinct groups of children with the symptom of grunting respirations were identified. The child's initial symptoms may be able to guide the selection of diagnostic tests. Grunting frequently indicates a serious illness and warrants thorough attempts to accurately diagnose and treat its cause.

▶ This report describes the causes of grunting. It even defines grunting: a repetitive low- to medium-pitched, short, explosive sound that is produced by vocal cord closure during expiration. This is an accurate definition of a grunt (please note that *Webster's* dictionary also includes under grunt, fish of the genera *Haemulon* and a U.S. infantryman in the war in Vietnam). The only animals that grunt are hogs and humans. That having been said, this report teaches us that there are many nonrespiratory causes of grunting in infants and young children. In addition to infection, in the latter category are included such peculiar etiologies as intussusception, abnormal ventriculo-peritoneal shunts, and corneal abrasions.

It's easy to understand why infants and children with cardiorespiratory problems grunt. Grunting prevents alveolar collapse, improves ventilation-perfusion inequities, and decreases alveolar and interstitial fluid. Grunting has been shown to increase the arterial oxygen tension by more than 10%, while reducing arterial carbon dioxide levels. Thus, grunting in certain con-

TABLE 1.—Clinical Signs and Symptoms in 51 Pediatric Patients With Grunting Respirations

Diagnostic category	Clinical signs/symptoms	Diagnoses	No. of cases
Cardiorespiratory disorders; $n = 29$ (57%)	Predominantly respiratory signs and symptoms: cough, tachypnea, respiratory distress, wheezing, stridor. With or without fever	Reactive airways disease	10
		Pneumonia, viral/bacterial	7
		Aspiration pneumonia	3
		Bronchiolitis	2
		Croup and pneumonia	1
		Hydrocarbon aspiration	1
		Foreign body in airway	1
		Myasthenia gravis and bronchiolitis	1
		Myocarditis	1
		Congenital heart disease and congestive heart failure	1
		Sickle cell disease—acute chest syndrome	1
Nonrespiratory infections; $n = 13$ (25%)	Fever > 38.5°C (usually > 40°C). Without significant respiratory tract signs or symptoms	Bacteremia/sepsis	6
		Viremia with high fever	3
		Meningitis, viral/bacterial	2
		Pyelonephritis	2
Nonrespiratory, noninfectious disorder; $n = 9$ (18%)	No respiratory tract signs or symptoms. No fever	Intestinal ileus	2
		Intestinal obstruction	1
		Sickle cell disease, painful crisis	1
		Intussusception	1
		Ventriculoperitoneal shunt malfunction	1
		Corneal abrasion	1
		Skull fracture and subdural hematoma	1
		Hemolytic anemia, acute autoimmune with abdominal pain	1

(Courtesy of Poole SR, Chetham M, Anderson M: Grunting respirations in infants and children. *Pediatr Emerg Care* 11:158–161, 1995.)

ditions related to the heart and lungs seems to make sense. On the other hand, why someone with a corneal abrasion or an intussusception should grunt is unclear.

P.S.: If you are really an aficionado of the grunt, recognize that the older child or adult who grunts is technically called a "grunter." A young child or infant who grunts is technically a "gruntling." Only time and a lot of investigation will ultimately reveal why grunters and gruntlings grunt. In the meantime, keep this differential diagnosis list (see above) available, and recall it the next time you see a young one showing this clinical sign.

To learn more about abnormal breathing, see the excellent review by Manning et al.[1]

Reference

1. Manning HL, et al: *N Engl J Med* 333:1547, 1995.

Cardiorespiratory Function Before and After Corrective Surgery in Pectus Excavatum

Quigley PM, Haller JA Jr, Jelus KL, et al (Pediatric Respiratory Sciences, Baltimore, Md; Johns Hopkins Univ, Baltimore, Md)
J Pediatr 128:638–643, 1996   11–18

Purpose.—Some anecdotal reports suggest that pectus excavatum (PE) is associated with exercise limitations that improve with corrective surgery. Others maintain that the deformity is cosmetic only and that psychological problems are the only indication for surgery. Patients with PE were studied to see whether they had any cardiopulmonary abnormalities and, if so, whether the abnormalities improved after surgical repair.

Methods.—Thirty-six adolescent patients with PE were studied, as were 10 age-matched, healthy controls. All subjects underwent pulmonary function and incremental exercise tests. The tests were repeated after surgical repair in 15 of the patients with PE and in 6 of the controls. All PE repairs were performed by a standard surgical technique.

Results.—Fifty-eight percent of the PE patients complained of exercise intolerance before surgery, although 92% exercised on a regular basis or played team sports. Preoperative testing showed a mean forced vital capacity of 81% of the predicted value in the patients with PE, compared with 98% for the controls. Chest CT scans in the patients with PE found that the ratios of internal transverse to anteroposterior diameters were inversely correlated with total lung capacity. There was no difference in the preoperative exercise workload between PE patients and controls.

Surgical repair of PE was not associated with any change in forced vital capacity as a percentage of the predicted value. After surgery, the PE patients exercised for a somewhat longer time and had a slightly higher oxygen pulse. There was no change in the test results for control subjects.

Conclusion.—Pectus excavatum is associated with mild restrictive lung disease in some patients, but pulmonary function is unchanged by surgical repair of the PE deformity. Cardiac function during exercise does appear to improve somewhat after PE repair, but the improvement is small and of unknown clinical significance. The benefits of PE repair to the average patient remain unclear.

▶ So, how do you answer the query of the next youngster who walks into your office with a PE and who wants to know if he or she should have the thing fixed? Chances are that the study abstracted will not give you any additional insights, except to reinforce the fact that improvements in cardio-pulmonary function, if any, should be expected to be modest. Thus, the surgical indications remain improvement in cosmesis and possible avoid-ance of, or improvement in, psychological problems related to a PE.

Exposure of the US Population to Environmental Tobacco Smoke: The Third National Health and Nutrition Examination Survey, 1988 to 1991

Pirkle JL, Flegal KM, Bernert JT, et al (Ctrs for Disease Control and Prevention, Atlanta, Ga)

JAMA 275:1233–1240, 1996

11–19

Background.—Environmental tobacco smoke (ETS) exposure is associated with acute and chronic health effects in nonsmokers. The prevalence of ETS exposure in the U.S. population and subpopulations has not been well defined. The Third National Health and Nutrition Examination Survey (NHANES III) involved a representative sampling of the civilian, noninstitutionalized U.S. population, with data collected from October 1988 to October 1991. The NHANES III included questions on tobacco exposure at home and at work and serum measurements of the main nicotine metabolite, cotinine. This report examines the exposure of the U.S. population to ETS using the NHANES III data.

Study Design.—The NHANES III was designed to evaluate a representative sample of the civilian, noninstitutionalized population based on a complex, stratified, multistage probability cluster sampling design. A home interview was followed by a physical examination in a mobile examination center. Information was obtained by questionnaire for all 16,818 participants aged 2 months and older. Measurements of serum cotinine were obtained for all 10,642 participants aged 4 years and older.

Findings.—Among children aged 2 months to 11 years, 43% lived with at least 1 smoker, and 37% of adult nonsmokers lived in a home with at least 1 smoker or reported ETS exposure at work. Serum cotinine levels indicated that exposure to ETS was even larger than reported. Among nonsmokers, 88% had cotinine detected in their serum. Both the numbers of smokers in the household and the hours of work exposure were significantly and independently associated with serum cotinine levels. Higher levels of serum cotinine were detected in children, blacks, and males. There was no consistent association between serum cotinine and dietary variables. Including both smokers and nonsmokers, 92% of this population had detectable levels of cotinine in their serum.

Conclusion.—Data from the NHANES III reveal widespread exposure to tobacco smoke in both the home and work environment in a representative sampling of the U.S. population. The measurements of serum cotinine levels demonstrate that 92% of the population over the age of 4 years has detectable levels of this nicotine metabolite in the blood. These serum cotinine measurements provide an objective baseline to which future measurements can be compared in monitoring exposure trends and the effectiveness of public health campaigns for reducing exposure to ETS.

▶ There are some pretty stiff statistics in the April 24, 1996, issue of *JAMA*, statistics having to do with tobacco. Take, for example, the article abstracted. It is mind boggling to think that over 90% of the population of the United States aged 4 years and older have detectable levels of cotinine in their blood, demonstrating exposure to environmental tobacco smoke. What are some of the other fast facts about tobacco learned during the past year?

1. Contrary to the tobacco industry's claims, reductions in spending on tobacco products will actually boost employment in all of the 8 nontobacco regions of the United States and will not diminish employment in the southeastern tobacco region to the extent that the tobacco industry estimates. If the tobacco industry went out of existence, some 220,000 jobs would be lost in the Southeast, balanced by a gain of about 355,000 jobs throughout the rest of the country. If you want to understand why, see the report by Warner et al.[1]

2. We may now know why tobacco is addictive. In a recently reported study, a team of researchers from Brookhaven National Laboratory found that the brains of living smokers have markedly less of the enzyme monoamine oxidase B (MAO B) compared with the brains of nonsmokers or former smokers.[2] This enzyme is involved in breaking down dopamine, a neurotransmitter that plays a role in movement as well as in feelings of pleasure, such as those associated with most substances of abuse, including cocaine, amphetamines, heroin, alcohol, and nicotine. Nicotine, itself, also stimulates the release of dopamine, resulting in a double whammy.

3. Among eighth and tenth graders in this country, the proportion of those who smoke has increased by one third since 1991. Some 19% of eighth graders and 28% of tenth graders now report such use. Since 1992, the smoking rate has risen by more than one fifth among high school seniors, with 34% now saying they smoke.[3]

4. If you ever wondered whether it is the Republican party or the Democratic party that receives more monetary contributions from the tobacco industry, wonder no more. Until about 1993, the Republicans and Democrats got about an equal number of bucks from the tobacco industry, but in 1995, the Republicans garnered almost 4 times as much. The reason for the switch appears to be the philosophical position of the Republican party against

government regulation. Whatever the reason, we see political candidates willing to make medically incorrect statements about tobacco.

5. If you were asked the question "Is the percentage of male physicians who smoke in Beijing equal to, lower than, or higher than that of non physician males who smoke?", how would you answer? According to a recent survey, 68% of male physicians in Beijing are smokers, a statistic that is 7 percentage points higher than for other males in China.[4]

While on the topic of queries, what nation has the highest production and consumption of tobacco? It is not the United States. It is China, where 40% of the world's manufactured tobacco is produced. A remarkably high percentage (17%) of total household income in cities such as Shanghai is used to buy cigarettes.[5] Two percent of China's arable land is used to grow tobacco, land that could be used to feed an ever-increasing population.

6. Lastly, recognize that most of us are supporting the tobacco industry. Simply look at your retirement portfolio. Investors in the top 15 United States mutual funds own 69,903,870 shares of tobacco stocks. What does your portfolio look like?

References

1. Warner KE, et al: *JAMA* 275:1241, 1996.
2. Faller JS, et al: *Nature* 379:733, 1996.
3. Editorial comment: *JAMA* 275:1218, 1996.
4. Skolnick AA, et al: *JAMA* 275:1220, 1996.
5. Editorial comment: *JAMA* 274:1232, 1995.

Use of a Helium-oxygen Mixture in the Treatment of Postextubation Stridor in Pediatric Patients With Burns

Rodeberg DA, Easter AJ, Washam MA, et al (Univ of Cincinnati, Ohio)
J Burn Care Rehabil 16:476–480, 1995   11–20

Objective.—Because the mixture of helium and oxygen—or "heliox"—is less dense than room air, it can flow with less turbulence past airway narrowings. As such, it decreases airway resistance while increasing gas exchange volume. More than 90% of patients requiring reintubation will have stridor as a manifestation of airway obstruction. The use of heliox for the treatment of postextubation stridor or retractions in children with burns was assessed.

Methods.—Eight children with burns who had postextubation stridor or retractions that did not respond to treatment with nebulized racemic epinephrine were studied. All were treated with heliox by using a face mask. The mean treatment time was 28 hours, and the initial helium concentration ranged from 50% to 70%. The helium concentration was adjusted downward to the lowest concentration that relieved stridor; when it was less than 50%, the helium was discontinued.

Results.—Just 2 of the 8 children treated with heliox had respiratory distress requiring reintubation. The duration of stridor before the start of heliox therapy was 10 and 24 hours in these patients, compared with a mean of 1 hour in those who did not require reintubation. The mean respiratory distress score decreased from 6.8 to 2.0 after the start of heliox therapy.

Conclusions.—In pediatric burn patients, heliox is an effective treatment for postextubation stridor that does not respond to nebulized racemic epinephrine. Heliox treatment should be started as soon as possible after the onset of stridor. Heliox may help in preventing respiratory distress and the need for reintubation.

▶ The principle by which helium-oxygen mixtures are effective in reducing stridor is fairly simple. You will recall as a youngster, at birthday parties, if you took a breath of helium, your voice would become high-pitched. What you were experiencing was a basic law of physics. When you inhale a gas that is of lower density than room air, the resistance associated with the flow of that gas becomes markedly reduced, thereby limiting the ability to form deep tones. Capitalizing on this phenomenon, years ago helium-oxygen mixtures were used to reduce airway resistance in those who might have, for whatever reason, airway narrowing. Initial reports by Barach, published 60 years ago, demonstrated that the use of heliox in patients with chronic obstructive pulmonary disease would produce clinical improvement.[1] Heliox has also been used for the treatment of postextubation stridor in patients in ICUs, in the emergency management of upper airway obstructions, to decrease the nonelastic work of breathing, and in the treatment of children with status asthmaticus and croup. All of these conditions have similar pathologies—narrowing of the airway with a resultant increase in airway turbulence and resistance.

Now for a lesson in physics and an explanation of exactly how heliox works. Airflow through large airways is turbulent, but this turbulence disappears as airway diameters decrease below 2 mm, about the level of the bronchioles. Graham's law states that the flow of gas in the large airways, where turbulent flow predominates, varies inversely with the square root of its density. When the large airways become narrowed, airflow becomes even more turbulent, a problem that is relievable by changes in gas density. The use of heliox is successful because it is a lighter gas than air; a mixture of 80% helium and 20% oxygen has one third the density of room air. Because heliox has a lower density, there is less airway turbulence, less airway resistance, and increased flow. These kinds of improvements lead to a decrease in the work of respiration, oxygen consumption, and carbon dioxide production. As you might expect, heliox is most beneficial in the treatment of large airway disease where turbulent airflow predominates.

Heliox doesn't work miracles in everyone with narrowed airways. For patients who require a lot of oxygen, you can't use as much helium mixed with oxygen, thus diminishing some of the effectiveness of heliox. The nicest part about heliox is that it is not associated with any significant adverse side effects because it is a totally inert gas. It has even been used as part of the management of respiratory distress syndrome in tiny preterm infants.[2]

This is the last entry in the Respiratory Tract chapter, so we'll close with a quiz. Name the 512th reason not to exercise. It's swimming-induced pulmonary edema and hemoptysis. Eight 18-year-olds were recently described to have had pulmonary edema and hemoptysis develop during a training exercise that consisted of a swimming time trial over a 2.4-km course in the open sea at a water temperature of 23°C. In anticipation of a high heat load with this exercise, the instructor had recommended that the recruitees drink a lot of water before exercise. Forty-five minutes into the exercise, shortness of breath and coughing up of blood occurred.[3] All these teenagers were documented to be hypoxemic with radiographic evidence of pulmonary edema. All, fortunately, recovered nicely, although 2 of the 8 experienced similar problems the next time they attempted to swim. Swimming is the 512th reason not to exercise.

References

1. Barach AL: *Proc Soc Exp Biol Med* 32:462, 1934.
2. Elleau C, et al: *J Pediatr* 122:132, 1993.
3. Weiller-Ravell D, et al: *BMJ* 311:361, 1995.

12 The Heart and Blood Vessels

Factors Prompting Referral for Cardiology Evaluation of Heart Murmurs in Children
McCrindle BW, Shaffer KM, Kan JS, et al (Hosp for Sick Children, Toronto)
Arch Pediatr Adolesc Med 149:1277–1279, 1995   12–1

Introduction.—A major part of pediatric cardiology entails evaluating heart murmurs. This practice is a demonstrably accurate and cost-effective way of detecting heart disease, but the increasing use of echocardiography by other providers holds the potential for altering referral patterns.

Study Plan.—Providers requesting an outpatient pediatric cardiology consultation during an 8-month period at Johns Hopkins Hospital were sent a questionnaire. Responses were received from 143 providers seeking 235 referrals.

Referral Practices.—Pediatricians constituted 84% of the providers requesting referrals; a large majority were general pediatricians. About 40% of the providers indicated that they sometimes ordered an echocardiogram before deciding whether to refer. Three fourths of visits prompting the decision to refer were for well-child care, and only 16% for acute illness. A newly recognized murmur was the most frequent reason for referral (Table).

Diagnosis.—More than 60% of the children referred were considered by their providers to have less than a 50% probability of having a cardiac defect. The providers were very accurate in estimating the likelihood of disease. A defect was relatively likely when a child was referred for an unusually loud or harsh murmur.

Discussion.—Factors other than clinical features often influence the decision of whether to refer a child to a pediatric cardiologist. It may no longer be the case that cardiologists are the gatekeepers for access to diagnostic echocardiography. Better education of both referring providers and parents will help ensure that heart disease will be detected and families reassured in a cost-effective manner.

▶ Given the evidence from this study and others that referring physicians are reasonably accurate in their assessment of a patient's likelihood of

"

TABLE.—Referral Factors

Factor	Physicians Choosing Response, %
Clinical features	
Murmur characteristics	
Newly recognized	51
Unusual loudness	27
Unusual harshness	22
Unusual persistence	21
Atypical location	15
Change in murmur previously heard	9
Other murmur characteristics	6
Other symptoms and signs	
Associated cardiac symptoms	12
Abnormal second heart sound	3
Presence of an associated click	2
Other signs	5
Other features	
Unusual parental anxiety	
About child's general health	7
About disease and murmurs	14
Parents requested the referral	6
Concern about medicolegal issues	13
Physician concerns	4
Positive family history of heart defects	3
Pre-sports participation evaluation	2
Poor social situation and/or compliance	1
SBE prophylaxis concerns	1

Abbreviation: SBE, subacute bacterial endocarditis.
(Courtesy of McCrindle BW, Shaffer KM, Kan JS, et al: Factors prompting referral for cardiology evaluation of heart murmurs in children. *Arch Pediatr Adolesc Med* 149:1277–1279, Copyright 1995, American Medical Association.)

having cardiac disease and that a minority of children eventually receive diagnoses of disease at cardiology consultation, there must be many non-clinical factors that have a major impact on the reasons pediatricians and family physicians refer children for cardiac evaluations.[1] Why are there so many unnecessary referrals? What are the major clinical factors that are responsible for referrals? One factor suggested by this study is a lack of continuity of primary care, with newly heard murmurs being a common reason that prompts referral of patients not well known to the pediatrician or family practitioner. Parental anxiety is a frequent nonclinical reason for referral, followed by medical-legal concerns.

To avoid the problem of a referral to a pediatric cardiologist, many pediatricians and family practitioners are opting for a middle-ground alternative. This involves sending a child in just for an echocardiogram without a consultation. Studies done to date suggest that this approach is *not* cost-effective. "Echo first, consult later" actually costs more in the long run than referring a child initially to the pediatric cardiologist, who is not likely to perform an echocardiogram (the most expensive part of the consult) if there is little indication for its need. The best approach, however, is for primary care physicians neither to refer nor to do an echocardiogram, but to use the clinical skills that they have been trained to use.

This report teaches us many things. First, referring physicians can reasonably accurately assess a child's likelihood of having a cardiac problem. Second, even if a child has a low probability of having cardiac disease, a physician will often refer that child to a pediatric cardiologist. Lastly, we should be spending more time during residency training not in evaluating cardiac disease, which we seem to be doing a good job of, but rather in teaching residents how to deal with parental anxiety and their own anxiety about our medical-legal system. The fault lies not in how we teach cardiology, but rather in how we teach interpersonal skills in a climate that is so litigious.

Reference

1. Rushford JA, et al: *BMJ* 305:1264, 1992.

Cardinal Clinical Signs in the Differentiation of Heart Murmurs in Children

McCrindle BW, Shaffer KM, Kan JS, et al (Johns Hopkins Univ, Baltimore, Md)
Arch Pediatr Adolesc Med 150:169–174, 1996   12–2

Background.—Pediatric cardiologists are often consulted to assess children with heart murmurs. The goal is to identify pathologic conditions in a cost-effective manner. The role of echocardiography in these evaluations has not been established definitively. In addition, it would be helpful to know which clinical features can be used by referring physicians to more accurately identify children who require such consultation. The diagnostic accuracy of clinical heart murmur assessment in children was investigated.

Methods.—Two hundred twenty-two consecutive children undergoing heart murmur assessments for the first time were studied. The median age of the patients was 1.9 years, with a range of 2 days to 18 years. Fifty-two percent were male. Five academic pediatric cardiologists performed the evaluations. The results of ECGs and echocardiograms were assessed.

Findings.—Thirty-three percent of the patients had cardiac disease. The sensitivity and specificity of clinical evaluation in identifying patients with pathologic murmurs were 92% and 94%, respectively. Its positive and negative predictive values were 88% and 96%, respectively. When diagnostic uncertainty was considered an indication for echocardiography, the sensitivity increased to 97% and the specificity to 98%. Diagnoses were missed only in children with trivial or minor lesions. Clinical features that independently predicted disease included murmurs that were pansystolic, grade 3 or more in intensity, most audible at the left upper sternal border, and harsh. The presence of an abnormal second heart sound and an early or midsystolic click also independently predicted disease (Table 2).

TABLE 2.—Association of Clinical Features With Confirmed Diagnosis of a
Cardiac Lesion

Clinical Feature	No. (%) With Cardiac Lesion	P
Age at encounter		
<3 mo	27/45 (60)	
3 mo– <1 y	23/43 (53)	
1– <4 y	10/62 (16)	<.001
4– <10 y	9/44 (20)	
10+ y	5/28 (18)	
Gender		
M	32/116 (28)	
F	42/106 (40)	<.04
Presence of symptoms		
Absent	63/192 (33)	
Present	11/30 (37)	.84
Family history of heart murmurs		
Absent	51/150 (34)	
Present	23/72 (32)	.88
Family history of heart anomalies		
Absent	48/132 (36)	
Present	26/90 (29)	.31
Presence of extracardiac anomalies		
Absent	72/213 (34)	
Present	2/9 (22)	.86
Presence of hepatomegaly		
Absent	66/208 (32)	
Present	8/14 (57)	.05
Presence of abnormal pulses		
Absent	71/219 (32)	
Present	3/3 (100)	.04
Presence of abnormal precordial activity		
Absent	61/207 (29)	
Present	13/15 (87)	<.001
Presence of an abnormal second heart sound		
Absent	59/202 (29)	
Present	15/20 (75)	<.001
Presence of an early or midsystolic click		
Absent	59/202 (29)	
Present	15/20 (75)	<.001
Intensity of murmur		
No murmur	1/5 (20)	
Grade 1	6/33 (18)	
Grade 2	32/139 (23)	<.001
Grade 3	30/40 (75)	
Grade 4	5/5 (100)	
Quality/pitch of murmur		
Vibratory	30/152 (20)	
Harsh	43/66 (65)	<.001
Timing of murmur		
Systolic ejection	43/176 (24)	
Continuous/diastolic	5/16 (31)	<.001
Pansystolic	25/26 (96)	
Point of maximal intensity of murmur		
R upper sternal border/neck	3/11 (27)	
Low to middle L sternal border/apex	45/149 (30)	.16
L upper sternal border	25/57 (44)	

(Continued)

TABLE 2 (cont.)

Clinical Feature	No. (%) With Cardiac Lesion	P
Presence of radiation of murmur		
Well-localized	25/108 (23)	
Radiation of murmur	49/114 (43)	<.003
Presence of a second murmur		
Single murmur	60/181 (33)	
Multiple murmurs	14/41 (34)	.95
Electrocardiographic findings		
Normal	59/188 (31)	
Equivocal	1/12 (8)	<.006
Abnormal	13/22 (59)	

(Courtesy of McCrindle BW, Shaffer KM, Kan JS, et al: Cardinal clinical signs in the differentiation of heart murmurs in children. *Arch Pediatr Adolesc Med* 150:169–174, Copyright 1996, American Medical Association.)

Conclusions.—Clinical evaluation by a pediatric cardiologist is adequate for distinguishing pathologic from nonpathologic murmurs in children. Echocardiography should be used only after careful assessment by a cardiologist and only when the diagnosis of cardiac disease is uncertain or positive. With improved clinical assessment skills for all providers, unnecessary referrals and the inappropriate use of diagnostic testing may be prevented.

▶ Table 2 shows the 6 cardinal signs that can be used to accurately and consistently diagnose an innocent murmur. Careful and complete characterization of a heart murmur is necessary. Murmurs that are pansystolic in timing represent a situation in which there is abnormal blood flow, inconsistent with an innocent murmur. Harsh murmurs are caused by the production of sounds of mixed frequencies associated with flow turbulence, findings again inconsistent with an innocent murmur. In terms of loudness, innocent murmurs are not grade 3 or more. Innocent murmurs are best heard at the apex of the heart and along the left lower sternal border. Any murmur heard outside of this area is more likely to be associated with some pathology. Careful auscultation in early systole and midsystole, together with the use of postural maneuvers, is necessary to detect the ejection click of a bicuspid aortic valve or the systolic clicks associated with mitral valve prolapse. Selective and focused auscultation of the second heart sound during all phases of the respiratory cycle is required to detect abnormalities in intensity or in the relative timing of the aortic and pulmonic closure components. Occasionally, an abnormally wide or fixed split of the second sound may be the only physical finding in a patient with an isolated atrial septal defect. Clearly, careful attention to these 6 cardinal clinical signs will help the noncardiologist to differentiate accurately the majority of heart murmurs in children.

The results of this study also confirm that clinical assessment by a pediatric cardiologist is adequate, without a chest radiograph, an ECG, or an echocardiogram, to differentiate between innocent and pathologic murmurs.

Echocardiography should be reserved for use by cardiologists after careful clinical assessment and only in instances of uncertainty or a positive diagnosis of cardiac disease. As noted in the previous commentary, the use of echocardiography directly by primary care physicians is probably cost-ineffective.[1] Echocardiograms ordered this way are frequently read by unseasoned individuals (frequently adult cardiologists unfamiliar with the practice of pediatric cardiology). Subtle normal variations are overread and frequently misattributed to cardiac pathology that isn't there. A high rate of "nondisease" results with this kind of approach.

The lessons from all this are simple. Learn the 6 cardinal signs of significant murmurs. When in doubt, don't do an echocardiogram. Refer the patient to a pediatric cardiologist, who is more likely than not to have a good set of ears. It will be cheaper for everyone in the long run.

Reference

1. Toews WH: *Pediatrics* 92:304, 1993.

Results of 12 Nationwide Epidemiological Incidence Surveys of Kawasaki Disease in Japan
Yanagawa H, Yashiro M, Nakamura Y, et al (Jichi Med School, Tochigi-ken, Japan; Japan Kawasaki Disease Research Ctr, Tokyo; Kurume Univ, Japan)
Arch Pediatr Adolesc Med 149:779–783, 1995   12–3

Objective.—Long-term epidemiologic trends in Kawasaki disease were examined by reviewing data from 12 nationwide surveys conducted throughout Japan at 2-year intervals, starting in 1970. All pediatric departments of hospitals having more than 100 beds were included.

Findings.—At the end of 1992, there were 116,848 cases of Kawasaki disease, with a male-female ratio of 1.38. Annual rates increased sharply up to 1979 and subsequently remained nearly flat, apart from outbreaks in 1979, 1982, and 1986 (Fig 3). Disease was more frequent in males and in infants younger than 1 year. The mortality rate was 0.3% overall, decreasing from 1% in 1974 to 0.04% in 1992. Recurrence rates ranged from 0.3% to 5%. Cardiac sequelae at all intervals were most prevalent in males and in young infants (Fig 6). Steroid treatment has largely been replaced by immune globulin (Fig 7).

Implication.—Although the seasonality of Kawasaki disease and its cyclical changes in incidence support a causal role for an infectious agent, the most recent incidence data argue against an infectious cause.

▶ We are fast approaching the 30th anniversary of the first case descriptions of Kawasaki disease. It was in 1967 that Dr. Kawasaki described the entity that now bears his name. Despite the passage of almost 3 decades, we continue to learn a lot about this fascinating entity. It is extremely likely that the disease did not exist to a great extent before the 1960s. The unusual increase in the incidence of Kawasaki disease, as seen in many countries, supports the hypothesis that Kawasaki disease has an infectious cause. Many argue against an infectious etiology, however. With the exception of the attack rate among siblings (this rate is higher than would be expected in the general population), data to date fail to support any particular agent as a cause. There have been no cyclical changes, nor has there been any recent seasonal clustering. Moreover, a recurrence rate for the disease of 4% is difficult to explain if the cause of Kawasaki disease is infectious. Even with these disclaimers, any betting person will put money down on a transmissible agent as being the etiology of Kawasaki disease.

As we near the close of this century, the fatality rate from Kawasaki disease continues to decrease; it is now less than 0.1%. Most likely, the improvement is a result of the widespread use of immunoglobulin and the better detection and treatment of coronary artery aneurysms with the widespread use of echocardiography.

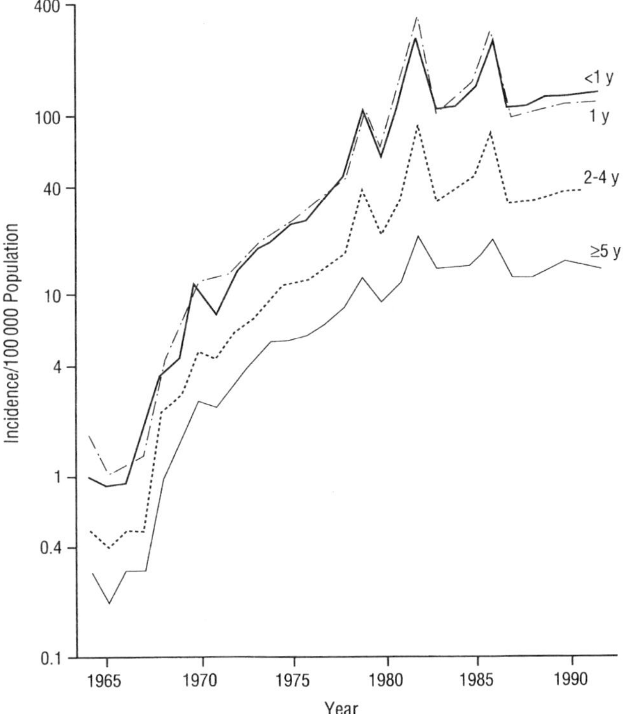

FIGURE 3.—Incidence rate per 100,000 population, by age and year. (Courtesy of Yanagawa H, Yashiro M, Nakamura Y, et al: Results of 12 nationwide epidemiological incidence surveys of Kawasaki disease in Japan. *Arch Pediatr Adolesc Med* 149:779–783, Copyright 1995, American Medical Association.)

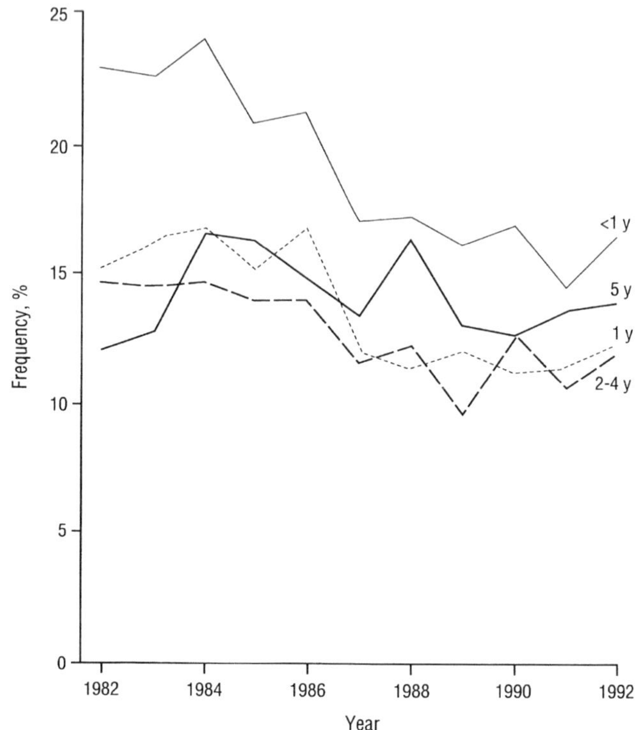

FIGURE 6.—Frequency of patients with heart sequelae, by age and year. (Courtesy of Yanagawa H, Yashiro M, Nakamura Y, et al: Results of 12 nationwide epidemiological incidence surveys of Kawasaki disease in Japan. *Arch Pediatr Adolesc Med* 149:779–783, Copyright 1995, American Medical Association.)

To learn more about the epidemiology of Kawasaki disease, see the article by Nakamura and associates[1]. For an excellent review on the diagnosis and management of children with Kawasaki disease, see the report by Gidding and associates.[2]

References

1. Nakamura Y, et al: *Acta Paediatr* 83:1061, 1994.
2. Gidding S, et al: *Heart Dis Stroke* 3:210, 1994.

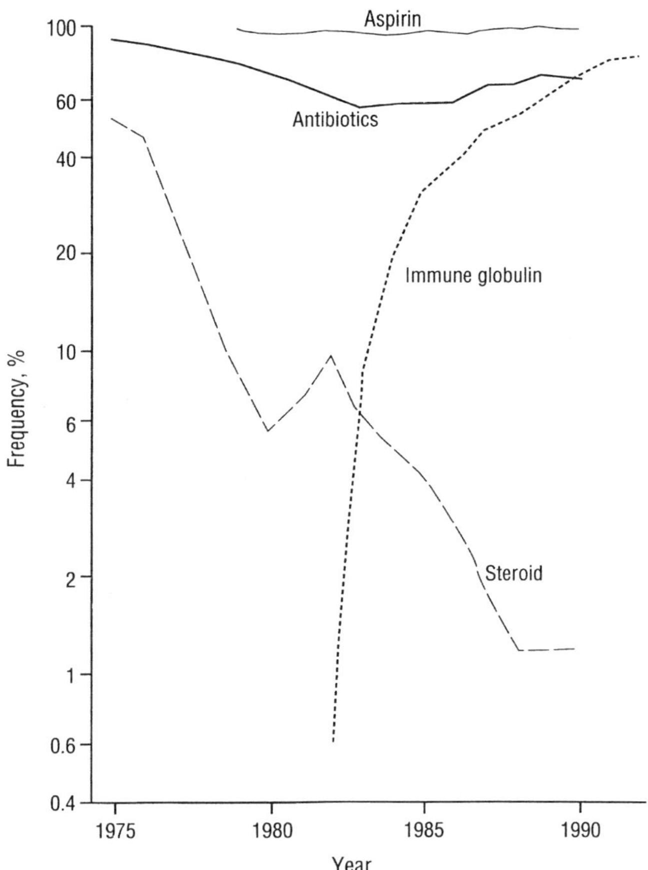

FIGURE 7.—Frequency of drug use, by year. (Courtesy of Yanagawa H, Yashiro M, Nakamura, et al: Results of 12 nationwide epidemiological incidence surveys of Kawasaki disease in Japan. *Arch Pediatr Adolesc Med* 149:779–783, Copyright 1995, American Medical Association.)

IV Gamma Globulin Treatment of Kawasaki Disease in Japan: Results of a Nationwide Survey

Yanagawa H, Yashiro M, Nakamura Y, et al (Jichi Med School, Tochigi-Ken, Japan; Japan Kawasaki Disease Research Ctr, Tokyo)
Acta Paediatr 84:765–768, 1995

12–4

Background.—Evidence suggests that IV gamma globulin (IVGG) treatment is effective against Kawasaki disease in Japan. However, the optimal dose and regimen continue to be debated. The use of IVGG therapy in Japan was described, and factors affecting pediatricians' decisions about the choice of IVGG regimen were identified.

Methods.—The pediatric departments of 2,652 hospitals were asked for information on IVGG administration for Kawasaki disease in 1993. A total of 1,826 hospitals, or 68.9%, responded. Data on 11,221 patients in

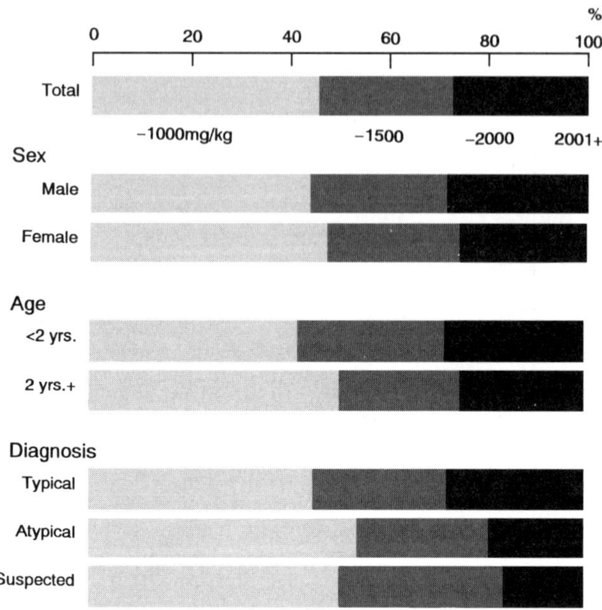

FIGURE 2.—Total dose of IV gamma globulin (*IVGG*) administration by sex and age (analysis of 8,958 patients treated with IVGG). (Courtesy of Yanagawa H, Yashiro M, Nakamura Y, et al: IV gamma globulin treatment of Kawasaki disease in Japan: Results of a nationwide survey. *Acta Paediatr* 84:765–768, 1995.)

whom Kawasaki disease was diagnosed in 1991 and 1992 were analyzed. A total of 8,958 patients, or 79.8%, received IVGG.

Findings.—The most common daily doses of IVGG were 200 mg/kg, given to 29.6% of the patients; 400 mg/kg, given to 18.7% of the patients; and 300 mg/kg, given to 12.9% of the patients. All of these dosage regimens were administered for 5 days. Total dose distributions were 1,000 mg/kg or less, used in 45.7% of the patients; 1,001–1,500 mg/kg, used in 27.3% of the patients; and more than 1,500 mg/kg, used in 23.8% of the patients (Fig 2). For all patients who received IVGG, treatment was begun in 53.8% by day 5 of illness, and in 86.1% by day 7 of their illness. Cardiac sequelae were more common in patients treated with IVGG (Fig 4).

Conclusions.—Nearly 80% of the patients were treated with IVGG, a significant increase from the numbers reported in surveys done in the 1980s. Treatment with IVGG appears to be more effective when it is begun on or before day 7 of the illness. The greater percentage of patients with cardiac sequelae in the IVGG group may have been because this group included more severely ill patients.

▶ The 30th anniversary of Kawasaki disease has arrived with 1997. The cause is still unknown. Interestingly, Dr. Kawasaki himself notes that there

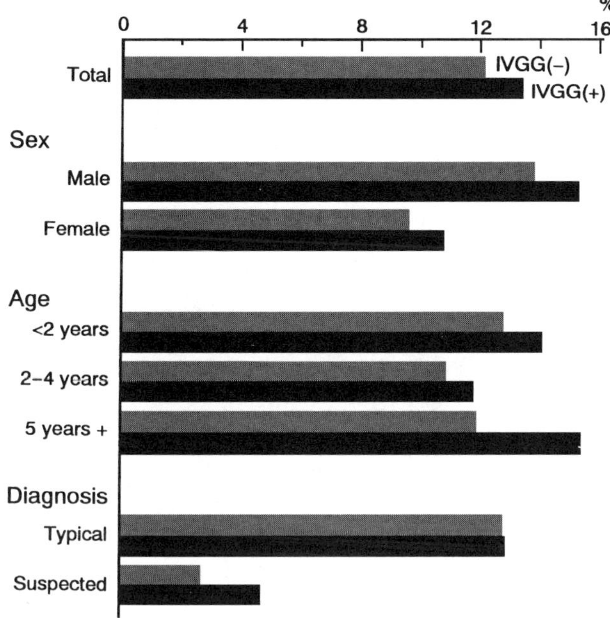

FIGURE 4.—Percentage of patients with cardiac sequelae by age, sex, and diagnostic criteria, according to IV gamma globulin (*IVGG*) administration. (Courtesy of Yanagawa H, Yashiro M, Nakamura Y, et al: IV gamma globulin treatment of Kawasaki disease in Japan: Results of a nationwide survey. *Acta Paediatr* 84:765–768, 1995.)

were rare case reports of autopsy findings of fatal cases described as infantile periarteritis nodosa long before his initial report. These earlier cases had exactly the same findings at autopsy as had been noted in children dying of Kawasaki disease. It might also be mentioned that in 1954, Bohman presented a case report in *Acta Paediatrica* entitled "Periarteritis nodosa in an infant of three months".[1] Is it possible that Kawasaki disease may actually be 42 years old?

The report abstracted tells us a great deal about the modern management of Kawasaki disease. The anti-inflammatory and antithrombotic effects of aspirin make it a suitable agent for the treatment of Kawasaki disease, and it was the main drug used before high-dose gamma globulin treatment was introduced. Today, the principal therapy in acute stage disease is, of course, high-dose gamma globulin with aspirin. A dosage of IVGG of 400 mg/kg/day for 4 or 5 days is commonly used, but studies from the United States suggest that a single large dose (2 g/kg) is a bit more effective and certainly shortens the hospital stay.[2]

What is most interesting about this report is that it verifies that Japanese investigators never shortchange on study design and implementation. Imagine 11,221 patients with a single disease diagnosed and treated within a 24-month period. As importantly, imagine that each and every one of those patients had complete and accurate records maintained to form the basis of this report. This is data management at its finest and should be the envy of us all.

To learn more about Kawasaki disease elsewhere in the world, see the report by Schiller et al.[3] Better yet, see a review article on this topic by Dr. Tomisaku Kawasaki himself.[4] The latter review is a modern medical classic.

References

1. Bohman M: *Acta Paediatr* 43:374, 1954.
2. Newburger JW, et al: *N Engl J Med* 324:1633, 1991.
3. Schiller B, et al: *Acta Paediatr* 84:769, 1995.
4. Kawasaki T: *Acta Paediatr* 84:713, 1995.

Guideline Maintenance and Revision: 50 Years of the Jones Criteria for Diagnosis of Rheumatic Fever
Shiffman RN (Yale School of Medicine, New Haven, Conn)
Arch Pediatr Adolesc Med 149:727–732, 1995   12–5

Objective.—The year 1994 marked the 50th anniversary of the Jones criteria for diagnosing rheumatic fever. The guidelines have been accepted worldwide but have been revised 4 times by committees of the American Heart Association. Each version of the Jones criteria was reviewed to determine precisely how the diagnostic criteria were modified, and to categorize the changes using the classification of knowledge-based maintenance activities formulated by Coenen and Bench-Capon.

TABLE 1.—Corrective Maintenance Applied to Classification of Manifestations of Rheumatic Fever

	Revision Year		
Manifestation	1944	1955	1965
Carditis	Major	Major	Major
Arthralgia	Major	Minor	Minor
Polyarthritis	NI	Major	Major
Chorea	Major	Major	Major
Subcutaneous nodules	Major	Major	Major
History of rheumatic fever	Major	Minor	Minor
Erythema marginatum	Minor	Major	Major
Evidence of preceding streptococcal infection	NI	Minor	*Necessary*
Fever	Minor	Minor	Minor
ESR, CRP, leukocytosis, prolonged PR interval*	Minor	Minor (split)*	Minor
Abdominal or precordial pain	Minor	NI	NI
Epistaxis	Minor	NI	NI
Pulmonary changes	Minor	NI	NI

Abbreviations: NI, not included; *ESR*, erythrocyte sedimentation rate; *CRP*, C-reactive protein.
* In 1955, the hematologic and ECG abnormalities were split into separate categories of minor manifestations.
(Courtesy of Shiffman RN: Guideline maintenance and revision: 50 years of the Jones criteria for diagnosis of rheumatic fever. *Arch Pediatr Adolesc Med* 149:727–732, 1995.)

TABLE 2.—Maintenance Activities Associated With Clinical Manifestations of Rheumatic Fever

| | Revision Year | | | |
Manifestation	1955	1965	1984	1992
Carditis	P	...	A	P, A
Arthralgia	C, P	P	P	...
Polyarthritis	C, P	...	P	P
Chorea	P	P	P	P
Subcutaneous nodules	P	P	P	...
History of rheumatic fever	C	...	...	...
Erythema marginatum	C, P	P	...	...
Evidence of preceding streptococcal infection	C	C	P	P, A
Fever	P	P	C	C
ESR, CRP, leukocytosis, prolonged PR interval	C, P	C, P	...	...
Abdominal or precordial pain	C	...	...	...
Epistaxis	C	...	...	...
Pulmonary changes	C	...	...	...

Abbreviations: C, corrective; P, perfective; A, adaptive; ESR, erythrocyte sedimentation rate; CRP, C-reactive protein.
(Courtesy of Shiffman RN: Guideline maintenance and revision: 50 years of the Jones criteria for diagnosis of rheumatic fever. *Arch Pediatr Adolesc Med* 149:727–732, 1995.)

Definitions.—*Corrective* maintenance identifies and corrects errors that result from identifying or encoding current knowledge. The need for this type of maintenance is recognized when incorrect conclusions are drawn from a given set of facts. *Perfective* maintenance modifies the knowledge base in response to user needs to render it more functional without making major changes in content. *Adaptive* maintenance alters the knowledge base to reflect new findings.

Observations.—The modifications that have been made in the Jones criteria are chiefly corrective and perfective. The original criteria failed to recognize that arthralgias and arthritis have different value when diagnosing rheumatic fever (Table 1). A number of corrective changes were made in an attempt to relate streptococcal infection to the diagnosis. The types of maintenance activities related to particular clinical manifestations of rheumatic fever are shown in Table 2. Examples of adaptive maintenance include the use of echocardiographic data to support a diagnosis of pericarditis, and the recognition that throat culture and rapid antigen testing have limited usefulness.

Implications.—The need for corrective and perfective maintenance may be lessened by making good use of existing knowledge at the time guidelines are published. Guidelines that are based on evidence and are properly structured should require minimal maintenance of this type. Adaptive maintenance may be anticipated by recording the quality of evidence or level of consensus supporting each recommendation.

▶ If you've never watched a football game and don't understand the meaning of the term "Monday morning quarterbacking," read this report. It is as good an example of Monday morning quarterbacking as you will ever find. If you are like this editor, you have a distaste for those who relish the use of the retrospectoscope. That is the feeling this article left with this reader. Some things in science are too precious to tinker with by trying to improve on them or even to explain them in greater detail than might have been done originally. The Jones criteria are a Stradivarius of medicine. It takes a fair degree of academic hubris to engage in an autopsy of these criteria. That having been said, there is something to be learned from any postmortem study, no matter how irreverently done.

So, what did we learn from this report? We learned that when T. Duckett Jones published his landmark article, "The diagnosis of rheumatic fever," in *JAMA* in 1944, he made some mistakes.[1] He did not include evidence of a preceding streptococcal infection in the original criteria, but then again, the link between group A streptococcal pharyngitis and rheumatic fever was just beginning to be recognized. That one problem aside, the other changes that have come about in subsequent revisions of the Jones criteria in 1965, 1984, and 1995 were enhancements to, not revisions of, the original criteria, enhancements in response to new knowledge.

The next half century is likely to be gentler and more deferential to the Jones criteria. The very fact that we haven't included an abnormal echocardiogram to the list of Jones criteria is evidence of that. With half a century of hindsight, most of us still consider Dr. Jones' achievement quite amazing.

Reference

1. Jones TD: *JAMA* 126:481, 1944.

Effect of Zidovudine and Didanosine Treatment on Heart Function in Children Infected With Human Immunodeficiency Virus
Domanski MJ, Sloas MM, Follmann DA, et al (Natl Heart, Lung, and Blood Inst, Bethesda, Md; Natl Cancer Inst, Bethesda, Md; Georgetown Univ Hosp, Washington, DC)
J Pediatr 127:137–146, 1995
12–6

Introduction.—More than 50% of adults infected with HIV have echocardiographic abnormalities. Children also have a high incidence of cardiac abnormalities. In HIV-infected children and adults, possible causes of heart disease include HIV itself, other viruses, malnutrition, cardiotoxic medicines, and zidovudine (azidothymidine; AZT). Other studies have been contradictory on the effect of AZT on the heart. The effect of AZT and didanosine on cardiac performance was studied in a group of 137 children infected with HIV.

Methods.—Echocardiograms, clinical records, and laboratory data from 137 HIV-infected children were retrospectively reviewed. The children were receiving AZT (52 children), didanosine (13 children), both drugs (1 child), or no antiretroviral therapy (71 children). Drug dosages varied, with AZT administered at 90–180 mg/m² every 6 hours, and didanosine administered at 90–180 mg/m² every 8 hours.

Results.—Children treated with AZT had a lower average fractional shortening than children who were not treated with AZT, despite correction of the echocardiographic results for HIV disease severity with markers such as CD4⁺ lymphocyte count, mode of acquisition of HIV, time since infection, and age. A nonlinear relation was present between days of AZT use and the decrease in fractional shortening. Children who had previously used AZT were 8.4 times more likely to have a cardiomyopathy than children who had never taken AZT. The development of a cardiomyopathy was not associated with didanosine.

Conclusion.—Development of cardiomyopathy may be associated with AZT in the treatment of HIV-infected children, whereas the risk of cardiomyopathy is not increased with didanosine. Serial cardiac examinations and echocardiograms should be conducted on all children receiving AZT, and the continued use of AZT in a child with cardiomyopathy should be carefully evaluated. Withdrawal of AZT should be considered in any child in whom cardiomyopathy develops, because of the association of AZT therapy with cardiomyopathy. This will depend on whether other HIV-related disease manifestations, such as neuroencephalopathy, are improving and whether alternate therapies are available.

▶ Cardiac abnormalities unrelated to AZT use can develop in children with HIV infection. Thus, it is important to determine that changes in cardiac function are not a consequence of HIV disease progression. Both AIDS and its treatment, AZT, damage the heart. Sorting out what causes what can be a complex issue. The fact that another drug (didanosine) used to treat HIV infection is not associated with comparable heart disease does suggest that AZT is cardiotoxic. Why AZT causes such odd effects isn't known. The theory is that this drug inhibits cardiac mitochondrial DNA replication.[1]

Concern about the role of AZT in the development of cardiomyopathy has led some investigators to recommend withdrawal of antiretroviral therapy in patients in whom symptomatic cardiac disease develops.[2] The conundrum is that if the cardiomyopathy seen in a child is actually a manifestation of HIV infection and not a result of AZT use, then a change in therapy would perhaps be wrong. Thus, the risk-benefit ratio of continuing AZT therapy must be carefully weighed in each patient and depends on whether other HIV-related disease manifestations (e.g., neuroencephalopathy) were improving and whether alternative therapies exist. One thing is for sure: this problem is of such significance that if HIV disease were cured tomorrow, a number of the kids treated thus far would be in need of a cardiac transplant.

References

1. Luginbuhl LL, et al: *JAMA* 22:2869, 1993.
2. Herskowitz A, et al: *Ann Intern Med* 116:311, 1992.

Diagnosis, Surveillance, and Epidemiologic Evaluation of Viral Infections in Pediatric Cardiac Transplant Recipients With the Use of the Polymerase Chain Reaction

Schowengerdt KO, Ni J, Denfield SW, et al (Baylor College of Medicine, Houston; Texas Heart Inst, Houston)

J Heart Lung Transplant 15:111–123, 1996   12–7

Introduction.—Cytomegalovirus and other viral infections cause major postoperative morbidity and mortality in heart transplant recipients. The traditional methods of diagnosing these infections, including peripheral viral cultures and serologic studies, are time-consuming and insensitive. There is no histologic technique by which to differentiate between viral myocarditis and acute cellular rejection. Polymerase chain reaction (PCR) was studied for its ability to diagnose viral infection in pediatric heart transplant recipients.

Methods.—A total of 129 right ventricular endomyocardial biopsy samples from 40 pediatric heart transplant recipients were analyzed. Polymerase chain reaction studies were performed to detect the presence of adenovirus, cytomegalovirus, enterovirus, herpes simplex virus, and parvovirus nucleic acid. The results were used to diagnose and follow the course of cytomegalovirus infection of cardiac tissue. Particularly in patients with unexplained late rejection or chronic rejection, the PCR findings were also used to detect other viral infections of the heart.

Results.—Positive results were noted in 32% of samples. Sixteen samples were positive for cytomegalovirus, 14 for adenovirus, 6 for enterovirus, 3 for parvovirus, and 2 for herpes simplex virus. Sixty-two percent of patients who were positive for viral genome had International Society for Heart and Lung Transplantation histologic scores of 3A or greater, which suggest the presence of mutifocal-to-severe rejection. The mean rejection frequency was not significantly different for PCR-positive vs. PCR-negative patients.

Conclusions.—For heart transplant recipients, particularly those with late-onset or chronic rejection, PCR may provide a rapid and sensitive indicator of postoperative viral infections of the heart. It may also be useful in monitoring the presence and course of cytomegalovirus infection. Multiple viral primers can be used for a better diagnostic evaluation and a better understanding of posttransplantation viral infections and the causes of late or chronic rejection.

▶ This article was selected, not because the average individual will need to know a great deal about how to diagnose viral infections of the heart in patients who have undergone cardiac transplantation, but rather because it shows how far along PCR technology has come and how it can assist us in circumstances that would otherwise represent serious diagnostic challenges. One of the latter circumstances arises in the postoperative heart transplant recipient. In patients who must undergo periodic myocardial biopsy to determine whether rejection is occurring, it is frequently difficult, if not impossible, to distinguish inflammatory changes of the heart muscle that result from viral infection as opposed to rejection. Viral cultures, serologic studies, and histopathologic studies lack sensitivity and specificity. Serologic testing is of no help when decisions have to be made immediately about instituting antiviral therapy. It was for such reasons that these investigators chose molecular techniques to detect the presence of viral genomes in cardiac tissue. They hypothesized that PCR could prove a rapid and sensitive means to detect viral genomes within myocardial tissue in heart transplant recipients. They were not wrong in their assumption. The use of PCR proved to be valuable both in the diagnosis and management of these patients. The authors clearly documented how molecular techniques can rapidly detect the presence of viral nucleic acid in tissue specimens.

More common than the problem of posttransplantation viral infection is the patient who has what appears to be a viral myocarditis unrelated to transplantation. Chow et al. and Hauck et al. have previously found that the ability to diagnose myocarditis in previously well patients using light microscopic analysis was only 50%.[1, 2] This low percentage can be bumped to 79% but requires as many as 17 different biopsy samples to be obtained from the heart. More recently, PCR technology has been applied to this broader category of patients and has been able to detect enteroviruses, the most common category of viruses that causes myocarditis in children and adults.

The best thing that you can do for a child with suspected viral myocarditis is to get him or her to a center that can perform an endomyocardial biopsy which includes PCR analysis. With such diagnostic tools now available, we can tailor specific antiviral therapies in a much more specific way than has ever been true in the past. We've said it before in the YEAR BOOK OF PEDIATRICS; it seems worthy of saying again: "PCR is the best thing to happen in medicine in a long time."

References

1. Chow LH, et al: *J Am Coll Cardiol* 14:915, 1989.
2. Hauck HA, et al: *Mayo Clin Proc* 64:1235, 1989.

Essential Hypertension Predicted by Tracking of Elevated Blood Pressure From Childhood to Adulthood: The Bogalusa Heart Study
Bao W, Threefoot SA, Srinivasan SR, et al (Tulane School of Public Health and Tropical Medicine, New Orleans, La; Tulane Natl Ctr for Cardiovascular Health, New Orleans, La)
Am J Hypertens 8:657–665, 1995   12–8

Objective.—Previous studies have shown that children have persistence, or tracking, of elevated blood pressure (BP) over time. However, little is known about whether high BP persists into adulthood and eventually develops into adult hypertension. These issues were addressed in a community-based study of a biracial population.

Methods.—The data were drawn from the Bogalusa Heart Study, a community study of the early natural history of arteriosclerosis and essential hypertension. For this analysis, a longitudinal cohort of 1,505 individuals was created from 2 cross-sectional surveys, 1 performed in 1973–1974 and 1 in 1988–1991. The cohort, aged 5–14 years at the time of the first study, consisted of 56% girls and 35% blacks. Tracking of BP from childhood to adulthood was assessed, including the ability of childhood BP to predict adult hypertension. A subsample of individuals were studied to find out whether multiple observations could enhance this predictive ability.

Results.—Childhood and adult BP measurements were significantly correlated, with variations by race, sex, and age. However, the correlations were unchanged after controlling for body mass index (BMI). About 40% of children with systolic and diastolic BP levels in the highest quintile still had BP levels in the highest quintile as adults. Childhood BP level was the best predictor of adult BP level, followed by change in BMI. In the second survey, clinically diagnosed hypertension was more likely in individuals whose childhood BP levels were in the top quintile: nearly 4 times more likely for systolic BP and 3 times more likely for diastolic BP. Forty-eight percent of the adults with hypertension had elevated systolic BP during childhood, and 41% had an elevated diastolic BP. African-Americans, individuals with a higher BP or BMI during childhood, and those who had gained more BMI from childhood to adulthood were more likely to have hypertension as young adults (Table 5). Multiple examinations between

TABLE 5.—Predictors of Essential Hypertension in Adults 20–31 Years of Age by Race and Sex in the Bogalusa Heart Study Cohort

Independent Variables*	White Males (n = 432)	White Females (n = 538)	Black Males (n = 218)	Black Females (n = 299)	Total (n = 1487)
Age (5-year difference)			1.3†	2.2†	
Baseline systolic BP (107 v 93 mm Hg)	2.6†	1.7	2.6‡	2.3‡	2§
Baseline diastolic BP† (68 v 57 mm Hg)	2.1				1.5†
Baseline BMI (19.1 v 15.3 kg/m^2)	1.5			1.6‡	1.3†
ΔBMI (9.8 v 7.5 kg/m^2)	1.7†	1.9‡	2.4‡		1.6‖
Black v white	—	—	—	—	2.4‖

Values are odds ratios, comparing high (75th percentile) vs. low (25th percentile) values.

* Independent variables included age, race, sex, baseline systolic and diastolic blood pressure (*BP*), baseline body mass index (*BMI*), and change of BMI from baseline to follow-up.

Variables entered the stepwise logistic regression model at $P \leq 0.15$. Baseline, 5–17 years of age; follow-up, 20–31 years of age.

† $P \leq 0.05$.

‡ $P \leq 0.01$.

§ $P \leq 0.001$.

‖ $P \leq 0.0001$; other values, $P \leq 0.07$.

(Reprinted by permission of Elsevier Science Inc. from Bao W, Threefoot SA, Srinivasan SR, et al: Essential hypertension predicted by tracking of elevated blood pressure from childhood to adulthood: The Bogalusa Heart Study. *Am J Hypertens* 8:657–665, Copyright 1995 by American Journal of Hypertension, Inc.)

surveys improved the ability to predict hypertension from earlier BP level; individuals with elevated BP levels at multiple time points were more likely to have hypertension as adults.

Conclusions.—Elevated BP levels in childhood persist over time, leading to hypertension in adulthood. Making repeated measurements of BP in childhood and adolescence can aid in predicting adult hypertension. Hypertension is also predicted by childhood obesity and weight gain during growth toward adulthood. Elevated blood pressure in children progresses for many years before the adult criteria for hypertension and hypertensive disease become clinically apparent.

▶ Bogalusa is fast becoming a more recognizable household name for a town in Louisiana than is New Orleans, all because of the Bogalusa Heart Study. When the Tulane National Center for Cardiovascular Health and the Tulane School of Public Health and Tropical Medicine launched the Bogalusa Heart Study more than 20 years ago as a long-term epidemiologic investigation of cardiovascular risk factors in children and young adults, who would have known that so much important data would be exuding from this population? Exude it does, and the wellspring of this data should continue for generations to come.

In the study abstracted above, more than 1,500 study subjects are being followed who were 5–14 years of age back in 1973. At follow-up, they ranged in age from 20 to 31 years. Thus there was a rich base of patients to examine, to find out what became of their BPs.

Persistence (tracking) of elevated BP over time has been well documented in children. However, few large-scale epidemiologic studies have shown the long-term persistence of elevated BP from childhood into adulthood, and more important, how the persistent elevation in BP ultimately develops into adult hypertension. This report fills in a missing piece in this knowledge void. Although several reports have shown that BP can be tracked for as long as 3–8 years in children and adolescents, this study shows that the same tracking can occur over a much longer period (at least 15 years), from childhood to adulthood. Childhood BP elevation does serve as a good predictor of elevated BP and hypertension in adulthood, especially when multiple observations are made. The study also shows that both childhood weight (obesity) and weight gain during growth toward adulthood independently predict future hypertension. These factors appear to be even more important than a parent history of hypertension, which explains only 1% of the variation of BP seen in children.

The people who work with the Bogalusa study tell us that we must measure BP. Such determinations most likely should be made at every medical examination. As more and more data are derived from the Bogalusa study, we'll likely know the best ways of modifying the behaviors of those at high risk to see whether we can prevent the serious problem of hypertension as is now seen in adults. To use the international vernacular, a milligram of prevention is worth a kilo of cure.

Heart Transplantation in Children With Congenital Heart Disease

Hsu DT, Quaegebeur JM, Michler RE, et al (Columbia Univ, New York)
J Am Coll Cardiol 26:743–749, 1995   12–9

Background.—Longer survival after heart transplantation has prompted a greater consideration of this treatment option for children with complex congenital heart disease. However, transplantation can be more complex and presents unique problems in this population, and some studies have reported higher mortality rates among children with congenital heart disease than among children with other indications for heart transplantation. The pretransplantation and posttransplantation courses of a series of children with and without congenital heart disease were described, and their outcomes were compared.

Methods.—During a 9-year period, 84 consecutive children undergoing primary heart transplantation were studied, including 37 patients with congenital heart disease and 47 patients with congestive heart failure secondary to other etiologies, primarily cardiomyopathy. Preoperative and postoperative variables and survival were compared in the 2 groups of patients.

Results.—Among the patients with congenital heart disease (mean age, 9.3 years), all but 5 had undergone previous cardiac surgery and 22 had undergone at least 2 previous cardiac procedures. Additional extracardiac procedures were performed at the time of transplantation in 23 of the patients with congenital heart disease. Of the 37 patients, 13 died after transplantation of donor heart failure, right heart failure secondary to pulmonary hypertension, postoperative hemorrhage, pulmonary hemorrhage, infection, rejection, and graft atherosclerosis (Table 4). Of the 25 survivors, 22 are performing age-appropriate activities. Comparisons of

TABLE 4.—Cause of Death in 13 Patients With Congenital Heart Disease

Cause of Death	No. of Pts
Donor failure	1
Right heart failure	1
Postoperative hemorrhage	2
Pulmonary hemorrhage	1
Infection (< 6 mo after transplantation)	3
Aspiration pneumonia	1
Fungal and CMV sepsis	2
Acute rejection secondary to improper cyclosporine dosage	1
Graft atherosclerosis	1
Infection (9 mo after transplantation)	1
Noncompliance with immunosuppressive protocol	2

Abbreviations: CMV, cytomegalovirus; *Pts,* patients.
(Reprinted with permission from the American College of Cardiology [*Journal of the American College of Cardiology,* 1995, 26:743–749].)

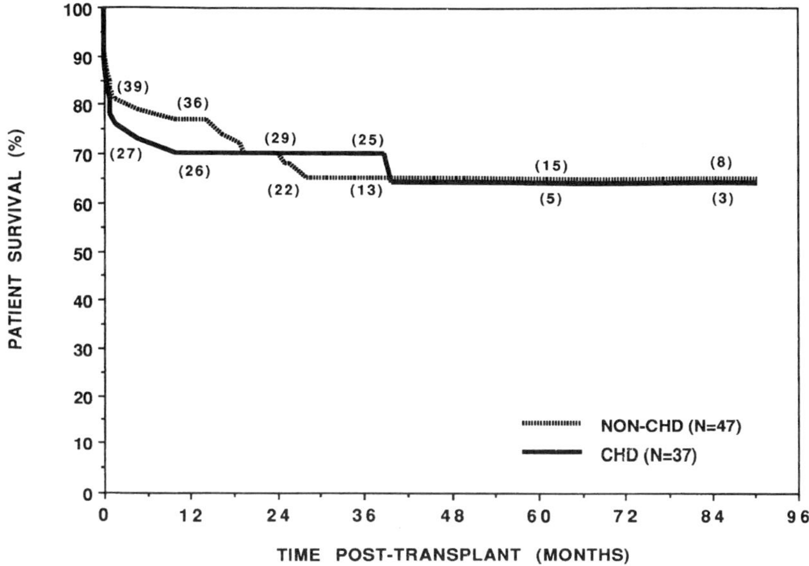

FIGURE 4.—Patient survival after transplantation in patients with and without congenital heart disease. *Abbreviation: CHD*, congenital heart disease. (Reprinted with permission from the American College of Cardiology [*Journal of the American College of Cardiology,* 1995, 26:743–749].)

the patients with and without congenital heart disease revealed no significant differences in pretransplant variables, including the age at transplant, sex, duration of congestive heart failure, inotropic medication treatment, or mean pulmonary vascular resistance index. There were no significant differences in survival (Fig 4), overall graft survival, or incidence of graft atherosclerosis or lymphoproliferative disorders. However, the patients with congenital heart disease had a significantly longer graft ischemia time and cardiopulmonary bypass time, and a greater incidence of postoperative infection.

Conclusions.—Although children with congenital heart disease require longer graft ischemia and bypass times and have a higher incidence of infection, their survival is similar to that of children with other cardiac diseases undergoing cardiac transplantation. Therefore, heart transplantation should be considered for children with congenital heart disease without other viable treatment options.

▶ If one draws an analogy between the engine in an automobile and the heart in a human being, one can understand the point of this report. Engines can be repaired, and indeed rebuilt, only so many times before a decision must be made about taking out the old one and putting in a new one. The only alternative is the scrap heap. As far as children with congenital heart disease are concerned, if surgery is not curative but merely palliative, there may be only so many times you can do an overhaul without seriously contemplating whether in the long run it would be best to simply replace the heart. We see that despite many prior surgical procedures, cardiac transplantation in children with congenital heart disease has the same success rates as in children who receive new hearts for disorders such as cardiomyopathy, where no prior surgeries have been performed.

The role of cardiac transplantation in children with congenital heart disease is now much clearer. Children who otherwise might have died as their heart eventually failed can now be given a new lease on life. Long-term survival rates, at 65%, are reasonably good after such surgeries. A youngster who survives 3 years after transplantation has a medium- to long-term prognosis that is excellent.

Ketoconazole to Reduce the Need for Cyclosporine After Cardiac Transplantation

Keogh A, Spratt P, McCosker C, et al (St Vincent's Hosp, Darlinghurst, NSW, Australia)

N Engl J Med 333:628–633, 1995

12–10

Introduction.—Ketoconazole has been used in combination with cyclosporine to reduce cyclosporine requirements. This is especially important given the high cost of cyclosporine treatment. Ketoconazole also has the potential to reduce infectious complications, decrease serum cholesterol, and reduce the amount of low-density lipoprotein–bound cyclosporine, increasing free cyclosporine levels. However, ketoconazole is hepatotoxic and may also result in resistant strains of certain yeasts and fungi. The efficacy and safety of low-dose ketoconazole in reducing cyclosporine

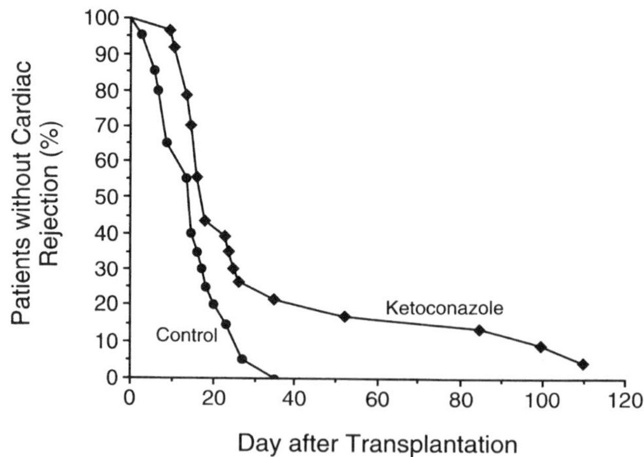

FIGURE 2.—Life-table analysis showing the occurrence of first episodes of cadiac rejection. Rejection occurred significantly less often and significantly later in the ketoconazole group than in the control group ($P = 0.04$). (Reprinted by permission of the *The New England Journal of Medicine,* from Keogh A, Spratt, P, McCosker C, et al: Ketoconazole to reduce the need for cyclosporine after cardiac transplantation. *N Engl J Med* 333:628–633, Copyright 1995, Massachusetts Medical Society.)

requirements were evaluated, and the effect of ketoconazole on infection and rejection rates after cardiac transplantation was determined.

Methods.—Forty-three cardiac transplant recipients were randomly assigned to treatment with either ketoconazole, 200 mg daily, or no ketoconazole (control patients), with treatment beginning on day 2 after transplant surgery. Immunosuppressive agents used included equine antithymocyte globulin, cyclosporine, azathioprine, and prednisolone. Methylprednisolone was given for cardiac rejection of grade 2 or higher (based on endomyocardial biopsy specimens); OKT3 monoclonal antibody or antithymocyte globulin were used for rejection that persisted after methylprednisolone therapy. Cyclosporine levels and cost of treatment were also determined.

Results.—At day 7, the cyclosporine requirements were reduced by 62% in patients receiving ketoconazole as compared with control patients. By day 28, a 68% reduction was observed, by 6 months, a 74% reduction, and by 12 months, cyclosporine requirements were reduced by 80%. At 1 year, actuarial survival in the ketoconazole group was 96% compared with 88% in control patients. The rate of cardiac rejection in the ketoconazole group was significantly lower compared with control patients (Fig 2). The interval between first and third rejection was also significantly longer in the ketoconazole group. The need for cytolytic treatment and total lymphoid irradiation were also lower in the ketoconazole-treated group, with 22% of ketoconazole patients and 35% of control patients requiring OKT3. Patients receiving ketoconazole also had a significantly lower overall rate of infection during the second and third months. The incidence of fungal infections was 9% in the ketoconazole group as compared with 40% in the control group. The cost of cyclosporine treatment was reduced from $6,640 to $1,130 per ketoconazole-treated patient during the first year, with a reduction to $950 in subsequent years.

Conclusion.—Combined ketoconazole-cyclosporine treatment after cardiac transplantation allowed for a reduction in cyclosporine dosage and cost, lower infection rates, and lower rates of transplant rejection. Although the effect of ketoconazole on cyclosporine has been known for some time, economic considerations have made the interaction more important. Ketoconazole is thought to inhibit the cytochrome P450 enzymes responsible for the metabolism of cyclosporine. Ketoconazole may also affect the absorption, excretion, volume of distribution, and protein binding of cyclosporine. Diltiazem, which also inhibits the metabolism of cyclosporine, has been investigated for its effect on cyclosporine dosage and cost.

▶ There are many reasons to think about using ketoconazole in patients who are receiving cyclosporine after transplantation. The article abstracted shows one fiscal reason this can be important.

The deliberate use of ketoconazole to reduce the need for cyclosporine is not new. Previous studies have shown that the requirement for cyclosporine can be reduced by as much as 88% using high doses of ketoconazole.[1] No toxic effects have been seen in more than 2 years of follow-up of combined use of these agents. Other theoretical advantages of ketoconazole include a reduction in the rate of infection because of the drug's broad antimicrobial effects. Additionally, a decrease in the level of low-density lipoprotein (LDL) cholesterol reduces the level of LDL-bound cyclosporine, leaving a higher level of free cyclosporine. A reduction in serum cholesterol levels could theoretically decrease any role that cholesterol might have in the development of coronary artery disease in transplant patients.

So why is the study abstracted important? It is important because there are possible disadvantages of ketoconazole. It is hepatotoxic, as is cyclosporine itself. Also, ketoconazole use has some concerned about the possible emergence of resistant strains of fungi and yeast. What this study from Australia does is attempt to show whether low-dose ketoconazole can still affect cost savings while being safer. Reduce cost it does! In adults, it saves an average of $100 per week. It causes no greater risk of hepatotoxicity or resistant infections. Astoundingly, the rate of rejection is much lower in the ketoconazole-treated patients, and if rejection does occur, the average time to rejection is twice as long.

Who can argue with something that saves money, does what it's supposed to do, and doesn't increase the risk of side effects? If you don't like ketoconazole, remember that grapefruit juice can also significantly reduce the requirements for cyclosporine, although fruit juice isn't much of an antimicrobial.[2]

References

1. Butman SM, et al: *J Heart Lung Transplant* 10:351, 1991.
2. Yee GC, et al: *Lancet* 345:955, 1995.

Blunt Impact to the Chest Leading to Sudden Death From Cardiac Arrest During Sports Activities

Maron BJ, Poliac LC, Kaplan JA, et al (Minneapolis Heart Inst Found; Dartmouth Med School, Lebanon, NH; Univ of North Carolina, Chapel Hill)
N Engl J Med 333:337–342, 1995   12–11

Background.—Although most cases of sudden death in young athletes result from unsuspected cardiovascular diseases, this is not always the case. Athletes with no structural cardiovascular disease or traumatic injury may die suddenly of cardiac arrest from a blow to the chest. This condition is known as cardiac concussion or commotio cordis. Twenty-five cases of sudden death resulting from a blunt impact to the chest in young sports participants were reported.

Findings.—The patients were identified by review of registry data and other sources, including news media reports. All but 1 of the patients were male; the age range was 3–19 years. All had cardiac arrest and collapsed immediately after an unexpected blow to the chest (Table 1).

Most of the injuries were inflicted by a projectile, such as a baseball or hockey puck. Sixteen occurred during organized competitive sports. In no

TABLE 1.—Clinical Data on 25 Victims of Blunt Impact to the Chest Resulting in Sudden Cardiac Death

Subject No.	Age (yr)/ Sex	Sport	Circumstances of Impact to the Chest	Collapse*	CPR in ≤3 Min	Chest Padding	Chest Contusion†
1	3/M	Baseball (R)	Struck by ball batted off T-ball stand 6–8 m (20–25 ft) away by 6-year-old brother near home	A	Yes	No	Yes
2	3/M	Baseball (R)	Struck by ball batted at close range (5 m [15 ft]) by 10-year-old brother in front yard of home	I	Yes	No	No
3	4/F	Softball (R)	Pitcher struck by ball batted at close range by 9-year-old sister in back yard of home	I	Yes	No	No
4	4/M	Baseball (R)	Strick by ball batted by father along the ground (30 m [100 ft]) that suddenly bounced up; in back yard of home	A	Yes	No	Yes
5	5/M	Baseball (R)	Struck by line-drive hit by adult friend on playground	I	Yes	No	No
6	6/M	Baseball (R)	Struck by ball thrown by mother (26 m [85 ft]) in 45-degree arc, in back yard of home	A	Yes	No	Yes
7	7/M	Baseball (R)	Struck by batted ball while standing 5 m behind and to the right of batter, an 8-year-old brother, in back yard of home	I	No	No	Yes
8	8/M	Baseball (C)	Batter struck by ball pitched 14 m (45 ft) by 12-year-old during batting practice	A	Yes	No	Yes
9	8/M	Baseball (C)	Batter struck by ball pitched 14 m by 9-year-old during game	I	Yes	No	No
10	9/M	Baseball (C)	Batter hit by ball pitched 12 m (40 ft) during game	A	Yes‡	No	No
11	9/M	Baseball (C)	Batter hit by ball pitched 12 m during game	A	Yes‡	No	Yes
12	10/M	Baseball (C)	Batter struck by ball pitched 14 m by 9-year-old during game	A	No	No	Yes

(Continued)

TABLE 1 (cont.)

13	10/M	Baseball (R)	Struck by batted line drive at 12 m while attempting to catch ball during school recess	I	Yes	No	Yes
14	12/M	Baseball (C)	Batter hit by ball ejected by pitching machine at 14 m	I	Yes	No	Yes
15	14/M	Lacrosse (C)	Goalie hit by shot on goal at 14 m during practice	I	Yes	Yes	Yes
16	14/M	Baseball (C)	Catcher hit by pitched ball at 18 m (60 ft) during game	A	Yes	Yes	No
17	15/M	Hockey (C)	Struck by puck from a forehand shot at 6 m (20 ft) during game	A	Yes	Yes	Yes
18	15/M	Hockey (C)	Struck by puck from forehand slap shot at 9 m (30 ft) during game	I	Yes	Yes	Yes
19	16/M	Baseball (C)	Hit by batted line drive at 30 m during batting practice	I	Yes	No	No
20	16/M	Karate (C)	Kicked sharply by opponent at close range during match	I	Yes	No	No
21	16/M	Softball (R)	Struck by batted ball at 27 m (90 ft) during family game in public park	A	No	No	No
22	16/M	Hockey (C)	Bodily collision with another player (i.e., body check) during game—shoulder thrust into left chest area of victim	A	Yes	Yes	No
23	18/M	Football (C)	Struck by helmet while tackling ball carrier during game	A	No	Yes	No
24	18/M	Baseball (C)	Struck near second base by ball thrown by catcher 37 m (120 ft) during pregame practice	A	No	No	No
25	19/M	Hockey (C)	Slashed with heel of hockey stick at close range during game	I	No	Yes	No

Abbreviations: R, recreational sport; C, competitive sport.

* A denotes a victim who demonstrated some activity after impact and before final collapse; I, instantaneous collapse.

† "Yes" indicates a contusion was present on the left precordium, probably representative of the site of impact.

‡ Victim was in a coma, with irreversible brain damage, 4 days (subject 11) or 9 days (subject 10) before death.

(Courtesy of Maron BJ, Poliac LC, Kaplan JA, et al: *N Engl J Med* 333:337–342, 1995.)

case did the chest impact seem excessive for the sport involved nor to have sufficient force to be fatal. Twelve of the victims collapsed immediately, and 13 were conscious and physically active for awhile. Nineteen of the victims received CPR within about 3 minutes; however, only 2 regained normal cardiac rhythm, and both of these patients died of irreversible brain damage. Twenty-eight percent of the victims were wearing protective chest padding when injured.

Discussion.—Blunt inpact to the chest can cause sudden death from cardiac arrest in young athletes. Most of these deaths probably result from a ventricular dysrhythmia induced by a sudden, blunt precordial blow. The impact most likely occurs at an electrically vulnerable phase of ventricular excitability. Hopefully, these findings will stimulate a better clinical understanding of commotio cordis as well as efforts to define its mechanism and to prevent it.

▶ It's difficult to think of any greater tragedy than the death of a healthy child or adolescent that results from participation in a sporting activity. It is similarly difficult to realize that baseballs, hockey pucks, football helmets, hockey sticks, karate kicks, and the human shoulder can be lethal weapons under certain circumstances. The forces involved with some of these deaths were not even extraordinary. A 6-year-old child was killed by a ball thrown by his mother who was some 85 feet away. A 3-year-old child died after being struck by a ball batted off a T-ball stand. The person batting was his 6-year-old brother.

As if all this isn't tragic enough, a fair percentage of these children and adolescents died while wearing "appropriate" protective gear. Most also had prompt resuscitations. Unfortunately, a prime feature of cardiac concussion is its irreversible nature in most individuals. There is only 1 report of a successful resuscitation of a victim after what appeared to be a cardiac contusion resulting in ventricular fibrillation.[1]

There is nothing new about sudden death in young athletes. The first record of such a death was that of the Greek soldier, Pheidippides, who collapsed at the completion of his legendary run from Marathon to Athens in 490 B.C., after delivering the message of victory over the Persians.

Sudden death from trauma to the heart represents only a very small fraction of the annual traumatic deaths in children and adolescents; most result from a failure to use seat belts or bicycle helmets, or are a result of firearms. The United States Product Safety Commission has followed deaths from cardiac contusion related to sporting activity for more than 20 years and still has not figured out a way to deal with this low-frequency, but nonetheless serious, problem in children and adolescents. In the meantime, children, adolescents, and their parents and coaches will have to decide for themselves what is the best protection while on the playing field or on the ice. Don't ask this editor his opinion about how to solve this problem.

Reference

1. Abrunzo T: *Am J Dis Child* 145:1279, 1991.

Supraventricular Tachycardia: Response to Cardioinversion

Heaton PAJ (Taranaki Base Hosp, New Plymouth, New Zealand)
Med J Aust 163:595–596, 1995   12–12

Background.—The recommended first-line treatment for supraventricular tachycardia in children consists of physical methods of increasing vagal tone, such as immersing the face in ice water and, for older children, the Valsalva maneuver. Vagal activity acts directly on the atrioventricular node, resulting in a reduction in tachycardia. A boy with recurrent episodes of supraventricular tachycardia unresponsive to conventional techniques of vagal stimulation but responsive to cardioinversion was described.

Case Report.—Boy, 7 years, had recurrent episodes of palpitations, lasting 1–2 hours, during a 2-month period. When 1 episode persisted for 6 hours, he was hospitalized. The presence of supraventricular tachycardia was confirmed on ECG. Facial immersion in ice water and carotid sinus massage did not decrease the tachycardia. The administration of IV adenosine had an immediate effect. Further evaluation led to the diagnosis of Wolff-Parkinson-White syndrome. Sotalel was prescribed but was stopped after 1 week because of excessive tiredness and coughing. Digoxin was then prescribed, but unrelenting nausea and anorexia necessitated the discontinuation of this medication too. Episodes of symptomatic tachycardia recurred once every 2 weeks, lasting for 30 minutes to 8 hours. Vagal stimulation by carotid sinus massage or by the Valsalva maneuver was ineffective. Verapamil therapy was initiated, but brief episodes of supraventricular tachycardia recurred periodically. During 1 episode, the boy's father became exasperated, picked up the boy by his heels, and held him upside down, which immediately restored a normal heart rate. Verapamil therapy was stopped. Since then, several episodes of supraventricular tachycardia have been instantly stopped by holding the boy upside down. There have been no adverse effects.

Conclusions.—Simple inversion appears to be an easy, safe, effective method for stopping supraventricular tachycardia in children. This technique may be more acceptable to children and their parents than other methods, such as facial immersion in ice water.

▶ There aren't many treatments that have not been tried to abort a run of supraventricular tachycardia (SVT). Most maneuvers are geared toward increasing vagal activity, which reduces tachycardia by direct action on the atrioventricular node. In infants, the diving reflex is stimulated by immersion of the face in cold water; immediate apnea is usually followed by bradycardia before restoration of normal sinus rhythm. Older children may be able to perform the Valsalva maneuver. Massage of the carotid sinus and compression of the eyeballs can work but occasionally can have fairly serious potential adverse effects. More than 1 eyeball has been ruptured in the name of better cardiac rhythm. Other less orthodox methods of managing supraventricular tachycardia include jumping off a ladder, firing a 12-gauge shotgun, and self-electrocution with an electric cattle fence.[1] Add to this list of unusual, if not bizarre, treatments of SVT, standing on your head.

The 7-year-old boy described had a particularly serious form of SVT secondary to Wolff-Parkinson-White syndrome. His arrhythmias were unresponsive to standard pharmacologic therapies. Also, ice water, Valsalva maneuvers, and carotid sinus pressure did nothing. Being picked up by his feet, on the other hand, worked.

Why being hung by one's feet works for this purpose is speculative at best. We do know that in such a position our blood pressure increases, resulting in some change in vagal tone.

There seems to be little harm in picking up a youngster by his feet as an alternative therapy for SVT. It certainly looks no more odd than pushing a child's face in a bowl of ice water. Unless you drop a youngster on his head, the child may actually enjoy this form of therapy. If nothing else, you'll get your workout for the day.

Reference

1. McKnight JA, et al: *BMJ* 297:1641, 1988.

13 The Blood

Estimated Risk of Transmission of the Human Immunodeficiency Virus by Screened Blood in the United States
Lackritz EM, Satten GA, Aberle-Grasse J, et al (Ctrs for Disease Control and Prevention, Atlanta, Ga; Orkand Corp, Atlanta, Ga; American Natl Red Cross, Rockville, Md)
N Engl J Med 333:1721–1725, 1995   13–1

Introduction.—The risk of transmission of HIV by blood transfusion decreased dramatically after initiating the screening of all blood donations for antibodies to HIV in 1985. There is a window of time when a recently infected donor is infectious before antibodies are detectable. The risk of HIV transmission from blood tested by contemporary HIV-antibody tests during the window period was estimated.

Methods.—Demographic and laboratory data were analyzed for more than 4.1 million blood donations obtained by the American Red Cross from 19 regions during 1992 and 1993. Results of HIV-antibody tests taken from 4.9 million donations from an additional 23 regions were also evaluated.

Results.—A total of 318 donations from the 19 regions were HIV-seropositive. Of these, 250 were from first-time donors and 68 were from repeat donors. The HIV-positive donors were more likely than HIV-negative donors to be young, male, black, and test positive on all other screening tests. In the 23 regions, 173 seropositive donations were made from 99 first-time donors and 74 repeat donors. The incidence rate of HIV for all donors in all 42 regions was 2.6 per 100,000 person-years. The probability of a donation made during the window period in the 19-region area was 1 in 360,000. The probabilities of such a donation being made by first-time and repeat donors, respectively, was 1 in 220,000 and 1 in 400,000. The probability of an HIV-positive donation being available for transfusion as a result of laboratory error was 1 in 2,600,000. It was estimated that 1.36 such donations could be made per year. In all 42 regions, the likelihood of a window-period donation was 1 in 450,000. Of the 318 HIV-positive units of blood, 133 were also seropositive on other screening tests. If the proportion of window-period donations were likewise seropositive for other tests, 42% would have been discarded. The estimated risk of an HIV-infectious donation being available for transfusion in the 42 regions ranged from 1 in 450,000 to 1 in 660,000.

Conclusion.—If the American Red Cross centers are representative of all United States blood centers, it is estimated that 18 to 27 of 12 million donations screened annually would be infectious for HIV. The estimated risk of transmitting HIV-positive blood is very small.

▶ The risk of transmission of HIV by blood transfusion remains a moving target. Currently this risk is almost completely the result of donations made during the "window period," when a recently infected donor is infectious but not detectable with HIV antibody surveillance. The probability of a donation during this period is related both to the duration of the window period and the incidence of HIV infection among blood donors. When HIV antibody screening began a little more than 10 years ago, the average length of this window period was thought to be 45 days.[1] With contemporary antibody assays to HIV types 1 and 2, the window period is averaging about 25 days. This shortening of the window period, as well as a lower incidence of HIV infection among blood donors (based on better counseling before donation and the questioning of prospective donors), means that the risk of receiving an HIV-infected transfusion has now decreased to 1 chance in 360,000. This means that there are an estimated 18–27 infectious donations available for transfusion in this country each year. That doesn't mean that 18–27 individuals would contract AIDS, because somewhere between 25% and 50% of transfusion recipients die of other causes within 24 months of receiving transfusions.

Is the risk of contracting HIV infection—1 chance per 360,000 transfusions—too high? The Food and Drug Administration certainly thinks so. It has recently recommended testing of all blood donations for HIV p24 antigen. On the basis of the estimated shortening of the window period by testing for p24 antigen, it is estimated that an additional 4–6 infectious units will be detected among the 12 million units donated nationally each year, units that would otherwise not be detected by antibody screening. Introduction of p24 antigen testing has been criticized, because to detect these 4–6 cases, several more millions of dollars a year will need to be spent on blood screening. Because 4–6 infectious units would result in only 2 or 3 cases of transfusion-related AIDS prevented, is this an appropriate way to spend our health care dollars?

One other way of reducing the risk of HIV infection from transfusions is to reduce the number of transfusions. Most hospitals across the United States now offer individuals the opportunity to donate their own blood before elective surgery, and surgeons are conserving their transfusion resources. With the advent of hematopoietic growth factors, the need for transfusions is further reduced. Computerized tracking and identification systems are decreasing sources of error related to transfusion. Given the difficulty of safeguarding human blood from the emergence of new infectious agents, and granted that noninfectious risk factors are rare but finite, blood has become one of the safest medical therapies around. Current data suggest that transfusion practice in the United States has become increasingly safe, particularly during the past decade. Today the risk from transfusion is less than the risk of being involved in a fatal accident sometime during one's lifetime.

To learn more about the safety of the U.S. blood supply, read the superb review on this topic by Sloand et al.[2]

References

1. Peterson L, et al: *Transfusion* 34:283, 1994.
2. Sloand EM, et al: *N Engl J Med* 274:1368, 1995.

Red Blood Cell Indices and Iron Status According to Feeding Practices in Infants and Young Children

Kim SK, Cheong WS, Jun YH, et al (Inha Univ, Seongnam, Korea)
Acta Paediatr 85:139–144, 1996

13–2

Objective.—Although the prevalence of iron deficiency anemia (IDA) has declined in the last 20 years, it is still the most common single-nutrient deficiency worldwide. Breast-feeding is generally thought to protect infants against IDA, but there is conflicting evidence on this point. The electronic counters used in modern laboratories permit practical determinations of hemoglobin concentration, red blood cell indices, and red blood cell distribution width (RDW) concurrently. This technology was used to examine the link between feeding practices and iron status in infants and young children.

Methods.—The study sample comprised 1,028 hospitalized infants and children 6 to 24 months of age, most with acute infectious or inflammatory diseases. Analyses of feeding history revealed that 299 children had been exclusively breast-fed for more than 6 months (group A); 608 had received iron-fortified formula since birth (group B); and 121 had been breast-fed for 5 to 6 months before being switched to iron-fortified formula (group C). Blood samples were obtained for measurement of hemoglobin, hematocrit, mean corpuscular volume (MCV), and RDW.

Results.—Thirty-five percent of children in group A were classified as anemic—based on a hemoglobin level of less than 10 g/dL—compared with 6% of those in group B and 7% of those in group C (Table 3). Nearly 40% of the children in group A had an MCV of less than 70 fL, compared with 7% of those in group B and 13% of those in group C. Eighty-two percent of anemic children had laboratory findings consistent with iron deficiency, which was usually suggested by the dietary history.

An MCV value of less than 70 fL was 90% sensitive for IDA, with a specificity of 54%. An RDW value of 15% or greater was 83% sensitive and 58% specific for RDW. The combination of MCV and RDW had a positive predictive value of 98%. Sensitivity was 62% for a serum ferritin concentration of less than 10 ng/mL and 72% for a transferrin saturation of less than 12%; specificities were 100% and 81%, respectively.

TABLE 3.—Incidence of Anemia in Exclusively Breast-fed (Group A), Formula-fed (Group B), and Switched From Breast-feeding (Group C) Groups

Age (mon)	Group A (%)	Group B (%)	Group C (%)	Total (%)
6 ~ 9	28/79 (35.4)	7/181 (3.9)	2/31 (6.5)	37/291 (12.7)
10 ~ 12	26/75 (34.7)	8/168 (4/8)	1/26 (3.8)	35/269 (13.0)
13 ~ 15	25/66 (37.8)	7/105 (6.6)	1/20 (5.0)	33/191 (17.2)
16 ~ 18	10/35 (28.6)	6/63 (9.5)	2/27 (7.4)	18/125 (14.4)
19 ~ 21	9/28 (32.1)	2/38 (5.3)	1/4 (25)	12/70 (17.1)
22 ~ 24	6/16 (37.7)	4/53 (7.5)	1/13 (7.6)	11/82 (13.4)
Total (%)	104/299* (34.8)	34/608† (5.6)	8/121 (6.6)	146/1,028 (14.2)

*$P < 0.001$ compared with groups B and C, respectively.
†$P < 0.5$ compared with group C.
(Courtesy of Kim SK, Cheong WS, Jun YH, et al: Red blood cell indices and iron status according to feeding practices in infants and young children. *Acta Paediatr* 85:139–144, 1996.)

Conclusion.—Iron deficiency anemia is common in infants and young children who have been exclusively breast-fed. When they reach the age of 6 months, these infants should receive iron-fortified weaning foods or an iron supplement. Screening for IDA can be made more accurate by combining hemoglobin measurement with MCV and RDW.

▶ These data are not very different from data from other studies showing that there is a substantial risk of the development of IDA after 6 months of age in solely breast-fed infants. As good as breast milk is, the mathematics are pretty straightforward: Compared with 250 mg/yr, the calculated amount of absorbed iron required during the first year of life, the total iron potentially incorporated by an exclusively breast-fed infant during a year of life is calculated to be just 57.3 mg/yr. To say this differently, despite the high bioavailability of breast milk iron, the necessary amount of iron just isn't there during the period of life (6–12 months) when infants are growing rapidly.

The data from this report also show something else important, i.e., that a hemoglobin determination by itself is an insensitive way to screen for iron deficiency in early childhood—not exactly news. What is new is the comparison of the relative sensitivity and specificity of other red cell parameters such as the MCV and RDW. The MCV is 90% sensitive and 54% specific. The RDW is 83% sensitive and approximately 60% specific. Put the 2 tests together (looking for an MCV less than 70 fL and an RDW equal to or greater than 15%), and you find a positive predictive value of 98%. If you are not familiar with the RDW, it is the standard deviation of MCV/mean MCV, a measure of variation in red cell size. In iron deficiency, the cells vary fairly markedly in size, and, thus, one expects to see a high RDW (greater than 15%).

It is this editor's opinion that not every healthy 9- to 12-month-old infant needs to be screened for iron deficiency. Those who have been receiving a formula with iron or who have received supplemental iron if they are breast-fed (assuming an accurate history) are quite unlikely to have iron deficiency.

Infants who have been breast-fed without supplemental iron, those who have received cow's milk, or those who have had more than their share of infections such as otitis media in the first year of life (such infections both inhibit the absorption of iron and its incorporation into heme) are at significant risk for iron deficiency and should be screened.

The data from this report reinforce what an adequate screen is. It is not a hemoglobin determination. It is a hemoglobin determination, MCV, and RDW looked at together. A normal hemoglobin value may exclude anemia, but it does not exclude other early hematologic signs of iron deficiency. Because iron deficiency sans anemia is thought to produce some, albeit modest, degree of cognitive and developmental impairment, we should be screening for it with MCVs and RDWs, not just hemoglobin concentrations or hematocrits. See Abstract 13–3, which also shows the inadequacy of the hematocrit in detecting iron deficiency.

Failure of Hematocrit to Detect Iron Deficiency in Infants

Kazal LA Jr (Baylor College of Medicine, Houston)
J Fam Pract 42:237–240, 1996   13–3

Background.—A hematocrit measurement is used routinely in infants to screen for iron deficiency, the most common nutritional deficiency in the United States. There are 3 stages of iron deficiency: iron depletion, decreased iron transport, and decreased hemoglobin production. The final stage of iron deficiency ancmia (IDA) is associated with behavioral, cognitive, and developmental deficits. To prevent these deficits, effective screening must identify iron deficiency in the earlier stages. A group of infants at righ risk for IDA were studied prospectively to evaluate the efficacy of screening with a hematocrit measurement.

Methods.—Infants aged 9–18 months attending clinics exclusively for low-income families for well-child visits were evaluated with measurements of both hematocrit and serum ferritin. Iron deficiency was defined by a serum ferritin level of less than 10 µg/L. Anemia was defined by a hematocrit of no more than 33%. Infants with both conditions were classified as having IDA.

Results.—Of the 321 infants studied, 6 (1.9%) were classified as anemic, 51 (15.9%) were classified as iron deficient, and no patients had both classifications. Serum ferritin levels and the hematocrit did not correlate (Table). The mean hematocrit in the patients with iron deficiency was in the normal range and was not significantly different from that in the patients without iron deficiency, as indicated by the serum ferritin level.

Conclusions.—Hematocrit measurement, the standard screening test for iron deficiency, was an inadequate indicator of iron deficiency in this group of infants from low-income, high-risk families. More attention is required for primary prevention of iron deficiency so that screening would be unnecessary.

TABLE.—Mean Hematocrit and Ferritin, by Race

Race	No.	Hct, % (SD)	Ferritin, μg/L (SD)
Hispanic	160	36.9 (2.1)	21.2 (15.8)
Black	138	37.3 (2.4)	23.1 (15.2)
White	8	37.1 (1.7)	22.8 (10.0)
Mixed/other	15	37.0 (2.2)	15.8 (4.2)
Total	321	37.0 (2.2)	21.8 (15.1)

Abbreviations: Hct, hematocrit; *SD,* standard deviation.
(Courtesy of Kazal LA Jr: Failure of hematocrit to detect iron deficiency in infants. *J Fam Pract* 42:237–240, 1996. Reprinted by permission of Appleton & Lange, Inc.)

▶ It's difficult to know exactly when in the history of medicine the hematocrit began to be used as a screening tool for the detection of IDA. This study demonstrates what other studies have shown. The hematocrit, although a simple screening test to perform, is quite insensitive. Screening tests should have high sensitivity. Specificity is not as important. Of the several hundred infants in this report, not a single one had IDA detected by the hematocrit, yet 16% had documented evidence of iron deficiency by serum ferritin assay. These results obviously raise a question about the most appropriate way to screen for iron deficiency.

The prevalence of IDA has declined across all socioeconomic groups, leading some to recommend selective screening of individual infants at high risk for iron deficiency instead of routine screening of all infants. Most agree that infants of low-income families should remain the exception to this rule. Infants of low-income families have 3 times the risk of iron deficiency as those above the poverty level, at least according to the Second National Health and Nutrition Examination Survey.[1]

Why is all this important and how should we screen for iron deficiency? The reason why it is important is that iron deficiency is still the most common nutritional deficiency in this country. The reason for detecting iron deficiency has nothing to do with anemia, but rather the fact that iron deficiency per se can cause behavioral, cognitive, and developmental disturbances.[2, 3] The trick is to detect iron deficiency before the late and infrequent last step in its progress, that of anemia. Serum ferritin, transferrin saturation, and free erythrocyte protoporphyrin (FEP) are typically considered diagnostic, but there are problems with each of these tests. Transferrin saturations are notoriously unreliable. Serum ferritin, besides being a measure of total body iron, is also an acute phase reactant and may be elevated in the presence of simple infections and inflammation. The FEP is not commonly available any longer (it used to be widely used to detect lead poisoning). One simple thing that may detect iron deficiency before its anemia stage is to perform a complete blood cell count and look for changes in the mean corpuscular volume and the red blood cell distribution width.

Given the absence of any perfect test to detect iron deficiency before the onset of anemia, the trick is primary prevention, not screening. Use infant foods fortified with iron. Avoid cow's milk. Breast milk is best but should be supplemented with iron starting at 4 months of age. The admonition against cow's milk should be for the entire first year of life.

In many respects, there's nothing terribly new in the article abstracted. Anyone who is still doing hematocrits as a screening test may find that it is now time to set aside this piece of laboratory antiquity. Given the frequency with which hematocrit tubes break either during blood sampling or in a centrifuge and the risk such breakage poses, there is probably little role any longer for the time-honored, but no longer revered, hematocrit. For the hematologists among us, this is a sad passing.

References

1. Filer LJ Jr (ed): *Dietary Iron: Birth to Two Years.* New York, NY, Raven Press, 1989, pp 19–56.
2. Lozoff B, et al: *N Engl J Med* 325:687, 1991.
3. Walter T, et al: *Pediatrics* 84:7, 1989.

Prevalence of Heterozygotes for Hemochromatosis in the White Population of the United States
McLaren CE, Gordeuk VR, Looker AC, et al (Moorhead State Univ, Minn; George Washington Univ Med Ctr, Washington, DC; Natl Ctr for Health Statistics, Hyattsville, Md; et al)
Blood 86:2021–2027, 1995   13–4

Background.—HLA-linked hemochromatosis is believed to be the most common genetic illness in whites. Previous research has estimated the prevalence of this disorder by identifying homozygotes in the population. However, not all homozygotes express the disease phenotypically; thus, the accuracy of these estimates is uncertain.

Methods.—Data from the second National Health and Nutrition Examination Survey were analyzed to determine the distribution of transferrin saturation values for the estimation of the prevalence of hemochromatosis heterozygotes in the United States population. The final analyses included 1,325 men and 1,547 women.

Findings.—After values for possible homozygotes were removed, 2 populations were identified for both men and women. When data were weighted to reflect the United States adult male population as a whole, a proportion of 850 per 1,000 comprised a population with a lower mean transferrin saturation of 29.7%, whereas 150 per 1,000 comprised a population with a greater mean transferrin saturation of 47%. Findings for the female population were comparable (Fig 1). Gene frequencies for men and women were estimated to be 0.081 and 0.070, respectively. These frequencies corresponded to the prevalences of homozygotes of 6.6 and 4.8 per 1,000, respectively.

Conclusions.—Two subpopulations were identified in this analysis of transferrin saturation data after the relatively small proportion of poten-

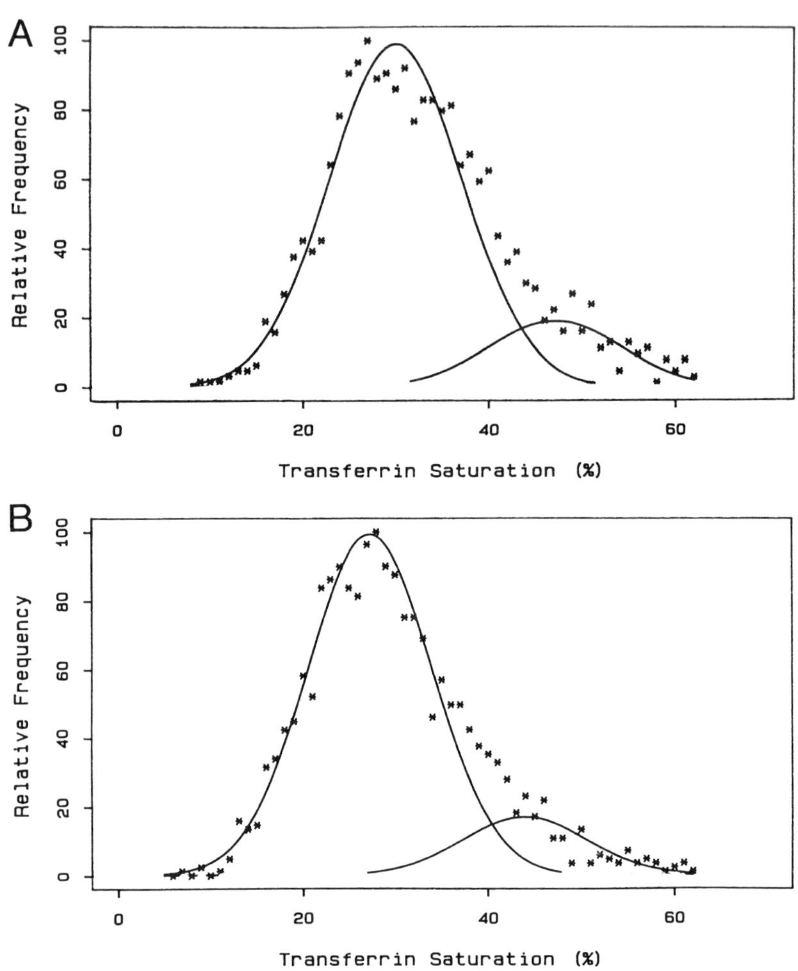

FIGURE 1.—Distribution of transferrin saturation values in (A) white men and (B) white women. Observed data are indicated with an *asterisk*. Fitted distributions are indicated with a *solid line*. The relative frequency indicates the proportion of subjects having transferrin saturation values within a given interval, relative to that of the interval containing the maximum frequency. For each interval the relative frequency is calculated by (frequency/maximum frequency) × 100. (Courtesy of McLaren CE, Gordeuk VR, Looker AC, et al: Prevalence of heterozygotes for hemochromatosis in the white population of the United States. *Blood* 86:2021–2027, 1995.)

tial homozygotes were excluded. One subpopulation consists of 85% of men and 87% of women in the U.S. population, with mean respective saturations of 29.7% and 27.0%. This group may predominately include individuals unaffected by the gene for hemochromatosis. In the second subpopulation, consisting of about 15% of men and 13% of women, mean transferrin saturations are abnormally high, at 47% and 44.7%, respectively. These individuals may be heterozygous for the hemochromatosis gene. Increased efforts for early diagnosis are justified.

▶ In case you think this editor has taken leave of his senses by selecting an article for inclusion in the YEAR BOOK OF PEDIATRICS that has nothing to do with pediatrics, you are wrong. The report abstracted has a lot to do with children. This study shows us that 5 or 6 adults per 1,000 have a homozygous form of hemochromatosis and that 7% to 8% of adults have a heterozygous form of the same disorder. If you remember the scenes from Dickens' *A Christmas Carol*, you will recall that Scrooge learned a great deal about himself by seeing what he was going to be like later in life. To say this differently, if adults have such a high frequency of hemochromatosis, so do the children for whom we provide care. Although it's not likely that children will get into major difficulty, if any, with respect to hemochromatosis, they may grow up to be adults who are compromised because of our lack of knowledge as pediatricians.

If pediatricians knew they were providing care to children who had hemochromatosis, they would be very careful in limiting access to unnecessary amounts of iron in the diet. Although heterozygotes for hemochromatosis who have no underlying hematologic disorder rarely develop iron overload states resulting in overt organ damage, kids and adults who are carriers have had marked iron overload develop if they have certain disorders, such as idiopathic refractory sideroblastic anemia, hereditary spherocytosis, pyruvate kinase deficiency, or porphyria.

The problem for providers of pediatric and adult health care is how to detect hemochromatosis. This report shows us that the average normal adult should have a serum iron saturation of about 30%. If that percentage is closer to 50%, it's likely that the individual has heterozygous hemochromatosis. If the serum iron saturation is above 65%, an individual is a homozygote, most likely in need of immediate treatment. As far as children are concerned, we don't know what the iron saturations are relative to the heterozygote and homozygote states of hemochromatosis. Thus, we are left in the dark, not knowing what to look for, but at least being aware that this entity exists.

The seeds of the problem caused by homozygous hemochromatosis are sown during the childhood years. The ill-fated harvest of that seeding will not come for many years, but it will come. Perhaps with additional investigations aimed at our pediatric population, we will know more about the relative importance of this interesting "adult" disease.

Discontinuing Penicillin Prophylaxis in Children With Sickle Cell Anemia
Falletta JM, for the Prophylactic Penicillin Study II (Duke Univ, Durham, NC; Children's Mercy Hosp, Kansas City, Mo; George Washington Univ, Washington, DC; et al)
J Pediatr 127:685–690, 1995   13–5

Rationale.—Infants and young children with sickle cell anemia are extremely vulnerable to bacteremia and meningitis secondary to *Strepto-*

coccus pneumoniae infection. Long-term penicillin prophylaxis carries a risk of accelerating the development of antibiotic-resistant strains of *S. pneumoniae*. Older preschool children seem to be less susceptible to pneumococcal bacteria.

Study Design.—Whether it is feasible to withdraw penicillin prophylaxis at age 5 years was determined. Children with sickle cell anemia who had received penicillin prophylactically for 2 years or longer up to age 5 years, and who also had received 23-valent pneumococcal vaccine between ages 2 and 3 years and again at the time of randomization, were eligible for the study. None of the patients had had documented bacteremia or meningitis caused by *S. pneumonia* or *Haemophilus influenzae* type b. Four hundred children were randomly assigned to receive either 250 mg of penicillin V potassium or a placebo tablet twice per day and were followed at 3-month intervals. The average follow-up was about 3 years.

Results.—Six children, 4 placebo recipients and 2 given prophylaxis, had systemic infection caused by *S. pneumoniae*. The relative risk was 0.5. Four of the causative strains were penicillin susceptible. Five children had bacteremia secondary to other organisms, 2 while receiving penicillin. None of the 4 deaths occurring after randomization resulted from infection. No serious adverse effects from penicillin prophylaxis were seen.

Conclusion.—Penicillin prophylaxis may safely be discontinued at age 5 years in children with sickle cell anemia who have not had severe pneumococcal infection, provided they are receiving comprehensive care.

▶ All the world loves a well-done study that gives us useful information indicating the best way to deal with a problem that previously had to be treated more with folklore approaches than with scientific ones. In the case of penicillin prophylaxis and sickle cell disease, there has been little to guide us in our timing of when to recommend discontinuation of penicillin prophylaxis as part of the prevention of pneumococcal infection. The report abstracted provides this information. After 5 years of age, children with sickle cell anemia who are receiving comprehensive care have a sufficiently low risk of acquiring pneumococcal bacteremia or meningitis that they no longer require prophylactic penicillin.

This does not mean that every child with sickle cell disease should have their penicillin stopped at 5 years of age. Cessation or continuation of prophylaxis to some older age should be based on an evaluation of multiple factors. Stopping penicillin treatment is reasonable *if* a child has not had prior, severe pneumococcal infection or a surgical splenectomy and is receiving comprehensive care. Such children must have received pneumococcal vaccine at appropriate times. Only if all of these caveats are met can one be reasonably secure in stopping penicillin at age 5 years. Otherwise, you are on your own when trying to decide when to stop penicillin prophylaxis.

A Comparison of Conservative and Aggressive Transfusion Regimens in the Perioperative Management of Sickle Cell Disease
Vichinsky EP, and the Preoperative Transfusion in Sickle Cell Disease Study Group (Children's Hosp Oakland, Calif; Univ of Washington, Seattle; Univ of California, San Francisco; et al)
N Engl J Med 333:206–213, 1995

13–6

Background.—Patients with sickle cell anemia are at high risk for perioperative and postoperative complications, with a perioperative mortality rate as high as 10% and a postoperative complication rate as high as 50%. As a preventive measure, the patients are generally given red blood cell transfusions. The transfusion regimens vary from conservative (enough to correct the anemia) to aggressive (enough to reduce the hemoglobin S level to less than 30%), and there is no consensus on the optimal approach. The rates of perioperative complications were compared among patients receiving either aggressive or conservative transfusion regimens, and the risk factors for perioperative complications were investigated in a prospective, randomized, multicenter trial.

Methods.—Between 1988 and 1993, 551 patients with sickle cell anemia undergoing 604 elective surgical procedures were randomly assigned to either an aggressive transfusion regimen (group 1), which maintained a preoperative hemoglobin level of 10 g/dL and a hemoglobin S level of $\leq$ 30%, or a conservative transfusion regimen (group 2), which maintained

TABLE 3.—Serious or Life-threatening Complications*

COMPLICATION	GROUP 1 (N = 303)	GROUP 2 (N = 301)
	% of operations	
Before, during or after surgery		
Miscellaneous intraoperative event	19	20
Acute chest syndrome	11	10
Fever or infection	7	7
Miscellaneous postoperative event	6	5
Painful crisis	5	7
Neurologic event	1	1
Renal complication	1	< 1
Death	1	0
Any complication	31	35
After surgery		
Acute chest syndrome	10	10
Fever or infection	7	5
Miscellaneous postoperative event	6	5
Painful crisis	4	7
Neurologic event	1	< 1
Renal complication	1	< 1
Death	1	0
Any complication	21	22

*Complications associated with transfusions are excluded here. The group numbers refer to operations.

(Reprinted by permission of *The New England Journal of Medicine*, from Vichinsky EP, and the Preoperative Transfusion in Sickle Cell Disease Study Group: A comparison of conservative and aggressive transfusion regimens in the perioperative management of sickle cell disease. *N Engl J Med* 333:206–213, 1995.)

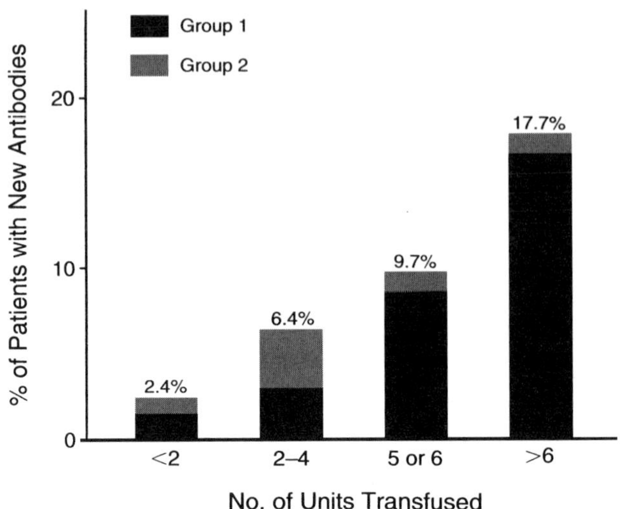

FIGURE 1.—Percentage of patients in whom new antibodies developed, according to the amount of blood transfused. (Reprinted by permission of *The New England Journal of Medicine*, from Vichinsky EP, and the Preoperative Transfusion in Sickle Cell Disease Study Group: A comparison of conservative and aggressive transfusion regimens in the perioperative management of sickle cell disease. *N Engl J Med* 333:206–213, 1995.)

a hemoglobin level of 10 g/dL regardless of the hemoglobin S level. All perioperative complications that occurred through the 30-day follow-up were classified as minor, serious, or life-threatening.

Results.—At the time of enrollment, average hemoglobin values were 8 g/dL in group 1 and 7.9 g/dL in group 2; these increased preoperatively to 11 g/dL in group 1 and 10.6 g/dL in group 2. The median hemoglobin S levels were 31% in group 1 and 59% in group 2 before surgery. A single transfusion was given to 77% of the patients in group 2, whereas in group 1, 57% received exchange transfusions and 30% received repeated transfusions. There was at least 1 complication in 31% of the group 1 procedures and 35% of the group 2 procedures, a nonsignificant difference. The most common complications were the development of new alloantibodies or transfusion reactions during the preoperative period and serious blood loss during the intraoperative period. Serious or life-threatening postoperative complications occurred in 21% of the group 1 procedures and 22% of the group 2 procedures and were most commonly the acute chest syndrome (Table 3). Multivariate analysis revealed that a higher surgical risk category and a history of pulmonary disease were independent predictors of the acute chest syndrome, and older age and more frequent hospitalizations in the previous year predicted painful crises. Overall, older age, CNS disease, prior alloimmunization, and a higher surgical risk category were risk factors for serious or life-threatening complications. The development of new alloantibodies was significantly more common in group 1 than in group 2 (10% vs. 5%) and was associated with the number of units transfused (Fig 1).

Conclusions.—The conservative and aggressive regimens are equally effective in preventing perioperative complications in patients with sickle cell anemia, but transfusion-related complications are reduced by 50% with a conservative regimen. However, even with optimal care, these patients are at high risk for perioperative complications.

▶ Until this report appeared, there had been no universal agreement on which approach, conservative or aggressive, is better suited to the surgical management of patients with sickle cell anemia when it comes to the issue of preoperative transfusions. Early reviews of operative mortality in patients with sickle cell anemia show death rates as high as 10% and the rate of postoperative complications as high as 50%.[1] The problems that may arise include perioperative hypoxia, hypoperfusion, and acidosis, which cause red blood cells to sickle, thus precipitating vasoocclusion and organ dysfunction. Because of this, most physicians have transfused red blood cells before surgery to reduce the proportion of sickle cells to less than 30%. This study performed by the Preoperative Transfusion in Sickle Cell Disease Study Group shows that what we have been doing probably is not necessary. The same levels of protection of a patient can be achieved merely by increasing the hemoglobin level to 10 g/dL. It does not seem necessary to decrease the hemoglobin S level to less than 30%. Merely raising the hemoglobin level with smaller amounts of blood seems to do the trick. Thus, a relatively small number of units of transfused blood can decrease sickling events in vivo.

There is an important point to be made about the results of this report. These patients with sickle cell disease were operated on in centers that had multidisciplinary teams. These centers had anesthesiologists who knew exactly what to expect in terms of complications of anesthesia in a patient with sickle cell disease. Unless there is some dire reason for a patient with sickle cell disease to be operated on in less than these optimal circumstances, everyone affected with this hemoglobinopathy should be afforded the benefit of surgery in an experienced institution. Anything less is not doing the patient a service. To learn more about the pathophysiology of sickle cell disease, see the report of the Meeting of Physicians and Scientists, University of Texas Health Science Center in Houston.[2]

References

1. Lubin NLC, et al: Sickle Cell Disease and Anesthesia, in: Gallagher TT (ed): *Advances in Anesthesia.* St Louis, Mosby, 1984, p 289.
2. Pathophysiology and management of sickle cell pain crisis. Report of a Meeting of Physicians and Scientists, University of Texas Health Science Center at Houston, Texas. *Lancet* 346:1408, 1995.

Isolating Fetal Nucleated Red Blood Cells From Maternal Blood: The Baylor Experience—1995

Simpson JL, Lewis DE, Bischoff FZ, et al (Baylor College of Medicine, Houston)
Prenat Diagn 15:907–912, 1995

13–7

Background.—Researchers are increasingly studying isolation and analysis of fetal cells in maternal blood as a noninvasive method of prenatal diagnosis. The authors have previously isolated fetal cells from maternal blood and used fluorescent in situ hybridization (FISH) for chromosome-specific probes to identify aneuploidy. More recent goals have been to achieve consistency in methodology and to determine sensitivity and specificity.

Methods and Findings.—Five glycophorin A (gly A) antibodies were evaluated systematically. All produced agglutination, which led to the abandonment of gly A antibody use for positive selection of fetal cells. Conversely, LDS-751 was found to be useful for nuclear selection. The use of flasks coated with goat antibodies against mouse antibodies was the best way to achieve CD45 negative selection. Using flow sorting for either $CD71^+$ cells or γ-globin–positive cells for positive selection, male fetal cells were detected in pregnancies in which the fetus was 46,XY in 10 of 18 and in 12 of 14 patients, respectively.

Conclusions.—Analysis of fetal cells from maternal blood may be more sensitive in detecting chromosomal abnormalities than analysis of tissue obtained by invasive techniques. Confirmation could be done by analysis of villi or amniotic fluid cells.

▶ If you as a practitioner of medicine think FISH is something you keep in a bowl, or have mostly on Fridays, or goes by the nickname Wanda, you have missed out on learning about one of the greatest advances in modern day medicine: fluorescent *in situ hybridization* (FISH). With FISH one can develop specific probes with fluorescence markers that identify chromosome segments of interest. Together with cell sorting, FISH allows, among other things, identification of small numbers of "foreign" cells in a population of many cells. For example, to answer the question, "Do fetal cells regularly circulate within maternal blood?" all one has to do is use a cell sorter and FISH (using a probe against a fetal marker) to find an infant's blood in the maternal circulation. The reason for including this article in the YEAR BOOK OF PEDIATRICS is pretty straightforward. With current technologies, including FISH, one can isolate and then analyze fetal cells in the maternal circulation. Such approaches have become an extraordinarily attractive method for non-invasive prenatal diagnosis, one being pursued by an increasing number of investigators.

The authors of this report were the first to detect fetal trisomy 18 and trisomy 21 by isolating fetal nucleated red blood cells and performing FISH for chromosome-specific probes. By 1993, 69 cases had successfully been analyzed in which there was detection of trisomy 18 or 21, done merely by taking a sample of mother's blood. No need for chorionic villus sampling or amniocentesis.

If you run across an article on prenatal diagnosis using maternal blood samples, pay attention to it. It is a technology that is truly the hottest thing going. Since 1987, the National Institute of Child Health and Development (NICHD) has sponsored collaborative investigations of the feasibility of isolating fetal cells from maternal blood for prenatal diagnosis. These studies have matured nicely, and since 1995, socioeconomic and demographic information has been obtained on all individuals undergoing such forms of prenatal diagnosis, with all data being accumulated in a central computer repository. The sensitivity and specificity of such noninvasive techniques are being compared to traditional invasive techniques such as chorionic villus sampling and amniocentesis.

Please do not consider this form of prenatal diagnosis to be, as yet, a procedure of choice. We still don't know the answers to a number of key questions. What is the optimal time during gestation to sample maternal blood? Is it possible that fetal cells may persist from prior pregnancies? What is the effect of potential confounding variables such as maternal and fetal blood types? Irrespective of these questions, the data to date tell us that we can assume for now that fetal cells can be recovered in a pregnant woman's circulation in 60% to 80% of cases. Preliminary data also suggest the possibility that fetal cells analyzed from maternal blood could be a more sensitive and certainly safer way to detect chromosomal abnormalities than analysis of tissue (e.g., villi) obtained by invasive methods.

The use of FISH extends well beyond prenatal diagnosis. It has been used to detect metastases from solid tumors using tumor-specific probes.[1] It can also help determine whether a leukemia has been cured or is merely in a quiescent stage.[2]

Many investigators are FISH'ing about these days, giving us new and valuable information on disease states that can be detected or monitored with molecular probes. Truly the age of Aquarius. To learn more about prenatal diagnosis by analysis of fetal cells in the maternal circulation, see the review of the topic by Bianchi.[3]

References

1. McManus AP, et al: *J Pathol* 176:137, 1995.
2. Martinez-Climent JA: *Leukemia* 9:1299, 1995.
3. Bianchi DW: *J Pediatr* 127:847, 1995.

The Changing Profile of Homozygous β-thalassemia: Demography, Ethnicity, and Age Distribution of Current North American Patients and Changes in Two Decades

Pearson HA, Cohen AR, Giardina P-JV, et al (Yale Univ, New Haven, Conn; Univ of Pennsylvania, Philadelphia; Cornell Univ, New York)
Pediatrics 97:352–356, 1996   13–8

Background.—The profile of patients with homozygous β-thalassemia is changing as treatment for this condition improves and the number of infants born with it decreases. The numbers, ages, ethnicities, and transfusion requirements of patients with homozygous β-thalassemia followed up at 48 medical centers in North America were documented.

Methods and Findings.—Mail questionnaires elicited information on patient age, clinical severity, and ethnicity. The response rate was 83%. Data were collected on a total of 518 patients, representing most such patients in North America. Eighty-three percent had transfusion-dependent thalassemia major (TM), and 14% had thalassemia intermedia (TI). The ethnicity of 62% was Greek or Italian (Table 2). The numbers of patients with TM in 5-year age intervals between 0 and 25 years were about equal. The number of patients older than 25 years fell markedly. Patients with TM were aged a mean 16.1 years. Sixty-six percent of the patients with TM of Italian or Greek ancestry were older than 16 years, whereas 77% of patients of other ethnicities were younger than 15 years. The 75 patients with TI had a higher mean age than patients with TM. Seventy-three percent of blacks with thalassemia and none of the Southeastern Asian patients had TI. The mean ages of patients with TM increased steadily over time, being 11.4 years in 1973, 14.2 years in 1985, and 16.1 years in 1993 (Fig 1).

Conclusion.—The increasing mean age and age distribution of North American patients with homozygous β-thalassemia show that modern treatments are effective. Also, only about 15 to 20 diagnoses in infants are made each year in North America. However, the immigration of non-

TABLE 2.—Ethnicity of Homozygous Patients With β-thalassemia (Major and Intermedia)

Ethnicity	N	%
Italian	229	44.2
Greek	92	17.8
Indian/Pakistani	56	10.8
Middle Eastern	47	9.0
Chinese	43	8.3
African-American	22	4.2
Southeast Asian	19	3.7
Other	10	1.9
Total	518	

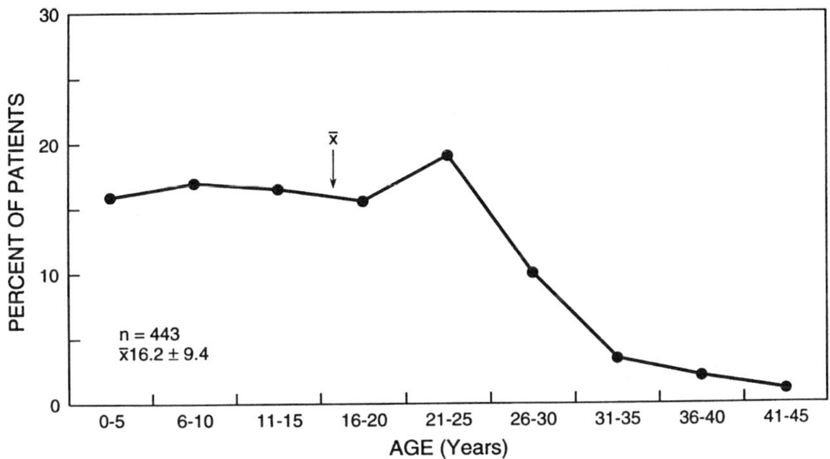

FIGURE 1.—Patients with thalassemia major reported by 40 North American medical centers. (Courtesy of Pearson HA, Cohen AR, Giardina P-JV, et al: The changing profile of homozygous β-thalassemia: Demography, ethnicity, and age distribution of current North American patients and changes in two decades. Reproduced by permission of *Pediatrics*, Vol 97, pp 352–356, Copyright 1996.)

Mediterranean ethnic groups with thalassemia has resulted in the presence of more, younger patients in the population. Increasingly, TM is becoming a disease of young adults.

▶ Shortly after the original description of TM by Cooley in 1925, it was recognized that the lives of patients with this disorder could be prolonged by transfusions of normal red blood cells. Early on, such transfusions were given infrequently because of the risk of iron overload, but beginning in the mid-1970s, they were given more often to maintain a patient's hemoglobin above 9.0–10.0 g/dL, in the so-called "hypertransfusion" range. Multiple blood transfusions inevitably produced transfusion-related hemosiderosis with resultant damage to endocrine organs, the heart, and the liver, causing death during the second and third decades of life. It was not until the early 1980s that effective chelation programs that used daily subcutaneous infusions of deferoxamine mesylate were widely implemented across the country. Such chelation is effective in producing negative iron balance. Regular therapy has been shown to prevent or slow the progression of cardiac dysfunction and to prolong life.

The increasing mean age of patients with TM in this report indicates that modern transfusion and chelation therapy do extend the life span of these patients. In 1973, only 16% of patients with TM were older than 20 years. In 1993, this increased to 33%. Despite this, very few current patients with TM are older than 35 years, probably reflecting the fact that effective chelation therapy has been widely used only for the past 10–15 years. Most older patients began therapy after they were 15 years of age, an age at which many may have already sustained some cardiac damage.

This report shows us the changing ethnicity of children with TM. Fewer patients of Greek and Italian background are receiving this diagnosis, presumably reflecting the fact that some parents are availing themselves of prenatal diagnosis techniques. Other families have chosen to have no children or to have elective abortions without prenatal diagnosis. In Italy and Greece, aggressive programs to screen for thalassemia carriers coupled with antenatal diagnosis have reduced the incidence of new cases of TM quite markedly. On our shores, there is an increasing percentage of new patients with TM among populations with non-Mediterranean ethnic backgrounds (Indian, Pakistani, Middle Eastern, Chinese, blacks, Southeast Asians, and others).

Read this study in detail. It teaches us that the aging of patients with TM has evoked new problems. Issues of sexuality and marriage produce major difficulties for some patients. Economic problems also have become evident. Young adults with TM are losing coverage on their parents' health insurance policies, and many have difficulty obtaining their own insurance because of their preexisting condition. Some are approaching lifetime insurance caps. We have also seen the social tragedy of bright, competent patients who have had to drop out of employment to qualify for medical coverage under social security. In a small but real number, HIV has developed as a consequence of transfusions some years back. As fewer patients with thalassemia are born and as their survival increases, TM is no longer exclusively a problem of children and adolescents but is a disease of young adults and even beyond.

Acquired Platelet Dysfunction With Eosinophilia in White Children
Poon M-C, Ng SC, Coppes MJ (Univ of Calgary, Alta, Canada; Subang Jaya Med Centre, Selangor, Malaysia)
J Pediatr 126:959–961, 1995   13–9

Background.—Acquired platelet dysfunction associated with eosinophilia occurs primarily in children indigenous to Southeast Asia and East India. The development of this disorder in 2 white boys who had lived in Malaysia for 12–18 months was described.

Case Report.—Boy, 6 years, was brought to a Calgary hospital because of a 4-week history of easy bruising. He was otherwise healthy and had not recently taken aspirin or other medications. He had been living in Malaysia for 1 year, returning to Canada 5 weeks previously for vacation. The boy had fallen and sustained unusually large bruises. The day before, he had had an abscessed tooth extracted and had continued oozing for 18 hours. On physical assessment, he was found to be healthy, with ecchymoses of his chest, back, and thighs. A hemogram revealed a leukocyte count of 9.5×10^9 cells/L with an absolute eosinophil count of 2.8×10^9 cells/L. Coagulation studies revealed a Template bleeding time of

17.5 minutes. The patient returned to Malaysia without specific treatment. During the next several months, the easy bruising spontaneously resolved. Ten months after his initial assessment in Canada, his leukocyte count was 7.3×10^9 cells/L with an eosinophil count of 0.3×10^9 cells/L.

Conclusions.—The 2 patients described in this paper had a mild, transient hemorrhagic disorder typical of acquired platelet dysfunction associated with eosinophilia. This disorder should be considered in children with easy bruising and eosinophilia who have visited Southeast Asia or East India.

▶ After reading about these 2 cases, I suddenly realized that I had seen a patient with a virtually identical clinical presentation. The difference was that the patient that I had seen was a citizen of the United States and had never traveled to a tropical or Southeast Asian country. This leads me to suspect that we may have been missing cases of acquired platelet dysfunction in association with eosinophilia in this country.

All of the children described thus far with this disorder have presented in similar ways. The chief complaint is easy bruising. The complete blood cell count shows normal numbers of platelets, but the eosinophil count is elevated. If you bother to do tests for platelet function, you will find them to be abnormal, particularly the bleeding times. What causes all of this is unknown. Given the predilection for the disorder to occur where it does, one might suspect that a parasitic infection is the underlying cause in some cases.

In any event, there isn't much one can do about the platelet dysfunction in children with this disorder. It would make sense to avoid agents such as aspirin or similar platelet-inhibiting drugs. The ultimate cure, as with so many things, is a tincture of time. With the passage of 6–12 months, everyone gets better.

Mortality in Patients With Hemophilia: Changes in a Dutch Population From 1986 to 1992 and 1973 to 1986

Triemstra M, Rosendaal FR, Smit C, et al (Vrije Universiteit, Amsterdam; Univ Hosp Leiden, The Netherlands; The Netherlands Hemophilia Society, Badhoevedorp)

Ann Intern Med 123:823–827, 1995   13–10

Background.—Survival among patients with hemophilia decreased sharply in the 1980s because of deaths from HIV infection or hepatitis. Patients with severe hemophilia are especially vulnerable. The overall percentage of Dutch hemophiliacs infected with HIV is about 13%, which is low compared with that in the United States and other European countries. A Dutch cohort of hemophiliacs followed up from 1986 to 1992

TABLE 4.—Standardized Mortality Ratios and Median Life Expectancies According to Severity of Hemophilia for Periods 1973–1986 and 1986–1992*

Variable	Severe Hemophilia		Moderate Hemophilia		Mild Hemophilia		Total	
	Standardized Mortality Ratio	Median Life Expectancy y	Standardized Mortality Ratio	Median Life Expectancy y	Standardized Mortality Ratio	Median Life Expectancy y	Standardized Mortality Ratio	Median Life Expectancy y
1973 to 1986								
All (n = 717)†	2.9	63	2.3	65	1.6	69	2.1	66
1986 to 1992								
All (n = 919)‡	4.0	61	2.6	65	1.1	74	2.0	68
Without AIDS (n = 907)	1.9	69	2.3	66	1.0	74	1.5	70
Without AIDS or liver disease (n = 902)	1.2	73	2.1	67	1.0	74	1.2	73

*Liver disease and AIDS were subsequently excluded from the analysis.
†A total of 7,788 person-years of follow-up.
‡A total of 5,753 person-years of follow-up.
(Courtesy of Triemstra M, Rosendaal FR, Smit C, et al: Mortality in patients with hemophilia: Changes in a Dutch population from 1986 to 1992 and 1973 to 1986. *Ann Intern Med* 123:823–827, 1995.)

was analyzed to determine the causes and rates of death, to document changes in mortality, and to distinguish hemophilia-related deaths from death caused by viral infections.

Methods.—The cohort included 919 males with hemophilia A or B who participated in a national survey on hemophilia in 1985. The median follow-up was 6.4 years, yielding 5,753 person-years of follow-up. The ages of patients at study entry ranged from 1 to 85 years. Data from this cohort were compared with data from a previous cohort follow-up from 1973 to 1986.

Findings.—Forty-five patients, or 5%, died between January 1986 and June 1992. The number of patients expected to die was 22.6, for an overall standardized ratio of 2.0. The median life expectancy in the earlier cohort was 66 years, compared with 68 years for the later cohort. When deaths from viral infection were excluded from the analysis, the life expectancy of this cohort was nearly equal to that of the general male population. One patient in the later cohort died of ischemic heart disease, compared with an expected 5.2. The strongest independent predictor of death was HIV infection. After adjusting for HIV infection, there were no other hemophilia-related risk factors correlated with the risk for death (Table 4).

Conclusions.—Death rates among hemophiliac patients have dramatically worsened in the past decade because of viral infections. In the absence of such infections, life expectancy apparently would have improved. The increase in deaths from viruses was most evident among patients with severe hemophilia, who are the primary users of clotting factor concentrates. Unless effective treatments are developed, the devastating consequences of hepatitis viruses and/or HIV infection will be seen for many more years.

▶ This study emanates from Holland. It would seem curious that an article from Europe dealing with hemophiliacs would be selected for inclusion in the YEAR BOOK OF PEDIATRICS, but when it comes to the long-term prognosis of children with hemophilia, Holland has many things to teach us.

In the United States, the majority of individuals with hemophilia have become HIV positive. Thus it is virtually impossible to tease out long-term consequences related to hemophilia that are not influenced by the concomitant presence of HIV infection. In Holland, on the other hand, the overall percentage of those infected with HIV is approximately 13%, a relatively small percentage compared with other European countries or the United States. A Dutch study, therefore, can examine mortality ratios, causes of death, median life expectancy, and age-adjusted relative risks associated with hemophilia, such as the presence of inhibitors and the use of factor VIII prophylaxis, in patients with or without HIV infection.

So, what do we learn? We learn that before 1960, hemophilia was characterized by excess mortality caused by hemorrhage, mainly intracranial. Once substitution therapy was introduced in the 1960s, there was a rapid decrease in hemophilia-related mortality. However, survival decreased sharply in the late 1980s because of deaths from HIV or hepatitis infections, particularly in patients with severe hemophilia. Because of the HIV infection problem, AIDS has become the predominant cause of death (more than 50% of deaths) among patients with hemophilia A in the United States. Additionally, the number of deaths from liver disease has increased more than threefold. Absent HIV infection (which usually means absent other viruses such as hepatitis B and C that can cause liver disease and death), this Dutch study shows us how well hemophiliacs are doing these days. If one does not become infected, survival to old age is now possible. We also see that individuals who receive prophylaxis rather than episodic factor replacement do much better. We learn that the terrible problem of inhibitors and early mortality that was seen in the 1970s and early 1980s is no longer a contributor to a significant increase in the risk of death. Additionally, we see that hemophiliacs have a lesser chance of dying of certain diseases. Take, for example, heart attacks. Hemophiliacs appear to have one fifth the chance of having a myocardial infection in comparison with age-match controls. It has been suggested that a high level of factor VIII activity is associated with an increased incidence of heart attacks because it predisposes patients to thrombosis. No patient with hemophilia, not even those on prophylaxis, runs consistently high levels of factor VIII.

In summary, the long-term prognosis for patients with hemophilia, if charted out, has a bimodal pattern. The prognosis for patients with HIV infection is bleak. The prognosis for those with hepatitis C infection is questionable. Estimates are that 50% of patients infected with hepatitis C will subsequently have chronic hepatitis, and that many of them will progress to cirrhosis. Absent AIDS and cirrhosis, the prognosis for the remainder of hemophiliacs is a life expectancy that will be almost normal. Unfortunately, many decades will pass before total mortality is no longer excessive. These are the decades in which those with HIV infection and liver disease will be dying. Because the currently available recombinant replacement products are HIV-free, given enough time, we will see a whole new generation of completely, or nearly completely, healthy hemophiliacs.

To learn more about the effects of factor VIII concentrates on the immune system of patients with hemophilia, see the article by Mannucci.[1] To see what the current issues are with regard to AIDS and hemophilia, see the summary by Evatt.[2] Finally, to get a good overview of the total management of a child with hemophilia, see the superb analysis of this topic by Aladort.[3]

References

1. Mannucci PM: *Thromb Haemost* 74:437, 1995.
2. Evatt BL: *Thromb Haemost* 74:36, 1995.
3. Aladort LM: *Thromb Haemost* 74:440, 1995.

Factor VIII Gene Inversions in Severe Hemophilia A: Results of an International Consortium Study

Antonarakis SE, Rossiter JP, Young M, et al (Geneva Univ, Switzerland; Johns Hopkins Univ, Baltimore, Md; Univ of Münster, Germany; et al)
Blood 86:2206–2212, 1995   13–11

Background.—Most mutations of the coagulation factor VIII gene, which are associated with hemophilia A, are found in a single family or a few unrelated families. Recently, a number of unrelated, severely affected patients had a common inversion of the gene that is mediated by the presence of 3 copies of a DNA sequence—sequence A. Unequal crossing over between 2 of the sequences leads to inversion of exons 1–22 and precludes the formation of intact factor VIII protein.

Objective.—A consortium study was conducted by 22 molecular diagnostic laboratories in 14 countries to determine the role of factor VIII gene inversions in severe hemophilia. A total of 2,093 patients had Southern blot studies for the presence of a factor VIII inversion. Including some mildly to moderately affected patients evaluated by some of the participating laboratories, a total of 2,560 patients were studied.

Findings.—A distal factor VIII gene inversion was identified in 35% of cases and a proximal inversion in 7%. Other abnormal or polymorphic patterns were found in 25 cases. All but 2% of 532 mothers of patients carrying gene inversions themselves carried the abnormal gene. Nine of 225 mothers of nonfamilial cases had de novo inversions in maternal germ cells. A de novo factor VIII inversion originated in germ cells of the maternal grandfather in 69 cases, and in the maternal grandmother in only 1 instance. Factor VIII inhibitors were only slightly more prevalent in patients with, than those without, gene inversions (20% vs. 16%).

Summary.—About one third of cases of severe hemophilia were associated with a distal inversion in the factor VIII gene. Inversions do not predispose strongly to the development of factor VIII inhibitors.

▶ This report was selected for inclusion in the YEAR BOOK, not because it is on your "must-read" list, but because the information it contains provides another stitch in the tapestry of what ultimately will be a full understanding of the genetics of hemophilia A. This entity is not a rare disorder. In this country, about 1 in 5,000 boys is affected. The gene for factor VIII was cloned about a decade ago, and since then many mutations have been described. Most of these are known as "private" mutations, that is, they have been found in 1 or only a few unrelated families. Recently, a common inversion of the factor VIII gene was identified in many unrelated patients with severe hemophilia. An inversion occurs when there is unequal crossing over between 2 abnormal gene sequences; in factor VIII hemophilia, gene inversion results in no intact factor VIII protein being produced. We see from this report that in excess of 35% of all factor VIII hemophilias are the result of such gene inversions.

These data are critical to our understanding of the genetic inheritance, carrier detection, and prenatal diagnosis of hemophilia. Although gene analysis is technically demanding in patients with hemophilia A (more so than for hemophilia B) because of the greater complexity of the factor VIII gene, the recent description of X-chromosome inversions as a cause of severe hemophilia in close to half of patients now permits us to readily detect these inversions in families with a very precise means of carrier detection.

Stay tuned for more stitches in the tapestry. In the meantime, to further your knowledge of the latest with respect to genes and hemophilia, see the references listed below.[1-4]

References

1. Peak EI: *Thromb Haemost* 74:40, 1995.
2. Thompson AR: *Thromb Haemost* 74:45, 1995.
3. Fallaux FJ, et al: *Thromb Haemost* 74:263, 1995.
4. Antonarakis SE: *Thromb Haemost* 74:322, 1995.

Survival in Families With Hereditary Protein C Deficiency, 1820 to 1993
Allaart CF, Rosendaal FR, Noteboom WMP, et al (Univ Hosp, Leiden, The Netherlands)
BMJ 311:910–913, 1995   13–12

Background.—Protein C is a natural clot-inhibiting factor that, when activated, renders factors Va and VIIIa inactive. In families with hereditary protein C deficiency, those heterozygous for the defect are at increased risk of venous thromboembolism. If these individuals have increased mortality as a result, prophylactic anticoagulation might be indicated.

Objective.—Whether anticoagulant therapy is warranted was studied by determining the mortality risk associated with the heterozygous state in 23 affected families registered in The Netherlands between 1820 and 1993. A total of 736 probands and relatives having a 50% or 100% genetic likelihood of being heterozygous were studied.

Findings.—No excess mortality was evident in the 206 proven heterozygotes and "obligatory transmitters" (those who definitely transmitted protein C deficiency). The standardized mortality ratio was 0.95 in this group (Fig 2) and 1.10 in 380 family members of unknown status who had a 50% genetic probability of being heterozygous.

Conclusion.—Heterozygous members of families with inherited protein C deficiency type I are not at increased risk of dying compared with the general population. Although prophylactic anticoagulation may prevent thrombotic events, it will not enhance survival.

▶ This editor found this report fascinating. It is important in its own right because it tells us a lot about protein C deficiency, but as importantly, it is the only study of its type that traces a genetic disorder back many generations (in this case, 173 years) to determine the impact of that genetic

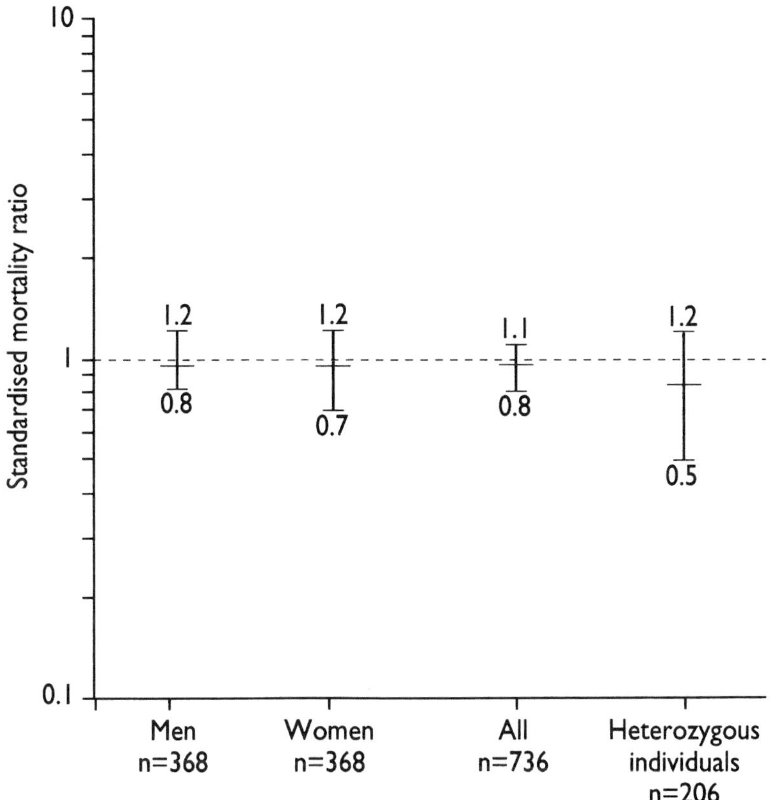

FIGURE 2.—Mortality for 368 men and 368 women with 50% or 100% genetic probability of being heterozygous for hereditary protein C deficiency type I and for 206 individuals with 100% probability of being heterozygous, on basis of DNA analysis or their place in pedigree. (Courtesy of Allaart CF, Rosendaal FR, Noteboom WMP, et al: Survival in families with hereditary protein C deficiency, 1820 to 1993. *BMJ* 311:910–913, 1995.)

disease on mortality rates. Only in a country such as The Netherlands, where careful record keeping has occurred for almost 2 centuries, could one undertake such an investigation.

By way of background, protein C deficiency (along with protein S deficiency, antithrombin III deficiency, and factor V Leiden deficiency) is a major cause of problems related to venous thrombosis. Protein C is a natural clotting inhibitor that in its activated form renders inactive certain clotting factors (Va and VIIIa). In families with symptoms of hereditary protein C deficiency in the heterozygotic form, there is an increased risk of superficial thrombophlebitis and deep vein thrombosis, both of which can be life-threatening because they can lead to pulmonary embolism. What is not known is whether routine prophylactic anticoagulant treatment of carriers of this disorder would reduce thrombotic events and prolong one's life. To investigate the effect of prophylactic anticoagulation on the survival of carrier individuals would require a long-term follow-up and would likely have many ethical problems associated with it. Hence the importance of this report, which shows that in families with a high prevalence of the carrier state (going back 170 years), there is no difference in mortality rates compared with the normal population.

Please note that these conclusions are based on individuals with the heterozygous form of protein C deficiency. Infants who are homozygous or doubly heterozygous for the deficiency frequently have life-threatening thrombotic complications. Such infants surviving the newborn period are likely to become children who will have an ongoing problem with an overly zealous clotting system.

Several recent reviews dealing with thrombotic complications in children are well worth reading.[1-3]

References

1. Andrew M: *Thromb Haemost* 74:415, 1995.
2. Less AJ: *J Pediatr Health Care* September/October 1995, p 222.
3. de Chalain T, et al: *Ann Plast Surg* 35:300, 1995.

Thrombosis in Otherwise Well Children With the Factor V Leiden Mutation
Sifontes MT, Nuss R, Jacobson LJ, et al (Univ of Colorado, Denver; Children's Hosp, Denver; Scripps Research Inst, La Jolla, Calif)
J Pediatr 128:324–328, 1996   13–13

Introduction.—Factor V Leiden mutation—an arginine-506–to–glutamine mutation associated with resistance to activated protein C—is the most common genetic defect associated with venous thrombosis. In a previous study, 70% of children with thromboses were found to have 1 or more hemostatic abnormalities. However, that study did not look for the factor V Leiden mutation. The relationship between factor V Leiden mutation and thrombosis in children was investigated.

Methods.—Fourteen children with thrombosis were screened for activated protein C resistance by determination of the normalized activated protein C sensitivity ratio. If the screening results were abnormal, factor V Leiden mutation was sought by DNA analysis. The DNA studies were also performed in the family members of children with activated protein C resistance.

Results.—The normalized activated protein C sensitivity ratio was abnormal in 3 of the 14 children. All 3 children had hyperlipidemia, and 1 had protein S deficiency. The DNA studies confirmed the presence of factor V Leiden mutation in all 3 children with positive screening results, and members of the family of each child also had the mutation.

Conclusion.—Venous thromboses in children may be associated with the factor V Leiden mutation. Other risk factors may be present as well. Screening for this mutation can be achieved by means of the normalized activated protein C sensitivity ratio, although DNA studies are needed to confirm the presence of the mutation.

▶ Here is another study dealing with factor V Leiden mutation. By now, the reader of the YEAR BOOK OF PEDIATRICS is wondering why this heretofore relatively obscure coagulation factor mutation is getting all the attention it has recently had. This mutation is the most common genetic defect associated with venous thrombosis. About 20% of adults with venous thrombosis and as many as 60% with thrombosis in families with unexplained problems have been identified as having this mutation—a mutation in which a protein is produced that is resistant to inactivation by protein C. These investigators from Colorado and California tell us that children—not just adults—who experience unusual clotting should be considered suspect for having the factor V Leiden mutation. When these data are put together with some recent information from Great Britain that shows that children who experience strokes are 5 times more likely to have factor V Leiden mutations, you have a pretty good argument for the importance of this clotting factor.[1] Lastly, if you see a patient with homocystinuria (such individuals are known to be at increased risk of thrombosis), you may wish to screen that patient for factor V Leiden, as the combination of homocystinuria and factor V Leiden can be quite lethal.[2]

There are ways to screen for factor V Leiden. The gene abnormality is present mainly in populations of Caucasian origin. It is not present among the Japanese or Chinese. The highest prevalence is found in areas of southern Sweden, where as many as 15% of the population are heterozygotes, with a fivefold to tenfold increased risk of thrombosis. A homozygote has a 100-fold increased risk. Whether general screening programs, say before surgery, would be beneficial is uncertain at this time. The possible exception to not screening is the adolescent who is white with a Nordic family background and who is about to be given oral contraceptives. We now know that the combination of oral contraception and heterozygous carriage of factor V Leiden carries with it a 35- to 50-fold increased risk of venous thrombosis.

As we learn more and more about factor V Leiden, we see that it has quickly become a major player among the causes of venous thrombosis in children and adolescents. In the absence of anything to tell us differently, we certainly should not be writing a prescription for an oral contraceptive without at least thinking about the possibility that the blond-haired, blue-eyed girl for whom that prescription is intended might have as much as a 15% chance of having factor V Leiden deficiency.

This commentary on factor V Leiden closes with a quiz: your diagnosis please. A 15-year-old previously in good health is seen by you for an orthopedic evaluation after an emergency department visit to an outlying hospital. The history is as follows: Three days earlier, the patient had competed in a wrestling match. He sustained no injury. The day after the match, he noticed some ecchymoses about the right arm and shoulder. The second day after the match, the shoulder was stiff and there was diffuse swelling of the right upper extremity. When you examine him, he has marked swelling from his shoulder to his fingers with a 3-cm difference in the diameter of the right biceps compared with the left biceps. His superficial veins are prominent. Motor and sensory function and pulses are normal. There is quite a bit of pain on movement of the arm. X-ray films of the arm and shoulder and a bone scan are all negative. What would you do next and why?

If you answered a venogram and digital venous imaging, you would be right. This boy has what is known as "effort thrombosis." The teenager in question was actually reported by Medler et al.[3] Studies of the teenager showed a total occlusion of the axillary and subclavian veins, which required 6 months of anticoagulation therapy before a return to normal functioning.

Athletes who use their arms in an overhead position, such as swimmers, baseball players, and tennis players, are predisposed to "effort thrombosis" syndrome. This position of the arm narrows the thoracic outlet compressing the subclavian vein while also stretching it. This will result in tears of the intima of the vein. Two types of athletes are particularly prone to this problem: the female athlete taking oral contraceptives and the dehydrated male wrestler (who tries to lose weight before an upcoming match). Presumably, the presence of factor V Leiden deficiency would only make this scenario more likely.

"Effort thrombosis" is the 497th reason not to exercise. The only good wrestling bout is when you wrestle with yourself about the decision to engage in such sporting activities.

References

1. Ganesan V, et al: *Lancet* 347:260, 1996.
2. Mandel H, et al: *N Engl J Med* 334:763, 1996
3. Medler RG, et al: *J Bone Joint Surg (Am)* 75-A:1071, 1993.

Activated Protein C Resistance in a Neonate With Venous Thrombosis
Kodish E, Potter C, Kirschbaum NE, et al (Case Western Reserve Univ, Cleveland, Ohio; Blood Ctr of Southeastern Wisconsin, Milwaukee; Med College of Wisconsin, Milwaukee)
J Pediatr 127:645–648, 1995   13–14

Introduction.—Resistance to activated protein C (APC) is the most common coagulation abnormality seen in patients with venous thrombosis. Resistance to APC has also been associated with a mutation resulting in the production of a factor V (FV) molecule, FV Leiden, which contributes to a prothrombotic state. All published reports of APC resistance and venous thrombosis have involved adults. A newborn with APC resistance and venous thrombosis was described.

Case Report.—A full-term infant boy was the third child of a 35-year-old mother. He had bilateral edema of the feet at 20 hours of life, which then extended to the thighs. Abdominal ultrasonography revealed a thrombus in the inferior vena cava extending between the midhepatic vein and the femoral veins. Thrombolytic therapy was initiated on day 3 after placement of a right pedal venous catheter and a left radial arterial line. Clot resolution progressed both clinically and ultrasonographically, and warfarin treatment began on day 11. Thrombolytic therapy was discontinued and oral warfarin therapy continued at home. Laboratory studies were performed with plasma from the infant and his family.

Methods.—Resistance to APC was assayed with an activated partial thromboplastin time reagent after dilution of the patient plasma samples with FV-deficient plasma. The FV Leiden mutation was detected by polymerase chain reaction and restriction enzyme *Mn1*I digestion. Patient results were compared with results of testing with plasma obtained from patients known to be either normal or heterozygous or homozygous for FV Leiden.

Results.—The infant and the mother both had abnormal APC resistance clotting results and were heterozygous for the FV Leiden mutation.

Discussion.—The lack of a history of venous thrombosis despite 3 pregnancies in the mother indicates the variable clinical penetrance of APC resistance and FV Leiden mutation. Thrombophilia in patients with heterozygosity may depend upon multiple genetic abnormalities combined with environmental factors. This is the first report of neonatal venous thrombosis associated with heterozygous FV Leiden status, occurring without predisposing environmental factors. It is recommended that all infants and children with thrombosis and their families be tested for APC resistance and/or FV Leiden mutation. In addition, because there is a 5% prevalence of the FV Leiden mutation, screening children with serious underlying illness or an indwelling catheter should be considered to identify those who should receive prophylactic therapy.

▶ This is a very important report. Its implications are extraordinary. Unfortunately, this report is likely to be overlooked by the average individual because of the myriad of reports available these days.

Why is this report so important? It is important because it tells us that 5% of the children we care for have a mutation in 1 of their coagulation factors (FV) that predisposes them at some time in life to a serious risk of venous thrombosis. The mutation these youngsters have results in the production of an abnormal FV molecule (named FV Leiden) with a glutamine substitution for arginine at amino acid 506. Arginine 506 is a cleavage site for APC. A mutation at this site results in inefficient activation of activated FV Leiden by APC. The prothrombotic state that exists in these individuals is presumed to be caused by this relative inability of APC to inactivate activated FV Leiden. The upshot of all this is that these youngsters have a tendency to be hypercoagulable. Although most excess clotting has been reported in adults, we see from this report that neonates are not immune to the problem.

So, what do we learn from this report? We learn that if there is no obvious cause for venous thrombosis in a child (such as sepsis, dehydration, or the presence of an indwelling catheter), we should look for other conditions that lead to hypercoagulable states. The list of causes of hypercoagulability includes protein C deficiency, protein S deficiency, antithrombin-III deficiency, homocystinuria, and autoimmune diseases, particularly those associated with anticardiolipin antibody. Add to the list APC resistance caused by a heterozygous state for FV Leiden, and you are well on your way to being very thorough in your evaluation of children who are prone to clotting. Assays exist for all of these entities. Many laboratories have panels that include these assays in case you forget what to ask for. The trick is to be thorough.

This is the last entry in the Blood chapter, so we'll close with a query having to do with those who practice hematology. The 1995 annual meeting of the American Society of Hematology took place in Seattle. The question is, as there is only 1 direct flight each day from the United Kingdom to Seattle, what percentage of all British hematologists were likely to have traveled on the same overseas flight to this meeting?

The answer to this query is that about 40% of all British hematologists traveled to the American Society of Hematology meeting on 1 of 2 flights during the days preceding the conference. So what? The "so what" has to do with what would happen if there were an airplane crash. There are just 400 hematologists in Great Britain. Although air crashes are quite rare, the impact on medical services in England by such a loss would have been enormous had a plane full of hematologists gone down.[1]

One could debate whether the loss of a gaggle of hematologists would seriously affect the health services of a country as large as Great Britain, but in 1994, the U.K. Department of Health and Social Services did stop 200 British orthopedic surgeons from flying in 1 plane to an international conference for fear of what would happen should that plane be lost. Please note that the United Kingdom had no objection when a similar number of British gastroenterologists took a plane to a world conference in Mexico that very same year.[2] Editorial comment: no comment.

References

1. Rees DC: *Lancet* 347:274, 1996.
2. Baron JH: *Lancet* 347:982, 1996.

14 Oncology

Childhood Cancer in the United States: A Geographical Analysis of Cases From the Pediatric Cooperative Clinical Trials Groups
Ross JA, Severson RK, Pollock BH, et al (Univ of Minnesota, Minneapolis; Univ of Florida, Gainesville)
Cancer 77:201–207, 1996   14–1

Background.—Cancer is second only to trauma as the leading cause of death in U.S. children younger than 15 years. The proportion of children with cancer treated at centers using up-to-date treatment protocols is not known. The proportion and geographic distribution of such patients at participating centers of the Children's Cancer Group (CCG) and the Pediatric Oncology Group (POG) were investigated.

Methods.—The study group consisted of 21,026 children younger than 15 years who received a diagnosis of cancer from 1989 through 1991. The observed number of cases were compared with the expected number determined from incidence rates obtained from the Surveillance, Epidemiology, and End Results (SEER) Program and population counts from the 1990 U.S. Census Bureau.

Findings.—About 94% of the children were seen at a POG and CCG member institution. A comparison of the observed-to-expected numbers of incident cases in 4 age groups showed an ascertainment rate of 100% in the birth to 4-year-old cohort, 93% in the 5- to 9-year-old cohort, 84% in the 10- to 14-year-old cohort, and 21% in the 15- to 19-year-old cohort (Table 3). The observed number of cases was significantly less than expected in some regions, such as areas of Idaho, Oklahoma, and Virginia. In parts of California and Florida, the observed number of childhood cancer cases was markedly greater than that expected (Fig 1).

Conclusions.—Most children with cancer in the United States receive state-of-the-art care at centers associated with the POG and CCG. For young children, the CCG and POG may be a mechanism of case ascertainment approximating a population-based series for the United States.

▶ The number of malignancies in children each year pales in comparison to that in adults. Recognize, however, that after trauma, childhood malignancy is the most common cause of death in children. Also, despite the higher cure rates seen in children compared with adults, a child who dies loses many

TABLE 3.—Age- and Site-specific Observed and Expected Values of Pediatric Cancer From January 1989 to December 1991 in the United States (Excluding Alaska and Hawaii)

Site	Age group (yr)	Observed		Expected		Observed/expected ratio	95% CI
		No.	%	No.	%		
Leukemia	0–4	3495	49.7	3135	44.2	1.11	1.08, 1.15
	5–9	1792	25.5	1631	23.0	1.10	1.05, 1.15
	10–14	1160	16.5	1235	17.4	0.94	0.88, 1.00
Lymphoma	0–4	370	14.1	264	5.7	1.40	1.26, 1.55
	5–9	668	25.5	673	14.5	0.99	0.92, 1.07
	10–14	947	36.1	1177	25.4	0.80	0.75, 0.86
Central nervous system/brain	0–4	1486	38.3	1497	32.8	0.99	0.94, 1.04
	5–9	1192	30.7	1381	30.3	0.86	0.81, 0.91
	10–14	871	22.4	800	17.6	1.09	1.02, 1.16
Neuroblastoma	0–4	1336	49.8	1164	88.2	1.15	1.09, 1.21
	5–9	139	5.2	91	6.9	1.53	1.28, 1.80
	10–14	48	32.5	17	1.3	2.82	2.07, 3.70
Soft tissue	0–4	523	38.1	410	30.0	1.28	1.17, 1.39
	5–9	332	24.2	192	14.0	1.73	1.54, 1.92
	10–14	294	21.4	304	22.2	0.97	0.86, 1.08
Kidney	0–4	941	72.9	893	67.5	1.05	0.99, 1.12
	5–9	284	22.0	325	24.5	0.87	0.77, 0.98
	10–14	49	3.8	59	4.5	0.83	0.61, 1.08
Bone	0–4	68	5.0	51	3.1	1.33	1.03, 1.68
	5–9	257	18.9	302	18.1	0.85	0.75, 0.96
	10–14	574	42.3	591	35.4	0.97	0.89, 1.05
Retinoblastoma	0–4	373	92.1	670	89.6	0.51	0.50, 0.62
	5–9	23	5.7	57	7.6	0.40	0.25, 0.59
	10–14	5	1.2	10	1.3	0.50	0.15, 1.05

(Courtesy of Ross JA, Severson RK, Pollock BH, et al: Childhood cancer in the United States: A geographical analysis of cases from the Pediatric Cooperative Clinical Trials Groups. *Cancer* 77:201–207, 1996. Reprinted by permission of Wiley-Liss, Inc., a division of John Wiley & Sons, Inc.)

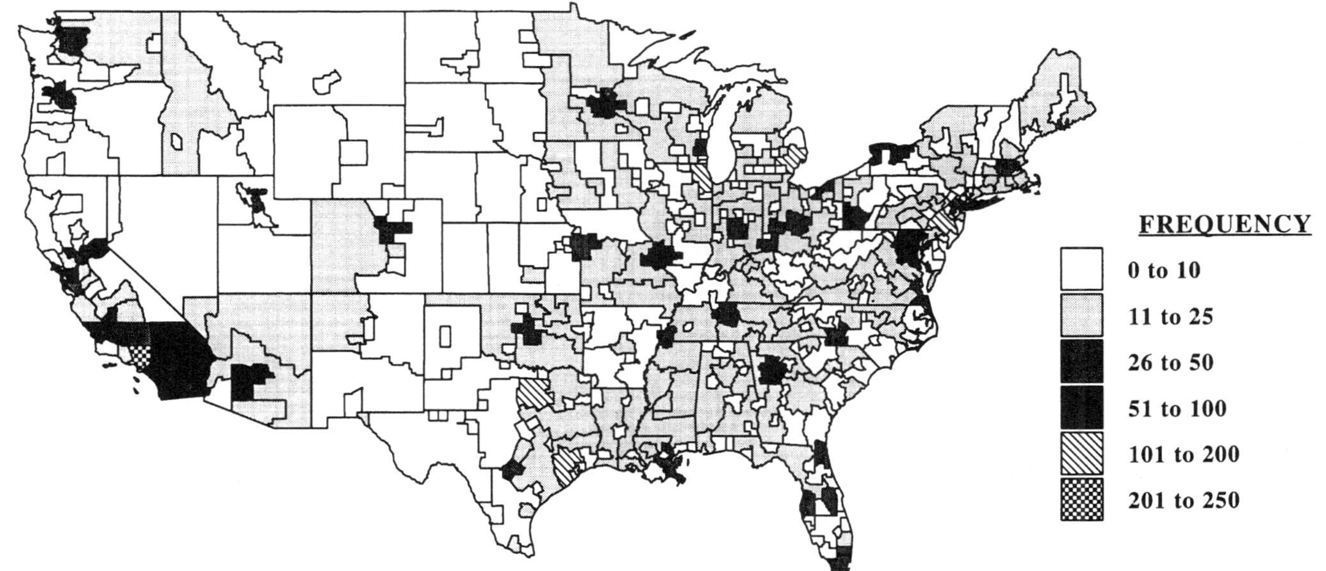

FIGURE 1.—Average annual number of expected cases of cancer (0–14 years of age) calculated using Surveillance, Epidemiology, and End Results Program incidence rates and 1990 population data (includes all cancer sites, sexes, and races combined). (Courtesy of Ross JA, Severson RK, Pollock B, et al: Childhood cancer in the United States: A geographical analysis of cases from the Pediatric Cooperative Clinical Trials Groups. *Cancer* 77:201–207, 1996. Reprinted by permission of Wiley-Liss, Inc., a division of John Wiley & Sons, Inc.)

more years of potential life compared with most adults who have malignancy. Ten thousand new cases translates to 100,000 years of life lost per year in children.

Many, if not most, of the major improvements in survivorship in children with malignancies have been the direct result of treatment using cooperative group protocols, particularly those of the POG and the CCG. This report shows encouraging conclusions: more than 90% of children nationwide younger than 15 years are being seen by pediatric cooperative group institutions.

In one sense, every child with a malignancy should be considered a national resource in the sense that each is capable of contributing knowledge that can lead to the potential cure of their illness. It is imperative that, except where circumstances otherwise cannot permit it, children should be treated at institutions that share the ability to design, implement, and report standardized treatments that answer important questions about childhood malignancy. Short of this, we will squander our already limited abilities to move quickly in finding the causes and potential cures of cancers in children.

Cancer in the Parents of Children With Cancer
Olsen JH, Boice JD Jr, Seersholm N, et al (Danish Cancer Society, Copenhagen; Natl Cancer Inst, Bethesda, Md)
N Engl J Med 333:1594–1599, 1995   14–2

Introduction.—The occurrence of neoplastic disease in the young suggests a role for heritable factors in causing cancer, and there is evidence from epidemiologic and clinical studies that close relatives of affected children themselves have an increased rate of cancer.

Objective.—To determine whether childhood cancer predicts an increased familial risk of cancer, 11,380 parents of Danish children with cancer were surveyed. The children were identified from records in the Danish Cancer Registry.

Findings.—The parents had a total of 1,445 cancers, compared with 1,496 expected on the basis of national incidence data. The standardized incidence ratio was 1.0 for mothers and 0.9 for fathers. Fathers had a standardized incidence ratio of 0.8 for lung cancer. There was no increase in cancer in parents of children having osteogenic or soft-tissue sarcomas. Excluding these cases, there was an apparent association between childhood leukemia and renal cancer, especially in mothers (Table 5). In addition, non-Hodgkin's lymphoma in children correlated with cancers of the brain and uterine cervix in mothers.

Discussion.—This survey revealed a limited number of specific associations between cancer in children and neoplastic disease in their parents.

TABLE 5.—Standardized Incidence Ratios for All Cancers Combined and Cancers at Selected Sites in the Parents of 5,155 Children With Cancers Other Than Osteogenic and Soft-tissue Sarcomas*

TYPE OF CANCER IN CHILD†	TYPE OF CANCER IN PARENT	MOTHERS			FATHERS		
		NO. OSERVED	NO. EXPECTED	SIR (95% CI)	NO. OBSERVED	NO. EXPECTED	SIR (95% CI)
Leukemia (n = 2067)	All sites	243	258.9	0.9 (0.8–1.1)	242	269.6	0.9 (0.8–1.0)
	Rectum	8	9.2	0.9 (0.4–1.7)	6	15.2	0.4 (0.1–0.9)
	Lung	18	15.7	1.1 (0.7–1.8)	37	52.5	0.7 (0.5–1.0)
	Kidney	12	5.5	2.1 (1.1–3.8)	12	8.9	1.4 (0.7–2.4)
	Leukemias	6	4.5	1.3 (0.5–2.9)	5	7.4	0.7 (0.2–1.6)
Lymphoma or other recitulo-endothelial neoplasm (n = 541)	All sites	87	70.2	1.2 (1.0–1.5)	73	73.6	1.0 (0.8–1.2)
	Cervix uteri	15	7.6	2.0 (1.1–3.3)	—	—	—
	Brain and nervous system	6	2.1	2.9 (1.1–6.3)	2	2.2	0.9 (0.1–3.3)
	Malignant lymphoma	0	1.4	0.0 (0.0–2.6)	1	2.1	0.5 (0.0–2.3)
Central nervous system neo-plasm (n = 1368)	All sites	153	166.4	0.9 (0.8–1.1)	184	173.8	1.1 (0.9–1.2)
	Rectum	5	5.9	0.9 (0.3–2.0)	19	9.8	1.9 (1.2–3.0)
	Brain and nervous system	6	4.9	1.2 (0.8–2.7)	7	5.3	1.3 (0.5–2.7)
Sympathetic nervous system neoplasm (n = 319)	All sites	29	25.1	1.2 (0.8–2.7)	22	25.7	0.9 (0.5–1.3)
Retinoblastoma (n = 178)	All sites	12	16.1	0.8 (0.4–1.3)	25	17.9	1.4 (0.9–2.1)
	Melanoma of skin	1	0.5	1.9 (0.0–11)	3	0.4	7.5 (1.5–22)
Renal tumor (n = 381)	All sites	44	43.0	1.0 (0.7–1.4)	33	49.5	0.7 (0.5–0.9)
	Kidney	0	0.9	0.0 (0.0–4.1)	3	1.6	1.9 (0.4–5.4)
Germ-cell, trophoblastic, or other gonadal neoplasm (n = 125)	All sites	13	12.6	1.0 (0.5–1.8)	14	13.1	1.1 (0.6–1.8)
	Lip	0	0.0	—	3	0.2	14.7 (3.0–43)
	Breast	3	3.2	0.9 (0.2–2.7)	0	0.0	—
	Cervix uteri	3	1.5	2.1 (0.4–6.0)	—	—	—
	Corpus uteri	0	0.7	0.0 (0.0–5.3)	—	—	—
	Prostate	—	—	—	0	0.9	0.0 (0.0–4.1)
	Ovary	0	0.8	0.0 (0.0–4.6)	—	—	—
	Testis	—	—	—	1	0.3	3.5 (0.0–20)
Carcinoma or other malignant epithelial neoplasm (n = 176)	All sites	25	27.9	0.9 (0.6–1.3)	10	12.8	0.8 (0.4–1.4)

*Parents of 51 children with hepatic tumors and 77 children with other and unspecified malignant neoplasms are not shown in this table because these groups were too small to yield meaningful results. Expected numbers of cancers are from national incidence rates adjusted for sex, age, and date of diagnosis.

†According to a classification scheme for childhood cancers (Birch JM, Marsden HB: *Int J Cancer* 40:620–624, 1987).

Abbreviations: SIR, standardized incidence ratio; *CI*, confidence interval.

(Reprinted by permission of *The New England Journal of Medicine*, from Olsen JH, Boice JD Jr, Seersholm N, et al: Cancer in the parents of children with cancer. *N Engl J Med* 333:1594–1599, Copyright 1995, Massachusetts Medical Society.)

There is no good evidence that the lack of a general association is a result of bias.

▶ You are what your genes make of you and what the environment modifies. With that as a given, this report asks a very important question: do parents who give birth to a child in whom a malignancy develops have an increased risk of malignancy themselves? It has been known for some time that an inherited susceptibility to tumors occurs for parents of children with bilateral retinoblastoma and for what is known as Li-Fraumeni syndrome, in which families are prone to breast cancer and malignancies of early life, such as childhood sarcoma. In fact, it has been suggested that mothers of children with sarcoma should be screened for breast cancer in early adulthood. Despite these bits and pieces of data, however, it hasn't been known whether the occurrence of childhood cancer can actually predict an increased familial risk of cancer; hence the importance of this report. Only in a few countries such as Denmark can you do a study where every child younger than 15 years born between 1943 and 1985 can be tracked to determine whether they have had a malignancy, and if so whether their parents have shown an increased risk of malignancy.

This report is comforting and disturbing at the same time. It shows that, in general, cancer in children should not, and cannot, be viewed as a general marker for an increased risk of cancer in parents of such children. If, however, you look at the data carefully by subgroups, further breakdown shows a significant association between breast cancer in mothers younger than 45 years and sarcomas in children younger than 3 years. The latter finding is consistent with the Li-Fraumeni syndrome. In general, parents may be able to breathe a sigh of relief that they themselves are not at increased risk except in very restricted circumstances.

While on the topic of cancer risk, were you aware that being a butcher carries with it a higher chance of having premalignant and malignant conditions? Butchers, for example, have more hand warts than individuals in any other profession (as high as a 34% prevalence). This excess of warts in butchers is mainly accounted for by human papillomavirus 7 (HPV 7). Worse yet, butchers who handle fresh meat rather than chilled meat have significantly higher incidences of squamous cell cancer of the lung than does the mean population at large. As a number of HPVs cause squamous cancers of various parts of the body, there may be a link between butchers' warts and malignancy.[1]

Reference

1. Benton EC: *Lancet* 343:1114, 1994.

Trends in Incidence of Testicular Cancer in Boys and Adolescent Men
Møller H, Jørgensen N, Forman D (Internatl Agency for Research on Cancer,
Lyon, France; Rigshospitalet, Copenhagen; Univ of Leeds, England)
Int J Cancer 61:761–764, 1995   14–3

Introduction.—Testicular cancer is most common among men in their
twenties through their forties, and epidemiologic studies have consistently

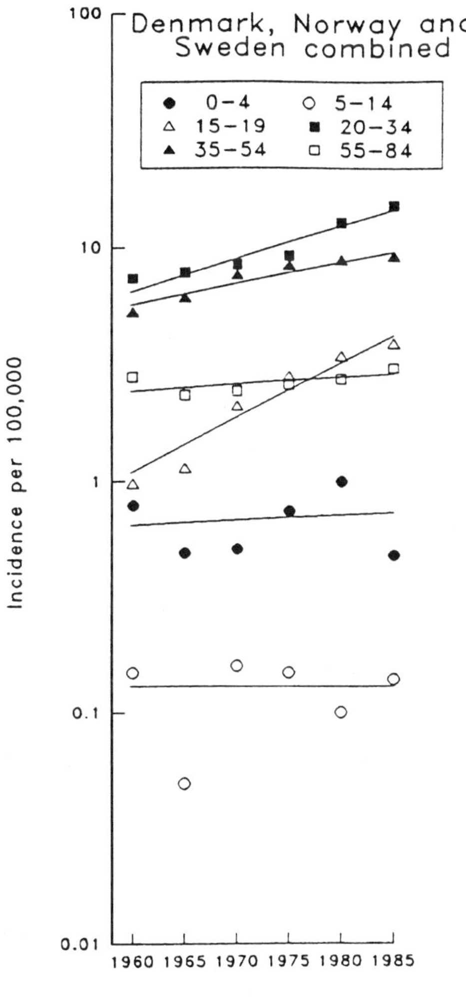

FIGURE 2.—Trends in incidence of testicular cancer (per 100,000) in the age groups 0–4, 5–14, 15–19,
20–34, 35–54, and 55–84 years in the combined population of Denmark, Norway, and Sweden,
1958–1987. (Courtesy of Møller H, Jørgensen N, Forman D: Trends in incidence of testicular cancer in
boys and adolescent men. *Int J Cancer* 61:761–764, Copyright© 1995. Reprinted by permission of John
Wiley & Sons, Inc.)

found increased age-adjusted incidence rates over time. However, few studies have examined trends in the incidence of testicular cancer among young boys, adolescents, and older men. The incidence of testicular cancer among young boys and adolescents in Nordic countries was studied and compared with corresponding data in adults.

Methods.—Registry data were used to assess the incidence of testicular cancer in Denmark, Norway, and Sweden from 1960 to 1985. Trends in the incidence of testicular cancer among boys from birth to 4 years of age and adolescents aged 15–19 years were evaluated and compared with those in adults. The data for the 3 countries were described separately and in combination.

Findings.—There were few cases of testicular cancer among young boys. However, the available data suggested that the incidence of testicular cancer in this age group has remained stable at around 0.5 per 100,000. In all 3 countries separately and combined, the incidence increased significantly over time in the 15- to 19-year, 20- to 34-year, and 35- to 54-year age groups (Fig 2). The average annual increase in these groups was 5.6%, 3.2%, and 2.1%, respectively. The incidence levels in young boys and adults were not correlated across populations.

Conclusions.—The incidence of testicular cancer has remained stable in young boys while increasing in older age groups, particularly adolescents. The findings suggest that testicular cancer in young boys may be etiologically distinct from that occurring in adults. The high average annual increase in the incidence of testicular cancer among adolescents may result from a secular trend toward younger age at puberty.

▶ There is really very little in the literature about the risk that young boys and adolescent males have of developing testicular malignancies. Sure, there is a great deal known about the risk of malignancy in those who have undescended testes, but the latter category of youngsters constitutes a distinct minority of those in whom testicular cancer develops. What we do know about testicular cancer is that it is very rare before puberty, but the incidence increases rapidly thereafter, probably indicating that male sex hormones are required for invasive tumor growth. The stages through which this malignancy progresses involve normal primordial germ cells, through the preinvasive stage of carcinoma in situ, to invasive cancer. The occurrence of testicular cancer predominantly in young men and the rarity of the disease in old men suggest that exposure to risk factors early in life, possibly in utero, are likely to be more important than exposures in adulthood. Indeed, the age incidence pattern is compatible with the hypothesis that there is a susceptible population of men, defined at or around birth, in whom testicular cancer will eventually develop.[1]

Testicular cancers occur in distinct age groups: an early incidence (albeit low) in young boys and again in adolescents and in young adult males in their 20s, 30s, and 40s. This study suggests that testicular cancer in young boys and in adult men may have different etiologies based on differences in histology and changing patterns of incidence. Adolescents act like young adult men.

What is the importance of this report? It tells us that adolescent males are the same as young men. They are at risk for testicular malignancy, and we should be training teenage boys in testicular self-examination. Everyone is aware that the age of onset of puberty has been decreasing in girls (from an age of menarche of 17 years in 1850 to 13 in 1970). Everything we know about boys suggests that they are entering puberty earlier as well.[2] It is precisely in this transition age of adolescence that there is a particularly high rate of increase in the incidence of testicular cancer. This again validates the concept that these malignancies result from a burst of hormonal stimulation that marks the movement to adulthood.

The trick in survivorship with testicular cancer is founded on the principle of early detection with self-examination. Alternatively, one could try to stay young forever because this is a disease of maturing. Bo Derek, Zsa Zsa Gabor, and Dick Clark, let your youthful genes be cloned.

References

1. Møller H: *Eur Urol* 23:8–15, 1993.
2. Roche AF: *Monogr Soc Res Child Dev* No. 179, Vol. 44, 1979.

Mass Screening and Age-specific Incidence of Neuroblastoma in Saitama Prefecture, Japan
Yamamoto K, Hayashi Y, Hanada R, et al (Saitama Children's Med Ctr, Japan; Univ of Tokyo; Natl Children's Hosp, Tokyo; et al)
J Clin Oncol 13:2033–2038, 1995   14–4

Background.—Neuroblastoma can have a markedly varied prognosis, depending on the patient's age and disease stage. Because infants have a better prognosis than children older than 1 year, it was hypothesized that mass screening of infants at the age of 6 months would improve the overall prognosis of the disease in the population. To test this hypothesis, the incidence of neuroblastomas in children younger than 15 years was studied during a 12-year period in Saitama Prefecture, Japan, during which mass screening was performed. The age-specific incidence of the tumor was analyzed.

Methods.—Mass screening of 6-month-old infants was initiated in June 1981 and involved the qualitative assessment of urinary vanillylmandelic acid (VMA) and later (after 1989) the measurement of VMA/creatinine (Cre) and homovanillic acid (HVA)/Cre by high-performance liquid chromatography. The numbers of children younger than 15 years with a diagnosis of neuroblastoma between January 1981 and December 1992 were obtained from the Prefectural Cancer Registry. The trends in annual age-specific incidence rates were analyzed for four 3-year periods.

Results.—Of the 491,908 infants screened during the study period, neuroblastomas were detected in 77 (Table 1). Overall, there were 199

TABLE 1.—Children Screened and Neuroblastoma Cases Detected in Saitama Prefecture From 1981 to 1992

Year	Target Population	Infants Screened* No.	Infants Screened* %	No. of Neuroblastome Cases Detected
1981	72,881	3,913	5.4	0
1982	71,794	18,881	26.3	0
1983	70,614	33,045	46.8	1
1984	69,184	34,240	49.5	3
1985	67,980	39,286	57.8	7
1986	65,618	43,180	65.8	5
1987	62,819	45,458	72.4	8
1988	63,121	48,717	77.2	4
1989	64,165	53,444	83.3	5
1990	62,077	55,179	88.9	12
1991	61,779	57,371	92.9	15
1992	64,331	59,194	92.0	17
Total	796,363	491,908	61.8	77

*Methods of screening are qualitative vanillylmandelic acid (*VMA*) from June 1981 to September 1989, and quantitative VMA/creatinine (*Cre*) and homovanillic (*HVA*) Cre from October 1989 to December 1992. Percentages are calculated as screened infants/target population × 100.

(Courtesy of Yamamoto K, Hayashi Y, Hanada R, et al: Mass screening and age-specific incidence of neuroblastoma in Saitama Prefecture, Japan. *J Clin Oncol* 13:2033–2038, 1995.)

children with a diagnosis of neuroblastoma during the same period. The detection rate was twice as high when diagnosed with quantitative measurements of VMA/Cre and HVA/Cre as when diagnosed with qualitative assessment of urinary VMA. There were significant increases in the annual incidence rates in the 4 periods for all children younger than 15 years (from $6.4/10^6$ to $20.1/10^6$), for children younger than 5 years (from $17.0/10^6$ to $64.1/10^6$), and for infants younger than 1 year (from $27.9/10^6$ to $260.4/10^6$).

Discussion.—The data suggest that the incidence rates of neuroblastoma increased among infants younger than 1 year because of improved detection methods, but that this increase was not accompanied by a decrease in the incidence rate in older children. Therefore, there may be a subset of neuroblastomas with a favorable biology that can be detected with screening in infants, but which would not be expressed clinically in older children. These findings suggest that mass screening will not affect the overall disease mortality.

▶ Although the Japanese have been quick to institute mass screening programs for the detection of neuroblastoma in infants younger than 1 year, we in the United States have been laid back, to say the least, in this regard. This difference in attitudes is not based on any debate about whether you can actually detect these tumors. Indeed, using high-performance liquid chromatography, one can readily measure elevated VMA and HVA in the urine of infants. That is not the concern. The reticence that has existed in the United States is based on the fact that many physicians believe that the Japanese are detecting a biologically different malignancy of little consequence.

The study abstracted actually validates the American opinion of neonatal screening for neuroblastoma. The study shows us that when you do detect a neuroblastoma in early infancy and take care of it, you actually do not decrease the overall incidence of new-onset neuroblastoma beyond the age of 1 year. In other words, tumors detected with screening are not those tumors that would have eventually gone on to express themselves later in infancy or childhood, but rather represent a unique malignancy for which one can seriously question the need for any detection or treatment. These investigators in Japan are probably correct when they suggest that there is a subset of neuroblastomas with a very favorable biology that can be detected by screening at 6 months of age but that would not be diagnosed clinically at an older age. This is probably a "new" disease entity, and screening for it will not reduce the overall mortality for the disease that occurs at an older age.

For an excellent review of neuroblastoma, see the recent article by Ater.[1]

Reference

1. Ater JL: *Pediatr Dent* 17:4, 1995.

Breast Cancer and Other Second Neoplasms After Childhood Hodgkin's Disease
Bhatia S, Robison LL, Oberlin O, et al (Univ of Minnesota, Minneapolis; Institut Gustave-Roussy, Villejuif, France; Hosp for Sick Children, Toronto; et al)
N Engl J Med 334:745–751, 1996   14–5

Background.—Patients treated for Hodgkin's disease in childhood have been reported to be at increased risk for second neoplasms. The incidence of second neoplasms in such patients was studied further, and specific factors associated with this risk were identified.

Methods.—A cohort of 1,380 children with Hodgkin's disease was followed for a median of 11.4 years. Eighty percent of the cohort was alive at the last contact.

Findings.—Eighty-eight second neoplasms occurred in the cohort, compared to an expected 4.4 in the general population, for a standardized incidence ratio of 18.1. The estimated actuarial incidence of any second neoplasm 15 years after diagnosis of Hodgkin's disease was 7%. Solid tumors occurred at an incidence of 3.9%. The most common solid tumor was breast cancer, with a standardized incidence ratio of 75.3. Its estimated actuarial incidence approached 35% in women by 40 years of age. A significantly increased risk of breast cancer was associated with older age at the time of radiation treatment in children and a higher radiation dose (Fig 2). Sixty-six percent of the solid cancers occurred in patients who had received both radiation and chemotherapy (Table 4).

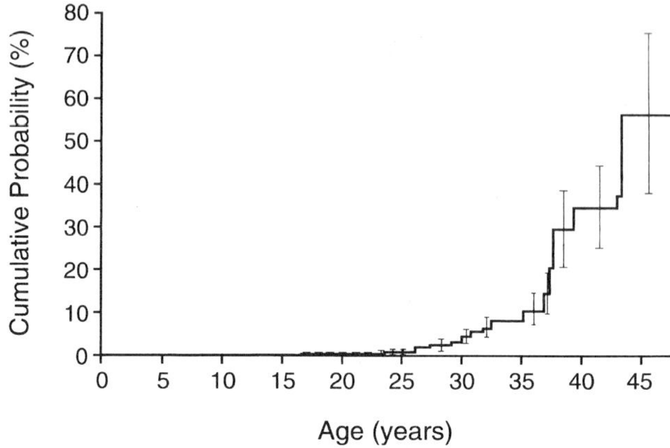

FIGURE 2.—Cumulative probability of breast cancer as a function of age in the cohort of female survivors of Hodgkin's disease in childhood. *Bars* indicate standard errors. (Reprinted by permission of *The New England Journal of Medicine*, from Bhatia S, Robison LL, Oberlin O, et al: Breast cancer and other second neoplasms after childhood Hodgkin's disease. *N Engl J Med* 334:745–751, Copyright 1996, Massachusetts Medical Society.)

Conclusions.—Patients treated with radiation for Hodgkin's disease in childhood are at high risk for the development of solid tumors, particularly breast cancer. Systemic breast cancer screening may be important for such women.

▶ This report teaches us a lot about the consequences of what we do when we treat children with malignancy. It also tells us that the follow-up of

TABLE 4.—Risks of Second Cancers According to the Type of Treatment for Hodgkin's Disease

Type of Cancer and Treatment	Observed Cases	Observed: Expected Cases (95% CI)	Cumulative Probability at 15 yr (95% CI) %
Leukemia			
Radiation	0	0	0
Chemotherapy	5	1091 (344–2256)	7.9 (1.0–14.8)
Radiation and chemotherapy	21	439 (270–645)	3.4 (1.8–4.9)
Non-Hodgkin's lymphoma			
Radiation	1	11 (0.01–44)	0.4 (0–1.2)
Chemotherapy	1	60 (0.02–235)	0.0
Radiation and chemotherapy	4	23 (6–50)	0.9 (0–1.9)
Solid tumors			
Radiation	15	11 (6–17)	3.3 (2.9–3.7)
Chemotherapy	1	5 (0.01–18)	2.9 (2.3–3.5)
Radiation and chemotherapy	31	13 (9–18)	4.6 (4.4–4.8)

Abbreviation: CI, confidence interval.

(Reprinted by permission of *The New England Journal of Medicine*, from Bhatia S, Robison LL, Oberlin O, et al: Breast cancer and other second neoplasms after childhood Hodgkin's disease. *N Engl J Med* 334:745–751, Copyright 1996, Massachusetts Medical Society.)

youngsters, particularly girls, with Hodgkin's disease, needs to be long, very long. Such patients have a variety of problems with secondary malignancies, the most common solid tumor of which is breast cancer. The women reported on had a risk of breast cancer 75 times greater than that seen in the general population. Moreover, the estimated cumulative probability of breast cancer among women in this series who survived childhood Hodgkin's disease is now approaching 35% by 40 years of age. Most previous studies of large populations of patients who were treated for Hodgkin's disease did not detect a significantly elevated risk of breast cancer. Most likely this was the result of inadequate long-term follow-up. This increased risk of breast cancer after treatment for Hodgkin's disease is closely related to the age at the time of radiation exposure. Sixteen of the 17 breast cancers occurred after Hodgkin's treatment that was given between 10 and 16 years of age. This age relationship suggests that the tumorigenic influence of radiation mainly affects proliferating breast tissue.

As of now, the number of deaths resulting from Hodgkin's disease itself significantly exceeds the number of deaths resulting from complications of therapy. This underscores the admonition that maintaining high cure rates remains the highest priority in the management of childhood Hodgkin's disease. At the same time, we need to develop strategies that maintain lifelong follow-up of treated patients to minimize the long-term risks of treatment, to improve the accuracy of our risk estimates, and to deal with the psychological and social consequences of surviving one disease only to face special risks for others.

This commentary closes with some good news and some bad news. The good news is that the concern about a relationship between breast-feeding and the occurrence of breast cancer (a concern raised some 70 years ago and persisting even now) has been laid to rest. A study of thousands of women for more than half a million person-years indicates that there is no important overall association between breast-feeding and the occurrence of breast cancer.[1] Feed your baby to your heart's content. Also good news is that radiation therapy that includes portals encompassing the breast tissue of adolescent males who are being treated for Hodgkin's disease does not have any long-term risk of the occurrence of breast cancer. The bad news is that boys are not off scot-free in this regard, however, because such boys are at exceptional risk for the development of premature coronary artery disease even if they have no other coronary risk factors.[2] As pediatricians, we need to be aware of this when we consign these youngsters over to adult care providers. We should remind the latter of this risk.

One final note regarding breast cancer. If you've ever been a flight attendant, recognize that you have been exposed to altitude radiation consisting of neutrons and gamma rays. A report examining the incidence of cancer among Finnish airline cabin attendants shows that they have a twofold increased risk of breast cancer.[2] Presumably you don't have to be on a Finnish air carrier to have this problem. United, American, and US Air flight attendants should be aware of this risk as well. Whoever said the friendly skies were all that friendly?

References

1. Jacobi A, et al: Dentition and its derangements. New York Medical College. Baillere Brothers, 1862.
2. Pukkala E, et al: *BMJ* 311:649, 1995.

Persistence of Circulating Blasts After 1 Week of Multiagent Chemotherapy Confers a Poor Prognosis in Childhood Acute Lymphoblastic Leukemia

Gajjar A, Ribeiro R, Hancock ML, et al (St Jude Children's Research Hosp, Memphis, Tenn; Univ of Tennessee, Memphis)
Blood 86:1292–1295, 1995   14–6

Background.—For children with acute lymphoblastic leukemia (ALL), the finding of an early response to therapy—as reflected by bone marrow status—predicts a favorable outcome. However, there are few data on the prognostic significance of early disappearance of blast cells from the peripheral blood. The prognostic significance of persistent circulating blast cells after 1 week of chemotherapy was evaluated retrospectively.

Methods.—The records were reviewed of all 358 children with previously untreated ALL who were enrolled in a risk-based therapy study. The presence of blast cells in the peripheral blood at the time of diagnosis and 1 week after the start of intensive induction chemotherapy was determined. Excluding 59 patients with no circulating blast cells at diagnosis and 2 with missing data, a total of 297 patients were studied. Multivariate

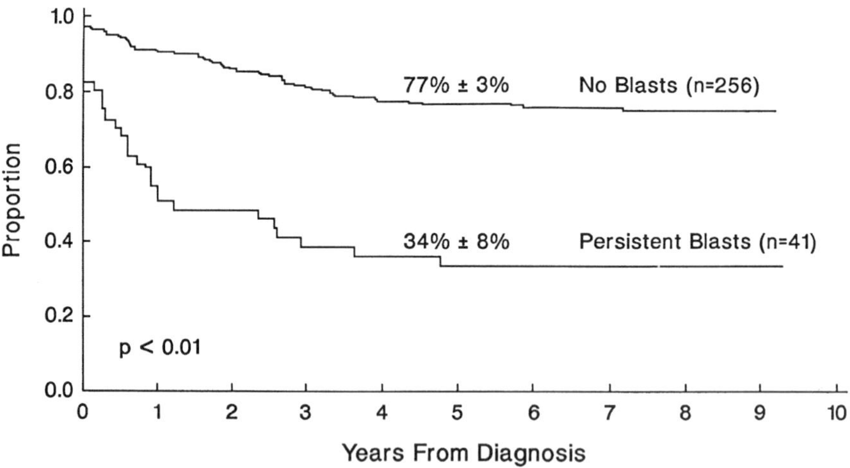

FIGURE 1.—Event-free survival according to the presence or absence of leukemic blast cells in peripheral blood at day 8 of remission induction therapy. (Courtesy of Gajjar A, Ribeiro R, Hancock ML, et al: Persistence of circulating blasts after 1 week of multiagent chemotherapy confers a poor prognosis in childhood acute lymphoblastic leukemia. *Blood* 86:1292–1295, 1995.)

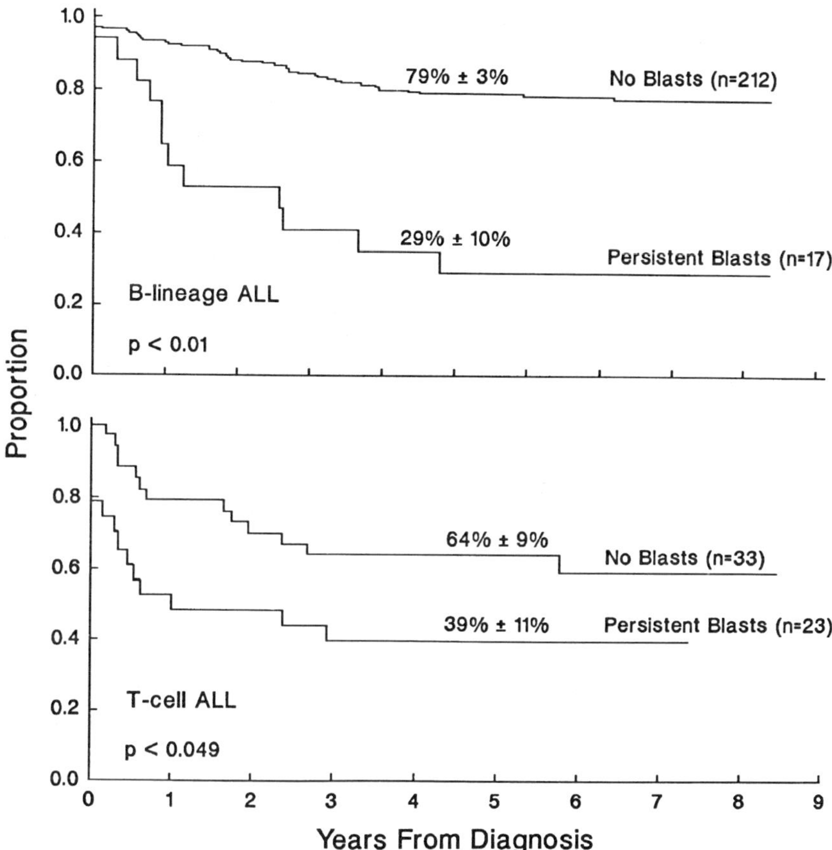

FIGURE 2.—Event-free survival in B-lineage and T-cell acute lymphoblastic leukemia (*ALL*) by the presence or absence of circulating blast cells at day 8 of remission induction therapy. (Courtesy of Gajjar A, Ribeiro R, Hancock ML, et al: Persistence of circulating blasts after 1 week of multiagent chemotherapy confers a poor prognosis in childhood acute lymphoblastic leukemia. *Blood* 86:1292–1295, 1995.)

analysis, including variables known to be associated with an unfavorable outcome, was performed to evaluate the prognostic significance of persistent circulating blast cells.

Results.—Fourteen percent of patients had persistent circulating leukemic blasts after 1 week of chemotherapy. A number of different adverse prognostic factors were more frequent in the "blast-positive" than in the "blast-negative" patients: a leukocyte count of greater than 50×10^9/L, a mediastinal mass, CNS leukemia, T-cell phenotype, lack of CD10 expression, and L2 morphology. Furthermore, 5-year event-free survival was only 34% in the blast-positive patients, compared with 77% in the blast-negative patients (Fig 1). For the overall group of patients, persistent blast cells were the most significant adverse factor, carrying a relative risk of 2.9. It was also the most significant adverse factor among patients with B-lineage disease, with a relative risk of 3.6 (Fig 2).

Conclusions.—For children with ALL, the persistence of blast cells in the peripheral blood after 1 week of intensive induction chemotherapy appears to be a poor prognostic factor. Detection of circulating blasts cannot identify all patients who will later have disease relapse. However, it does offer a simple, noninvasive approach to identifying patients who might benefit from early modification of therapy.

▶ Determining prognostic features in a child with newly diagnosed ALL is one of the most critically important activities of the pediatric oncologist. For patients with a favorable prognosis, protocols are designed to reduce acute and long-term side effects by avoiding unnecessarily toxic treatment. For patients with high-risk leukemia, there must be more intensive therapy. Effective risk-based therapy produces complete remission in 95% of patients. Even with appropriate risk assignment, 25% of children will subsequently relapse. That is why reports such as this are so important, because they tell us that early in the course of a child's disease, failure to clear blast cells from the circulation is a bad prognostic feature and that such children must be moved to aggressive chemotherapy regimens to achieve the best long-term outcome. Such patients most likely have aggressive, inherently resistant disease and would therefore benefit from alternative therapeutic strategies.

The findings of this report must be correlated with the fact that bone marrow examination, performed at day 14 of remission induction therapy, remains the clinical "gold standard" for assessment of early treatment response for American studies of childhood leukemia. The ultimate value of using the presence or absence of peripheral blast cells 7 days from the start of therapy in predicting long-term response remains to be determined. That's what future chemotherapy protocols will be all about. Stay tuned.

The Discriminating Value of Serum Lactate Dehydrogenase Levels in Children With Malignant Neoplasms Presenting as Joint Pain
Wallendal M, Stork L, Hollister JR (Natl Jewish Ctr for Immunology and Respiratory Medicine, Denver; Univ of Colorado, Denver)
Arch Pediatr Adolesc Med 150:70–73, 1996   14–7

Background.—Although joint pain is common in children, the cause can be difficult to determine. Limb pain is the initial complaint in 10% to 20% of children with leukemia, some children with early leukemia and limb pain will have normal blood studies, which may delay the diagnosis. Many of these patients are referred to pediatric rheumatologists for evaluation of suspected collagen vascular disease. The serum lactate dehydrogenase (LDH) level was investigated as an indicator of malignant neoplasms in children with musculoskeletal complaints and normal blood studies.

Methods.—The retrospective study included 12 patients who initially received a diagnosis of a rheumatic form of arthritis—mainly juvenile rheumatoid arthritis (JRA)—but were later proven to have a malignant

TABLE 1.—Laboratory Values in 12 Patients With Malignant Neoplasms and 24 Patients With Juvenile Rheumatoid Arthritis

	Group	
Values	Malignant Neoplasm	Juvenile Rheumatoid Arthritis
Hematology		
Hemoglobin, g/L	124 ± 17 (n=11)	117 ± 17 (n=24)
White blood cell count, ×10⁹/L	9.1 ± 5 (n=11)	11.6 ± 6 (n=24)
Platelets, ×10⁹/L	425 ± 185 (n=10)	481 ± 155 (n=22)
Erythrocyte sedimentation rate mm/h	41.5 ± 18.5 (n=10)	46.9 ± 31.0 (n=24)
Serum chemistry		
Uric acid, μmol/L (mg/dL)	260 ± 60 (4.4 ± 1.0) (n=12)	180 ± 70 (3.0±1.2) (n=24)
Aspartate aminotransferase, U/L	20 ± 10 (n=10)	22 ± 32 (n=22)

Note: Values are expressed as mean ± standard deviation.

(Courtesy of Wallendal M, Stork L, Hollister JR: The discriminating value of serum lactate dehydrogenase levels in children with malignant neoplasms presenting as joint pain. *Arch Pediatr Adolesc Med* 150:70–73, Copyright 1996, American Medical Association.)

neoplasm. The cancer diagnosis was delayed because of normal blood counts and elevated sedimentation rates. Most of the patients with malignant neoplasms had acute lymphocytic leukemia (ALL); the mean time to correct diagnosis was 16 weeks. Serum LDH levels and other findings were compared with those of 24 patients whose final diagnosis was JRA.

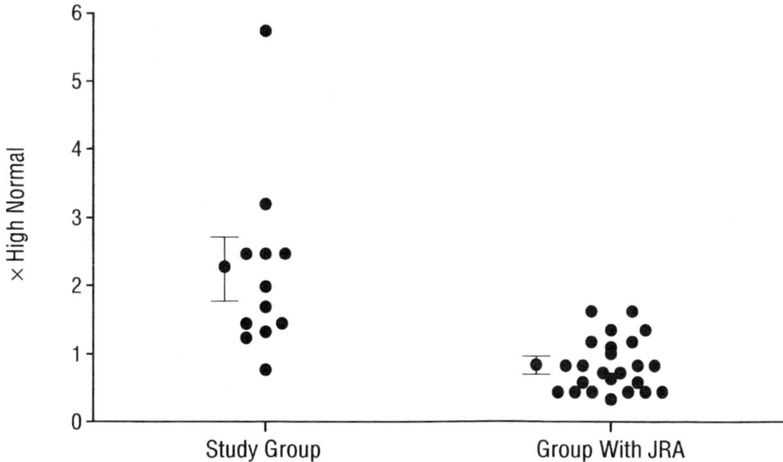

FIGURE.—Serum lactate dehydrogenase values are shown as a ratio of high normal for the individual laboratory. The mean ± standard error for the study group is 2.2 ± 1.3; for the group with juvenile rheumatoid arthritis, it is 0.8 ± 0.3. (P = 0.004, Mann-Whitney U test). (Courtesy of Wallendal M, Stork L, Hollister JR: The discriminating value of serum lactate dehydrogenase levels in children with malignant neoplasma presenting as joint pain. *Arch Pediatr Adolesc Med* 150:70–73, Copyright 1996, American Medical Association.)

TABLE 2.—Clinical Features of Patients With Malignant Neoplasms

Patient/ Sex/Age at Onset, y	Neoplasm, Duration of Symptoms Before Diagnosis, wk	Current Status
1/F/9	ALL, 8	7 y off treatment
2/M/15	ALL, 20	3 y off treatment
3/F/2	ALL, 12	15 mo off treatment
4/M/4	ALL, 12	4 y off treatment
5/F/11	ALL, 4	3 y off treatment
6/F/7	ALL, 28	2 y off treatment
7/M/4	ALL, 12	In remission after bone marrow transplant for marrow relapse
8/F/14	ALL, 12	Deceased
9/M/13	Squamous cell carcinoma, 48	Deceased
10/M/12	Ewing's tumor, 12	Deceased
11/M/3	Stage IV neuroblastoma, 10	3 y off treatment
12/F/2	Stage IV neuroblastoma, 8	Deceased

Abbreviation: ALL, acute lymphocytic leukemia
(Courtesy of Wallendal M, Stork L, Hollister JR: The discriminating value of serum lactate dehydrogenase levels in children with malignant neoplasms presenting as joint pain. *Arch Pediatr Adolesc Med* 150:70–73, Copyright 1996, American Medical Association.)

Results.—The 2 groups were similar in their initial hemoglobin levels, white blood cell and platelet counts, erythrocyte sedimentation rates, uric acid levels, and aspartate aminotransferase levels (Table 1). However, serum LDH levels were a mean of 2.2 times high normal (95% confidence interval, 1.33 to 3.00) in the patients with malignant neoplasms vs. 0.8 times high normal (0.67 to 0.94) in the patients with JRA (Figure). The serum LDH level was within the range of normal in just 1 patient with cancer and above normal (but not as high as in the cancer group) in 4 patients with JRA. Outcomes were good for the patients who had ALL but poor for those with metastatases of other malignant neoplasms (Table 2).

Conclusion.—The serum LDH level may be helpful in distinguishing malignant neoplasms from rheumatic disease in some patients whose symptoms and other laboratory tests do not clarify the diagnosis. Patients suspected of having JRA who have an elevated LDH level should undergo further tests for malignancy, which may permit an earlier diagnosis. The sensitivity and specificity of serum LDH determination must be evaluated prospectively.

▶ This is one article that all who provide care to pediatric patients should read. Even though we are trained to know that some of the signs and symptoms of a malignancy may mimic JRA, children continue to be missed, sometimes until it is too late. A child seen with joint pain should be considered worrisome because a subgroup of those with ALL, and occasionally other forms of cancer, will have limb or joint pain as the heralding symptom of their disease and at a time when peripheral blood counts and blood smears are still completely normal. Studies have shown that as many as 75% of leukemia patients seen with severe bone pain have normal hemoglobin levels, 50% have normal white blood cell counts, and 50% have normal platelet counts. More than one third of such patients have no circulating blast cells. Because of the nonspecific or absent hematologic abnormalities, a diagnosis of leukemia is frequently delayed for weeks or months. Worse yet, some of these children are mistakenly thought to have an autoimmune form of arthritis and are treated with steroids. Such mistreatment can convert a good leukemia prognosis to an unfavorable one.

So, how can one tell if a malignancy is a cause of joint or extremity pain? It is not easy. A couple of years back, we learned from a very important report that pain that awakens a child in the middle of the night is quite suggestive of a malignancy rather than JRA.[1] From the report abstracted here, we learn that serum LDH levels give us a valuable clue as well. The LDH is more likely to be normal in JRA and elevated in malignant neoplasms that present with joint pain. Other routine tests beyond the complete blood cell count and LDH are much less helpful. An elevation in sedimentation rate is common to both diagnoses. Relief after medical therapy for rheumatic disease can also be misleading because the majority of children with malignant neoplasms diagnosed as an arthritis improve with antirheumatic agents.

This study reinforces the importance of considering malignant neoplasm in the differential diagnosis of arthritis in a child. Normal blood smears and blood cell counts may be misleading, leading to serious delays in diagnosis. Until some readily available specific marker for a malignant cell is identified in children with ALL, we are left with the history, a physical examination, and LDH levels as being the most helpful discriminators in such children with normal blood counts. Not even uric acid levels distinguish those with malignancy.

Reference

1. Ostrov BE, et al: *J Pediatr* 122:595, 1993.

Obesity After Successful Treatment of Acute Lymphoblastic Leukemia in Childhood
Van Dongen-Melman JEWM, Hokken-Koelega ACS, Hählen K, et al (Erasmus Univ, Rotterdam, The Netherlands)
Pediatr Res 38:86–90, 1995   14–8

Background.—Research has shown that many survivors of childhood acute lymphoblastic leukemia (ALL) are overweight or obese. Excessive weight gain has been documented in particular during the first year after antileukemic treatment is completed. Although most authorities believe that this weight gain is the result of cranial irradiation, others think that corticosteroid medication may be an important factor.

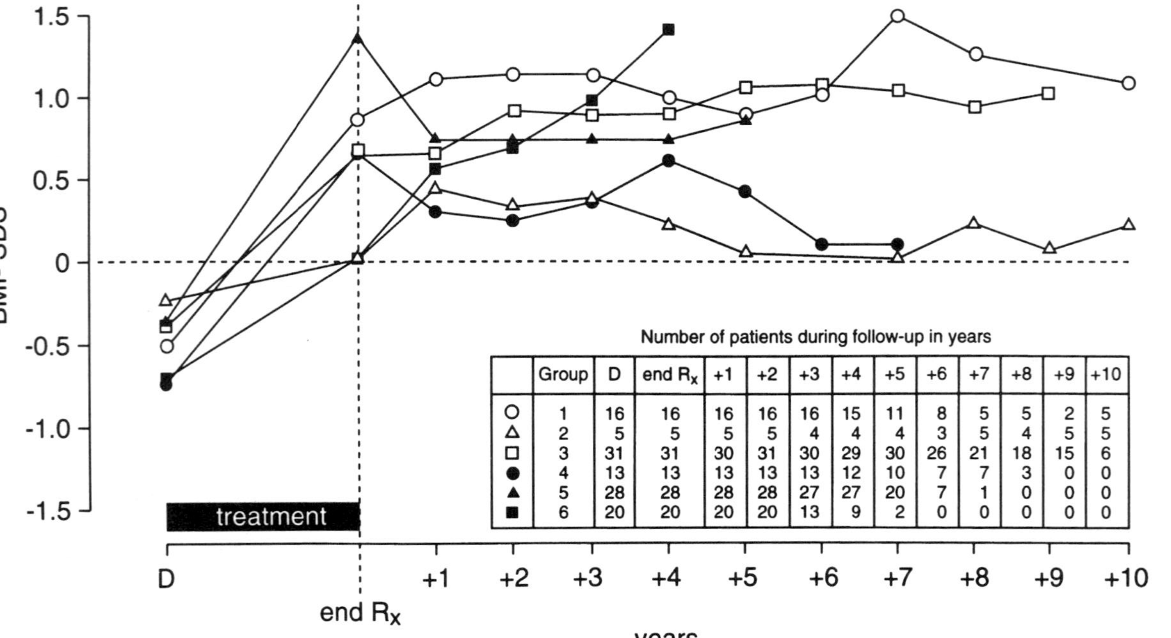

Number of patients during follow-up in years

	Group	D	end R_x	+1	+2	+3	+4	+5	+6	+7	+8	+9	+10
○	1	16	16	16	16	16	15	11	8	5	5	2	5
△	2	5	5	5	5	4	4	4	3	5	4	5	5
□	3	31	31	30	31	30	29	30	26	21	18	15	6
●	4	13	13	13	13	13	12	10	7	7	3	0	0
▲	5	28	28	28	28	27	27	20	7	1	0	0	0
■	6	20	20	20	20	13	9	2	0	0	0	0	0

FIGURE 1.—*Abbreviations: BMI*, body mass index; *SDS*, SD scores; *D*, diagnosis; *R_x*, treatment. Body mass index–SDS in 113 children up to 13 years from acute lymphoblastic leukemia diagnosis. Time points for the different treatment protocols were excluded if < 30% of patients were evaluated or if data were obtained from ≤ 3 patients. *Open symbols*, treatment regimens with cranial irradiation; *closed symbols*, treatment regimens without cranial irradiation. (Courtesy of Van Dongen-Melman JEWM, Hokken-Koelega ACS, Hählen K, et al: Obesity after successful treatment of acute lymphoblastic leukemia in childhood. *Pediatr Res* 38:86–90, 1995.)

Methods.—One hundred thirteen children treated for ALL were assessed up to 10 years after the completion of treatment with or without cranial irradiation and with different modes of corticosteroid medication. The patients were 58 boys and 55 girls, aged 6 months to 15 years at diagnosis. Criteria for inclusion were complete first remission for 2 years or more after treatment cessation and no evidence of CNS or constitutional chromosomal abnormality. Corticosteroid therapy was included in all treatment regimens. Fifty-two patients received cranial irradiation as well.

Findings.—The prevalence of overweight was increased after treatment. This increase persisted over time. Weight gain did not differ between patients treated with or without cranial irradiation (Fig 1), demonstrating that corticosteroid therapy rather than cranial irradiation may explain weight gain in these children. Dexamethasone was associated with significantly increased weight after treatment completion. Forty-four percent of the children receiving combined prednisone and dexamethasone had obesity as a late effect, which was the highest prevalence in the study. Sex and age at diagnosis were unassociated with increases in weight.

Conclusions.—Protocols with cranial irradiation are not associated with more weight gain than protocols without cranial irradiation. The highest prevalence of obesity after treatment completion occurred in children treated with corticosteroids and without irradiation. The use of corticosteroids may therefore have a greater effect on weight gain than irradiation-induced pituitary dysfunction.

▶ With more than 80% of children with ALL surviving these days, there is increasing emphasis on the late effects of antileukemic therapy. One effect appears to be obesity. This retrospective study, representing one of the largest single institutional reviews on weight of patients surviving ALL, clearly shows that obesity is a late effect for children who are successfully treated. Just as important, this investigation also gives us insight into factors that may account for the increase in weight. It has been suggested that cranial irradiation may cause damage to the hypothalamic-pituitary axis, resulting in a decreasing growth rate and a tendency toward excess body weight. This study did not show any such relationship. The protocols with the highest prevalence of obesity were those associated with steroid use and with no irradiation. This finding implies that the use of corticosteroids has a more dominant effect on weight gain than anything else. One would think that once steroids were stopped, the weight problem would resolve. Apparently not. It remains unclear why this increase in weight continues long after chemotherapy (including steroids) is stopped.

Thus, the inevitable conclusion is that obesity is both an early and late side effect of antileukemic therapy. Obesity can affect both boys and girls. Knowing this should allow early institution of counseling and dietary manipulation to minimize this long-term complication.

Magnetic Fields and Childhood Cancer: A Pooled Analysis of Two Scandinavian Studies

Feychting M, Schulgen G, Olsen JH, et al (Karolinska Institutet, Stockholm; Albert-Ludwigs-Univ, Freiburg, Germany; Danish Cancer Society, Copenhagen)

Eur J Cancer 31A:2035–2039, 1995   14–9

The Studies.—The first indication that residential exposure to magnetic fields of 50–60 Hz might be a risk factor for childhood cancer came in 1979. Two Scandinavian case-control studies evaluating the relationship between childhood cancer and exposure to magnetic fields from power lines, reported in 1993, found an increased risk of leukemia in exposed children. One of the studies also claimed an increased risk of lymphoma. The magnetic fields were estimated from the configuration of power lines and the load on the lines at various intervals before diagnosis.

Objective.—The original data from these studies, each of which included a limited number of cases, have been pooled to enlarge the database. The Swedish study was based on about 127,000 children living within 300 m of a 220- or 440-kV power line from 1960 to 1985. The Danish study is based on the entire Danish population younger than 15 years, followed from 1968 through 1986. National cancer registries in both nations were surveyed to identify cases of leukemia, lymphoma, and CNS tumor.

Findings.—Calculated magnetic field levels of 0.2 µT and higher carried a relative risk of 2.0 for childhood leukemia. The relative risk for exposure to field levels of 0.5 µT and higher was 5.1 (Table 3). The risk of lymphoma was increased for intermediate exposure levels only, but there were only 2 exposed cases in the group with highest exposure. There was no indication of an association between magnetic field exposure and CNS tumors.

Conclusion.—Scandinavian children exposed residentially to high magnetic fields appear to be at increased risk of leukemia.

▶ This story, which attempts to link power lines and magnetic fields to the occurrence of childhood cancer, seems to have no final chapter. We're approaching 20 years since the first description suggesting a link between residential exposure to magnetic fields and malignancy in children.[1] As recently as 1993, results from 2 Scandinavian studies investigating the relationship between magnetic fields from power lines and childhood cancer showed elevated relative risks of leukemia among children exposed to such fields.[2, 3] One of these studies also found an increased risk of lymphoma. These 2 studies took advantage of the population registry system in Scandinavian countries that makes it possible to avoid problems with selection bias. They also used a novel approach to exposure assessment, in that magnetic fields were tabulated based on power line configuration and load on the power lines for different points in time before diagnosis. The study abstracted extends these findings by adding more patients from Scandina-

TABLE 3.—Cancer Risk in Relation to Cumulative Lifetime Magnetic Field Exposure, Adjusted for Age, Sex, and Country

Diagnosis	µT-years	Swedish study				Danish study				Combined study			
		No. Cases	No. Controls	RR	95% CI	No. Cases	No. Controls	RR	95% CI	No. Cases	No. Controls	RR	95% CI
Leukemia	≤0.09	21	336	1		829	4760	1		850	5096	1	
	0.1–0.9	11	180	1.4	0.6–3.0	1	18	0.4	0.0–2.7	12	198	0.9	0.5–1.8
	≥1.0	6	38	3.6	1.3–9.8	3	10	1.9	0.5–7.1	9	48	2.5	1.1–5.4
Lymphoma	≤0.09	10	336	1		245	4760	1		255	5096	1	
	0.1–0.9	8	180	1.3	0.5–3.5	4	18	4.0	1.3–11.8	12	198	2.0	0.9–4.3
	≥1.0	1	38	0.8	0.1–6.5	1	10	1.7	0.2–13.1	2	48	1.2	0.3–5.3
Central	≤0.09	18	336	1		621	4760	1		639	5096	1	
nervous	0.1–0.9	14	180	1.2	0.6–2.5	1	18	0.4	0.1–3.1	15	198	1.2	0.6–2.2
system	≥1.0	1	38	0.4	0.0–3.0	2	10	1.5	0.3–6.8	3	48	0.8	0.2–2.7
tumor													
Combined	≤0.09	49	336	1		1695	4760	1		1744	5096	1	
group	0.1–0.9	33	180	1.3	0.8–2.1	6	18	1.0	0.4–2.4	39	198	1.2	0.8–1.9
	≥1.0	8	38	1.5	0.6–3.4	6	10	1.7	0.6–4.7	14	48	1.6	0.8–2.9

Abbreviations: RR, relative risk; *CI*, confidence interval.
(Courtesy of Feychting M, Schulgen G, Olsen JH, et al: Magnetic fields and childhood cancer: A pooled analysis of two Scandinavian studies. *Eur J Cancer* 31A:2035–2039, Copyright 1995, with kind permission from Elsevier Science Ltd, The Boulevard, Langford Lane, Kidlington 0X5 1GB, UK.)

vian oversight investigations. The main finding of the report was an elevated relative risk for childhood leukemia in relation to calculated exposures to magnetic fields. The study also confirmed an added risk for lymphoma, albeit based on very small numbers.

Thinking there is a last word on the topic of magnetic fields as a cause of leukemia is about as wishful a form of thinking as is possible. Nonetheless, Levallois took on the formidable task of doing a meta-analysis of all of the literature from the past 10 years that has examined the possibility of a causal relationship between exposure to electromagnetic fields and childhood leukemia.[4] The conclusion: On the basis of epidemiologic findings to date, as well as on the analysis of their strengths and limitations and on the discussion of classical criteria for causal inference, it appears that the 50- to 60-Hz magnetic fields emanating from electrical wiring cannot be dismissed as a possible causal factor for childhood leukemia. The evidence is even stronger when the results of recent epidemiologic studies are taken into account. The public health impact of possible effects of exposure to electromagnetic fields is difficult to assess. Nonetheless, given the large number of children exposed to electromagnetic fields, such an impact could be extraordinarily significant. The concept of prudent avoidance, as proposed some years ago here in the United States, has actually been implemented in Sweden.[5]

The real issue with all studies relating power lines and malignancy has to do with whether firm conclusions can be drawn. What do we as physicians and what do other public health providers draw in terms of conclusions? To be honest about it, the small number of exposed cases makes it extremely difficult to form strong conclusions about a dose-response pattern. A focus on highly exposed individuals and future studies seems to be the right way to go.

If you were a school physician and were asked to advise a school board about whether a new school can be safely constructed near power lines, you probably would be hard pressed to make a firm statement. In Sweden and Denmark, where these studies were performed, officials have concluded that restricting exposure to high-voltage installations does limit public health risks.

References

1. Wertheimer N, et al: *Am J Epidemiol* 109:273, 1979.
2. Olsen JH, et al: *BMJ* 307:891, 1993.
3. Feychting M, et al: *Am J Epidemiol* 138:467, 1993.
4. Levallois P: *Am J Prev Med* 11:263, 1995.
5. Anonymous: No EMF limits in Sweden in near future. *EMF Health Safety Dig* 12:16, 1994.

15 Ophthalmology

Can Non-ophthalmologists Screen for Retinopathy of Prematurity?
Saunders RA, Bluestein EC, Berland JE, et al (Med Univ of South Carolina, Charleston)
J Pediatr Ophthalmol Strabismus 32:302–304, 1995   15–1

Purpose.—Survival beyond the newborn period is becoming more common among low–birth weight infants, with a corresponding increase in the incidence of retinopathy of prematurity (ROP). Because of the complicated clinical courses of these infants, it is not always possible to perform a detailed examination of the peripheral retina. Also, appropriate specialists may not be available in the community for infants who are transferred before complete maturation of the retinal vessels. Some simplified method of screening the posterior pole vessels by a nonophthalmologist would increase the chances of identifying infants at risk for ROP. The ability of nonophthalmologists to identify retinal blood vessel abnormalities associated with ROP was evaluated.

Methods.—Fifty infants with birth weights of less than 1,600 g who were examined at 32–40 weeks after conception were studied. Each infant was evaluated by nonophthalmologist examiners—fourth-year medical students, pediatric residents, and nurse practitioners—who graded the ophthalmoscopic appearance of the posterior pole vessels as normal or abnormal. The teaching mirror of the indirect ophthalmoscope was used in 121 of these examinations and the direct ophthalmoscope in 179. At the same time, indirect ophthalmoscopy was performed by an ophthalmologist who examined the posterior pole vessels for abnormalities. This was followed by a peripheral fundus examination in both eyes.

Results.—The examinations performed by the nonophthalmologist examiners had a testing sensitivity of 96% using direct ophthalmoscopy and 92% using indirect ophthalmoscopy. The difference was nonsignificant. The results from these 2 techniques were combined, yielding a Clopper-Pearson 95% sensitivity confidence interval of 82% to 99% for the identification of abnormal arterioles and venules. The point estimate was 95%. Diagnostic reliability was similar for the nurse practitioners, medical students, and pediatric residents.

Conclusions.—Nonophthalmologist examiners can correctly identify vascular abnormalities of the posterior pole in premature infants. With proper training, these clinicians could perform screening examinations to identify premature infants with vascular abnormalities that place them at risk for ROP. The patients could then be promptly referred for complete ophthalmologic examination with peripheral funduscopy.

▶ The overall meaning of the data from this report is that nonophthalmologists can do a fairly good job of detecting ROP. Perhaps they are not as good as ophthalmologists, but they aren't half bad either.

This report comes none too early. As the number of low–birth weight (less than 1,500 g) infants surviving the newborn period continues to increase, the incidence of ROP is also increasing. Currently, about 50,000 infants born in the United States each year require screening examinations for ROP. They often have prolonged hospital courses with periods of clinical instability. Detailed examination of the eyes is not always possible, nor is an appropriate specialist consistently available in community nurseries for follow-up examinations of infants who have been transferred back from neonatal ICUs. Additionally, outside the United States, little or no screening is done because of a lack of adequately trained ophthalmologists. Throw all this together and you can see the importance of a simplified method of screening the retina of a preterm infant by a nonophthalmologist.

As good as these data are, we have to decide whether we are willing to miss 4% to 6% of retinal disease by having nonophthalmologists do the screening and also whether we can accept overdiagnosing 30% of patients. Actually, these numbers aren't terrible by any means because the nonophthalmologists in this study were nurse practitioners, medical students, and residents who had been given a "crash" course on how to examine the eyes of tiny newborns. With additional practice and training, the agreement between such unseasoned individuals and the expert pediatric ophthalmologist would be expected to improve substantially.

Are we as pediatricians and neonatologists willing to assume such responsibilities, particularly in an era of managed care in which we are increasingly expected to do more and to do it well? Frankly, there is nothing magical about an eye exam, even in a 1,200-g newborn. A generous dose of patience mixed with an anecdote for the fear of missing something would go a long way toward establishing the necessary competence to accomplish what these authors are suggesting.

Severe Retinopathy of Prematurity in Infants With Birth Weights Less Than 1250 Grams: Incidence and Outcome of Treatment With Pharmacologic Serum Levels of Vitamin E in Addition to Cryotherapy From 1985 to 1991
Johnson L, Quinn GE, Abbasi S, et al (Univ of Pennsylvania, Philadelphia)
J Pediatr 127:632–639, 1995   15–2

Background.—Cryotherapy significantly reduces the incidence of unfavorable outcome in eyes with severe retinopathy of prematurity (ROP). However, many eyes will still have an unfavorable structural outcome, and

TABLE 2.—Threshold Retinopathy of Prematurity (ROP) Treated With Cryotherapy

Study group	Treatment	Normal	Macular heterotopia	Retinal fold or worse
Pennsylvania Hospital (n = 17) 1985–1991	Vitamin E plus Cryotherapy	71% (n = 12)	12% (n = 2)	18% (n = 3)
CRYO-ROP (n = 207) 1986–1987	Cryotherapy only	38% (n = 79)	36% (n = 74)	26% (n = 54)

Note: Appearance of posterior retina at age 3½ years in infants with birth weight less than 1,251 g. Multiple chi-square analysis: CRYO-ROP vs. Pennsylvania Hospital, *P* = 0.03.

(Courtesy of Johnson L, Quinn GE, Abbasi S, et al: Severe retinopathy of prematurity with birth weights less than 1250 grams: Incidence and outcome of treatment with pharmacologic serum levels of vitamin E in addition to cryotherapy from 1985 to 1991. *J Pediatr* 127:632–639, 1995.)

about half will have an unfavorable functional outcome. Thus, some alternative or additional form of treatment is needed. Vitamin E is a biological antioxidant vitamin. The effects of vitamin E prophylaxis and treatment were assessed in cryotherapy-treated infants with ROP.

Methods.—Starting on the day of birth, all infants with birth weights of 1,250 g or less who were treated at 1 hospital received vitamin E supplements using standard preparations. For infants with immature retinal vasculature or ROP of stage 2 or less, vitamin E was given to achieve a target serum level of 23–58 μmol/L. For those with prethreshold ROP, the target was 58–81 μmol/L. If threshold ROP was diagnosed, the infants received an investigational new α-tocopherol preparation, given parenterally, to achieve a pharmacologic serum E level of 93–116 μmol/L. Cryotherapy to 1 or both eyes was performed within 3 days of the diagnosis of threshold ROP, at the discretion of the retinal specialist. The 4-year visual outcomes and structural findings (Table 2) were compared with 42-month outcomes in the previously reported Multicenter Trial of Cryotherapy for ROP (CRYO-ROP).

Results.—Of 450 infants who survived to 3 months of age, ROP developed in 22. Treatment to achieve pharmacologic serum E levels was given in all 22 patients. In addition, 17 received cryotherapy: 10 in 1 eye and 7 in both eyes. Risk of poor visual outcomes in the cryotherapy-treated infants was at least equal to that of 187 infants from the CRYO-ROP trial. This was so on the basis of birth weight, gestational age, percentage of zone 1 ROP, and the mean interval from appearance of ROP to the diagnosis of prethreshold ROP. The latter interval was only 4 days in the current study compared with 10 days in the CRYO-ROP trial. However, progression of retinopathy beyond the prethreshold stage was slower and visual outcomes were better for infants receiving both cryotherapy and vitamin E. The mean number of days between the diagnoses of prethreshold and threshold ROP was 12½ days in the current study vs. 10½ days in the CRYO-ROP trial. The mean extent of extraretinal neovascularization at threshold was 8 vs. 10 sectors, respectively (Table 4). Favorable visual acuity was present in 76% of infants receiving cryotherapy plus

TABLE 4.—Risk Factors for Unfavorable Outcome After Threshold Retinopathy of Prematurity (ROP) in Infants Weighing <1,251 g at Birth Who Were Treated With Cryotherapy

	Birth weight (gm)	Gestational age (wk)	Location threshold ROP zone 1	Interval ROP onset to prethreshold (days)	Interval prethreshold to threshold (days)	Age onset threshold ROP (wk)	Extent of stage 3+ ROP (sectors)
Pennsylvania Hospital: vitamin E + cryotherapy (n = 17; 1985–1991)	731 ± 162	25.7 ± 2.0	18%	4.1 ± 6.6 (0* to 28)	12.5 ± 13.0 (0* to 49)	11.3 ± 2.1	7.9 ± 2.5
CRYO-ROP cryotherapy (n = 207; 1986–1987)	800 ± 165	26.3 ± 1.8	10%	10.2† (5.8 to 14.7)	11.0† (6.9 to 15.6)	11.3 ± 2.4	9.7 ± 2.2

Note: Data are reported as mean ± SD.

*In 1 infant (birth weight, 492 g; gestational age, 26.5 weeks) the first appearance of retinopathy, at age 9 weeks, was reported as bilateral "Rush" ROP in zone 1 (threshold). The left eye was treated with cryotherapy. Functional outcome was favorable in both eyes.

†Standard deviation could not be computed from reported data; statistical analysis was deferred.

(Courtesy of Johnson L, Quinn GE, Abbasi S, et al: Severe retinopathy of prematurity in infants with birth weights less than 1250 grams: Incidence and outcome of treatment with pharmacologic serum levels of vitamin E in addition to cryotherapy from 1985 to 1991. *J Pediatr* 127:632–639, 1995.)

vitamin E vs. 48% for those receiving cryotherapy only. The percentage of patients with a structurally normal posterior pole was 71% vs. 38%, respectively.

Conclusions.—The addition of vitamin E prophylaxis and treatment to cryotherapy may decrease the severity and sequelae of threshold ROP in low–birth weight infants. A large multicenter clinical trial is needed to confirm the results of the current, small case series. Vitamin E nutrition and treatment may prove to be an important addition to the available surgical therapies for ROP.

▶ This editor has been hearing about vitamin E as part of the management of preterm infants since the start of his residency in the late 1960s. It's quite clear that vitamin E is hardly a panacea for what ails preterm infants. Nonetheless, we continue to see reports such as the one abstracted that seem to indicate that vitamin E can lend a modest margin to the success rate with which we can prevent or mollify retinal disease. From 1978 to early 1981, 6 controlled clinical trials of vitamin E prophylaxis, conducted in the United States and Canada, showed that vitamin E might be effective in lessening the severity of ROP. In the Baylor trial (1979–1980) of physiologic doses of vitamin E as prophylaxis for ROP, there again was some evidence that vitamin E might be of help. The data from the report abstracted are essentially the same as earlier data suggesting that vitamin E may be useful.

A word of warning is important when using vitamin E. Use doses of vitamin E that are at or near physiologic amounts. To say this differently, use amounts necessary to maintain vitamin E levels in the normative range. When huge pharmacologic doses are used, trouble can brew. An increased incidence of sepsis and delayed-onset necrotizing enterocolitis may be seen, particularly if vitamin E has been used very early on when immunologic function is considerably less than at 2 or 3 months of age.

Overall, it is obvious that vitamin E doesn't produce the fountain-of-youth effect that was once hoped for. Nonetheless, it does play an important role as a free radical scavenger. The trick is not to overdose on it or to expect too much. Please consider vitamin E to be just 1 variable in a complex equation that defines the risk of ROP.

Risk Factors for Acanthamoeba Keratitis in Contact Lens Users: A Case-control Study
Radford CF, Bacon AS, Dart JKG, et al (Moorfields Eye Hosp, London; Inst of Ophthalmology, London)
BMJ 310:1567–1570, 1995   15–3

Background.—Acanthamoebas are free-living amoebas in the air, dust, and water. The cysts of these amoebas are resistant to antimicrobial agents, including solutions currently used for contact lens disinfection. The relative risks of acanthamoeba keratitis associated with different lens types and the importance of lens type, disinfection regimens, and other risk factors were investigated.

Methods.—Thirty-five patients with acanthamoeba keratitis and 378 control subjects were enrolled in a case-control study. The control subjects were lens users without lens-related disease. Questionnaires eliciting information on lens use and hygiene practices were completed.

Findings.—Compared with conventional soft lens wearers, users of daily-wear disposable lenses had a crude relative risk of 49.45 for acanthamoeba keratitis. In a multivariate analysis, this increased risk was found to be primarily caused by lack of disinfection and the use of chlorine-based disinfection. No other significant associations were identified.

Conclusions.—Major risk factors for the development of acanthamoeba keratitis include failure to disinfect daily-wear soft contact lenses and the use of chlorine release lens disinfection systems, which have little protective effect against the organism. These are particularly common risks among disposable lens users. More than 80% of acanthamoeba keratitis may be avoided if lens disinfection systems effective against the organism were used.

▶ Most of us tend to think of amoebas as invading our gut, not our eyes, but indeed they may find their way into both. When it comes to the latter, they can wreak havoc. Although an uncommon cause of keratitis, amoebas in the eyes can initiate a potentially devastating corneal infection. Although this report is from London, we in the United States are seeing the emergence of a similar problem. The problem seems to be related to the use of daily-wear disposable lenses, which are now documented to be associated with a greatly increased risk of acanthamoeba keratitis.

Actually, it isn't just the daily-wear disposable lenses themselves that are the culprits. Only a relatively small excess risk of acanthamoeba keratitis is specifically associated with the use of these kinds of lenses. The real problem is that these lenses are considered to be "low care," which translates to some people as being "no care." Also, to ease care, at least in England, many use the simple chlorine release system of contact lens maintenance. Chlorine disinfectants, as opposed to other chemical disinfectants, do not work well against amoebic cysts, which can survive 10 times the concentration of chlorine used in many eye care systems. Amoebas are hardy, surviving the effects of high concentrations of chlorine that would have long since "done in" HIV.

The key messages are as follows:

- Failure to disinfect soft contact lenses and the use of chlorine disinfection systems are major factors accounting for the increase worldwide in cases of acanthamoeba keratitis.

- More than 80% of acanthamoeba infections could be eliminated by daily disinfection of reused lenses with systems effective against the organism.

- Disinfection systems ineffective against acanthamoeba should not be licensed for use here or anywhere.

Photoscreening for Amblyogenic Factors

Ottar WL, Scott WE, Holgado SI (Univ of Iowa, Iowa City)
J Pediatr Ophthalmol Strabismus 32:289–295, 1995   15–4

Introduction.—It is very important to detect amblyopia and amblyogenic factors in children, yet most available screening techniques are ineffective for use in preverbal children. In photoscreening, a flash photograph of the individual's eye is taken and the light reflected from the retina is analyzed to identify possible refractive errors, strabismus, and/or media opacities. The eccentric photoscreener known as the Medical Technology Inc. (MTI) Photoscreener is being marketed for the detection of amblyogenic factors in this age group. The sensitivity, specificity, and accuracy of the MTI Photoscreener were evaluated in healthy young children.

Methods.—The MTI Photoscreener was used to evaluate 1,003 healthy children aged 6–59 months. Each photograph was examined to measure the pupil and bright crescent size using the measurement tool supplied with the camera. Differences in crescent size were compared to detect anisometropia and astigmatism (Figs 2 and 3). The findings of 949 children were compared with those of a complete, cycloplegic ophthalmologic examination.

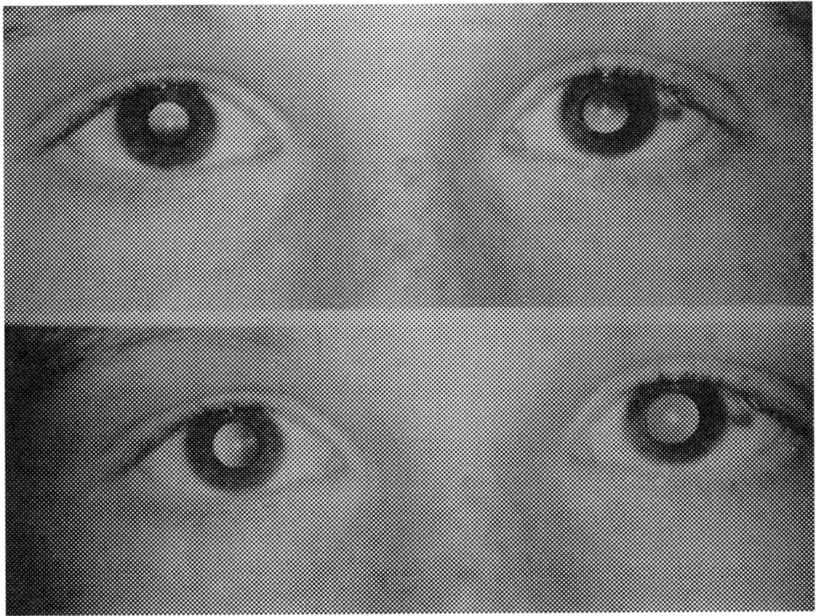

FIGURE 2.—Photoscreening picture of a subject with a difference in crescent location between the eyes. This is an example of anisometropia. **Upper photograph:** *right eye,* 3.0-mm myopic crecent in a 5-mm pupil; *left eye,* 3.0-mm hyperopic crescent in a 5.5-mm pupil. **Lower photograph:** *right eye,* 3.0-mm myopic crescent in a 5.5-mm pupil; *left eye,* 1.0-mm hyperopic crescent in a 6.0-mm pupil. (Courtesy of Ottar WL, Scott WE, Holgado Sl: Photoscreening for amblyogenic factors. *J Pediatr Ophthalmol Strabismus* 32:289–295, 1995.)

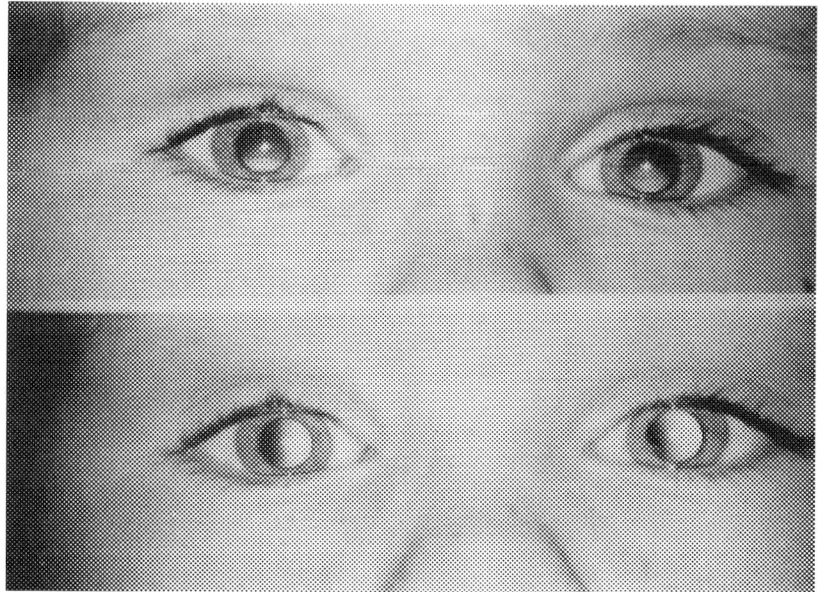

FIGURE 3.—Photoscreening picture of a subject with a difference in crescent size between the **upper and lower photograph.** This is an example of astigmatism. **Upper photograph:** *right eye,* 0.5-mm hyperopic crescent in a 6-mm pupil; *left eye,* 2.0-mm hyperopic crescent in a 6-mm pupil. **Lower photograph:** *right eye,* 3.0-mm hyperopic crescent in a 6-mm pupil; *Left eye,* 4.5-mm hyperopic crescent in a 6-mm pupil. (Courtesy of Ottar WL, Scott WE, Holgado Sl: Photoscreening for amblyogenic factors. *J Pediatr Ophthalmol Strabismus* 32:289–295, 1995.)

Results.—One hundred ninety-two patients failed the clinical eye examination, most commonly because of astigmatism, hyperopia, and myopia. The MTI Photoscreener had a sensitivity of 82% in correctly identifying the presence of an amblyogenic factor. The specificity in identifying the absence of any such factor was 91%, and the overall agreement rate in detecting normal and abnormal results was 89%. The Photoscreener examination had a positive predictive value of 69% and negative predictive value of 95%. No cases of strabismus or media opacities were missed.

Conclusions.—In preverbal children, the MTI Photoscreener is an accurate and reliable device for the detection of amblyogenic factors. The test is easily performed, inexpensive, and easy to interpret. It shows promise as a mass-screening tool for amblyogenic factors.

▶ This report was selected for inclusion in the YEAR BOOK OF PEDIATRICS to demonstrate how far along screening processes have developed to detect common childhood eye disorders. Among the most important consequences of a variety of eye problems is the development of amblyopia, which occurs in as many as 3% to 5% of children. The need for early detection of this problem is widely recognized and is the reason current vision screening methodologies have been developed. The technique that these authors used relies on an instant film photoscreener, the MTI Photoscreener. As the report indicates, the MTI Photoscreener has a high degree of sensitivity and specificity along with good accuracy in detecting strabismus, corneal and lens opacities, and refractive errors, all without the need for a detailed ophthalmologic examination. The equipment used has a rechargeable battery and can be used to screen many youngsters in a short period. The value of such methodologies is that they do not require pharmacologic dilation of the pupil. This can be done by having the children tested in a darkened room.

If you are not familiar with such screening methods to detect common eye problems in children, read this article in detail.

16 Dentistry and Otolaryngology

Planning for the Children of Your Current Pediatric Dental Patients
Waldman HB (State Univ of New York, Stony Brook)
J Dent Child 62:418–425, 1995

16–1

Objective.—By the year 2020, there will be an increase of 8.1 million children, and the increase will not be uniform across the country or across different ethnicities. At the same time, the number of dentists will be declining. Census figures were reviewed, as were projections from the American Dental Association, to develop an estimate of the number of pediatric dentists that will be needed.

Methods.—It was assumed that each state's present ratio of number of pediatric dentists to number of children is to be maintained, that all pediatric dentists older than 40 years in 1991 will not be practicing in 2020, and that all pediatric dentists younger than 40 years will still be practicing in 2020.

Changing Numbers of Children.—The numbers of children will decrease in the New England and Middle Atlantic states and increase everywhere else, particularly in the Pacific states.

Pediatric Dentists.—Only 28% of pediatric dentists were younger than 40 years in 1991. There were 5.1 pediatric dentists per 100,000 children younger than 18 years in 1993 (Table 3). Between 1993 and 2020, it will take 2,537 new pediatric dentists to treat the population of children. By 2020 there will be a total of 2,869 pediatric dental graduates in this country, 120 fewer than will be needed. Women in pediatric training programs increased from 45% in 1984 to 62% in 1993, but they tend to work fewer hours than men.

Conclusion.—The number of new pediatric dentists that will be needed is based on conservative estimates. These dentists will not necessarily distribute themselves according to the needs of the pediatric population. The dentist-to-patient ratio is expected to continue to decline. Manpower planning is necessary to optimize the dentist-to-patient ratio by evaluating service needs, evolving payment mechanisms, and disease patterns, and comparing them to the "production" of pediatric dental graduates.

TABLE 3.—Total Number of Private Practice Pediatric Dentists, Number Younger Than 40 Years in 1991, Ratio Per 100,000 Children Younger Than 15 Years, and Numbers Needed in 2020 by Region and State

| Region & State | 1991 | | 1993 | 2020 | |
	Total number	Number under age 40	Number pediatric dentists per 100,000 children	Total number ped. dentists needed to maintain 1993 ratio	Number of "new" pediatric dentists needed
New England	232	62	8.7	225	163
Connecticut	71	21	10.7	73	52
Maine	9	3	3.5	8	5
Massachusetts	121	32	10.2	111	79
New Hampshire	11	3	4.6	11	8
Rhode Island	14	3	7.0	13	10
Vermont	6	0	4.9	6	6
Middle Atlantic	449	152	5.8	446	294
New Jersey	110	32	6.8	120	88
New York	196	75	5.2	192	117
Pennsylvania	143	45	5.9	135	90
South Atlantic	460	128	4.8	529	401
Delaware	18	3	12.0	20	17
Dis. of Columbia	15	7	15.4	14	7
Florida	131	37	4.9	152	115
Georgia	73	20	4.7	88	68
Maryland	81	22	7.5	98	76
North Carolina	49	13	3.4	55	42
South Carolina	34	7	4.2	38	31
Virginia	62	19	4.6	71	52
West Virginia	7	1	2.0	6	5
East South Central	188	54	5.5	201	147
Alabama	50	8	5.5	58	50
Kentucky	44	14	5.5	44	30
Mississippi	24	7	3.9	24	17
Tennessee	69	25	6.5	74	49
East North Central	445	134	4.7	454	320
Illinois	125	4	4.8	133	129
Indiana	82	21	6.7	85	64
Michigan	63	17	2.9	66	49
Ohio	117	38	4.9	112	74
Wisconsin	59	16	5.2	58	42
West North Central	178	54	4.4	183	129
Iowa	38	11	6.2	36	25
Kansas	17	2	2.9	19	17
Minnesota	41	12	4.0	42	30
Missouri	47	15	4.1	49	34
Nebraska	25	9	6.7	26	17
North Dakota	4	2	2.8	4	2
South Dakota	5	3	2.9	5	2
West South Central	313	94	4.7	374	280
Arkansas	26	9	4.9	28	19
Louisiana	55	14	5.3	60	46
Oklahoma	27	4	3.7	30	26
Texas	205	67	4.7	257	190
Mountain	143	40	4.0	179	139
Arizona	29	6	5.5	31	25
Colorado	52	16	6.6	60	44
Idaho	9	2	3.3	11	9
Montana	7	2	3.7	8	6
Nevada	13	5	4.3	17	12
New Mexico	13	3	3.2	17	14
Utah	16	6	2.9	21	15
Wyoming	4	0	3.4	5	5
Pacific	541	109	5.6	763	654
Alaska	5	1	3.0	6	5
California	418	87	5.6	598	511
Hawaii	27	8	10.5	40	32
Oregon	39	8	5.9	51	43
Washington	52	5	4.4	69	64
United States	2,948	825	5.2	3,362	2,537

Note: Totals may differ as a result of rounding. Number of pediatric dentists and number younger than 40 years as presented in the American Dental Association publication.

(Courtesy of Waldman HB: Planning for the children of your current pediatric dental patients. *J Dent Child* 62:418–425, 1995.)

▶ In some respects, our dental colleagues are way ahead of us in terms of workforce planning. For example, take the article abstracted, which attempts to fine-tune the requirements for pediatric dental practitioners. It does this by making assumptions about how many children will need to be cared for between now and the year 2020. An understanding of this report has direct implications for pediatricians because the report gives accurate information from the U.S. Census Bureau about the projection of increases in number of children over the next 2½ decades. The Bureau tells us that between 1993 and 2020, there will be an increase of 8.1 million children (a 14.2% increase) younger than 15 years. The changes in numbers of children will not be uniform, however, throughout the country, ranging from decreases of 135,000 children in Pennsylvania and 89,000 children in Massachusetts and Ohio, to an increase of 1.1 million children in Texas and 3.2 million in California. In addition, the population changes will vary by race and ethnic origin. It is estimated that by 2020, California will have the largest white, Asian-American, and Hispanic populations. New York will have the largest black population, and Arizona will have the largest Native American population. Each of these populations has varying workforce requirements in terms of dental providers.

This overall increase in the general and child population is occurring at a time when we are seeing marked decreases in the overall numbers of dentists in this country. This decrease is expected to result in the lowest ratios of dentists to overall population that have been recorded throughout this century.[1]

How all this shakes out is pretty straightforward. If you do the math and assume that you would like to maintain the current ratio of number of pediatric dentists to number of children younger than 18 years, then by 2020 a total of 3,414 pediatric dentists will be needed. This includes 825 current pediatric dentists younger than 40 years of age, 2,123 "new" dentists to replace all current pediatric dentists older than 40 years, and 466 "new" pediatric dentists for the additional children.

Will our dental schools and pediatric dental residencies meet these goals? The answer is likely yes, especially because interest in pediatric dentistry appears now to be at an all-time high. Children deserve to be cared for by those who are best trained to provide that care, assuming cost-effective equivalency. By some time in elementary school, you have only 1 set of teeth to last you for the rest of your life. We should be supportive of our pediatric dentistry colleagues, for they, perhaps like us, are at risk in the competitive world of care providers. Neither pediatricians nor pediatric dentists are on the endangered species list, at least not at the present time. To prevent this from happening, we must be willing to demonstrate that what we do is of high quality and worth the quality.

Reference

1. Waldman HB: *Ill Dent J* 63:99, 1994.

Nursing-bottle Syndrome: Risk Factors

Muller M (Conferences des Universités, Nice, France)
J Dent Child 63:42–50, 1996

Introduction.—Nursing-bottle syndrome involves a rapidly destroyed primary dentition. A group of children with nursing-bottle syndrome were studied to identify socioeconomic, medical, nutritional, and oral hygiene risks associated with the syndrome.

Methods.—A total of 139 children younger than age 6 years were seen with nursing-bottle syndrome during a 30-month period. Their parents completed a questionnaire that requested information on the family demographics, the child's medical history, nutritional habits, and the history of tooth brushing and fluoride administration.

Results.—The parents of the affected children typically had low socioprofessional status and were more often of white than black ethnicity. There were an average of 2.66 children in these families, but 27.34% of the children were the only child in the family. In families with multiple children, the other children were also frequently affected. A medicinal

TABLE 4.—Child's Position in Family, Health Status, Diet, Oral Hygiene, and Fluoride Ingestion by the Affected Children According to Ethnic Origin

	Ethnic origins	Total	Male	Female
Affected children		139	77	62
Affected child's position in family				
	Only child	38	23	15
	Eldest	13	8	5
	Middle	30	17	13
	Youngest	58	29	29
Children suffering from serious illness		39	20	19
Children without severe illness		100	57	43
Breast-fed < 8 months		74	39	35
Breast-fed > 8 months		10	6	4
No breast-feeding		55	32	23
Sweetened pacifier		7	4	3
Chocolate		1		1
Misuse of baby bottle (2)		90	54	36
Medicinal syrup consumption (1)		3	2	1
(1) and (2)		38	17	21
Oral hygiene frequency	Never	30	20	10
	< 1t/d	9	5	4
	1 t/d	49	30	19
	2 t/d	44	19	25
	3 t/d	7	3	4
Tooth brushing by	Nobody	30	20	10
	Child	72	36	36
	Mother	37	21	16
Fluoride tablet consumption	Never	58	37	21
	1 t/d	44	24	20
	2 t/d	36	16	20
	3 t/d	1		1

(Courtesy of Muller M: Nursing-bottle syndrome: Risk Factors. *J Dent Child* 63:42–50, 1996.)

syrup, taken for an average of more than 1 week per month for at least 1 year, was a significant risk factor. The use of sweetened baby bottles was reported for 92.68%, with sweetened milk being the most common sweetened liquid reported. Feeding while falling asleep was reported for 109 children for an average of 32.45 months. No teeth cleaning was reported for 21.58% of the children. Among those with a tooth-brushing history, brushing began at the age of 2.45 years, with ethnicity-associated variation. Of the affected children, 58% had never used fluoride supplements, and the dosage was often inappropriately low in the remaining patients (Table 4).

Conclusions.—Interdisciplinary cooperation is necessary to prevent the occurrence of nursing-bottle syndrome. Risk-prone families must be taught proper oral hygiene methods. The appropriate dosage and form of fluoride should be prescribed and applied. Pediatricians should limit the prescription of sucrose-based syrups, particularly for bedtime treatment. If they are necessary, a fluoridated toothpaste or mouthwash should also be prescribed. Parents should be advised to limit the use of bottles containing a liquid with sucrose, fructose, or lactose and to give a bottle only with the child held in the arms, never in bed. The use of a cup is recommended after the age of 6 months.

▶ The entity known as nursing-bottle syndrome has been with us for some time. The earliest descriptions of it are from the mid-1800s.[1] Breast-feeding that is prolonged beyond the normal age for weaning is also a known risk factor for this dental disease. In addition to bottle-feeding and extended breast-feeding, other risk factors include falling asleep with a pacifier covered with honey or jam and the regular use of syrups for therapeutic reasons during chronic or recurring illnesses.

The study abstracted attempts to tell us additional specific risk factors for nursing-bottle caries. At-risk children are from families with an average of 2.66 children. Low or moderately low parent socioeconomic status is fairly common. This is not a universal finding, however. Also at risk is the youngster with no siblings. The "only" child is the one to whom nothing is refused, including that which gets into his or her mouth. Thus, having a lot of children or very few children in a family appear to be risk factors for nursing-bottle caries. Lastly, failure to brush is a significant contributor to this problem. Would you believe that by the age of 2½ years, 20% to 25% of children in this series had never seen the working end of a toothbrush?

Care of one's primary dentition goes a long way to make for a healthy mouth and one's permanent teeth. One is never too young to use fluoride. A bit of Pepsodent wouldn't hurt either.

As an aside, are you aware of what the most natural of toothbrushes is? It's the chewing stick, *Salvadora persica*.[2] In fact, chewing sticks have been used for more than 7,000 years. The Babylonians were documented to have used them. They were later used by the Greek and Roman emperors and have been used by Jews, Egyptians, and many other peoples over the ages. Today they may be found in Africa, Asia, the middle Mediterranean region, and South America. *Salvadora persica* is a small tree or shrub with a crooked trunk. Its stems and roots are spongy and can be easily crushed between the teeth. Such chewing sticks contain trimethylamine, salvadorine, chloride, fluoride (in large amounts), silica, sulfur, vitamin C, and small amounts of tannins, sapomins, flavenoids, and sterols. In many parts of the world, chewing sticks are a good alternative to a toothbrush as a means of preventing oral and dental disease. They clean all the teeth, not those that just see the brushes of a toothbrush.[3] With this novel form of cleaning one's teeth, parents of kids who fail to brush their teeth can now chew them out, both figuratively and literally.

References

1. Michaels KB, et al: *Lancet* 347:431, 1996.
2. Missouris CG, et al: *Lancet* 408, 1996
3. Almas K, et al: *World Health Forum* 16:206, 1995.

Effects of Current and Former Pacifier Use on the Dentition of 24- to 59-month-old Children
Adair SM, Milano M, Lorenzo I, et al (Med College of Georgia, Augusta; Danbury, Conn; Manila, The Philippines)
Pediatr Dent 17:437–444, 1995   16–3

Introduction.—It has long been recognized that nonnutritive sucking has soothing effects in infants. However, pacifier use has also been associated with malocclusions. In an attempt to normalize arch development and minimize malocclusion, pacifiers and nursing-bottle nipples have been developed that more closely resemble the shape of the mother's breast during feeding. The effects of both types of pacifiers on dentition were studied in children aged 24–59 months, and compared in those with current, former, or no pacifier use. In addition, ethnic patterns of pacifier use were compared.

Methods.—Dental examinations were performed on 218 children between the ages of 24 and 59 months without digit sucking habits. A parent completed a questionnaire that requested information on ethnicity, the type of pacifier used, the hours per day of pacifier use, and the ages at which a pacifier was used. Occlusion was compared between pacifier users and children who had never used pacifiers, between current and former pacifier users, and between users of conventional pacifiers and users of functional exercises.

Results.—Compared with the children who had not used pacifiers, children with a history of pacifier use had a significantly greater mean overjet and a significantly greater incidence of Class II primary canine relationships, distal step primary molar relationships, openbites, and posterior crossbites. There were no significant differences between the users of conventional pacifiers and the users of functional exercises in the mean overjet or the incidence of openbite or posterior crossbites. However, the users of functional exercisers were significantly more likely to have class II

TABLE 6.—Differences in Pacifier Use and Occlusion Between African-Americans ($n = 55$) and European-Americans ($n = 60$)

Parameter	African-Americans	European-Americans	Significance (P)
Mean age at start of habit months (SD)	2.4 (2.4)	2.3(2.8)	0.924†
Mean use per day hours (SD)	6.5 (4.3)	6.7 (3.5)	0.739†
Mean duration of use months (SD)*	15.1 (10.9)	23.7 (11.5)	< 0.001†
Mean time since discontinuation months (SD)*	24.5 (16.6)	18.4 (16.0)	0.047†
Overjet, mm mean (SD)	2.1 (1.5)	2.7 (1.5)	0.019†
Occurrence (%) of overjet ≥4 mm	16.4	21.7	0.644‡
Occurrence (%) of openbite	10.9	21.7	0.139‡
Openbite, mm mean (SD)	2.8 (1.9) (N = 6)	2.8 (1.5) (N = 13)	0.939†
Occurrence (%) of one or two Class II canines	16.2	19.7	0.600‡
Occurrence (%) of distal step molars	4.5	15.0	0.009‡
Occurrence (%) of posterior crossbite	5.5	23.3	0.008‡

*Among those who had discontinued habit: African-American, $n = 47$; European-American, $n = 48$.
†t-test of independent groups.
‡Fisher's exact test.
(Courtesy of Adair SM, Milano M, Lorenzo I, et al: Effects of current and former pacifier use on the dentition of 24- to 59-month-old children. *Pediatr Dent* 17:437–444, 1995.)

primary canines and distal step molars. The number of hours of use per day did not correlate with any of the occlusions. However, children with prolonged use were more likely to have openbites and posterior crossbites.

European-Americans and African-Americans began pacifier use at similar ages and had similar patterns of hours of pacifier use per day. However, African-American children discontinued pacifier use significantly sooner, had a smaller mean overjet, and had a lower incidence of distal step molars and posterior crossbites (Table 6)

Conclusions.—Pacifier use results in significant occlusions in all 3 planes, with no benefit associated with the use of functional exercisers. A longer duration of pacifier use can increase the occurrence of anterior openbite and posterior crossbite. The patterns of pacifier use were similar in African-American and European-American infants, except that the African-American children tended to discontinue pacifier use sooner.

► Pacifiers, or as the British call them, dummies, have been around a long time. The soothing effects on infants and young children of nonnourishing sucking have been apparent to caretakers for some centuries. For example, reference to sucking such objects appeared in the German medical literature in the late 15th and early 16th centuries.[1, 2] Winter described the use in 1801 of a linen "sucking bag" containing milk, sugar, and bread used to feed and comfort children. In 1996, current data suggest that somewhere between 60% and 95% of children have used pacifiers in this country, the variation depending on local customs.

Pacifiers can cause no end of dental problems, particularly with malocclusions. Anterior openbites have been reported in as many as 75% of children who have used pacifiers for prolonged periods of time. Other difficulties, such as crossbites and increased overjet, are also common, as is an increased prevalence of what is known as Class II canines (a.k.a., Bela Lugosi variants). As you might suspect, binkie manufacturers have attempted to design pacifiers and nursing bottle nipples to more closely imitate the shape of a mother's breast as it is in an infant's mouth during feeding. One such product, the Nuk Functional Orthodontic Nursing Nipple and Orthodontic Pacifier/Exerciser was introduced in this country in the late 1950s. It has been promoted as allowing a more natural arch development because it encourages muscular movements that closely approximate those seen with breast-feeding. Some time ago, Adair et al. demonstrated, in a study of 54 pacifier users and 25 controls, no clinically significant differences in the dental problems of children using such specifically designed functional exerciser pacifiers in comparison to conventional pacifiers.[3] In the study abstracted, the comparison of 2 similar pacifier groups also shows no support for the purported advantages of functional exercisers over conventional pacifiers. Curiously, babies using functional exercisers tended to maintain their pacifier habit for a substantially shorter time yet demonstrated no lesser incidence of dental problems.

Parents who allow their infants and toddlers to use pacifiers to an excessive degree must recognize the long-term problems that can be created. If you don't want your child to have a malformed mouth and wind up getting a lot of x-ray examinations and orthodontia, go easy on the binkies. By the way, do you know the dose effect of a single dental radiograph? Not much. The average exposure to the face and lens of the eye per dental radiograph is just 0.001–0.003 Gy. It takes an average dose of 2.0–3.0 Gy to produce redness of the skin and the face, more than 1,000 times the diagnostic x-ray exposure per single radiograph. Thus, your dentist is not likely to do harm to your face unless he or she goes whole hog and orders 30 views of each of your teeth.[4]

References

1. Ravn JJ: *Community Dent Oral Epidemiol* 2:316, 1974.
2. Winter GB: *Int Dent J* 30:28, 1980.
3. Adair SM, et al: *Pediatr Dent* 14:13, 1992
4. Daffner RH, et al: *JAMA* 273:503, 1995.

Premature Loss of the Maxillary Primary Incisors: Effect on Speech Production
Gable TO, Kummer AW, Lee L, et al (Children's Hosp Med Ctr, Cincinnati, Ohio)
J Dent Child 62:173–179, 1995   16–4

Background.—Dental caries—most often caused by the nursing bottle—sometimes necessitates extraction of the maxillary anterior teeth in children younger than 5 years of age. The few studies of such children suggest that premature loss of the missing maxillary primary central and lateral incisors may lead to residual speech problems. The effects of premature extraction of the maxillary incisors on the development of speech were studied further.

Methods.—The study included 26 children who had had their 4 maxillary primary incisors extracted by the age of 5 years. They were tested at a mean age of 9 years 5 months, at which time all had their maxillary permanent incisors in place. The children underwent a hearing and dental screening, along with an articulation evaluation. This included an assessment of the production of all consonant sounds and 3 consonant blends, and of articulation at the sentence level. Twenty-six children with normal exfoliation of the maxillary primary incisors were studied for comparison.

Results.—The 2 groups of children were not significantly different in their articulatory abilities: about half of the children in each group produced articulation errors. In both groups, sibilant distortions and fricative substitutions were the most common types of errors. The number of errors was decreased in older children—very few articulation problems remained for children who were 10 years of age. Articulation was for the most part normal even for individuals with malocclusion.

Conclusions.—Children who undergo premature extraction of the maxillary incisors do not appear to have any lasting difficulties with speech. By the time they are 10 years of age, most of these children will have normal speech. With further research, it may be possible to identify special characteristics of children who fail to acquire normal speech sounds after early loss of teeth and thus to predict early speech problems.

▶ It may be unfortunate, but it does happen that children younger than 5 years of age must have their anterior teeth extracted because of dental caries. This report tells us that when the 4 maxillary incisors have to be removed, a youngster may be in for a problem with his or her speech. Eventually, however, things do turn out all right. Studies of approximately 700 children with normal exfoliation of their incisors reveal that most will manage to produce normal sounds, and most of those who have sound distortions will self-correct their errors when the missing teeth are replaced.[1] For children who have their teeth forcibly removed, once permanent dentition erupts, speech generally does return to normal, at least by 10 years of age.

The article includes a couple dozen sentences that illustrate how to demonstrate speech problems in those who have no front teeth. If you have a child at home who is 6 years old and is now lacking the requisite number of baby teeth, try some of these sentences out on him or her. It will teach you what these investigators were looking for. The transient speech impediment that comes with having missing front teeth is no fun for kids. It is the sort of predicament of which songs are written: "All I Want for Christmas is My Two Front Teeth."

While on the topic of dentistry, are you aware of what dentists' incomes are doing in an era of health care reform? The income of dentists, which had been on a slide until the late 1980s, has really turned around. This change is based on the fact that the dentist-to-population ratio reached a peak in 1987 and has declined since then (dental school graduate numbers were 5,056 in 1983, but only 3,778 in 1993). Results from the 1993 American Dental Association Survey of Dental Practice-Specialists in private practice (1992 data) indicate that the average net income from private pediatric dental practice was $145,020, compared with the average net income of $153,700 for all independent dental specialists.

Reference

1. Snow K, et al: *J Speech Hear Disord* 26:209, 1961.

Treatment of Resistant Oral Aphthous Ulcers in Children With Acquired Immunodeficiency Syndrome
de Asis MLB, Bernstein LJ, Schliozberg J (Albert Einstein College, Bronx, NY)
J Pediatr 127:663–665, 1995   16–5

Background.—Aphthous ulcers of the oral cavity, pharynx, and esophagus are a problem in adult patients with AIDS. If not appropriately treated, the ulcers may persist or recur and cause significant pain and dysphagia. They also may involve areas of the gastrointestinal tract. These lesions may be equally important in children with AIDS, who may rapidly become dehydrated and malnourished.

Clinical Aspects.—Oral prednisone was used to treat resistant oral aphthous ulcers in 4 pediatric patients with AIDS, all of whom had pain and dysphagia. Oral intake was limited by the ulcers in all patients, who initially failed to respond to a 0.1% dexamethasone rinse when tried for 3–5 days. The 2 biopsy specimens demonstrated chronic inflammatory changes.

Treatment and Outcome.—The patients received prednisone orally in a dose of 1–5 mg/kg daily for up to 2 weeks, within which time all the ulcers healed (Table). Two patients had recurrent aphthous ulcers after 4–6 months, which responded to a second course of prednisone. Three of the

TABLE.—Characteristics and Clinical Course

Patient No.	Age (yr)/ gender	Total CD4+ lymphocyte count	Current HIV-related illness	Previous treatment	Duration of ulcer before prednisone treatment (days)	Prednisone dose (mg/kg/day)	Time to ulcer resolution (days)
1	9/M	11	Mycobacterium avium-intracellulare; herpes simplex	Dexamethasone rinse (0.1%); IV acyclovir	14	1 (2 divided doses)	7
2	4/F	16	None	Antibiotic/ dexamethasone rinse; oral acyclovir	21	2 (2 divided doses)	7
3	6/F	10	None	Oral acyclovir; dexamethasone rinse (0.1%)	14	2 (1 dose/day)	5
4	3/M	176	None	Dexamethasone rinse (0.1%; oral acyclovir	7	5 (1 dose/day)	11

(Courtesy of de Asis MLB, Bernstein LJ, Schliozbergh J: Treatment of resistant oral aphthous ulcers in children with acquired immunodeficiency syndrome. *J Pediatr* 127:663–665, 1995.)

patients were receiving the antiretroviral agent didanosine, but their ulcers did not improve when the drug was withdrawn.

Conclusion.—A brief course of oral prednisone is an effective treatment for refractory aphthous ulcers in children with AIDS.

▶ The onset of mouth ulcers in a youngster with AIDS can have devastating effects. The pain and swallowing difficulty, which often persist for weeks, can lead to profound weight loss. Anything, literally anything, that can be done to terminate this problem is welcome, even if it involves "big league" therapies such as high-dose prednisone. Before resorting to systemic steroids, however, the ulcers must be identified as aphthous lesions. Therefore other causes such as herpes simplex, cytomegalovirus, tuberculosis, fungi, and malignancy must be ruled out by culture, biopsy, or both. When aphthous ulcers are limited to the oral cavity, topical corticosteroid therapy (0.1% dexamethasone rinse) may be sufficient, but if the lesions persist, systemic therapy in the form of corticosteroids may be necessary.

Why immunocompromised patients, and some normal people, have recurrent aphthous ulcers is yet to be determined. Predisposing factors such as trauma, nutritional deficiencies (folic acid, iron, vitamin B_{12}, and zinc), endocrine disorders, emotional stress, and allergic reactions have all been implicated, in addition to serious underlying immunodeficiency problems. If treatment with high-dose systemic steroids makes you squirrelly, 3 other forms of therapy have been reported to be effective on occasion. These include cimetidine, levamisole, and thalidomide.[1-3]

Even if you don't care for a child with AIDS, much less a child with AIDS and aphthous ulcers, surely you have cared for other children with aphthous ulcers or had some personal experience with them. The report abstracted is important not just because of its implications for children with AIDS, but because it tells us a great deal more about the nature of aphthous ulcers, their cause, and the wide variety, of treatment options that exist. Suffer not, there are therapies that can now help.

References

1. Feder HM, et al: *Pediatr Infect Dis J* 8:186, 1989.
2. Glick M, et al: *J Am Dent Assoc* 123:61, 1992.
3. Youle M, et al: *BMJ* 298:432, 1989.

Looking a Gift Horse in the Mouth: Effects of Cornstarch Therapy and Other Implications of Glycogen Storage Disease on Oral Hygiene and Dentition
Farrington FH, Duncan LL, Roth KS (Med College of Virginia, Richmond)
Pediatr Dent 17:311–314, 1995   16–6

Background.—Cornstarch treatment effectively prevents hypoglycemia in patients with glycogen storage disease, eliminating the need for nightly nasogastric intubation. However, in patients with compromised resistance

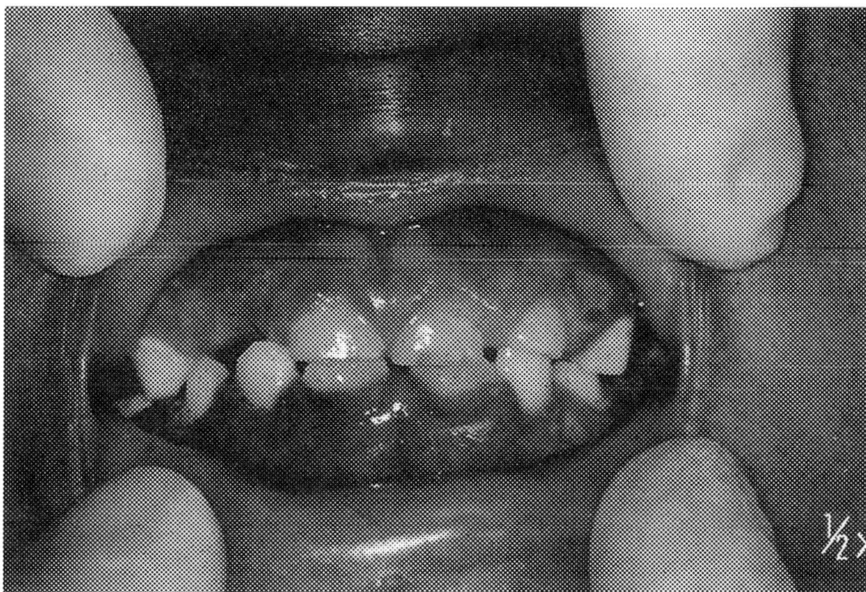

FIGURE 1.—Plaque and materia alba around gingival margin of teeth with resultant decalcification and smooth surface caries development. (Courtesy of Farrington FH, Duncan LL, Roth KS: Looking a gift horse in the mouth: Effects of cornstarch therapy and other implications of glycogen storage disease on oral hygiene and dentition. *Pediatr Dent* 17:311–314, 1995.)

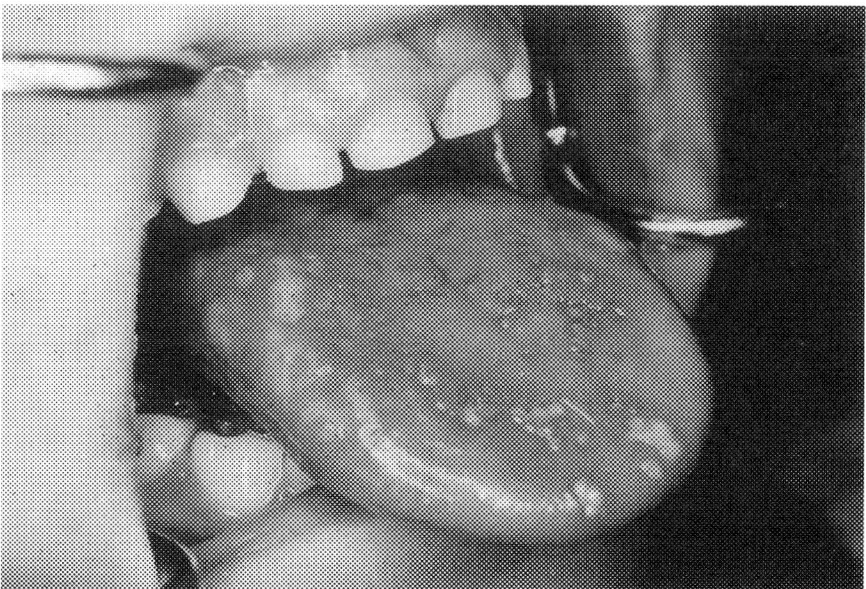

FIGURE 2.—Herpetiform lesions on the tongue. (Courtesy of Farrington FH, Duncan LL, Roth KS: Looking a gift horse in the mouth: Effects of cornstarch therapy and other implications of glycogen storage disease on oral hygiene and detition. *Pediatr Dent* 17:311–314, 1995.)

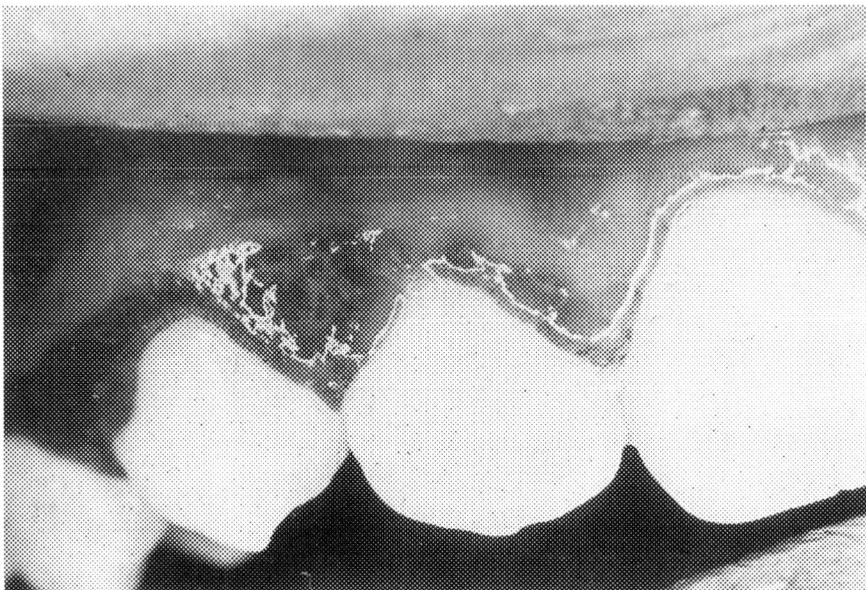

FIGURE 3.—Acute marginal gingivitis and herpetic-type lesions noted above the marginal tissue. (Courtesy of Farrington FH, Duncan LL, Roth KS: Looking a gift horse in the mouth: Effects of cornstarch therapy and other implications of glycogen storage disease on oral hygiene and dentition. *Pediatr Dent* 17:311–314, 1995.)

to pyogenic organisms, such treatment can have significant implications for oral hygiene and dentition. A child with type IB glycogenosis, in whom cornstarch treatment and frequent pyogenic infections resulted in major oral health problems, was described.

Case Report.—Girl, 6 months, had type I glycogen storage disease diagnosed clinically. Specific assessments at 16 months of age documented type IB disease. At 8 months of age, the patient began having recurrent otitis media, possibly caused by the partial obstruction from the nasogastric tube. Treatment consisted of a variety of antibiotics. Cornstarch therapy was begun at 18 months, earlier than recommended, because of problems with continuous nasogastric feeding. She did well on the cornstarch regimen. From 18 to 21 months of age, she had acute and chronic bouts of otitis media that required almost constant antibiotic treatment. Multiple episodes of oral thrush resulted, which adversely affected her oral intake. By 23 months of age, significant gingivitis was noted, compounded by an ineffectual leukocytic response. Bilateral myringotomy, performed at 25 months of age, relieved her middle ear problems and produced a dramatic improvement in her general health, appetite, and growth. At 42 months of age, she began having increased mouth breathing and breathing obstruction. At 51 months of age, tonsillectomy and adenoidectomy were performed, with the removal of "huge, obstructing" tonsils. Subsequently, her general health and development, to the age of 9 years and 9 months, have been good.

The patient's initial dental referral was at 18 months of age because of oral pain and recurrent soft-tissue ulcers. The ulcers recurred every 30 days. These lesions were diminished with treatment, but the child was seen again at 21 months of age because of oral ulcers with right-sided facial swelling. Many ulcers were observed on the lips, gingiva, tongue, mucobuccal fold, and palate (Figs 1–3). Oral hygiene was poor, and the teeth were continually coated with white milky plaque from cornstarch. However, there was no evidence of dental caries. At 30 months of age, plaque removal revealed extensive enamel decalcification. Occlusal and interproximal decay were found in several posterior teeth. Tooth extractions were necessary.

Conclusions.—This is the first report of the effects of cornstarch treatment on dentition in children with glycogen storage disease. Pediatricians must be aware of these adverse effects. Close cooperation among the pediatrician, dentist, otolaryngologist, and anesthesiologist is essential to safely perform procedures that are otherwise routine. Prolonged dental chair anesthesia is a threat to these patients' survival.

▶ Cornstarch is a gift to those with glycogen storage disease, particularly type I (von Gierke's disease). Youngsters with this disorder require a constant supply of glucose; otherwise lactic acidosis and hypoglycemia may develop. One of the easiest ways to supply glucose in a steady fashion is to administer cornstarch on a regular basis, particularly before retiring. Pancreatic amylase slowly digests the starch to yield glucose. With this form of therapy, life-threatening episodes of low blood sugar can be avoided.

As this article tells us, the administration of cornstarch for these purposes is like looking a gift horse in the mouth. The case study shows how devastating to one's oral hygiene the combination of von Gierke's disease and its treatment can be. The disease itself is associated with an increased susceptibility to pyogenic infections as a result of leukocyte dysfunction. The latter results from the cumulative effect of impairments in white blood cell metabolism caused by the metabolic defect. Add to this problem the fact that cornstarch is readily converted to glucose in the mouth by salivary amylase and you have a perfect setup for tooth and gum disease.

Not everybody in a primary care practice takes care of infants or children affected by a storage disease requiring cornstarch therapy. We all can, however, learn from the information provided by this report. It teaches us a great deal about the pathophysiology of oral hygiene–related diseases.

Lasty, recognize that cornstarch can cause problems other than just those in the mouth. Many of us substitute cornstarch for talcum powder for use in the diaper area. Should an infant inhale cornstarch, it can be as dangerous as talcum powder to the lungs. Reports have been published of the onset of acute respiratory distress requiring intubation secondary to cornstarch inhalation.

Oral Sequelae of Chronic Neutrophil Defects: Case Report of a Child With Glycogen Storage Disease Type 1b

Dougherty N, Gataletto MA (Albert Einstein College of Medicine, New York)
Pediatr Dent 17:224–229, 1995   16–7

Introduction.—Individuals with glycogen storage disease (GSD) type 1b, in whom glycogen is deposited in the liver rather than being metabolized to glucose, may have neutropenia and dysfunctional neutrophils. As a result, they are at risk of early and marked periodontal breakdown, as well as frequent oral ulcerations.

Case Report.—Boy, 3 months, was seen with diarrhea, dehydration, failure to thrive, and massive hepatomegaly. A liver biopsy specimen showing fatty infiltration and more than 10% glycogen prompted enzyme tests, which demonstrated GSD type 1b. The infant was mildly retarded functionally. He had both hypoglycemic and central seizures. Neutropenia as marked as 100 cells/mm^3 was present throughout the patient's life. Crohn's disease was diagnosed at 14 years of age and controlled with prednisone In late adolescence, a cardiomyopathy developed and progressed, leading to death resulting from presumed congestive heart failure and pulmonary edema at 21 years of age. The patient had had generalized alveolar bone loss at an early age and subsequently had

TABLE.—Conditions Exhibiting Neutrophil Disorders With Oral Manifestations

Condition	Neutrophil Disorder	Oral Manifestation
	⇊chemotaxis	Severe periodontal disease,
Chediak-Higashi disease	⇊phagocytosis	ulcerations
Papillon-Lefèvre syndrome	⇊chemotaxis	Severe periodontal disease
Infantile genetic agranulocytosis	Neutropenia	Gingival inflammation, ulcerations
Cyclic neutropenia	Neutropenia	Gingival inflammation, ulcerations
Benign chronic neutropenia	Neutropenia	Gingival inflammation, ulcerations
Down syndrome	⇊chemotaxis	Periodontal disease
Diabetes mellitus	⇊chemotaxis	Periodontal disease
Job's syndrome (hyper-immunoglobulin E)	⇊chemotaxis	Gingival inflammation, ulcerations
Chronic granulomatous disease	⇊cell killing	Gingival inflammation, ulcerations
Juvenile periodontitis	⇊chemotaxis	Periodontal disease
Chron's disease	Neutropenia ⇊chemotaxis	Ulcerations
GSD type 1b	Neutropenia ⇊chemotaxis	Severe periodontal disease, ulcerations

Abbreviation: GSD, glycogen storage disease.
(Courtesy of Dougherty N, Gataletto MA: Oral sequelae of chronic neutrophil defects: Case report of a child with glycogen storage disease type 1b. *Pediatr Dent* 17:224–229, 1995.)

progressive periodontal disease and chronic gingival inflammation. The remaining teeth had been extracted at 14 years of age.

Discussion.—Apart from local factors, a number of generalized disorders may be associated with oral mucosal inflammation, alveolar bone loss, and chronic oral ulcers in children (Table). Strict oral hygiene is indicated in all cases, although effective oral treatment may, in a given patient, depend on the level of neutrophil impairment.

▶ This article was selected to remind us that a whole variety of acquired and inherited neutrophil disorders can present with oral manifestations as a key component of a patient's signs and symptoms. The table shows the conditions that manifest in this way when the neutrophil is absent, moves poorly, or fails to kill organisms. There are 2 ways to use this list. If you see a child who has an unexplained inflammation that occurs periodically in his or her mouth, think white blood cell disorders and the potential causes of those disorders. Contrarily, if you take care of a child with any of the conditions included on the list, don't be surprised if mouth problems develop because of white cell blood disorders.

Does Clicking in Adolescence Lead to Painful Temporomandibular Joint Locking?
Könönen M, Waltimo A, Nyström M (Univ of Helsinki)
Lancet 347:1080–1081, 1996   16–8

Objective.—Clicking of the temporomandibular joint (TMJ) during active mandibular movement is common in adolescents and young adults. The cause of such clicking is unknown, but it has been assumed to predispose to the rare problem of closed locking of the TMJ. The ability of TMJ clicking to predict closed locking was assessed.

Methods.—One hundred twenty-eight young Finnish adults participated in the 9-year longitudinal study. Each subject was examined and interviewed at age 14 years for the presence of clicking and other TMJ disorders. The evaluations were repeated when the subjects were 15, 18, and 23 years old.

Results.—The prevalence of self-reported TMJ clicking increased from 11% to 31% from 14 to 23 years of age. Similarly, the prevalence of examiner-recorded clicking increased from 11% to 34%. However, the clicking did not follow any discernible pattern, and only 2% of subjects had clicking consistently. There were no cases of TMJ locking.

Conclusion.—Clicking of the TMJ is common in young people, its prevalence increasing from adolescence to young adulthood. However, this study found no association between TMJ clicking and TMJ locking. Even conservative treatment for TMJ clicking should, therefore, be undertaken cautiously.

▶ There are some interesting findings in this report. The prevalence of TMJ clicking appears to triple between the ages of 14 and 23 years. More importantly, however, when the jaws of adolescents click, this is not a harbinger of worse things to come, such as painful TMJ locking. Dysfunction of the TMJ does not evolve from such clicking.

Treatment of TMJ clicks has become a cottage industry. The cottage industry has mushroomed such that it could go public on the stock market. With this report and others that are now emerging, watch for a depression in this industry. Temporomandibular joint clicks just aren't worth taking stock in.

Sleeping Positions and Dental Arch Dimensions in Children With Suspected Obstructive Sleep Apnea Syndrome

Pirilä K, Tahvanainen P, Huggare J, et al (Univ of Oulu, Finland; Univ of Aarhus, Denmark)
Eur J Oral Sci 103:285–291, 1995
16–9

Background.—Little research has been done on children's sleeping position patterns and their relationship to dentofacial development. Possible associations between sleep patterns and dental arch dimensions were investigated.

Methods.—Twenty-seven children aged 3–10 years were included in the study. All were thought to have the obstructive sleep apnea syndrome (OSAS). Polysomnographic and videotape recordings were obtained under laboratory conditions. The apnea index and the relative time spent sleeping on the back were calculated on the basis of polysomnographic recordings. The videotapes were viewed to classify sleep and head postures (Fig 2). Dental arch morphology was examined using plaster casts.

Findings.—Sleeping primarily on the back was associated with a decreased maxillary intercanine width. Prolonged head extension during sleep and overjet were inversely correlated. Dental arches were larger in children with apnea index scores exceeding 4 (Table 1).

Conclusion.—Sleeping on the back apparently leads to a more posterior tongue position, which decreases its molding effect on the anterior dental arch. Because nasopharyngeal airway obstruction in children with OSAS may result in an anterior tongue position to ensure a free airway passage, lingual pressure on the dental arches will be increased, causing their dimensional increase.

▶ When the campaign was launched to teach parents and care providers about the need for otherwise healthy babies to sleep in the supine position to reduce the risk of sudden infant death syndrome (SIDS), none of us were aware of some of the secondary consequences of such a sea change in the

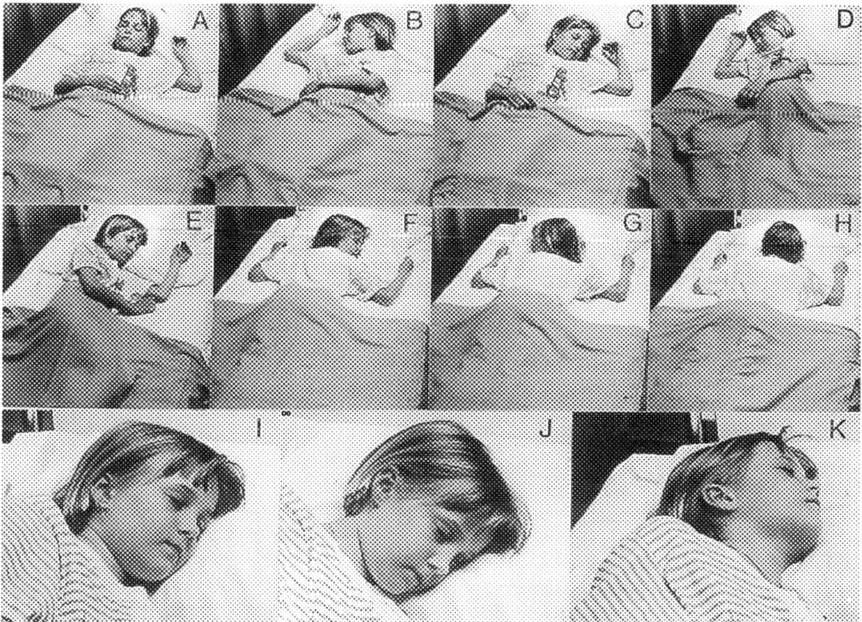

FIGURE 2.—Categorized sleep positions (letters refer to Table 1). **A:** supine, head straight; **B:** supine, head to the right; **C:** supine, head to the left; **D:** right side position; **E:** left side position; **F:** prone, head to the right; **G:** prone, head to the left; **H:** prone, head straight; **I:** head neutral; **J:** head flexed; **K:** head extended. (Courtesy of Pirilä K, Tahvanainen P, Huggare J, et al: Sleeping positions and dental arch dimensions in children with suspected obstructive sleep apnea syndrome. *Eur J Oral Sci* 103:285–291, 1995.)

way infants are put down at night. We now know (see Chapter 11) that although the risk of SIDS is definitely reduced by having children sleep in the supine position, supine-sleeping infants do not sleep as well. Also, supine-sleeping infants tend to have rounder heads, sometimes misshapen to the point of confusion with the possibility of craniosynostosis. Now we see in the article abstracted that how an infant sleeps determines how its mouth grows. Sleeping predominantly on the back causes a reduced maxillary width. Sleeping on the back apparently causes a more posterior tongue position, reducing its molding effect on the anterior dental arch. Is it possible that we are raising a generation of children with round heads and narrow mouths? Anthropologists in millennia to come may look back upon the 1990s and chuckle a bit about the long-term consequences—the ripple effect, as it were—of something as simple as a change from the prone to the supine infant sleep position.

Most of us, infants included, spend a third or more of our lives in sleep, apparently, increasingly on our backs. As pediatric care providers, we should recognize that immature bones are moldable and that the growth of bones is most intense at night, as growth hormone is secreted mainly during that period. Changing from bottoms up to bottoms down can cause more than just a lower incidence of SIDS. As an aside, one wonders why some smart

TABLE 1.—Means and Standard Deviations for Variables Depicting the Dental Arch, Sleep Positions, Head Positions, and Apnea Index

	n	X	SD
Dental arch (in mm)			
Overjet	27	3.4	1.59
Overbite	27	1.2	1.77
Intercanine width (max)	27	28.1	2.53
Bimolar width I (max)	27	33.2	2.26
Bimolar width II (max)	27	27.6	1.95
Arch length (max)	27	20.4	1.42
Intercanine width (mand)	22	23.3	2.32
Bimolar width (mand)	23	29.4	2.45
Arch length (mand)	23	16.2	1.37
Sleep positions (in %)			
Position A; supine	26	5.7	10.67
Position B; supine	26	13.3	15.32
Position C; supine	26	10.6	13.30
Position D; side	26	24.3	16.68
Position E; side	26	24.9	19.78
Position F; prone	26	6.7	10.09
Position G; prone	26	10.7	17.38
Position H; prone	26	1.0	4.62
Supine (A+B+C;from Video)	26	29.6	25.20
Supine (from PSG)	24	38.4	29.62
Head positions (in %)			
Neutral I	26	61.5	20.05
Flexed J	26	8.6	11.46
Extended K	26	25.3	21.01
Apnea index			
AI	26	1.7	1.87

Abbreviations: *PSG*, polysomnography; *AI*, apnea index.
(Courtesy of Pirilä K, Tahvanainen P, Huggare J, et al: Sleeping positions and dental arch dimensions in children with suspected obstructive sleep apnea syndrome. *Eur J Oral Sci* 103:285–291, 1995.)

person, capitalizing on the fact that growth hormone is secreted at night and that bones can be made to stretch, has not done a study to make short youngsters grow. If you want your kids to be tall, hang them upside down at night to sleep like a bat. A little vertical hanging, a little growth hormone pulse and maybe we could be raising a generation of giants—makes about as much sense as sleeping supine.

Use of Nasal Continuous Positive Airway Pressure as Treatment of Childhood Obstructive Sleep Apnea

Marcus CL, Davidson Ward SL, Mallory GB, et al (Johns Hopkins Univ, Baltimore, Md; Childrens Hosp Los Angeles; St Louis Children's Hosp; et al)
J Pediatr 127:88–94, 1995   16–10

Objective.—Although the majority of children with obstructive sleep apnea (OSA) can be treated successfully with tonsillectomy and adenoidectomy, some continue to have problems after surgery. The use of continuous positive airway pressure (CPAP) in these children has become more popu-

TABLE.—Predisposing Conditions for Obstructive Sleep Apnea in
94 Children

Predisposing condition	n (%)
Obesity	25 (27)
Craniofacial anomalies*	23 (25)
Idiopathic (total)	17(18)
T & A performed	16 (17)
T & A not performed†	2 (2)
Trisomy 21	12 (13)
Neuromuscular disease	5 (5)
Mental retardation and	
cerebral palsy	5 (5)
Pharyngeal flap surgery	4 (4)
Arnold-Chiari malformation	2 (2)
Other‡	1 (1)
Pending T & A	1 (1)

Abbreviation: T & A, tonsillectomy and adenoidectomy.

*Chromosomal anomalies ($n = 3$), Pierre Robin syndrome ($n = 3$), achondroplasia ($n = 2$), Treacher Collins snydrome ($n = 2$), pyknodysostosis ($n = 2$), maxillary hypoplasia ($n = 2$), Crouzon syndrome, Binder syndrome, incontinentia pigmentosa with maxillary hypoplasia, Apert syndrome, congenitally small nasopharynx, fibrous dysplasia of the mandible.

†Includes patient with cystic fibrosis.

‡Tracheomalacia after tracheal reconstruction in child who had tracheostomy because of laryngeal papillomatosis.

(Courtesy of Marcus CL, Davidson Ward SL, Mallory GB, et al: Use of nasal continuous positive airway pressure as treatment of childhood obstructive sleep apnea. *J Pediatr* 127:88–94, 1995.)

lar, although the numbers are still low. The use of CPAP in the treatment of childhood OSA was studied retrospectively.

Methods.—Data from questionnaires sent to 11 pediatric sleep disorder centers in the United States, France, and Canada were analyzed.

Results.—Data were obtained from 9 centers on 94 patients (64% male), including 3% who were younger than 1 year, 29% who were 1–5 years old, 36% who were 6–12 years of age, and 32% who were aged 13–19 years. The most frequent indications for CPAP were obesity, craniofacial abnormalities, idiopathic conditions, and trisomy 21 (Table). The use of CPAP was successful in 81 patients and unsuccessful in 1. Compliance was inadequate in 12 patients. The median CPAP level required was 8 cm H_2O, and 10 patients required supplemental oxygen. There were no significant differences in CPAP requirements with age. Changes in CPAP were necessary in 21 patients. Side effects included nasal symptoms and mask fit problems. All centers recommended adenoidectomy and tonsillectomy as first-line treatment for OSA. Problems with CPAP funding were encountered by 64% of sleep centers.

Conclusion.—Continuous positive airway pressure is safe, effective, and well tolerated in children with OSA, particularly as an alternative to surgery. The biggest problem encountered with the use of CPAP in both children and adults is poor compliance. A CPAP trial and prospective study are recommended.

▶ Despite the myriad of data about how successful CPAP can be when used to treat adults with OSA, other than the 1 early report by Guilleminault et al.,[1] there have been no controlled case series studying this problem until the one abstracted above appeared. We see that CPAP can work when other treatments fail. Because OSA is a significant cause of morbidity in children with complications including failure to thrive, cor pulmonale, developmental delay, and even death, having one more treatment option is something that should be considered highly desirable. Although the majority of children with OSA respond to tonsillectomy and adenoidectomy, a percentage of these children persist with obstruction after surgery. Furthermore, there is a whole cadre of children in whom tonsillectomy and adenoidectomy does not work: those with craniofacial anomalies, neuromuscular weakness, and obesity. All of these children might benefit from CPAP.

The big problem with CPAP, of course, is that both adults and children dislike it. Compliance at times is miserable. Reasons for poor compliance include inconvenience, discomfort, side effects, a feeling of claustrophobia, and expense. On the other hand, because the last-ditch alternative to CPAP in many patients is either tracheostomy or the disastrous side effects of OSA, parents and kids sometimes can become highly motivated. They will buy into the concept of CPAP, hoping that with time and growth the problem will resolve.

The conclusion of this report is pretty straightforward. The use of CPAP is safe. In many kids, it is well tolerated. It is an effective therapy even for the very young and some developmentally disabled children. Therapy with CPAP is a perfectly satisfactory alternative to tracheostomy in patients who have not responded to tonsillectomy and adenoidectomy. If nothing else, it does buy the time needed for airway growth.

One last comment about OSA. Take a clue from the adult literature about some of the secondary consequences of OSA. Adult men with OSA have a 50% increase in the incidence of nocturia.[2] Apparently, OSA alters the release of atrial natriuretic peptides leading to an increased urine volume and frequency. Treatment of OSA in adults with CPAP ablates this secondary consequence of airway blockage. It is possible that infants, toddlers, and children experience this as well? Could OSA be a significant cause of enuresis? Think about it.

References

1. Guilleminault C, et al: *Pediatrics* 78:797, 1986.
2. Dalhstrand C, et al: *Lancet* 347:270, 1996.

Two New Otolaryngologic Findings in Child Abuse
Drake AF, Makielski K, McDonald-Bell C, et al (Univ of North Carolina, Chapel Hill; Univ of Washington, Seattle)
Arch Otolaryngol Head Neck Surg 121:1417–1420, 1995   16–11

Introduction.—Child abuse may be evidenced by a number of head and neck abnormalities including caustic burns and ingestion, traumatic

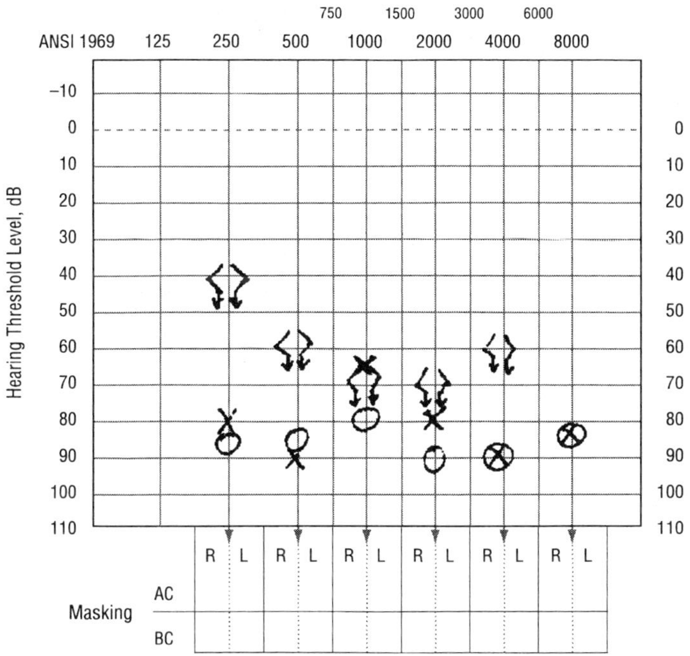

Speech Audiometry

Ear	Speech Receptor Threshold	Speech Discrimination	MCL	UCL (Tolerance)	Masking Level in Opposite Ear
Right	30 dB	100% @ 60 dB			55 dB
Left	25 dB	100% @ 60 dB			55 dB
Free Field	dB	% @ dB			
	dB	% @ dB			

CASE 4.—Initial audiogram of hearing loss. (Courtesy of Drake AF, Makielski K, McDonald-Bell C, et al: Two new otolaryngologic findings in child abuse. *Arch Otolaryngol Head Neck Surg* 121:1417–1420, 1995.)

alopecia, and various injuries to the ears, nose, and pharynx. Two new associations were described: functional hearing loss and hoarseness secondary to vocal nodules.

Observations.—Four children known to be at risk of abuse had apparently had vocal nodules develop from excessive crying and screaming, causing hoarseness. Four other children, 3 of whom had no other evidence of abuse when first seen, had functional hearing loss. It may be that an incident in the child's life attracts attention to hearing and that some secondary gain is derived from apparent hearing loss. Failure to pass a school hearing test may be the first suggestion of a problem. An audiogram will show exaggerated hearing thresholds for pure tones but normal speech reception thresholds (Case 4). Functional hearing loss may be superimposed on a true organic hearing loss.

Conclusion.—Abuse should be considered when a child is seen with functional hearing loss or early-onset vocal nodules.

▶ The spectrum of manifestations of child abuse does not seem to have a limit. Now we learn of 2 more: functional hearing loss and hoarseness secondary to vocal cord nodules. Why neither of these signs has been reported before is curious because both seem to be fairly obvious clinical indicators of possible abuse. An unusual amount of crying can cause vocal nodules. Nodules cause hoarseness. Pseudohypoacusis, or functional hearing loss, is actually not unusual in children. It is thought that an incident in a child's life attracts his attention to hearing, and the child subsequently derives some secondary gain from appearing to have hearing loss. There isn't anything that can be more traumatic than a single or multiple episodes of abuse. The tip-off that loss of hearing is functional comes when the audiogram shows exaggerated hearing thresholds for pure tones in the presence of normal speech reception thresholds. A trained audiologist can distinguish between true hearing loss, a problem of auditory perception, and nonorganic hearing loss.

Not every child with a hoarse cry, nor every child who feigns an episode of hearing loss, will be an abused child. Nonetheless, now that these clinical manifestations of child abuse have been reported, it is incumbent on all of us to know that an association between them and a potential serious problem can exist.

Characteristics of Objects That Cause Choking in Children
Rimell FL, Thome A Jr, Stool S, et al (Children's Hosp of Pittsburgh, Pa; Alfred I DuPont Inst, Wilmington, Del; Inchcape Testing Services Risk Analysis and Management, Moonachie, NJ)
JAMA 274:1763–1766, 1995   16–12

Objectives.—Young children often place household and other common objects in their mouths and, as a result, are at risk of choking and dying. Epidemiologic aspects of this problem were examined in a series of 165 children undergoing endoscopy after aspirating or ingesting a noncaustic foreign body. Another 449 children whose deaths from choking on a man-made object were reported to the Consumer Product Safety Commission in a 20-year period also were analyzed. Objects causing death were analyzed using computerized models of the pediatric aerodigestive tract.

Findings.—More than two thirds of bronchoscopies were done for suspected food aspiration but yielded food items in only about 60% of cases. Nuts were the most common offender. Three of 18 children who aspirated nonfood items were older than 3 years. Coins constituted more

TABLE 2.—Types of Objects Causing Children's Choking Deaths, January 1972 through January 1992*

Type of Product	Children Asphyxiated, No. (%)
Children's products	
Balloons	131 (29)
Balls	58 (13)
Marbles	26 (6)
Other toys	92 (20)
Total	307 (68)
Other products	
Hardware	32 (7)
Coins	14 (3)
Household	35 (8)
Other nonchild	61 (14)
Total	142 (32)
Total	449 (100)

*From the US Consumer Product Safety Commission, Directorate for Epidemiology, Division of Hazard Analysis, January 1972 through January 1992. The balloons category includes 2 latex gloves that were given to young children in physician offices and later caused asphyxiation. The household category includes pins (2); office supplies such as paper clips, pen caps, or chalk (19); pieces of glass bulbs (2); and paper products (12).

(Courtesy of Rimell FL, Thome A Jr, Stool S, et al: Characteristics of objects that cause choking in children. *JAMA* 274:1763–1766, Copyright 1995, American Medical Association.)

TABLE 5.—Diameter of Computer-simulated Ring Allowing Passage of Long Dimension of 101 Three-dimensional Objects Causing Children's Deaths by Asphyxiation*

Diameter of Virtual Ring, cm	Length, No. (%) (n=101)
≤0.63	2 (2)
1.27	6 (6)
1.9	32 (32)
2.54	6 (6)
3.17	27 (27)
3.81	10 (10)
4.44	3 (3)
5.08	5 (5)
5.71†	1 (1)
6.35	6 (6)
6.98	1 (1)
7.62	2 (2)
8.25	0
8.89	0
9.52	0
10.16	0
Total	101 (101)

*Data from Inchcape Testing Services Risk Analysis and Management, Moonachie, NJ. Numbers in "Length" column represent numbers of objects that passed through computer-simulated ring of that diameter.

†Length of the Small Parts Test Fixture. Objects intended for use by children younger than 3 years must be larger than 3.17 cm in diameter or 5.71 cm in length to be approved for interstate commerce.

(Courtesy of Rimell FL, Thome A Jr, Stool S, et al: Characteristics of objects that cause choking in children. *JAMA* 274:1763–1766, Copyright 1995, American Medical Association.)

than half of the 105 foreign bodies removed from the cricopharyngeus or esophagus. Balloons were the most common object causing death, accounting for 29% of cases (Table 2). Older children were likelier than those younger than 3 years to choke on conforming objects. Approximately three fourths of children who died of choking on either a spherical or nonspherical object were younger than 3 years. The diameters of computer-simulated rings through which objects passed are given in Table 5.

Discussion.—Children younger than 3 years are the likeliest to incur injury or die from a foreign body in the aerodigestive tract. Conforming objects such as balloons are the most dangerous objects. Spherical objects may cause asphyxiation even if they meet current standards. Of note is that 2 deaths occurred when children visiting a clinician choked on an examination glove.

▶ This report contains much new information. It is well worth reading in detail. It shows us that although kids continue to aspirate food (particularly pieces of hot dog) and coins, an equally greater risk is the aspiration of balloons. Almost one third of all deaths from aspiration of foreign bodies result from a balloon blocking the airway. What is unique about balloons is that they are a particularly prominent cause of morbidity and mortality in the child older than 3 years (presumably a child younger than 3 years doesn't have the strength to expand a balloon). In older children, airway blockage by balloons accounts for 60% of deaths caused by foreign-body choking.

The Consumer Product Safety Commission regulates products to prevent them from killing children. Balloons have long been exempted from such regulations, however. It's hard to imagine that even product warnings will solve the problem of kids dying from inhaling balloons. Baker and Halperin give us some solutions that might minimize these kinds of risks.[1] They note that Mylar balloons and inflatable paper balloons, such as those used by Japanese children, would not be expected to block a child's airway. It has also been suggested that balloon manufacturers could solve this choking problem by putting a plastic ring of approximately 4 cm in diameter inside a balloon to prevent airway blocking. Additionally, it has been proposed that balloons could be designed with ridges or bumps that would allow air to flow between the surface of the airway and an aspirated latex balloon. One might even think about putting a bittering agent into the latex of a balloon so that children will have little desire to keep them in their mouths very long.

Lastly, this editor would make 1 more recommendation about balloons that might minimize their risk. Physicians and nurses should not blow up examining gloves and give them to kids. Such gloves (when they burst) have caused problems.

Reference

1. Baker SP, Halperin K: *JAMA* 274:1805, 1995.

Use of Dexamethasone in the Outpatient Management of Acute Laryngotracheitis
Cruz MN, Stewart G, Rosenberg N (Children's Hosp of Michigan, Detroit; Wayne State Univ, Detroit)
Pediatrics 96:220–223, 1995
16–13

Purpose.—Previous reports have shown that administration of a single IM dose of dexamethasone, 0.6 mg/kg, shortens the duration and severity of acute viral laryngotracheitis—or croup—in hospitalized patients. The use of dexamethasone in outpatients with moderately severe croup was studied.

Methods.—The double-blind trial included 38 patients who came to the emergency department (ED) with acute viral croup, a croup score of at least 2, and a disposition of discharge. The median patient age was 19 months and median croup score, 3. The patients were randomly assigned to receive either dexamethasone, 0.6 mg/kg given intramuscularly, or an equal volume of saline before discharge from the ED. Patients with structural abnormalities, patients who had received steroids in the preceding 24 hours, as well as those who required β-agonist therapy, more than 1 racemic epinephrine treatment, or hospitalization were excluded. One, 7, and 10 days after discharge, the parents were asked by telephone whether they had sought any additional treatment for the child's condition. They were also asked to rate how well they thought the child was doing at 24 hours and how long it took the croup to resolve completely.

Results.—The 2 groups were similar in the number of patients requiring racemic epinephrine. Of the 5 patients who sought additional medical attention, 4 were in the placebo group. Twenty-one percent of the placebo group sought further medical attention, compared with 5% of the dexamethasone group, although this difference was not significant. At 24 hours, significantly more patients in the dexamethasone group had scores indicating improvement: 84% vs. 42%. The number of days to resolution was not significantly different.

Conclusions.—Giving dexamethasone to outpatients with viral croup yields a reduced severity of illness within 24 hours. The use of dexamethasone before ED discharge should be considered for children with moderately severe viral croup.

▶ This is another report on the use of dexamethasone in the management of patients with croup. This is another report that supports the use of steroids in patients with moderate or more severe croup. The important aspect of this study is that it looked only at patients who were able to be managed as outpatients. Several previous studies related to the use of steroids examined patients who were sick enough to be hospitalized.

The steroid and croup story has been milked for all it is worth. It is time to call a halt to additional studies. The stuff works, and no one should be embarrassed about using it.

The Incidence of Gastroesophageal Reflux in Recurrent Croup

Waki EY, Madgy DN, Belenky WM, et al (Children's Hosp of Michigan, Detroit)

Int J Pediatr Otorhinolaryngol 32:223–232, 1995   16–14

Background.—Perhaps half of all healthy infants less than 2 months of age exhibit gastroesophageal reflux (GER). By age 18 months, a majority of infants are asymptomatic. Pathologic reflux has been associated with a number of respiratory disorders, including asthma, apnea, recurrent pneumonia, bronchitis, and chronic coughing. It is conceivable that infants with GER who aspirate the gastric contents into the trachea will be vulnerable to recurrent croup or crouplike symptoms.

Objective and Methods.—A chart review was carried out for 262 patients admitted in 1985–1991 with a diagnosis of croup or viral laryngotracheobronchitis. All of them had documented prodromal symptoms, stridor, and a barking cough. Sixty-six patients had 2 or more episodes of croup necessitating hospitalization. Six of the latter patients were studied prospectively by magnified airway tomography, barium video-esophagraphy, scintiscanning for GER, direct laryngoscopy, and bronchoscopy under general anesthesia. In addition, tracheobronchial washings were examined histopathologically.

Findings.—Fifteen of 32 patients with recurrent croup (47%) were found to have GER at an average age of 6 months. The average interval between episodes was 3 months. The incidence of GER was 63% in patients having 3 or more recurrences of croup. Those with GER tended to be younger than other patients and to have a shorter interval between episodes of croup. Asthma was diagnosed in 44% of patients with recurrent croup. In one fourth of cases, an anatomical airway abnormality was implicated as a significant factor. The findings and outcomes in the 6 prospectively studied infants are summarized in Table 3.

Recommendation.—Young children who have 2 or more episodes of croup necessitating admission to the hospital should be studied for GER and airway abnormalities.

▶ Some studies are too good to be buried in journals that are not seen by those who could best use the reported findings for the greatest benefit of children. To say this differently, who would expect that a pediatric care provider, such as a pediatrician, would be reading the *International Journal of Pediatric Otorhinolaryngology?* Those who might have missed this report would have missed a critical addition to our understanding of the causes of recurrent croup. Infants and toddlers who have 2 or more episodes of croup have a 50% (or greater) probability of having GER as the potential cause. Because GER is easily diagnosed with esophageal pH monitoring, we have solved, in part, one of the great dilemmas of pediatrics: why some children have recurrence of their croup.

The list of complications associated with GER continues to grow. That list includes bronchospasm, asthma, stridor, apnea, recurrent pneumonia/bron-

TABLE 3.—Summarized Clinical Course of 6 Infants With Recurrent Croup

Patients	Age at episodes of croup	Diagnosis	Diagnostic procedures	Management and outcome
DA	7,16,21,23 month	GER with tracheal aspiration*	MAG airway-mild subglottic narrowing GER scan-mild GER to distal esophagus Endoscopy-erythema and edema of tracheal mucosa, blunted carina LLMI-251	Treatment with metoclopramide Resolution of stridor with a 5-month f/u Recurrent croup briefly after medication discontinued for 1 week
NS	7,9,12,14,18 month	GER with tracheal aspiration* Mild, SGS Asthma, S/P coarctation of aorta repair*	MAG airway-limited abduction, TVC GER scan-normal Endscopy-mild Grade I SGS, mild mild level tracheomalacia, erythema and edema of tracheal mucosa, blunted carina LLMI-275	Continued treatment with Albuterol, given Metoclopramide with dramatic improvement of wheezing and coughing with a 6-month f/u.
AT	3,5,9,13 month	Mild SGS GER (Dx-pH probe) and failure to thrive Asthma*	CXR-reactive airway or viral pneumonia MAG airway-fixed narrowing at glottis and possible subglottic narrowing Endoscopy-mild Grade I SGS LLMI—29	Increased current treatment to maximum dosage of Metoclopramide, Ranitidine and Albuterol No change in wheezing and coughing with a 3-month f/u
DP	4,5,7 month	Laryngomalacia* Mild SGS* Bronchopulmonary dysplasia Asthma*	GER scan-GER to mouth, delayed gastric emptying Endoscopy-laryngomalacia, mild Grade I SGS LLMI—11	Treated with Metoclopramide No change in stridor with a 4 month f/u
JR	36,38 month	Asthma*	MAG airway-limited motion TVC Endoscopy-normal LLMI—3	Continued treatment with Albuterol No change in wheezing with a 2-month f/u
CL	3,7,13 month	Posterior glottic stenosis*	MAG airway-limited abduction TVC GER scan-minimal GER to distal esophagus Endoscopy-posterior glottic stenosis LLMI—21	Observed, episode of URI with stertor with a 1-month f/u

*Diagnosis after workup.

Abbreviations: CXR, radiograph of chest, *GER scan*, gastroesophageal reflux scintiscan; *LLMI*, lipid-laden macrophage index; *MAG airway*, magnification HI-KV radiograph; *SGS*, subglottic stenosis; (Cotton, Grading Scale).

(Reprinted from Waki EY, Madgy DN, Belenky WM, et al: The incidence of gastroesophageal reflux in recurrent croup. *Int J Pediatr Otorhinolaryngol* 32:223–232, 1995 with kind permission from Elsevier Science Ltd, The Boulevard, Langford Lane, Kidlington OX5 1GB, UK.)

chitis, chronic cough, and even torticollis (Sandifer's syndrome). Add to this list recurrent croup and you see why spitting up isn't as simple for some infants as it is for others.

Ambulatory Tonsillectomy and Adenoidectomy

Gabalski EC, Mattucci KF, Setzen M, et al (North Shore Univ, Manhasset, NY)
Laryngoscope 106:77–80, 1996
16–15

Introduction.—The rising cost of health care has strongly influenced the trend toward outpatient surgeries. Controversy exists over the adequacy of postoperative care for patients undergoing tonsillectomy and adenoidectomy in an ambulatory setting. The incidence of complications during the first week after tonsillectomy with and without adenoidectomy was investigated prospectively in 534 consecutive patients between the ages of 16 months and 14 years.

Methods.—After surgery, the occurrence of fever, protracted emesis, and bleeding were recorded during the fifth postoperative hour in all patients and in 175 of the 534 patients in the sixth postoperative hour. Nurses telephoned patients' homes on the first postoperative day to ask about the occurrence of complications since discharge. Physicians were questioned regarding complications requiring follow-up care during the first postoperative week.

Results.—No adverse events were recorded in the fifth postoperative hour. In the sixth postoperative hour 1 patient had a low-grade fever of 38.0°C, no patients had postoperative bleeding, and no patients had emesis (Table 2). The complication rate for the sixth postoperative hour was 0.19%. One patient was seen in the emergency department during the eighth postoperative hour and was treated for bleeding from the tonsillar bed. Another patient seen in the emergency department for possible bleeding was found to have no bleeding. No treatment was required. The overall complication rate for the first week was 0.37% (2 of 534). There were no deaths.

TABLE 2.—Complications After Ambulatory Tonsillectomy With or Without Adenoidectomy

Time After Surgery	Number of Patients	Complications		
		Bleeding	Emesis	Fever
Hour 5	534	0	0	0
Hour 6	175	0	0	1
Hour 24	534	1	0	0
Day 7	534	0	0	0

(Courtesy of Gabalski EC, Mattucci KF, Setzen M, et al: Ambulatory tonsillectomy and adenoidectomy. *Laryngoscope* 106:77–80, 1996.)

Conclusion.—Tonsillectomy with and without adenoidectomy has a low postoperative morbidity rate when performed in an ambulatory setting. It is suggested that, with meticulous surgical technique and strict patient observation in the immediate postoperative period, patients undergoing tonsillectomy and adenoidectomy can safely be discharged home after a minimum of 4 hours of recovery room observation.

▶ This institutional review of 534 consecutive patients younger than 15 years of age who underwent ambulatory tonsillectomy with or without adenoidectomy demonstrates the art of otolaryngologic fine-tuning. The investigators studied patients ranging in age from 16 months to 14 years. They examined the complications that occurred. They concluded that not only are ambulatory tonsillectomy and adenoidectomy safe (which has been shown in numerous other studies), but also that you can cut the postoperative waiting time/observation time down to just 4 hours. In an era of managed care, a one-third reduction in the use of postoperative services does not represent a minor amount of dollars, particularly because tonsillectomy and adenoidectomy are among the most frequently performed procedures in this country. What few additional data there are regarding this subject show that children find this surgical experience more acceptable if they can recover at home rather than in a hospital.

Regardless of the reason for the shift from the inpatient setting to the ambulatory surgical unit, controversy still exists regarding the adequacy of postoperative care for patients treated on an outpatient basis. As far as tonsillectomy and adenoidectomy are concerned, vomiting, fever, and bleeding are the things to watch out for. Hemorrhage, obviously, is the most dangerous potential problem. The reported incidence of hemorrhage after tonsillectomy has ranged from 0.1% to 8.1%.[1] As far as vomiting is concerned, please note that the anesthesiologist who took care of these study patients at North Shore University Hospital in Manhasset, New York, reduced the frequency and duration of postoperative vomiting by evacuating the gastric contents with a nasogastric tube to remove irritating blood. Not all anesthesiologists do this.

It is difficult to imagine, even in an era of cost containment, that anyone will be looking for a shorter postoperative stay than 4 hours for children who have undergone such a tonsillectomy and adenoidectomy. As a medical student, this editor performed outpatient tonsillectomies years ahead of the time when it again became fashionable to do so. The patients were Philadelphia policemen who, if they took too many sick days for sore throats, were referred to the ear, nose, and throat clinic at the Philadelphia General Hospital. The ambulatory tonsillectomy consisted of being seated in an upright chair with one's head strapped back and mouth taped open followed by a curettage out of the tonsils, all too frequently by a medical student. A few hours later, they were out the door, never to return again with a complaint of a sore throat. True story.

Hopefully we will see no more articles of this type. If we do, one can see the title now: "The 10-Minute T and A, a.k.a. the Drive-Through Tonsillectomy and Adenoidectomy."

Reference

1. Patel RI, et al: *Anesthesiology* 77:A38, 1992.

Peritonsillar Abscess: Incidence, Current Management Practices, and a Proposal for Treatment Guidelines

Herzon FS (Univ of New Mexico, Albuquerque)
Laryngoscope 105(Suppl 74):1–17, 1995

16–16

Background.—Peritonsillar abscess (PTA), a common abscess of the head and neck, has no definitive guidelines for management. The relative merits of different surgical approaches and medical treatments, as well as diagnostic assessment, are still debated. Thus some patients may not be receiving the best care at a reasonable cost. The surgical, medical, diagnostic, and cost factors of PTA management were investigated.

Methods.—Three methodological approaches were used. In the first, outcomes of a cohort of 123 patients with PTA treated with needle aspiration as the initial surgical drainage were documented. In the second, the results of a national survey of PTA management practices of 2,000 randomly selected members of the American Academy of Otolaryngology–Head and Neck Surgery were analyzed. In the third, various components of the treatment regimen for PTA were assessed in 4 meta-analyses.

Findings.—In the cohort study, the acute resolution rate for PTA was 96%. In the survey study, with a 73% response rate, 96% of the respondents reported treating an average of 7 PTAs per year. Needle aspiration, incision and drainage, or abscess tonsillectomy was used for initial drain-

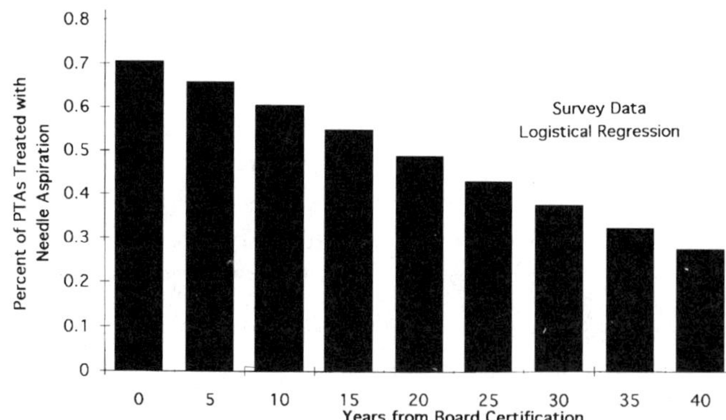

FIGURE 3.—Plot of years from board certification vs. percent of peritonsillar abscesses *(PTAs)* treated with needle aspiration. A logistical regression was used to evaluate the use of needle aspiration as a drainage procedure for PTA on the basis of data gathered in the national survey. There was a significant decrease in the use of needle aspiration to drain PTAs by practitioners as their years from board certification increased. (Courtesy of Herzon FS: Peritonsillar abscess: Incidence, current management practices, and a proposal for treatment guidelines. *Laryngoscope* 105(Suppl 74):1–17, 1995.)

TABLE 3.—Respondents' Use of Antibiotics to Treat Peritonsillar
Abscess (PTA)

Antibiotic	Percent*
Penicillin	62%
Cephalosporins	21%
Clindamycin	20%
Amoxicillin	14%
Amoxicillin/clavulanate potassium	11%

* Percentage of surveyed respondents who at some time use the specified antibiotic to treat PTA.
(Courtesy of Herzon FS: Peritonsillar abscess: Incidence, current management practices, and a proposal for treatment guidelines. *Laryngoscope* 105(Suppl 74):1–17, 1995.)

age (Fig 3). Sixty-two percent used penicillin to treat PTAs (Table 3). The incidence of PTA among patients 5–59 years old treated by the practitioners responding to the survey was 30.1 per 100,000 person-years, or about 45,000 cases per year. The meta-analysis demonstrated a needle aspiration success rate of 94% in patients with PTA. The recurrence rate ranged from 10% to 15%. Penicillin-resistant microorganisms were found in 0% to 56% of the patients with PTA. The rate of previous oropharyngeal infections associated with PTA ranged from 11% to 56%. In the United States, the 10% recurrence rate for PTA was significantly lower than the 15% rate worldwide.

Conclusions.—Based on these findings, a set of clinical guidelines was proposed (Fig 4). Needle aspiration should be the first surgical drainage procedure done for all patients with a PTA other than those with indications for abscess tonsillectomy. Treatment should be rendered in an outpatient setting, and penicillin should be given to all patients who are not allergic to it. Patients should also receive adequate pain medication. Examining the abscess contents for microorganisms does not appear to be of benefit. About 30% of the patients with PTA will have relative indications for tonsillectomy. Implementing these guidelines would cost about $62 million annually, resulting in a potential savings of about $89 million compared with the projected cost based on current treatment practices (Table 8).

▶ This is one powerhouse of a report. Although he gives us no new data, Dr. Herzon has managed to synthesize in one relatively brief manuscript what 2,000 members of the American Academy of Otolaryngology–Head and Neck Surgery do as part of their management of PTA, and there are some surprises here. First, however, it might be worthwhile to review some basic facts about PTAs. A conservative (low) estimate of the number of cases of PTA treated each year in the United States and Puerto Rico is about 45,000. This is probably a low estimate because it is based on reports from ear, nose, and throat (ENT) physicians, and not every case of PTA is seen by a head and neck specialist. Despite the large number of cases, controversy surrounds virtually every aspect of this disease. Dilemmas exist regarding the optimal surgical approaches, if any, to the drainage of the abscess, medical therapies, and diagnostic evaluation. The 3 different procedures used to drain

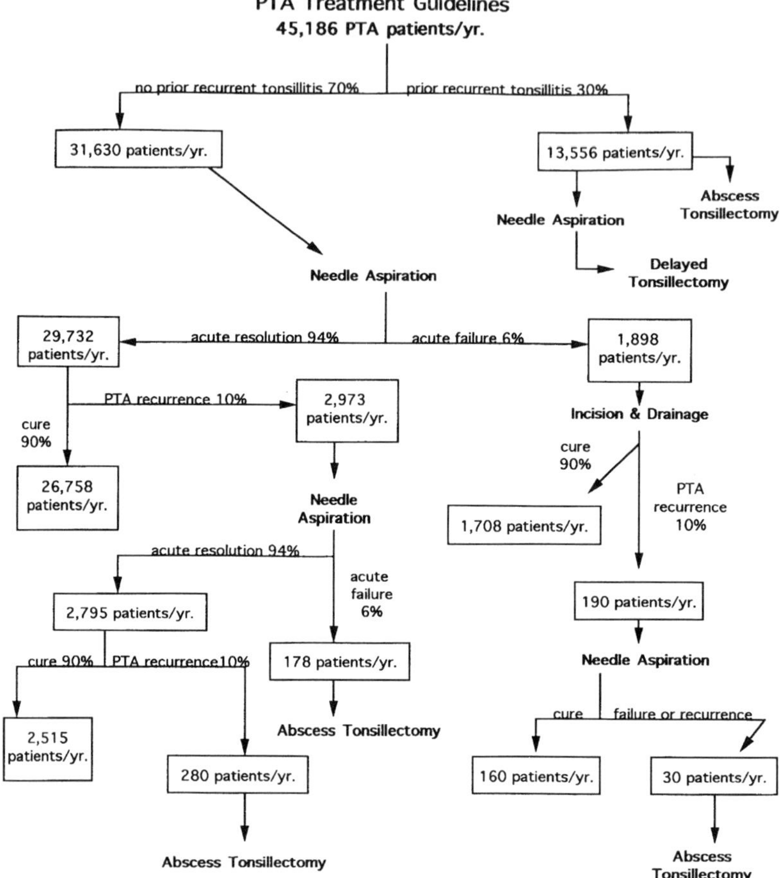

FIGURE 4.—Peritonsillar abscess *(PTA)* treatment guidelines. Data illustrated were derived from 3 sources: clinical series of patients with PTA; the national survey of members of the American Academy of Otolaryngology-Head and Neck Surgery *(AAO)*; and the meta-analyses of the success rate for needle aspiration, incidence of recurrent PTA, number of patients with penicillin-resistant microorganisms isolated from PTA, and association of tonsilitis with PTA. Number of PTAs treated annually by members of AAO was derived in following way. Average number of PTAs treated each year by practitoners was determined and multiplied by 6,884, the number of active members of AAO. Rate of prior recurrent tonsilitis (30%), the sole indication for tonsillectomy, was derived from variable rates reported in meta-analysis of prior tonsillitis associated with PTA and from data in present clinical series. Range of rate of prior oropharyngeal infection was 11% to 56%, and 30% was chosen as a conservative estimate of actual rate of prior recurrent tonsillitis, as this rate could not be determined with precision. (Courtesy of Herzon FS: Peritonsillar abscess: Incidence, current management practices, and a proposal for treatment guidelines. *Laryngoscope* 105(Suppl 74):1–17, 1995.)

PTAs include needle aspiration, incision and drainage, and abscess tonsillectomy. None of these surgical interventions has been singularly identified as the optimal drainage procedure for PTAs.

So what do we learn from this report? We see that the vast majority of cases can be managed with needle aspiration as the sole initial surgical drainage procedure. It resolves PTAs (along with antibiotics) in 96% of cases. Needle aspiration has several distinct advantages. It is relatively

TABLE 8.—Peritonsillar Abscess (PTA): Estimated Annual National Treatment Costs Using Needle Aspiration as the Primary Initial Surgical Drainage

	Patients	Cost/Patient	Cost
Patients without indications for tonsillectomy			
Needle aspiration	31,630	$ 200	$ 6,326,000
Needle aspiration—recurrence	2,973	$ 754	$ 2,242,600
Needle aspiration—failure	1,898	$ 375	$ 711,750
Patients with indications for tonsillectomy			
Needle aspiration—delayed tonsillectomy	11,658	$3200	$37,305,600
Abscess tonsillectomy*	1,898	$3600	$ 6,832,800
All patients treated for PTA			
Hospitalization	6,326	$1400	$ 8,856,456
Total estimated national cost	45,186	$1378	$62,275,206

*It is estimated that approximately 14% of the patients with prior indications for tonsillectomy will be treated by abscess tonsillectomy.

(Courtesy of Herzon FS: Peritonsillar abscess: Incidence, current management practices, and a proposal for treatment guidelines. *Laryngoscope* 105(Suppl 74):1–17, 1995.)

simple; the procedure can be performed by non–head and neck specialists; it does not require specialized equipment; and it is relatively inexpensive. Why it is not used by all ENT physicians is fairly straightforward. The survey abstracted shows a strong association between full incision and drainage, instead of needle aspiration, by older, as opposed to younger, board-certified ENT physicians. It's hard to break habits.

Even more controversial is whether abscess tonsillectomy is necessary as part of the management of PTA. Those who espouse tonsillectomy state the following benefits: tonsillectomy is the only way to drain the abscess completely; it eliminates the possibility of recurrent PTA or further tonsillitis; and it decreases hospitalization time and shortens the total period that patients are disabled. Whether the latter is true has been heavily debated. The recurrence rate of PTA that is managed with needle aspiration and antibiotics appears to be low (10%), which calls into question the need for a preventive role for tonsillectomy.

In conclusion, we've certainly come a long way in the treatment of PTAs. Only about 1 of 7 children with PTAs is hospitalized, and usually for a stay of under 2 days. Needle aspiration can be done as an outpatient. Six percent or fewer of cases will fail to resolve and will require incision and drainage for cure. Only about 10% of cases will recur, and these are the ones that probably would benefit from abscess tonsillectomy. A minimalist approach to this interesting infection works and saves time and dollars. Discuss this report with the ENT specialist that you rely on. In an era of managed care, it's nice to see that conservative approaches are both cost-effective and the optimal treatment for your patient.

There is a pearl that you should remember when dealing with a child who may have a strep pharyngitis/tonsillitis. If you are in a place where you can't readily do a culture or a fast strep screen, you can at least smell the child. Were you aware that children with a suspicious smell to their breath have a 4.33 times increased probability of having streptococcal infections?[1] The positive predictive value for strep of a suspicious smell is 72.7%; the negative predictive value of the absence of smell is 77.8%; the sensitivity of smell as a diagnostic test for streptococcal infection is 60%; the specificity of smell as a diagnostic test for streptococcal infection is 86%. Not all that bad for a sniffer. The schnozzola beats out most laboratory tests any day of the week.

Reference

1. Nakar S, et al: *Lancet* 343:729, 1994.

Changes in the Core Tonsillar Bacteriology of Recurrent Tonsillitis: 1977–1993
Brook I, Yocum P, Foote PA Jr (Georgetown Univ, Washington, DC; North Florida Regional Hosp, Gainesville)
Clin Infect Dis 21:171–176, 1995   16–17

Background.—Patients with recurrent pharyngotonsillitis caused by group A β-hemolytic streptococci (GABHS) are a continuing clinical challenge. Sometimes tonsillectomy is performed as a last resort to prevent recurrent infection. Penicillin may lose its effectiveness in these patients because its repeated use can change the tonsillar microflora, resulting in the selective survival of β-lactamase–producing bacteria (BLPBs), which degrade penicillin and protect both themselves and GABHS. The microbiology of recurrently infected tonsils during 3 periods in 16 years was reviewed to assess the changes in tonsillar flora over time.

Methods.—The aerobic and anaerobic organisms were isolated from the core tonsillar tissue of tonsils removed from 150 children with recurrent GABHS tonsillitis during 3 periods: 1977–1978 (period 1), 1984–1985 (period 2), and 1992–1993 (period 3). The chromogenic cephalosporin analogue 87/312 method was used to determine the β-lactamase activity of all the isolates.

Results.—Each tonsil had mixed flora, with a mean of 7.8 organisms (3.7 aerobes and 4.1 anaerobes) per tonsil in period 1, 8.3 organisms (3.9 aerobes and 4.4 anaerobes) in period 2, and 8.1 organisms (3.9 aerobes and 4.2 anaerobes) in period 3. The most common aerobic organisms in all periods were α-hemolytic streptococci, *Staphylococcus aureus*, and *Moraxella catarrhalis*. *Haemophilus influenzae* type b was found in 24% of the patients in period 1, 76% in period 2, and 12% in period 3 (in response to the introduction of the vaccine). *H. influenzae* non–type b was found in 4% of the patients in period 1, 10% in period 2, and 64% in period 3. In all 3 periods, the most common anaerobic organisms were *Peptostreptococcus* species, pigmented *Prevotella* and *Porphyromonas* species, *Fusobacterium* species, and *Bacteroides* species. β-lactamase–producing bacteria were found in 74% of the patients in period 1, 92% in period 2, and 94% in period 3. The number of BLPBs per tonsil also increased with succeeding periods. Several aerobic and anaerobic organisms demonstrated increasing β-lactamase production over time.

Discussion.—The core of recurrently inflamed tonsils contains polymicrobial aerobic and anaerobic flora. The common and increasing presence of BLPBs supports the theory that repeated penicillin therapy may select for these organisms. Bacterial isolates and their resistance patterns in recurrently inflamed tonsils should be monitored continuously to determine appropriate antimicrobial therapy.

▶ These investigators are the historical gurus of bacteria that lie deep within our tonsils. They are believers that one of the reasons recurrent tonsillitis caused by GABHS continues at a fairly high frequency is the failure of penicillin to work because of deeply imbedded microflora that are β-lactamase producing. Indeed there are many studies of tonsils removed at the time of surgery that demonstrate such bacteria within the core of tonsils. The debate over the years is whether such β-lactamase–producing organisms are really the cause of recurrent tonsillitis. This report does not reopen this issue but rather examines during a 16-year period whether there have been changes in core tonsillar flora. Both the rate of recovery of β-lactamase–producing bacteria and the number of these organisms per tonsil have increased over time. Specifically, β-lactamase–producing strains were detected in 74% of tonsils early in the 16-year period with an increase to 92% in the second portion of the 16-year period.

Some practitioners take these data to heart and go beyond the use of penicillin for patients with recurrent tonsillitis secondary to GABHS. They treat for the type of organism that produces the enzyme that incapacitates penicillin. Clindamycin or a combination of amoxicillin and clavulanic acid are such drugs. Although second- and third-generation cephalosporins are more efficacious than penicillin against many of the organisms that lie within tonsils, they are less effective than clindamycin or amoxicillin/clavulanic acid against anaerobic β-lactamase–producing bacteria. With the use of penicillin, current data suggest that a child will become strep culture negative in 24 hours 86% of the time.[1] This also tells us that such kids should be kept out of school for 1 day after start of treatment.

The answers are not in about the role of core tonsillar bacteria as a cause of recurrent tonsillitis. This is not to say that before tonsils are removed, one might not attempt a trial of antibiotics appropriate to dealing with these kinds of bugs. You'll have to be the judge because there is very little guidance from the literature on this topic.

Reference

1. Snellman LW, et al: *Pediatrics* 91:1166, 1993.

A Pacifier Increases the Risk of Recurrent Acute Otitis Media in Children in Day Care Centers

Niemelä M, Uhari M, Möttönen M (Univ of Oulu, Finland)
Pediatrics 96:884–888, 1995
16–18

Background.—In addition to acknowledged risk factors for acute otitis media (AOM), use of a pacifier reportedly increases the risk. Whereas most risk factors for acute otitis are difficult to control, pacifier use could readily be avoided by educating parents.

Objective.—During a 15-month period, episodes of AOM were monitored prospectively in 845 white children attending 20 day-care centers.

Results.—At least 1 episode of AOM occurred in 45% of the children monitored, and 11% had more than 3 attacks. In children younger than 2 years, the prevalence of multiple attacks of AOM was 29.5% in those who used pacifiers and 20.6% in those who did not (Fig 2). Pacifier use increased the annual incidence rate of AOM from 3.6 to 5.4 in children younger than 2 years, and from 1.9 to 2.7 in those aged 2–3 years. Among children younger than 3 years, adenoidectomy was done more often in those using pacifiers, but there was no significant difference in the number

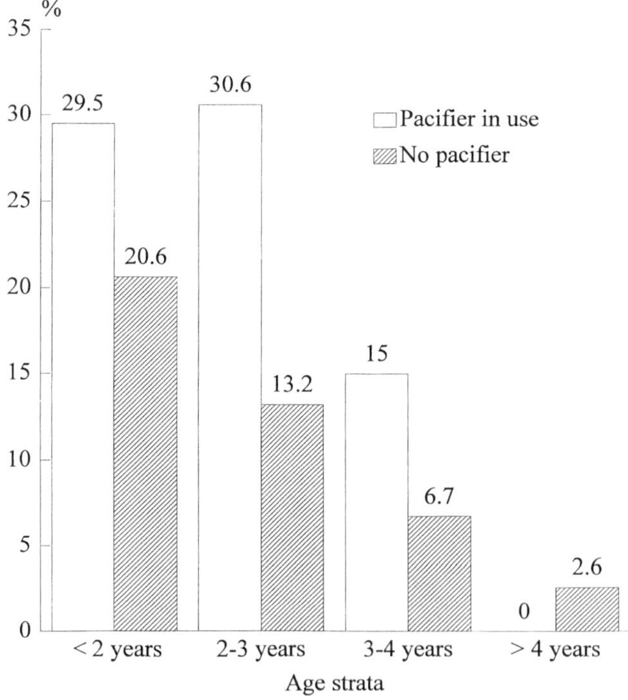

FIGURE 2.—Proportions of children with more than 3 attacks of acute otitis media during the monitoring period, by the use of pacifiers. (Courtesy of Niemelä M, Uhari M, Möttönen M: A pacifier increases the risk of recurrent acute otitis media in children in day care centers. Reproduced by permission of *Pediatrics*, Vol. 96, pp 884–888, Copyright 1995.)

of tympanostomies. After adjusting for age and time of monitoring, AOM correlated significantly with the time for which a pacifier had been used but not with thumb sucking.

Implications.—Use of a pacifier may have caused one fourth of the episodes of AOM in children younger than 3 years. It is suggested that pacifier use be limited to the first 10 months of life, when infants need most to suck and AOM is relatively infrequent.

▶ It is hard to deny the apparent link between pacifier use and an increased incidence of otitis media, particularly when, as this study shows, there are 5.4 episodes of otitis media per year per child younger than age 2 years who uses a pacifier (which is significantly higher than in those who do not).

Why pacifiers pose such a problem is not known. Sucking on a pacifier does increase the discharge of saliva, presumably an important medium for the spread of infectious agents from person to person. Frequent sucking on a pacifier could be harmful to the functioning of the eustachian tube. Sucking on a pacifier during a respiratory infection with a blocked nose may increase the reflux of nasopharyngeal secretions into the middle ear cavity. It has been shown that with increased intranasal pressure, secretions can enter the middle ear cavity via the eustachian tube and remain there for up to 10 minutes, even in healthy children.[1]

If there is any message that we should take home from this report, it is not that pacifiers should be removed from all children. There is a strong need for sucking on the part of every infant, particularly during the first 6 months of life. Beyond this time, however, the use of a pacifier tends to be more of a habit, perhaps producing a feeling of security. Before this report appeared, excessive pacifier use beyond the first half year of life was merely considered a harmless habit, perhaps causing minor malocclusions that would regress spontaneously. It is true that pacifier use is less harmful to the teeth than thumb sucking, but if the data from this report are to be believed, the use of a pacifier is responsible for about 25% of all attacks of otitis media in children younger than 3 years (at least in the construct of this investigation). The authors suggest that pacifiers should be restricted to the first 10 months of life, after which weaning should occur.

This editor would like to see more data linking pacifier use to an increased incidence of otitis media. In the meantime, it seems worthy to also focus on those entities known to increase the risk of otitis media: parental smoking and failure to breast-feed. Encouraging breast-feeding and snuffing out the butts would go a long way toward reducing the prevalence of otitis media.[2] Chucking the binky might as well; we'll see.

To learn more about managing otitis media in these changing times, see the excellent commentary on this topic by Jack Paradise.[3]

References

1. Wittenborg MH, et al: *Am J Roentgenol* 89:1194, 1963.
2. Aniansson G, et al: *Pediatr Infect Dis J* 13:183, 1994.
3. Paradise JL: *Pediatrics* 96:712, 1995.

Lateral Sinus Thrombosis Associated With Otitis Media and Mastoiditis in Children
Garcia RDJ, Baker AS, Cunningham MJ, et al (Massachusetts Gen Hosp, Boston; Massachusetts Eye and Ear Infirmary, Boston)
Pediatr Infect Dis J 14:617–623, 1995   16–19

Introduction.—Since the advent of antibiotics, lateral sinus thrombosis (LST) has been an uncommon complication of otitis media and mastoiditis. Three pediatric patients were affected in a 5-year period, prompting a literature review from 1960 to the present.

> *Case Report.*—Boy, 7 years, became febrile and had rhinorrhea and pain in the right ear, followed by dizziness, vomiting, and frontal headache. His temperature was 105.6°C. Right otitis media and tonsillitis were observed. Group A *Streptococcus* was grown from the blood. When fever persisted, an MR study demonstrated soft tissue density in the right middle ear and mastoid, as well as thrombosis in the right lateral and sigmoid sinuses and the proximal part of the right internal jugular vein. Tympanostomy tubes were placed, and antibiotic therapy given for *Staphylococcus aureus* infection. Heparin was given for 9 days when it was replaced by coumadin. The patient progressively improved and remained afebrile as the otorrhea resolved. He was left with a mild bilateral conductive hearing loss. Vascular MRI indicated some evidence of recanalization of the proximal part of the internal jugular vein. Anticoagulation therapy was continued for 6 months. Otitis media recurred 2 years later after the tubes had extruded. After adenoidectomy and tube replacements, the boy was well.

Clinical Review.—Including the present case, 58 patients have been described since 1960, 33 with otomastoiditis and 25 with otitis media alone. The most prominent clinical features were headache, fever, otorrhea, and otalgia; less frequent but more focal findings included papilledema, abducens nerve palsy, and vertigo. Both the white blood cell count and erythrocyte sedimentation rate were increased. Only 21% of patients had positive cultures. Mastoid radiographs were abnormal in all but 2 of 23 patients examined. Eight of 19 CT studies predicted LST. Radiopharmaceutical flow studies and MRI also were helpful in detecting changes of LST.

Management and Outcome.—All patients received systemic antibiotics, and all but 3 were operated on. Patients commonly received 2 antibiotics, often chloramphenicol combined with a penicillin. More than 80% of patients underwent mastoidectomy with subtemporal decompression. Only 4 patients had the internal jugular vein ligated. Otitic hydrocephalus was diagnosed in 26% of patients, and 5 patients had meningitis. Three had septic embolism. Three fourths of patients recovered completely by the time of discharge. Hearing loss developed in 8% of patients. All 3 patients who died (5%) were among a group of South African children who often were initially seen with advanced disease.

Conclusions.—Morbidity and deaths from LST have declined significantly in recent decades. Intravenous antibiotics alone may suffice in some cases, but it is not yet possible to predict which patients can avoid surgery.

▶ The causes of LST are fairly limited. The most common cause is an infection (such as an extension of otitis media). Noninfectious etiologies include traumatic or nontraumatic intracranial hemorrhage in newborn infants. Lateral sinus thrombosis has also been reported in Behçet's disease.

This review indicates that a high degree of suspicion is necessary when pursuing a diagnosis of LST because the most common clinical findings are similar to those seen in children with otitis media or mastoiditis. Headache, a most common symptom, is not typical for otitis media alone in children. The finding of a headache, together with findings of papilledema, sixth cranial nerve palsy, and vertigo should alert one to the possibility of LST.

Diagnosis is by MRI, and management requires the use of both antibiotics and, in some instances, surgery. The sinus itself is typically needled. If there is free blood return, no further intervention may be required. If there is no blood return, sinus incision with an attempt at thrombus removal is generally considered.

The overall mortality rate observed in this review was 5%. Fortunately, there are no reported pediatric deaths in the United States medical literature. This favorable outcome in children should not allow us the luxury of failing to diagnose this dreadful complication early. The next time you see a child with otitis media who has a splitting headache, worry.

Streptococcus pneumoniae Colonization in the Young Child: Association With Otitis Media and Resistance to Penicillin

Zenni MK, Cheatham SH, Thompson JM, et al (Vanderbilt Univ, Nashville, Tenn)
J Pediatr 127:533–537, 1995   16–20

Objectives.—A group of 215 healthy infants and children younger than 6 years who were receiving comprehensive care at a medical center clinic were studied to determine the frequency of pneumococcal colonization and whether colonization increased their risk of otitis media. In addition, the susceptibility of *Streptococcus pneumoniae* isolates to penicillin was studied.

Findings.—Of 842 nasopharyngeal cultures, 44% were positive for *S. pneumoniae*. Two thirds of the culture-positive children had more than a single positive culture. Positive culture results increased with advancing age. Thirty-seven percent of the isolates exhibited resistance to penicillin; of these, 28% were highly resistant and 66% were intermediately resistant (Table 1). Resistant isolates were much more frequent in children given antibiotics in the past month. Acute otitis media was diagnosed more often

TABLE 1.—Susceptibility of Penicillin-Resistant *Streptococcus pneumoniae* Isolates in the Clinic Population

Antimicrobial agent	No. isolates	Resistant to penicillin (MIC $\geq$0.1 µg/mL) Percent of isolates		
		Susceptible	Intermediately resistant	Highly resistant
Ampicillin	134	21	79	0
Amoxicillin/clavulanate	134	100	0	0
Cefuroxime	134	69	2	29
Cefaclor	134	39	7	54
Ceftriaxone	134	38	31	31
Rifampin	134	99	0	1
Chloramphenicol	134	96	0	4
Tetracycline	134	92	1	7
Trimethoprim-sulfamethoxazole	134	7	40	53
Erythromycin	134	83	1	16
Clindamycin	34*	100	0	0

*Only 34 isolates were tested with this antibiotic because it was added to the MIC plates during the study.
Abbreviation: MIC, minimum inhibitory concentration.
(Courtesy of Zenni MK, Cheatham SH, Thompson JM, et al: *Streptococcus pneumoniae* colonization in the young child: Association with otitis media and resistance to penicillin. *J Pediatr* 127:533–537, 1995.)

during visits in which *S. pneumoniae* was isolated from a nasal wash (27% vs. 16%). Resistant isolates were not more prevalent in children with otitis.

Implications.—These children probably are representative of many seen in pediatric practices nationwide. It should not be difficult to determine whether vaccination with conjugate pneumococcal vaccines would effectively combat colonization and reduce the risk of invasive disease.

▶ Penicillin-resistant *S. pneumoniae* has been found in this country for the past 22 years. The percentage of such resistant *S. pneumoniae* ranges from 5% (Centers for Disease Control and Prevention reports) to more than 25% (in certain day-care center surveys). The report abstracted attempts to determine whether there is a linkage between resistant organisms in the nasopharynx and the frequency of otitis media. The findings are a good news/bad news story. The good news is that children with acute otitis media and recurrent otitis media are not disproportionately colonized with resistant *S. pneumoniae*. The bad news is that the presence of penicillin-resistant organisms does correlate significantly with unresolved otitis media.

How does all this translate into what we should be doing for children with middle ear infection? Friedland and McCracken have strongly recommended that amoxicillin should continue to be the first-line therapy for otitis media, even in areas with high rates of antibiotic resistance.[1] When first-line therapy fails, the dilemma of what constitutes good alternative therapy then comes into play. The overwhelming majority of penicillin-resistant organisms in the report abstracted appear to be also resistant to trimethoprim-sulfamethoxazole (TMP-SMX). These same organisms also have high rates of resistance to cephalosporins. The organisms are susceptible to tetracycline, chloramphenicol, and ciprofloxacin. The toxic effects of these drugs in young children, however, prohibit their routine use in an outpatient setting.

A drug that is effective for penicillin-resistant organisms would be clindamycin, but this drug has not been well evaluated as part of the treatment for otitis media. Erythromycin might be another good alternative, although some organisms are resistant to this agent. The authors of the report abstracted suggest that the best approach in patients with otitis media that is refractory to first-line antibiotics may be to perform tympanocentesis and then to tailor antibiotic coverage to the laboratory susceptibilities of the organism recovered. This recommendation seems to make good sense.

So, what should we be doing to organize our thinking about the overall approach to otitis media in a time of bacterial resistance? Some authors have recommended withholding antimicrobial treatment entirely in some or all cases of acute otitis media unless symptoms persist or worsen.[2] Most do not accept this approach. Why let a child suffer when it is well known that antibiotics will usually produce prompt symptomatic improvement? Do we want to see a return of the high complication rates of mastoiditis and other suppurative complications of otitis media by failing to initially use antibiotics— Probably not. It seems reasonable to recommend that we use simple and inexpensive antibiotics as the first-line therapy for acute initial episodes of otitis media. A 10-day course of amoxicillin costs only about $6; TMP-SMX would cost even less. On the other hand, amoxicillin-clavulanate and cefaclor cost 10 times as much. For children with recurrent otitis media, this editor concurs with the recommendation of Paradise,[3] who says that sustained antimicrobial prophylaxis should be avoided; instead, periodic prophylaxis during upper respiratory tract infections and, when needed, tube placement are more appropriate alternatives in a time of emerging antibiotic resistance.

One of Murphy's laws states that nature frequently sides with therapies that are homeopathic. Our historical approach to otitis media, using broad-spectrum antibiotics, has violated that law. We may now be paying the price in terms of antibiotic resistance for tinkering with nature's principles.

References

1. Friedland IR, McCracken GH Jr: *N Engl J Med* 331:377, 1994.
2. Cunningham AS: *Contemp Pediatr* 11:17, 1994.
3. Paradise JL: *Pediatrics* 96:712, 1995.

Molecular Analysis of Bacterial Pathogens in Otitis Media With Effusion
Post CJ, Preston RA, Aul JJ, et al (Univ of Pittsburgh, Pa; East Tennessee State Univ, Johnson City)
JAMA 273:1598–1604, 1995   16–21

Background.—Our limited understanding of the cause and pathogenesis of otitis media with effusion (OME) has made it difficult to develop rational treatment approaches. A number of different infectious agents

TABLE 2.—Comparison of Culture and Polymerase Chain Reaction (PCR) Results From 97 Pediatric Middle Ear Effusions Analyzed for *M. catarrhalis, H. influenzae,* and *S. pneumoniae*

Bacteria	No. (%) of PCR-Positive, Culture-Positive Specimens	No. (%) of PCR-Positive, Culture-Negative Specimens	No. (%) of PCR-Negative, Culture-Negative Specimens	No. (%) of PCR-Negative, Culture-Positive Specimens	Total Culture-Positive Specimens*	Total PCR-Positive Specimens*	χ^2†	P
M catarrhalis	5 (5.2)	40 (41.2)	52 (53.6)	0 (0)	5 (5.2)	45 (46.4)	38.0	< .001
H influenzae	21 (21.6)	32 (32.9)	44 (45.3)	0 (0)	21 (21.6)	53 (54.6)	30.0	< .001
S pneumoniae	5 (5.2)	24 (24.7)	68 (70.1)	0 (0)	5 (5.2)	29 (29.9)	22.0	< .001
One or more of the target species	28 (28.9)	47 (48.4)	22 (22.7)	0 (0)	28 (28.9)	75 (77.3)	45.0	< .001

*1 df comparing total culture-positive specimens with total PCR-positive specimens.
†McNemar's test.
(Courtesy of Post CJ, Preston RA, Aul JJ, et al: Molecular analysis of bacterial pathogens in otitis media with effusion. *JAMA* 273:1598–1604, Copyright 1995, American Medical Association.)

may be involved in OME, but conventional culture techniques are not always adequate to identify these pathogens. The ability of polymerase chain reaction (PCR) to detect bacterial DNA in culture-negative middle ear effusions in children was assessed.

Methods.—Ninety-seven middle ear effusions were obtained from children undergoing myringotomy and tube placement for chronic OME. All children were treated on an outpatient basis, and all had had OME for longer than 3 months. The children's mean age was 42 months. The diagnosis was made by validated otoscopy and tympanometric evaluation. In all the children, multiple courses of antimicrobial therapy had been ineffective.

The effusion specimens were analyzed by both culture and PCR. The PCR-based detection systems were developed for *Moraxella catarrhalis, Haemophilus influenzae,* and *Streptococcus pneumoniae.* Differences in the percentage of positive test results on PCR vs. culture for these 3 organisms were assessed in blinded fashion.

Results.—Twenty-nine percent of effusion specimens tested positive by both culture and PCR for 1 of the 3 pathogens. In addition, 48% of specimens were PCR positive but culture negative for 1 of these 3 species. Overall, 77% of effusion specimens were PCR positive for *M. catarrhalis, H. influenzae,* or *S. pneumoniae* (Table 2). Dilutional experiments suggested that the average culture-negative effusion contained more than 10^4 bacterial genomic equivalents.

Conclusions.—In many children with culture-negative middle ear effusions, PCR-based assays can detect the presence of bacterial DNA. Although this does not prove the presence of active infection, the large number of bacterial genomic equivalents observed suggests an active process. If the findings are borne out by further study, they may influence antimicrobial treatment regimens, as well as the bacterial species and subtypes chosen for vaccine development.

▶ What a high-tech world we live in! Bacteria have nowhere to hide when it comes to PCR probes. Organisms that can't even be cultured can be unmasked with DNA technology. In this report we see that PCR-based systems do reveal the presence of bacterial DNA in a fairly high percentage of sterile middle ear effusions. Given our heretofore limited understanding of the etiology and pathogenesis of OME, any new information, such as this, is welcome, even though we don't know exactly what it means.

The pathogenesis of OME most likely is multifactorial. These factors include an immature anatomy, initiating viral infections that induce eustachian tube dysfunction, retrograde movement of bacteria from the oropharynx into the middle ear cavity, and host physiologic and immunologic variables. If the data from this report are reproducible, the PCR results for *H. influenzae* indicate that this pathogen may play a role in more than half of all cases of OME. The critical question, however, is whether PCR-positive, culture-negative results reflect the persistence of DNA from old infections, and nothing more. The authors say that it is unlikely that the data reported reflect the amplification of residual DNA from an earlier episode of otitis media, because animal-model experiments clearly demonstrate that purified bacterial DNA, co-inoculated with infectious organisms, does not persist for more than 2 days. To say this differently, the detection of amplifiable DNA in pediatric OME specimens suggests that viable bacteria are present in the middle ear, either at the time of sampling or within days of sampling.

In the final analysis, the data from this report suggest (but do not prove) that bacteria are present in culture-negative specimens from the middle ear of children with OME. Nonetheless, where there's smoke, and there certainly is a lot of that, there probably is fire—enough smoke and fire to set off an alarm. That alarm should signal us to stay tuned for further developments in this fascinating area.

Randomized Trial of the Efficacy of Trimethoprim-sulfamethoxazole and Prednisone in Preventing Post-tympanostomy Tube Morbidity

Daly KA, Giebink GS, Lindgren B, et al (Univ of Minnesota, Minneapolis; Park Nicollet Med Ctr, Minneapolis)
Pediatr Infect Dis J 14:1068–1074, 1995   16–22

Background.—Some children with chronic otitis media with effusion (OME) continue to have otorrhea and inflammation despite myringotomy and tympanostomy tube placement. Previous studies have documented short-term resolution of OME with prednisone and/or trimethoprim-sulfamethoxazole (TMP/SMX) treatment. It was hoped that combination treatment at the time of tube placement would delay the recurrence of otitis, prevent tube extrusion, and avoid the need for repeated intubation.

Study Plan.—Eighty children aged 6 months to 8 years were entered into the study when undergoing myringotomy and intubation for chronic OME. Middle ear effusion had been present for at least 8 of the past 12 weeks. Immediately after intubation, children were assigned to receive active treatment or placebo. Prednisone was given in a dosage of 1 mg/kg daily for 1 week, followed by the same dose on alternate days for a second week. Treatment with TMP/SMX suspension was given in respective daily doses of 8 and 40 mg/kg in 2 divided doses. Otoscopy was done 3 weeks and 3, 6, 9, and 12 months after surgery.

Results.—Actively treated children retained a functioning tympanostomy tube longer than placebo recipients (Fig 1). Rates of repeated intubation in the first year did not, however, differ significantly. Otitis media was present at 2 or more of the 5 first-year visits in 44% of actively treated children and 56% of those given placebo. Otorrhea was comparably frequent in the 2 groups.

Conclusion.—In children with chronic OME who undergo myringotomy and tube placement, 2 weeks of treatment with prednisone and TMP/SMX lowers the risk of tubal obstruction or extrusion for the first 3 months.

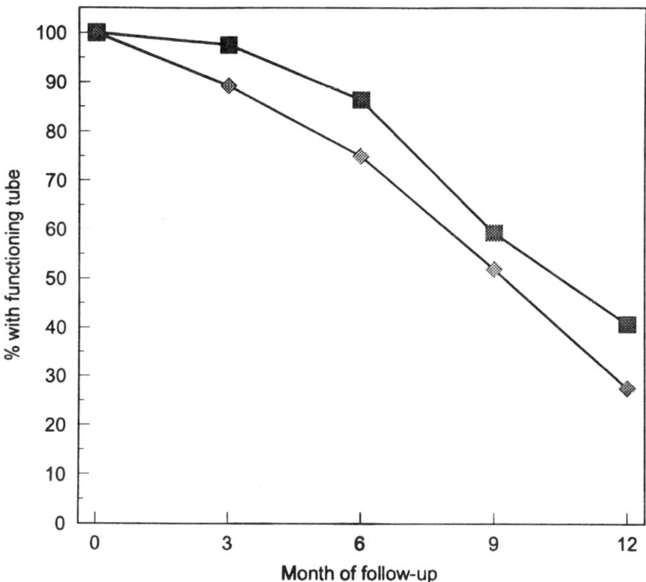

FIGURE 1.—Kaplan-Meier survival curves comparing duration of a functioning tube in active drug and placebo subjects during the first 12 postoperative months ($P = 0.02$, generalized Wilcoxon). *Squares,* active drug; *diamonds,* placebo. A functioning tube was defined as a patent tube in the tympanic membrane. (Courtesy of Daly KA, Giebink GS, Lindgren B, et al: Randomized trial of the efficacy of trimethoprim-sulfamethoxazole and prednisone in preventing post-tympanostomy tube morbidity. *Pediatr Infect Dis J* 14:1068–1074, 1995.)

▶ This paper, as far as this editor knows, is the first to examine posttympanostomy tube placement treatment with anti-inflammatory and antibiotic drugs. The rationale for this is the possibility that a combination of steroids and antibiotics will reduce middle ear inflammation, decrease early tube obstruction and extrusion, and reduce otitis media morbidity after surgery. The results of this study are pretty straightforward. Two weeks of treatment with prednisone and TMP/SMX does reduce the likelihood of tube obstruction and extrusion for about 12 weeks after surgery (but *not* longer than that).

It strikes this editor that, as interesting as these findings are, the results are not good enough to recommend such an approach. All of us must weigh potential risks against expected benefits in deciding on the therapies we prescribe. Relatively few these days are using antibiotics as a prophylaxis against recurrent otitis media, a trend that has resulted from the demonstration that prophylactic antibiotic use significantly increases the chance of the emergence of resistant organisms. Using steroids and antibiotics after surgery for placement of tympanostomy tubes seems to present a similar risk.

Let's face it, some good ideas just don't pan out.

Practice Variations Among Pediatricians and Family Physicians in the Management of Otitis Media

Roark R, Petrofski J, Berson E, et al (Univ of Colorado, Denver)
Arch Pediatr Adolesc Med 149:839–844, 1995   16–23

Introduction.—Otitis media is one of the most common childhood illnesses, accounting for almost 20% of all office visits for children 5 years and younger and resulting in expenditures of approximately $5 billion annually in the United States. Pediatricians and family physicians practicing in Colorado were surveyed to determine their practice patterns in the diagnosis and treatment of persistent and recurrent otitis media.

Methods.—The survey presented the physicians with 2 hypothetical cases: a 13-month-old boy with a persistent, asymptomatic middle ear infusion and a 15-month-old boy with recurrent otitis media. Physicians were asked to indicate which Medicaid codes they would use and to choose from a variety of management options. The survey was answered by 142 family physicians and 114 pediatricians, 65% of whom were in private practice.

Results.—Based upon responses for the 6-, 9-, and 12-week visits combined, most pediatricians and family physicians would use pneumatic otoscopy to identify an effusion and two thirds would use tympanometry (Table 1). Referral for audiologic testing was highest (25%) at the 12-week visit. More costly antibiotics were prescribed at a higher rate by family physicians (50%) than by pediatricians (33%) (Table 2). Overall, 54% of physicians would treat for 10 days. Family physicians were more likely than pediatricians to administer an oral decongestant at the 6-week visit (43% vs. 14%), and were 3 times more likely than pediatricians to refer children for ventilating tube surgery at the 9-week visit (Figure). The 2 groups concurred in their management of recurrent episodes of acute otitis media: 54% of respondents would start antibiotic prophylaxis, 23% would schedule follow-up visits, and 20% would consider both preventive treatment and follow-up unnecessary. Persistent effusions were often coded by physicians as acute otitis or as unspecified otitis media.

Conclusion.—Practice patterns for treating children with persistent and recurrent otitis media varied considerably. Compared with pediatricians, family physicians treated more often with high-cost antibiotics, despite

TABLE 1.—Use of Diagnostic Techniques Among Family Physicians and Pediatricians to Identify Middle Ear Effusion

	Family Physicians	Pediatricians	Combined
No. of visit responses	376	323	699
Diagnostic techniques, %			
Pneumatic otoscopy	88	91	90
Tympanometry	63	70	66
Audiology	9	12	11

(Courtesy of Roark R, Petrofski J, Berson E, et al: Practice variations among pediatricians and family physicians in the management of otitis media. *Arch Pediatr Adolesc Med* 149:839–844, Copyright 1995, American Medical Association.)

TABLE 2.—Antibiotic Selection for Management of Persistent Middle Ear Effusion Among Family Physicians and Pediatricians

	Family Physicians	Pediatricians	Combined
No. of treatment courses	152	151	303
Antibiotic selection, % of courses			
High cost*			
Amoxicillin+clavulanate potassium	18	21	20
Cefaclor†	22	7	15
Cefixime†	10	5	8
Low cost			
Amoxicillin	22	23	22
Erythromycin+sulfisoxazole	10	8	9
Sulfamethoxazole-trimethoprim	12	13	12
Sulfisoxazole	5	22	12
Erythromycin	1	0	1
Cephalexin	1	1	1
Total	100	100	100

*Family physicians > pediatricians (χ^2 = 8.89; odds ratio, 2.0 [95% confidence interval, 1.24–3.30]; P < 0.001).
†Family physicians > pediatricians (χ^2 = 14.9; odds ratio, 3.03 [95% confidence interval, 1.67–5.56]; P < 0.001).
(Courtesy of Roark R, Petrofski J, Berson E, et al: Practice variations among pediatricians and family physicians in the management of otitis media. *Arch Pediatr Adolesc Med* 149:839–844, Copyright 1995, American Medical Association.)

evidence of greater efficacy, and were 3 times more likely to refer patients for ventilating tube surgery. The coding inconsistencies observed indicate that claims data cannot distinguish between patients with recurrent acute otitis media and those with persistent otitis.

▶ This report would be without blemish except for 1 important fact: none of us really knows the very best way to manage otitis media. That having been said, it is probably safe to say that using amoxicillin plus clavulanate potassium, cefaclor, or cefixime does suggest that those who approach otitis media in this manner—both pediatricians and family practitioners—need to be educated. True, family practitioners, by a factor of 1.5, tend to use more expensive, but not necessarily more effective, therapies; however, if you read the data carefully, you will see that many pediatricians do as well.

None of this is a minor issue. Approximately $5 billion is expended annually in the United States for services related to the diagnosis and management of otitis media. Of this total, $2 billion is spent for surgical services, chiefly for placement of ventilating tubes. Anything, literally anything, that can be done to define better management and referral approaches that can be used effectively by both pediatricians and family practitioners (and other health providers as well) will be welcomed. A penny invested in research, in this regard, will have a many buck yield.

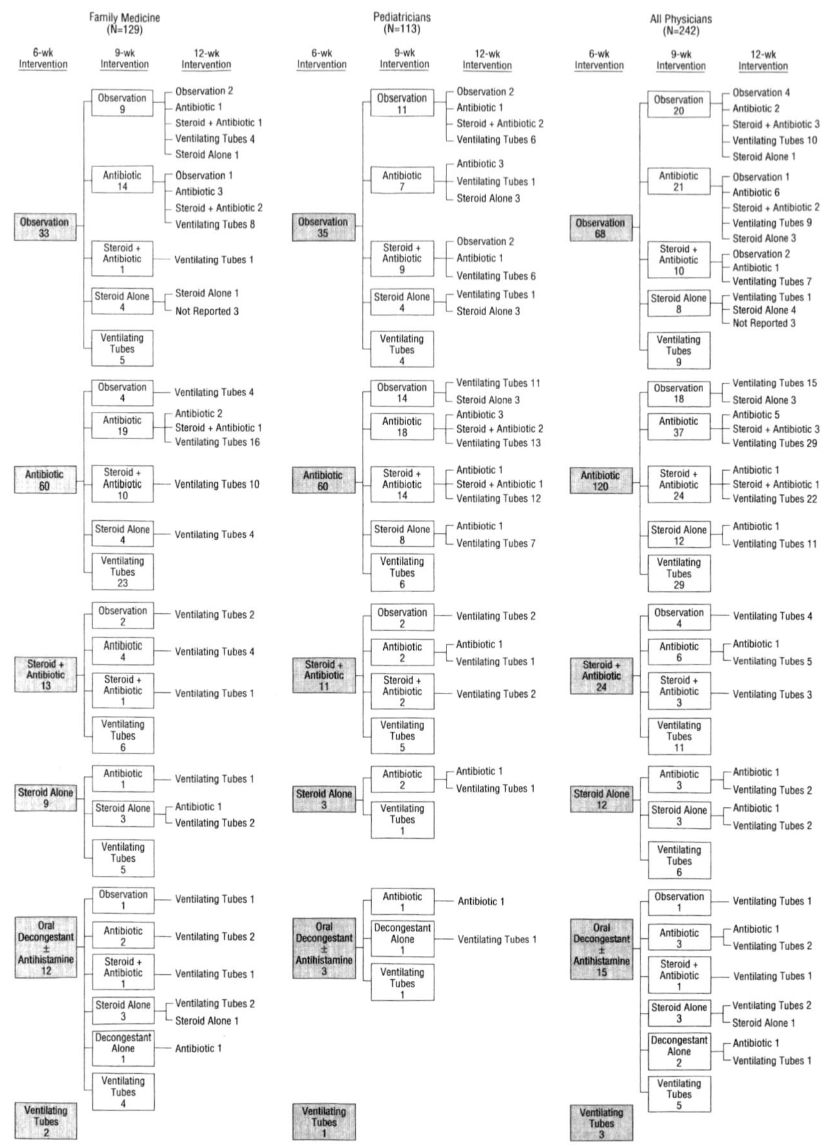

FIGURE.—Interventions selected to manage persistent middle ear effusions. (Courtesy of Roark R, Petrofski J, Berson E, et al: Practice variations among pediatricians and family physicians in the management of otitis media. *Arch Pediatr Adolesc Med* 149:839–844, Copyright 1995, American Medical Association.)

Efficacy of 20- Versus 10-day Antimicrobial Treatment for Acute Otitis Media

Mandel EM, Casselbrant ML, Rockette HE, et al (Children's Hosp of Pittsburgh, Pa; Univ of Pittsburgh, Pa)
Pediatrics 96:5–13, 1995   16–24

Rationale.—After a conventional 10-day course of antimicrobial treatment of acute otitis media (AOM), the clinician often must decide how to manage those children who have persistent middle ear effusion (MEE), as well as how to prevent recurrences of AOM. Often the choice is viewed as either continuing the same agent—often amoxicillin—or changing to another antimicrobial effective against β-lactamase–producing organisms, which frequently will be more expensive.

Patients.—A trial was undertaken in children 7 months to 12 years of age who were seen at an otitis media research clinic or in a private practice and received a diagnosis of AOM.

Methods.—A total of 267 children were randomly assigned to receive amoxicillin for 20 days; amoxicillin alone for 10 days and combined with clavulanate for 10 days longer; or amoxicillin followed by placebo. A double-blind design was used. Tympanocentesis was performed at the outset, and the children were reevaluated at intervals up to 3 months after entry to the trial. The groups were well matched for age and clinical characteristics.

Results.—Ultimately treatment failed in 9% of children who had 3 episodes of AOM during the 3-month study. In children with persistent MEE at day 10, both amoxicillin alone and combined treatment reduced

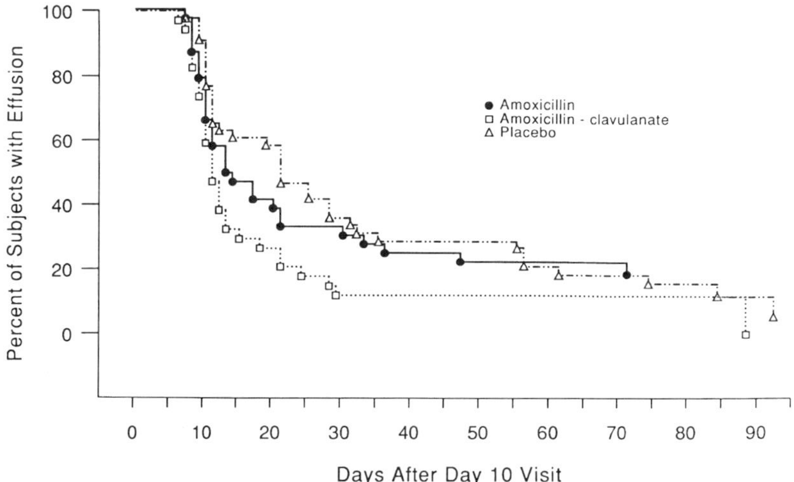

FIGURE.—Time after the day 10 visit until clearance of middle ear effusion for children with effusion at the day 10 visit. (Courtesy of Mandel EM, Casselbrant ML, Rockette HE, et al: Efficacy of 20- versus 10-day antimicrobial treatment for acute otitis media. Reproduced by permission of *Pediatrics*, Vol 96, pp 5–13, Copyright 1995.)

the time needed for effusion to resolve (Figure). Bilateral effusions took longer to resolve than those limited to 1 side. About three fourths of children in all treatment groups were free of effusion at their last visit. There were no significant differences in rates of recurrent AOM. Side effects were most prevalent (18%) in children given both amoxicillin and clavulanate.

Implications.—It is not yet clear whether prophylaxis is equally effective in preventing acute otitis in children with and those without MEE. If it is more effective when effusion is absent, combined treatment for 20 days might be advantageous, but it must be weighed against the greater expense entailed as well as an increased risk of side effects.

▶ Another report from the institution that has told us more about otitis media and what to do about it than probably any other institution on this planet. In this study, investigators in Pittsburgh focus on the optimal length of time for antibiotic treatment of AOM. Standard textbooks tell us that we should be using a 10- to 14-day course of treatment, but this length of time is probably based more on tradition than science. Such recommendations were originally generated for management of streptococcal pharyngitis. More recent studies have focused on the possibility that otitis media can be effectively managed with fewer than 10 days of antibiotics.

What this report specifically addresses is whether you can minimize the number of children who have MEEs with longer (more than 10 days) courses of therapy as part of the initial management of AOM. The investigators found that doubling the time of antibiotic therapy did reduce the number of MEEs when children were examined shortly after discontinuation of an antibiotic therapy. This advantage quickly disappeared within a few weeks. Add to all of this the concern about increased emergence of antibiotic-resistant bacteria and it's easy to conclude that anything longer than 10 days of antibiotic use as part of the initial management of AOM is senseless if the child has become symptom-free. Furthermore, it doesn't seem reasonable to reexamine a child who is free of symptoms immediately after you have concluded a course of antibiotics. Wait 30–60 days to allow MEEs to clear up. If an MEE is present for 3 months or more, one might then think about restarting antibiotics in an attempt to postpone or avoid the need for surgical intervention.

In an era of cost containment, these recommendations resonate well. Better yet, they are based on good, sound, scientific data. Obviously, for a few highly selected children with histories of recurrent AOM, antimicrobial prophylaxis immediately after the initial course of antibiotics may be reasonable because prophylaxis is effective in the prevention of recurrent AOM in some children.

As important as this report is, it fills in only 1 piece of the overall puzzle related to otitis media. Given all of the blanks that exist in our management portfolio, one can be fairly certain that there will be more and more written about the best ways to handle otitis media and its complications.

This is the last entry in the Dentistry and Otolaryngology chapter, so we close with a quiz. As an adolescent reaches adulthood, is there any part of the body that continues to enlarge throughout adulthood? The answer to the query is, it depends. If you are a man, it could well be that your ears grow. Did you ever notice that, as he approached the century mark, George Burns developed quite big ears? Go back and look at pictures of him when he married Gracie. Smaller, weren't they? If you're a nonbeliever, just look at Walter Matthau. It has been conclusively shown that long ears predict longevity, and the evidence is that as we get older, our ears get bigger.[1,2]

Your guess is as good as this editor's as to why the ears continue to grow. Is it because those who grow old with long ears have tugged on them many times for good luck? Is it that the ears are like other parts of the anatomy and sag with age, giving the appearance of being bigger? Perhaps the explanation is even more simple. Those who have grown old have heard a lot in life. They've simply had an ear full.

References

1. Heathcote JA: *BMJ* 311:1668, 1995.
2. Asai Y, et al: *BMJ* 312:582, 1996.

17 Endocrinology

Children Born Small for Gestational Age: Do They Catch Up?
Hokken-Koelega ACS, De Ridder MAJ, Lemmen RJ, et al (Erasmus Univ, Rotterdam, The Netherlands)
Pediatr Res 38:267–271, 1995   17–1

Objective.—In most cases, the cause of intrauterine growth retardation is unknown. Previous studies have found that full-term infants born small for gestational age (SGA) with no underlying disorder exhibit catch-up growth during the first years of life. However, the reported percentages of children who fail to show catch-up growth vary significantly. Postnatal growth and predictors for catch-up growth were studied in 724 SGA infants.

Methods.—A total of 423 premature and 301 full-term SGA infants whose birth length was less than the third length percentile (P3) for gestational age were studied. All had been admitted to 1 of 3 Dutch neonatology units during an 8-year period; infants with identified causes of growth retardation and those with neonatal or later complications were excluded. The infants were followed up through their first 2 years of life to

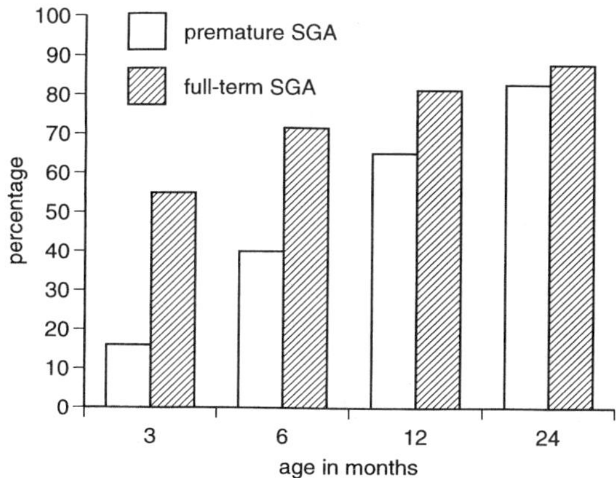

FIGURE 1.—Percentage of small-for-gestational-age (*SGA*) infants with postnatal catch-up growth to a height ≥ P3 at various ages. Data are given for premature (*white bars*) and full-term (*hatched bars*) infants of the total study group. (Courtesy of Hokken-Koelega ACS, De Ridder MAJ, Lemmen RJ, et al: Children born small for gestational age: Do they catch up? *Pediatr Res* 38:267–271, 1995.)

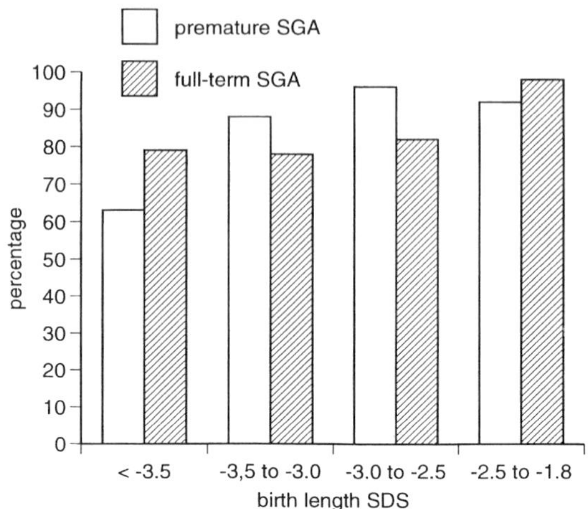

FIGURE 2.—Percentage of small-for-gestational-age (*SGA*) infants with postnatal catch-up growth to a height ≥ P3 for various subgroups of birth length standard deviation score (*SDS*). Data are given for premature (*white bars*) and full-term (*hatched bars*) infants from 1 of the 3 neonatology units. (Courtesy of Hokken-Koelega ACS, De Ridder MAJ, Lemmen RJ, et al: Children born small for gestational age: Do they catch up? *Pediatr Res* 38:267–271, 1995.)

describe their postnatal growth. In addition, predictive factors for catch-up growth—defined as a height of P3 or greater—were sought.

Results.—Catch-up growth was observed by 2 years of age in 82.5% of premature SGA infants and 87.5% of full-term SGA infants (Fig 1). For premature SGA infants, birth length standard deviation score (SDS) was a more sensitive predictor of catch-up growth than birth weight SDS (Fig 2). However, birth weight SDS was the best predictor of catch-up growth in full-term infants. Catch-up growth was not significantly related to gestational age, multiple birth, or sex. If the children were still at less than P3 in length at 3 or 6 months of age, the actual length SDS at that age was positively associated with catch-up growth. Weight gain during the first 6 months was positively associated with catch-up growth in SGA premature infants.

Conclusions.—About 85% of healthy SGA infants will show catch-up growth by 2 years of age. Predictive factors for catch-up growth were identified; for premature SGA infants, measures to optimize weight gain might improve the chances of catch-up growth. Children who were born SGA and show no signs of catch-up growth by 2 years of age should be investigated further.

▶ This is the first study to describe postnatal growth in a large number of uncomplicated premature infants who were born SGA. Small for gestational age in this study means having a birth length below the 3rd percentile for gestational age. The results show that 60% of full-term SGA infants who fail to catch up before 6 months of age will not attain catch-up growth at 2 years of age. Premature SGA infants with very severe intrauterine growth retardation (birth length less than 3.5 SDs) have the highest percentage (36%) of no catch-up growth equal to or greater than the 3rd percentile at 2 years of age. Fortunately, most SGA infants (term and preterm) do show catch-up growth during the first years of life. In fact, if you look at kids who are short later in life, SGA infants do not contribute a large proportion to such a population, at least under normal circumstances. To say this differently, if a full-term SGA child fails to appropriately catch up by 2 years of age, it may be worthwhile to institute the same sort of evaluation you would in a toddler who was not born SGA. You may want to do a thyroid screen, check for growth hormone deficiency, or for uncommon disorders such as celiac disease.

A Single-sample, Subcutaneous Gonadotropin-releasing Hormone Test for Central Precocious Puberty

Eckert KL, Wilson DM, Bachrach LK, et al (Stanford Univ, Calif)
Pediatrics 97:517–519, 1996   17–2

Background.—Central precocious puberty (CPP) is diagnosed by demonstrating pubertal levels of sex steroids and gonadotropins in response to gonadotropin-releasing hormone (GnRH) stimulation. The standard IV GnRH test has recently been shortened with no apparent decline in accuracy. A rapid, subcutaneous, single-sample GnRH test was studied for the diagnosis of CPP.

Methods.—The study included 22 girls, 8 years of age or younger, with evidence of precocious puberty. All patients received a 100 µg subcutaneous dose of GnRH in the clinic, followed 40 minutes later by a single measurement of serum luteinizing hormone (LH). No more than 2 weeks later, the girls underwent a standard IV GnRH stimulation test, with serum LH measurements performed at 0, 20, 40, and 60 minutes. An immunochemiluminometric assay was used to make the LH determinations, with a serum level of 8 IU/L or greater indicating CPP.

Results.—There was no difference in the mean peak LH levels after IV vs. subcutaneous GnRH injection. The LH levels measured after subcutaneous testing were significantly correlated with those measured after IV testing ($r = 0.88$). Both tests diagnosed CPP in 7 patients and excluded it in 14. The remaining patient had a negative result on subcutaneous testing but a positive result on IV testing.

Conclusions.—The mean and individual GnRH-stimulated LH levels obtained by rapid subcutaneous and rapid IV testing are similar in children with signs of precocious puberty. Thus the rapid subcutaneous GnRH test is valid for use in confirming the diagnosis of CPP. This test may also be useful in evaluating gonadotropin suppression in children receiving GnRH analogue therapy for CPP.

▶ All the world loves a simple, hopefully cheap, shortcut to a diagnosis. For children who are being evaluated for the potential of having CPP, what is described in this article may be just the answer.

The IV GnRH stimulation test is considered the standard test of reference for confirming CPP. Precocious puberty is usually defined as the presence of pubertal development in girls younger than 8 years of age and in boys younger than 9 years of age. The diagnosis of CPP includes documentation of pubertal levels of sex steroids and gonadotropins in response to GnRH stimulation. With IV GnRH administration, 20–40 minutes later, you will see a rise in LH levels. This study shows that giving GnRH subcutaneously works just as well for diagnostic purposes as giving it any other way. An LH value of 8 IU/L or more after subcutaneous GnRH defines CPP. There is no need to examine other substances such as follicle-stimulating hormone.

There are other alternatives to what is described above in terms of diagnosing CPP. These alternatives include urinary gonadotropin measurement, basal serum gonadotropin measurement, and IM administration of GnRH. Among all the options, SQ GnRH seems the easiest and least expensive.

The decision to treat a child with CPP relies not just on these biochemical tests, however. It relies also on other criteria including bone age, growth velocity, and the rapidity of growth suppression. Therefore, each patient should be considered for treatment of CPP on an individual basis. If all this seems confusing to you, get a consultation. Call 1-900-END-OCRIN.

To learn more about various approaches to the diagnosis and management of precocious puberty, see the fascinating article by Balducci et al.[1] Also, if you aren't certain whether a boy has entered puberty, the surest and most accurate way to find out is by measuring a testis. A boy with a testicular volume of 3 cc or greater, hair or no hair, is in puberty.[2] If you don't know how to determine testicular volume, buy a Prader orchidometer. If you can't afford the latter, practice on grapes of varying sizes. You can easily measure the volume of a grape by submersing it in a full container of water and measuring the amount of water that spills out. Wax the grapes and you can use them time after time. You may need a few jumbo variety, because the average tanner five male is somewhat larger than your average Napa Valley seedless grape. If you are sans grapes in your part of the country, try the same thing with Jelly Bellies. They, too, come in all sizes and don't even need to be waxed for repetitive use.

References

1. Balducci R, et al: *J Clin Endocrinol Metabol* 79:582, 1994.
2. Biro FM, et al: *J Pediatr* 127:100, 1995.

Neurophysiologic Studies and Cognitive Function in Congenital Hypothyroid Children

Weber G, Siragusa V, Rondanini GF, et al (Univ of Milan, Italy)
Pediatr Res 37:736–740, 1995   17–3

Background.—Although early replacement therapy has limited the most serious effects of congenital hypothyroidism (CH) on neuropsychological development, some children with a normal intelligence quotient (IQ) may nevertheless have subtle psychomotor abnormalities that may reflect minimal brain damage.

Objective.—The effects of replacement treatment were evaluated in 15 children and adolescents with CH who had been detected by neonatal screening and started on treatment before age 2 months (group A) and in 11 other patients in whom CH was diagnosed clinically before the advent of screening and who began replacement treatment after age 2 months and as late as 5 years of age (group B). Twenty healthy children and adolescents served as a control group.

Methods.—In addition to IQ testing, the auditory P300 wave response was recorded, and the long-latency somatosensory evoked potentials (LL-SEPs) analyzed.

Findings.—The group A patients were significantly younger than those in group B, but the 2 groups were well-matched with the control subjects for age. All patients with CH had normal serum levels of free thyroxine after 3 months on replacement therapy. Group B patients had significantly lower global and performance IQ scores than did those in group A. Neurophysiologic abnormalities were found in 82% of group B patients but also in 47% of those in group A who were detected by neonatal screening and had normal mental development. Compared with control subjects, LL-SEPs were significantly increased in both groups of patients with CH.

Interpretation.—Some children with CH may have subtle damage of the CNS despite receiving replacement therapy from an early age. It is not clear whether this results from a prenatal event or whether such postnatal factors as delayed replacement therapy or an adverse psychosocial environment may be important.

▶ It is not unexpected that infants with CH that has been undetected by neonatal screening programs will have lower IQ scores than screened patients. As this report indicates, the difference in IQ is remarkable between these 2 groups of infants. Nonetheless, even with the best of screening programs and the early institution of thyroid replacement, infants grow up to be toddlers and children who have about a 50% chance of not being normal in the sense that 1 or more neurophysiologic tests, should they be done, will be abnormal.

These data are not new. They are worthy of being reported because they remind us that although most states require neonatal screening for CH, this alone is not a perfect tool for the prevention of long-term problems. As of now, we have no method that can be reasonably used to detect and treat prenatally. Absent that, the best we can do is start replacement therapy at the earliest postnatal moment possible.

Significance of Elevated Serum Thyrotropin During Treatment of Congenital Hypothyroidism

Heyerdahl S, Kase BF (Rikshospitalet, Oslo, Norway)
Acta Paediatr 84:634–638, 1995
17–4

Background.—Serum thyrotropin (TSH) often remains elevated after treatment in children with congenital hypothyroidism. Because optimal treatment is crucial to normal mental development, it is important to determine whether elevated TSH is a sign of undertreatment or an indication that the feedback mechanism on TSH secretion is immature. Data from a study of 49 children with congenital hypothyroidism were analyzed for time to normalization of initially elevated TSH levels; the relationship between elevated TSH levels during treatment, the dosage of serum thyroxine T_4, and the serum T_4 concentration; and the possibility that elevated TSH levels result from noncompliance with treatment.

Methods.—In 46 children, the mean pretreatment serum T_4 concentration was 39.5 nmol/L, and the mean age at the start of treatment was 18.5 days. Three children had treatment postponed because transitory hypothyroidism was suspected. Levels of TSH greater than 10 mU/L during treatment were considered elevated. Noncompliance with medication was determined by review of medical records, laboratory results, and parent interviews.

Results.—The initial mean dosage of L-thyroxine (L-T_4) was 8.5 μm/kg/day. Normalization of TSH, indicated by serum concentrations less than 10 mU/L, was achieved in 71% of serum samples obtained 15–21 days after the start of treatment. Within 3 months of treatment, 36 of 42 children with samples analyzed for TSH had normalized TSH levels. The 6 children whose levels remained elevated during the first 3 months of treatment had a lower mean dosage of L-T_4 prescribed at 6 weeks of age than the children with normalized TSH levels. All 6 children responded with normal TSH levels once their dose of L-T_4 was increased. When the children were 6 years old, 77% of parents said they forgot to give the medication less than once a month, 16% forgot once a month, and 7% said they never forgot. An occasional missed dose did not significantly affect L-T_4 dosage, serum T_4, or TSH levels. No other evidence of noncompliance was found.

Conclusion.—Elevated TSH levels in these children with congenital hypothyroidism were related to L-T_4 dosage and serum T_4 levels rather than to noncompliance with treatment. Normalization of TSH levels usually occurs rapidly with treatment, and elevated levels are most likely to indicate undertreatment.

▶ Anyone who has treated an infant or child with congenital hypothyroidism knows the problem being referred to in this report. Some youngsters, when given thyroid hormone replacement, continue to have elevated serum TSH levels. Do these kids need more thyroid replacement, or do some children have an immature feedback mechanism that does not shut down TSH production? The latter scenario would theoretically require nothing more to be done about it.

We learn from this report that TSH levels can be normalized rapidly after institution of thyroid hormone replacement. We also learn that it requires above-average amounts of thyroid hormone to suppress TSH production. The mean serum T_4 level associated with an elevated TSH level was generally within the upper half of the normal range, whereas the mean serum T_4 level combined with a TSH level of less than 10 mU/L is in fact fairly high, especially during the first 6 months of life. Recent American and European guidelines recommend an initial dosage of thyroid replacement of 10–15 µg/kg/day of L-T_4.[1, 2] These dosages are higher than those that were suggested some years ago and should be adequate to suppress TSH levels. Nonetheless, TSH levels should be monitored fairly regularly.

The therapy for children with congenital hypothyroidism may be more difficult to optimize than generally recognized. Early normalization of TSH levels should be the aim. Although elevated TSH levels seem to be a sign of undertreatment, we still don't know whether TSH levels can or should be normalized in every case. If you have a child who has high TSH levels despite high–normal T_4 values, it's probably time to get on the horn with your consultant endocrinologist. Intelligence quotient points, once lost, are very hard to recover subsequently.

Test your knowledge about the management of the infant with a low T_4 level with the following clinical scenario: a full-term male was born after an uncomplicated pregnancy and delivery. His growth parameters at birth were unremarkable. He was discharged from the nursery on a soy formula at his parents' request because of a family history of intolerance to cow's milk in several siblings. During the first week of life, he experienced poor feeding, floppiness, and somnolence. On day 8 of life, a newborn thyroid screen confirmed the presence of primary hypothyroidism, and treatment was begun with standard doses of T_4. A technetium thyroid scan showed evidence of an ectopic thyroid (lingual) gland. After a month, the baby's TSH remained markedly elevated. His T_4 doses were increased. Thyroid tests continued to show lack of TSH suppression. A new prescription for a different variety of T_4 was given. By 49 days of age, his TSH remained high despite all efforts to bring it down with T_4. What is going wrong here? If you answer that the soy formula is the culprit, you are correct.

A soybean diet may have goitrogenic effects. Soy diets apparently are associated with a large enough fecal mass that they waste a fair amount of iodine that is ingested. Furthermore, there is something in soy, probably a glycopeptide, that blocks iodine uptake by the thyroid. The net effect is that before 1960, there were several notable cases of goiters occurring in infants who were exclusively fed soy formula. The problem resolved when these infants were switched to a cow's milk formula. Since commercial manufacturers began supplementing soy formulas with iodine in 1959, no further cases of soy formula–induced goiters have been reported. Note, however, that there are now 3 children with congenital hypothyroidism who were unable to be adequately managed with thyroid replacement because of being fed soy-based formulas.[3]

The lesson: when giving thyroid replacement to a sick infant, stick with breast milk or a cow's milk–based formula, otherwise you and the baby will be soy sorry.

References

1. Working Group on Congenital Hypothyroidism of the European Society for Pediatric Endocrinology: *Eur J Pediatr* 152:974, 1993
2. American Academy of Pediatrics: *Pediatrics* 91:1203, 1993.
3. Chorazy PA, et al: *J Pediatr* 126:148, 1955.

The Relation of Transient Hypothyroxinemia in Preterm Infants to Neurologic Development at Two Years of Age

Reuss ML, Paneth N, Pinto-Martin JA, et al (Columbia Univ, New York; Michigan State Univ, East Lansing; Univ of Pennsylvania, Philadelphia)
N Engl J Med 334:821–827, 1996

17–5

Background.—Many preterm infants have transient hypothyroxinemia, which has generally been viewed as a condition with no long-term sequelae that does not require thyroid hormone replacement. However, recent studies have suggested that hypothyroxinemia in newborns may be associated with later problems in motor and cognitive development. The possible link between hypothyroxinemia in premature infants and subsequent motor and cognitive abnormalities was investigated in a historical cohort study.

Methods.—The cohort included 463 subjects from a population-based study of the late sequelae of neonatal brain hemorrhage. All had birth weights of 2,000 g or less, were born at or before 33 weeks' gestation, and had records making available data on blood thyroxine values during the first week of life. Mental development assessments were performed at 2 years of age in 400 children. Correlations were sought between the blood thyroxine values in the first week of life and the presence of disabling cerebral palsy and mental development scores at age 2 years. Severe thyroxinemia was defined as a blood thyroxine level of more than 2.6 standard deviations below the mean.

Results.—The blood thyroxine concentration increased with gestational age for infants born after 29 weeks' gestation. The risk of disabling cerebral palsy was significantly increased for infants with severe hypothyroxinemia, compared with those without thyroxinemia (odds ratio, 10.8) after adjustment for gestational age. In addition, the mean mental development score at age 2 years was 15 points lower for the infants with severe hypothyroxinemia. The risk of disabling cerebral palsy associated with severe hypothyroxinemia remained elevated (odds ratio, 4.4) after adjustment for gestational age and various other prenatal, perinatal, and neonatal variables, including the presence of brain lesions. A 7-point reduction in the mean mental development score persisted as well.

Conclusion.—Severe hypothyroxinemia in preterm infants appears to be related to problems in neurologic and mental development at age 2 years. Studies of treatment to increase neonatal thyroxine concentration could help determine whether the relationship is a causal one and whether treatment can prevent the neurologic and developmental sequelae.

▶ Until this report appeared, transient low levels of thyroid hormones had been thought to be a common benign occurrence in preterm infants. Transient hypothyroxinemia has been viewed as an innocent developmental phenomenon, an expression of immaturity of endocrine regulatory systems, or a side effect of unrelated illnesses. Whatever the cause, it has been largely viewed as a laboratory phenomenon of no particular interest or consequence, at least until this study appeared. Severe hypothyroxinemia in preterm infants can be an important cause of neurologic problems, including mental retardation. Additionally, there is a fourfold increase in the risk of disabling cerebral palsy.

As disturbing as this report is, even more disturbing is the fact that given the information provided, we do not have a clue as to what we should be doing with these tiny preterm infants. Should all of them be monitored with thyroid studies? Should all get maintenance doses of thyroid hormone? What size study would be necessary to tell us whether these therapeutic interventions really did anything? Who is going to do such a study? Who is going to pay for it? Will it be done in our lifetimes? Your guesses are as good as this editor's! To learn more about pituitary-associated neurologic and developmental abnormalities and neonatal thyroid function, see the excellent overview of this topic by Vulsma and Kok.[1]

As an aside, it's interesting to note that preterm babies and those who exercise too much share one thing in common: both can experience transient disorders of their hypothalamus and pituitary glands. Recognize, however, that not all exercise produces this type of disregulation. For example, who is more likely to run into problems with hypothalamic disregulation: the teenage athlete who engages in serious long-distance running, the teenage athlete who is a highly competitive oarswoman, or the teenage athlete who participates in women's competitive judo? Actually, for all three, pushing 20 should have been exercise enough. All 3 types of athletes could get into trouble with "hypothalamic shut down," but those who participate in women's competitive judo appear to be at greatest risk. Judoists have significantly lower ovarian hormonal activity and hypothalamic/pituitary activity than do oarswomen or long-distance runners. The combination of exercise, low body fat, low body weight, loss of weight, and stress turns off the key that regulates the pituitary gland.[2] Please note that not all female judoists experience this problem. Those who don't exercise a lot, who don't strictly diet, and who have a more cavalier attitude about their performance may have physically fit bodies, but they are at significantly less risk for the secondary medical complications of excessive exercise. They also probably don't win as often. "Judoist pituitary," the 521st reason not to exercise.

References

1. Vulsma T, Kok JH: *N Engl J Med* 334:821, 1996.
2. Nader S: *Lancet* 347:920, 1966.

The Use of the hCG Stimulation Test in the Endocrine Evaluation of Cryptorchidism

Davenport M, Brain C, Vandenberg C, et al (Hosp for Sick Children, London)
Br J Urol 76:790–794, 1995   17–6

Introduction.—The presence or absence of functional testicular tissue is commonly evaluated using the human chorionic gonadotropin (hCG) stimulation test. Some isolated reports have indicated that the testosterone response to hCG was absent with intra-abdominal testes or that persisting testosterone production occurred with anorchia. The hCG stimulation test was reviewed in a series of 31 prepubertal boys with impalpable testes to confirm or refute its value.

Methods.—All boys received age-dependent daily doses of hCG: less than 1 year, 500 units; 1–10 years, 1,000 units; and older than 10 years, 1,500 units. Blood samples were obtained before the first dose and 24 hours after the final dose. All boys underwent a full surgical exploration.

Results.—Boys were grouped according to surgical findings: group 1 (8 boys)—anorchic; group 2 (14 boys)—bilateral intra-abdominal testes or normal volume; and group 3 (9 boys)—either a unilateral intra-abdominal testis only or with bilateral dysplastic testes, which were either intra-abdominal or intracanalicular (but impalpable) and were typically excised. Eight boys with anorchia and 1 with bilateral atrophic intra-abdominal testes had no response to hCG. Findings indicated that 22 boys responded to hCG stimulation testing and had testes whose size was related to the degree of testosterone elevation (Table 1). Positive and negative predictive

TABLE 1.—Value of the hCG Test in Predicting Bilateral Anorchia in 31 Boys With Bilateral Impalpable Testes

Threshold testosterone level	*Anorchia*	*Other*
<Twofold rise	8	1*
>Twofold rise	0	22
Peak <5 nmol/L	8	7
Peak >5 nmol/L	0	15

*11-year-old (basal testosterone = 0.7 mol/L; unchanged by IV hCG), basal follicle-stimulating hormone = 5 IU/L and basal luteinizing hormone < 1 IU/L). Surgical findings: bilateral atrophic intra-abdominal testes, which were both excised. No histologic examination was available.

(Courtesy of Davenport M, Brain C, Vandenberg C, et al: The use of the hCG stimulation test in the endocrine evaluation of cryptorchidism. *Br J Urol* 76:790–794, 1995.)

values for the hCG test were 89% and 100%. There was a significant quantitative difference in testosterone response between 14 boys with bilateral intra-abdominal testes of normal volume and 9 boys with an otherwise reduced volume of testes.

Conclusion.—The hCG stimulation test is an accurate predictor of anorchia. A good response to hCG suggests bilateral intra-abdominal testes of sufficient size for orchidopexy. Patients with no response to hCG do not need formal surgical exploration for confirmation.

▶ One of the great pediatric dilemmas is what to do with an infant boy or toddler in whom no testes can be palpated. Is a testis present or is the child one of those rare patients who have anorchia? This report attempts to tell us whether we can use the hCG test in the evaluation of such boys without palpable testes.

Anorchia is a fairly uncommon entity. Only about 1 in 200 boys with undescended testes actually has no testes or testicular tissue at the time of surgical exploration. Anorchia is the result of a vascular catastrophe to the testes occurring after 12 weeks' gestation. For a male phenotype, male genitalia must develop under the influence of testosterone in the first 3 months of life. The absence of any testes at all and testosterone early in gestation would lead to a female phenotype.

It is important to know whether true anorchia is present. If the diagnosis of anorchia can be established, an unnecessary surgical exploration will be avoided. Nonoperative approaches to determine the presence or absence of testes have not been well accepted. Computed tomography and MRI are not particularly sensitive. Laparoscopy is probably the investigation of choice at this time. Its disadvantages are pretty straightforward. It requires an invasive procedure and general anesthesia.

An alternative approach is an examination of the testosterone response to hCG. Functional testicular tissue in prepubertal boys will secrete testosterone in response to gonadotropin irrespective of the position of the testes. This is the basis for the interpretation of the hCG test.

Is the hCG test perfect? No. Is it a reasonably good test? Yes. Its sensitivity is 100%. The problem is one of a lack of specificity. If there is no testosterone response to hCG, it does not necessarily mean that no testicular tissue is present. Boys with dysplastic testes may have a poor response to hCG. Other findings may sort this out. Children with dysplastic or atrophic testes (and hence a poor response to hCG) have a tendency to have other congenital anomalies. The child with true anorchia does not. Micropenis, as an example, may be seen in boys with dysplastic testes but virtually is never seen in those with anorchia. Thus the presence of other anomalies should lead one to suspect that a dysplastic testis is present.

This report clearly shows us that the hCG stimulation test (because of its low specificity) is not the sine qua non for the diagnosis of anorchia. The authors believe, however, that the investigation of boys with bilateral impalpable testes should include a 3-day hCG stimulation test. In their opinion, those showing no response to hCG do not require surgical exploration to confirm this. Apparently they believe that severely dysplastic testes that cannot produce testosterone do not require formal surgical exploration. That is not the opinion of many others, because such testes can undergo malignant degeneration if left unattended.

So, what is the conclusion of this report? The conclusion to this editor is pretty straightforward. The hCG test seems superfluous. A negative response to hCG doesn't mean that a testis isn't present; a testis that could undergo malignant degeneration may be. A good response to hCG means you're going to operate to find the testis. Either way, it would seem that laparoscopy and/or surgical exploration is going to happen. It seems that simple. No hormone apparently will replace a surgeon's hands when it comes to organs as valuable as testes.

Slipped Capital Femoral Epiphysis Associated With Endocrine Disorders

Loder RT, Wittenberg B, DeSilva G (Univ of Michigan, Ann Arbor)
J Pediatr Orthop 15:349–356, 1995   17–7

Introduction.—Slipped capital femoral epiphysis (SCFE) has been associated with obesity and subtle hormonal imbalances, but the exact etiology of the disorder is unknown. Because few data are available on that subset of children with SCFE and definite endocrine disorders, 85 such patients were retrospectively studied.

Patients and Methods.—Seventy-nine of the patients were identified in a literature review, and 6 were treated at the study institution between 1975 and 1993. Information collected included primary endocrine diagnosis, time of diagnosis of SCFE relative to the time of diagnosis of the endocrine disorder, duration of symptoms, and treatment. The SCFE was classified as acute or chronic, and slip severity as mild, moderate, or severe.

Results.—The 85 patients had a total of 128 SCFEs. Primary endocrine diagnoses were hypothyroidism in 34 patients, growth hormone deficiency in 21, panhypopituitarism in 9, craniopharyngioma with undescribed endocrine deficiencies in 6, hypogonadism in 4, hyperparathyroidism, growth hormone excess, and multiple endocrine neoplasia IIb in 3 patients each, and Turner's syndrome and optic nerve glioma in 1 patient each (Table 1). The primary endocrine disorder was diagnosed at a mean age of 13.2 years and the first SCFE at 15.3 years. Mean bone age and chronological age, known for 53 hips, differed significantly (11.6 vs. 16.5 years, respectively). Time of diagnosis for the 2 disorders was known for 81 patients. In 44, the endocrine disorder was diagnosed first; in 33, the disorders were diagnosed simultaneously; and in 4, the SCFE was diagnosed before the endocrine disorder. Seventy-four hips were chronic, 13 were acute, and 13 asymptomatic. Slip severity, known for 82 hips, was mild in 48, moderate in 20. and severe in 12; 2 were pre-slips. The first SCFE was diagnosed in a child as young as 7 years, but only those with hypothyroidism or growth hormone deficiency were younger than 10 years at the time of SCFE diagnosis. None of the patients in whom the

TABLE 1.—Patients With Endocrine-associated Slipped Capital Femoral Epiphyses (SCFEs)

Source Author(s)/(yr)	No. of patients	No. of SCFEs	No. of patients with particular endocrine disorders								
			↓ T4	↓ GH	↓ Pit	Cp	↓ GN	↑ PTH	↑ GH	Men IIb	Misc.
University of Michigan (1993)	6	9	1	1	1	—	—	1	—	1	1*
Wells et al. (1993)	9	18	4	—	4	—	1	—	—	—	—
Prasad et al. (1990)	3	5	—	3	—	—	—	—	—	—	—
Bone et al. (1985)	1	2	—	—	—	—	—	1	—	—	—
Nishi et al. (1985)	1	1	1	—	—	—	—	—	—	—	—
Rappaport and Fife (1985)	16	17	—	16	—	—	—	—	—	—	—
Heyerman and Weiner (1984)	7	10	7	—	—	—	—	—	—	—	—
McAfee and Cady (1983)	1	2	—	—	1	—	—	—	—	—	—
Hennessy and Jones (1982)	1	1	1	—	—	—	—	—	—	—	—
Carney et al. (1981)	2	4	—	—	—	—	—	—	—	2	—
Fisher et al. (1980)	1	2	1	—	—	—	—	—	—	—	—
Jayakumar (1980)	2	3	2	—	—	—	—	—	—	—	—
Al-Aswad et al. (1978)	1	1	1	—	—	—	—	—	—	—	—
Hirano et al. (1978)	4	4	4	—	—	—	—	—	—	—	—
Reeves et al. (1978)	1	2	—	—	—	—	—	—	1	—	—
Zubrow et al. (1978)	1	2	1	—	—	—	—	—	—	—	—
Crawford et al. (1977)	5	7	5	—	—	—	—	—	—	—	—
Ogden and Southwick (1977)	5	8	2	—	1	1	1	—	—	—	—
Heatley et al. (1976)	4	8	—	—	1	2	—	—	—	—	1†
Hirsch and Hirsch (1976)	1	1	—	—	—	—	1	—	—	—	—
Moorefield et al. (1976)	3	5	2	—	—	1	—	—	—	—	—
Rennie and Mitchell (1974)	1	1	—	1	—	—	—	—	—	—	—
Chiroff et al. (1974)	1	2	—	—	—	—	—	1	—	—	—
Fidler and Brook (1974)	2	4	—	—	—	2	—	—	—	—	—
Primiano and Hughston (1971)	1	1	—	—	—	—	1	—	—	—	—
Epps and Martin (1963)	1	1	1	—	—	—	—	—	—	—	—
Goldman et al. (1963)	1	2	—	—	—	—	—	—	1	—	—
Löfgren (1953)	2	4	—	—	1	—	—	—	—	—	—
Benjamin and Miller (1938)	1	1	1	—	—	—	—	—	1	—	—
Total	85	128	34	21	9	6	4	3	3	3	2

Abbreviations: ↓ T4, hypothyroidism; ↓ GH, growth hormone deficiency; ↓ Pit, panhypopituitarism; Cp, craniopharyngioma with undescribed endocrine deficiencies; ↓ GN, hypogonadism; ↑ PTH, hyperparathyroidism; ↑ GH, growth hormone excess; MEN IIb, multiple endocrine neoplasia IIb.
* Turner's syndrome.
† Optic nerve glioma.
(Courtesy of Loder RT, Wittenberg B, DeSilva G: Slipped capital femoral epiphysis associated with endocrine disorders. *J Pediatr Orthop* 15:349–356, 1995.)

TABLE 2.—Comparisons Between Different Groups of Patients With Slipped Capital Femoral Epiphysis (SCFE) and Endocrine Disorders

Parameter	All children	Endocrine disorder					Craniopharyngioma		
		Hypo-thyroidism (group I)	Growth hromone deficiency (group II)	Other endocrine disorders (groups III)	p (I vs. II)	p* (I vs. II vs. III)	No	Yes	p
Sex (F/M)	37/43	19/15	6/9	12/19	0.31	0.33	30/30	7/13	0.24
Age at Dx of endocrine disorder (yrs)	13.2 ± 6.2	12.3 ± 6.7	13.2 ± 3.9	14.2 ± 6.8	0.27	0.28	12.9 ± 5.7	14.3 ± 7.8	0.44
Age at Dx of SCFE (yrs)	15.3 ± 5.3	13.7 ± 4.7	14.8 ± 3.2	17.4 ± 6.1	0.018	0.0014	14.8 ± 4.8	16.8 ± 6.4	0.17
Atypical age at Dx of SCFE (<10 yrs/>16 yrs)	8/21	3/4	5/5	0/12	1.0	0.00	7/15	1/6	0.63
Bone age (yrs)	11.4 ± 3.1	9.8 ± 2.7	9.5 ± 0	13.9 ± 1.6	0.65	0.0001	10.7 ± 2.9	14.3 ± 1.9	0.004
Unilateral/bilateral	27/42	18/16	2/3	7/23	0.66	0.025	26/32	1/10	0.04
Right/left (unilaterals only)	13/14	9/9	0/2	4/3	0.49	0.68	12/14	1/0	0.48
Symptomatic/asymptomatic	79/6	30/4	20/0	29/2	0.28	1.0	61/4	18/2	0.62
Symptomatic—chronic/acute	48/7	25/2	4/0	19/5	1.0	0.22	42/6	6/1	1.0
Symptom duration (mos)	5.2 ± 10.5	5.3 ± 6.0	1 ± 0	5.8 ± 14.7	0.038	0.047	5.5 ± 10.9	0.8 ± 0.9	0.89
Slip severity (slip/pre-slip)	48/2	23/1	2/0	23/1	1.0	1.0	38/2	10/0	1.0
Slip severity (mild/moderate and severe)	28/20	16/7	2/0	10/13	1.0	0.078	23/15	5/5	0.72

Height percentile (>5th/<5th)	19/26	7/15	0/2	12/9	1.0	0.075	16/23	3/3	0.68
Weight percentile (>95th/<95th)	16/34	4/9	8/7	4/18	0.027	0.076	6/28	10/6	0.003
Endocrine Dx (different/same as SCFE)	48/33	10/23	17/0	21/10	0.0000	0.25	31/31	17/2	0.0027
Endocrine Dx when different (before SCFE, after SCFE)	44/4	10/0	17/0	17/4	†	0.031	27/4	17/0	0.28
Time between endocrine and SCFE Dx (yrs)	2.2 ± 4.8	1.5 ± 3.7	1.8 ± 2.8	3.4 ± 6.6	0.004	0.046	2.1 ± 5.2	2.7 ± 3.2	0.57
SCFE Dx (before/during hormonal Rx)	30/35	20/10	1/12	9/13	0.0006	0.61	26/24	4/11	0.14
Time between hormonal Rx and SCFE (mos)	29 ± 51	65 ± 122	16 ± 18	31 ± 40	0.27	0.63	38 ± 68	18 ± 20	0.28
Follow-up (yrs)	4.2 ± 4.4	3.7 ± 4.0	1.9 ± 0.7	5.0 ± 4.9	0.92	0.72	4.2 ± 4.6	4.2 ± 3.7	0.82

Abbreviations: Dx, diagnosis; *Rx*, therapy.

* For categorical data, we combined groups I and II and reported the difference between this combined group and group III.

† No *P* value is possible because both groups being compared had no occurrences of the primary endocrine disorder being diagnosed after SCFE.

(Courtesy of Loder RT, Wittenberg B, DeSilva G: Slipped capital femoral epiphysis associated with endocrine disorders. *J Pediatr Orthop* 15:349–356, 1995.)

SCFE was diagnosed first were hypothyroid or growth hormone deficient. In all hypothyroid patients, the first SCFE developed before or during hormonal supplementation; in 92% of those with growth hormone deficiency, the first SCFE developed during or after hormone supplementation (Table 2). Ninety-one hips were known to have been treated surgically and 9 medically.

Conclusion.—Endocrine-associated SCFE showed a slight male predominance and a wide age range at diagnosis. The most common endocrine disorders were hypothyroidism and growth hormone deficiency, both of which were associated with younger age at diagnosis. Because bilaterality was common (61%), prophylactic treatment of the opposite hip should be considered in children with an endocrine disorder and a unilateral SCFE.

▶ Slipped capital femoral epiphysis is a fascinating disorder. All of us are trained to recognize that some children with it will have endocrine disorders, albeit a minority of affected children. This report tells us which endocrine disorders we should think about and tells us the timing of the relationship between the onset of endocrine and bony symptoms. Recognize, however, that only about 5% of children with SCFE will have an endocrine disturbance.

So what should you do the next time you see a child in whom you make a diagnosis of SCFE? Should you do an endocrine evaluation in everyone? Probably not. Assuming that the remainder of the physical examination is entirely normal and that physical growth including sexual maturation is on par with the child's chronological age, you're probably on safe territory simply following the youngster. Be aware, however, that if you do miss an endocrine disturbance, a child who has a unilateral SCFE has a 60% to 100% chance of having trouble with the opposite hip unless you do something about the underlying disorder. The trick is to keep an awareness of the association between one's glands and one's bones and to act on that awareness when there is a suspicion that a hormonal irregularity is present.

Brief Report: Short Stature Caused by a Mutant Growth Hormone
Takahashi Y, Kaji H, Okimura Y, et al (Kobe Univ, Japan; Kobe Children's Hosp, Japan)
N Engl J Med 334:432–436, 1996   17–8

Introduction.—Established causes of growth hormone–dependent short stature include primary pituitary disease, pituitary deficiency secondary to hypothalamic dysfunction, and insensitivity to growth hormone. A child with short stature related to a mutant growth hormone was described.

> *Case Report.*—An infant boy had a birth weight of 2,250 g and birth length of 39 cm after 41 weeks of gestation. At the age of 4.9 years, he had a height of 81.7 cm, which was 6.1 SDs lower than the mean for his age and sex. His bone age was 2 years. His basal

serum immunoreactive growth hormone concentrations were 7–14 ng/mL, which increased to 200 ng/mL afer prolonged growth hormone treatment. Treatment also increased his rate of linear growth from 3.9 to 6 cm/yr. Growth hormone bioactivity was subnormal (Table 1) and demonstrated an additional abnormal peak upon isoelectric focusing of the serum. Analysis of genomic DNA with polymerase chain reaction (PCR) amplification revealed the presence of a mutation in the *GH-1* gene, which sequencing revealed was a heterozygous single-base substitution resulting in the substitution of cysteine for arginine at codon 77. Comparisons of the wild-type and mutant growth hormone showed equal immunoreactivity. However, the mutant growth hormone had less than half of the bioactivity of the wild-type growth hormone when incubated with serum lacking growth hormone and prolactin and in the presence of recombinant human growth hormone–binding protein. The mutant growth hormone did not stimulate tyrosine phosphorylation and inhibited this activity in the wild-type growth hormone.

Discussion.—A single heterozygous missense mutation in the growth hormone gene was found to be a cause of severe growth retardation in a child. The mutant growth hormone demonstrated a higher affinity for growth hormone–binding protein and growth hormone receptor than the

---

TABLE 1.—Clinical Characteristics of the Proband and His Family*

CHARACTERISTIC	FATHER	MOTHER	ELDER SISTER	PROBAND	YOUNGER SISTER
Age (yr)	37	33	7	5.6	2.7
Height (cm)	168.7	162.2	127.1	84.8	88.4
SD†	−0.2	1.2	1.7	−6.1	−0.5
Serum growth hormone (ng/ml)					
Basal	1.4	0.2	1.6	7.0	0.2
Peak after insulin-tolerance test	23.7	NT	NT	38.0	NT
Bioactivity‡	1.0 ± 0.2	0.8 ± 0.4	1.2 ± 0.3	0.6 ± 0.2	1.0 ± 0.5
Serum IGF-I (ng/ml)	140	170	160	38	150
Normal	100–315	79–383	86–460	35–293	31–191
Serum IGF-binding protein 3 (µg/ml)	1.9	1.8	3.4	1.6	1.9
Normal	3.4 ± 1.1	3.3 ± 1.0	2.4 ± 0.8	2.4 ± 0.8	2.0 ± 0.6
Serum growth hormone-binding protein (pmol/liter)§	107	194	314	70	136

* Plus-minus values are means ± SE.

† Number of standard deviations above or below the mean for age and sex.

‡ Bioactivity is expressed as the ratio of bioactivity to immunoradiometric activity. The values are the means ± SE of 3 or more samples. The mean value in 30 normal subjects was 1.0 ± 0.2.

§ The normal value is 222 ± 115 pmol/L in men and 180 ± 92 pmol/L in women.

Abbreviations: NT, not tested; *IGF-I*, insulin-like growth factor I.

(Reprinted by permission of *The New England Journal of Medicine*, from Takahashi Y, Kaji H, Okimura Y, et al: Brief report: Short stature caused by a mutant growth hormone. *N Engl J Med* 334:432–436, Copyright 1996, Massachusetts Medical Society.)

wild-type growth hormone, resulting in both the inability to activate the growth hormone receptor itself and the inhibition of wild-type growth hormone activity.

▶ In a society that relishes normality, being unusually short is no laughing matter. This brief report by Takahashi et al. from Japan shows us one more treatable cause of short stature: a mutant growth hormone. Understanding what goes on with these children actually teaches us a great deal about the various ways in which children grow.

After birth, the manner in which we grow is largely dependent on pituitary growth hormone (regulated by what is known as the *GH-1* gene). Growth hormone results in the generation of insulin-like growth factor I (IGF-I). Growth hormone itself is regulated by growth hormone–releasing hormone, which is inhibited by the hormone somatostatin. Both growth hormone–releasing hormone and somatostatin are produced in the hypothalamus. The *GH-1* gene is located on chromosome 17 and exists among a family of growth hormone genes on the same chromosome. The other growth hormone genes largely relate to the production of placental hormones that regulate growth in fetuses.

What Takahashi and co-workers have described is a mutation in the growth hormone gene that causes the biological inactivation of growth hormone. The resultant growth hormone appears immunologically present but just doesn't work. Zvi Laron, in a superb review of growth hormone, reminds us of when we should suspect that a child may have a defect of genetic origin that results in short stature.[1] A genetic defect should be suspected in a child with short, obese parents who have small hands and feet, a history of delayed puberty, and the appearance of early aging. Newborn infants who are short (less than 48 cm in length for boys and 47 cm for girls), obese, have sparse hair, and have hypoglycemia should be examined for a molecular defect in the genes for growth hormone or its receptor. Affected boys may also have a micropenis. A molecular defect should also be suspected in infants or children who have marked growth retardation (height more than 4 SDs below the mean for age and sex) and a small face, a protruding forehead, sparse hair, a high-pitched voice, and severe retardation in skeletal maturation. In the absence of a lesion in the hypothalamic-pituitary region, as assessed by MRI, the finding of the lack of an increase in serum growth hormone after the administration of growth hormone–releasing hormone is proof of a defect in the release of growth hormone from the pituitary. In this case, a gene deletion should be suspected. A mutation in the growth hormone molecule, like that reported by Takahashi et al., should be suspected when serum growth hormone concentrations appear normal or elevated and serum IGF-I concentrations are low but increase with the administration of exogenous growth hormone. A molecular defect in the growth hormone receptor is most probable when serum growth hormone concentrations are high and serum IGF-I concentrations are low and do not increase after the administration of growth hormone.

If one obtains a detailed family history, performs a thorough examination, and monitors newborn infants who are small, and if one obtains detailed information about growth patterns of infants and children who are growing slowly, it should be possible to diagnose and treat in early childhood abnormalilties such as the ones described. It's not as complex as it might first appear. In fact, it's so logical that one wonders why most of us are so hesitant to approach these children ourselves. If you need more help with this topic, see the excellent overview on growth hormone insensitivity by Rosenfeld and the abstract that follows.[2]

References

1. Laron Z: *N Engl J Med* 334:463, 1996.
2. Rosenfeld R: *N Engl J Med* 333:1145, 1995.

Mutations of the Growth Hormone Receptor in Children With Idiopathic Short Stature

Goddard AD, for the Growth Hormone Insensitivity Study Group (Genentech Inc, South San Francisco; Univ of Göteborg, Sweden)
N Engl J Med 333:1093–1098, 1995   17–9

Background.—Many otherwise normal children of short stature secrete normal amounts of growth hormone (GH), but their target cells may not respond normally to GH because of either a defective GH receptor or abnormal intracellular mediators of GH signaling. Many affected children have low serum levels of GH-binding protein, suggesting that they may have an abnormal GH-receptor gene.

Objective and Methods.—The coding region of the GH gene was analyzed for mutations in 14 children with idiopathic short stature who had subnormal serum concentrations of GH-binding protein. The DNA was isolated from Epstein-Barr virus–transformed peripheral blood lymphocytes and directly from fresh lymphocytes. Genomic fragments of the GH-receptor gene were amplified by the polymerase chain reaction technique, and single-strand conformation polymorphisms of the reaction products were analyzed. Mutations were confirmed by sequencing the polymerase chain reaction products.

Results.—Four of the 14 children had mutations in the part of the GH-receptor gene coding for the extracellular domain of the receptor. None of 24 normal individuals exhibited such mutations. One of the 4 affected children was a compound heterozygote; 1 mutation reduced receptor affinity for GH, and a second one may alter some function other than ligand binding. The other 3 children had a single mutation in one allele of the gene. Two of these mutations substituted single amino acids in a structurally conserved receptor domain, and 1 mutation introduced a premature termination codon.

Conclusion.—Some children with idiopathic short stature who have findings consistent with partial insensitivity to GH are found to have mutations in the GH-receptor gene that may compromise receptor function.

▶ Children who are short pose unique problems to the generalist pediatrician and to the pediatric endocrinologist. Among these children are the enigmatic youngsters who have perfectly normal GH production and yet are still short. This phenomenon has become known as insensitivity to GH, the classic form of which is the very dramatic entity known as Laron dwarfism, originally reported 30 years ago.[1] Laron dwarfism is inherited as an autosomal recessive trait and is characterized by severe postnatal growth failure resulting from molecular defects in the GH receptor and its inability to bind GH. In the abstract above, Goddard and co-workers describe the intriguing finding that heterozygotes for such GH-receptor mutations may also have growth failure. By screening an extensive database of children identified as having "idiopathic" short stature who had normal serum GH responses to pharmacologic stimulation, they identified 14 children with short stature who had a receptor mutation consistent with being a heterozygote for the entity that in its homozygote form would be known as Laron dwarfism.

We are now challenged with an interesting task. How many children who are short carry the single-gene defect for GH-receptor mutations? Do they constitute a high percentage of children who, when treated with GH, fail to respond adequately in comparison with truly GH-deficient short children? Time will sort all this out. In the meantime, be aware that being short is much more than simply potentially having a deficiency of GH. Even if GH is present, its receptor may be mutated, producing what looks like GH deficiency when none is actually present.

To learn more about the use of growth hormone, see the guidelines concerning its use that were recently published by the Lawson Wilkins Pediatric Endocrine Society (A report of the drug and therapeutics committee of the Lawson Wilkins Pediatric Endocrine Society).[2] Ten very concrete guidelines and recommendations concerning the use of growth hormone are presented. They make good sense. Before embarking on serious consideration of growth hormone treatment for a child who's not growing well, recognize, however, that prepubertal children grow in fits and starts, and don't be too disappointed if you see a child who is slowing down at a particular time of the year. In northern climates, the greatest growth velocity is seen in prepubescent children during the spring months. They grow at an average of 8.15 cm per year at that time. During the fall months, however, this drops off by nearly 40% to 5.06 cm per year.[3]

If the way children grow seems difficult to remember, actually it's quite simple. Just recall that kids grow the same way grass grows. More rapidly in the spring and slow in the fall. In fact, children are quite a bit like grass, except that they don't need Scot's Turf Builder, or do they?

References

1. Laron Z: *Endocrinology* 3:21, 1963.
2. Lawson Wilkins Pediatric Endocrine Society: *J Pediatr* 127:857, 1995.
3. Jelander L, et al: *Acta Paediatr* 83:1249, 1994.

The Prevalence of Severe Growth Hormone Deficiency in Adults Who Received Growth Hormone Replacement in Childhood

Nicolson A, Toogood AA, Rahim A, et al (Christie Hosp, Manchester, England)
Clin Endocrinol (Oxf) 44:311–316, 1996   17–10

Background.—The few studies reassessing growth hormone (GH) status in young adults given GH treatment for childhood GH deficiency have focused on the incidence of "transient GH deficiency." This study determined how many patients receiving GH replacement therapy in childhood still have GH deficiency in adulthood severe enough for GH replacement treatment.

Methods.—Eighty-eight patients were included in the retrospective analysis. The investigation included the peak GH responses to provocative stimuli performed at diagnosis of GH deficiency in childhood and at growth completion after GH therapy had been stopped.

Findings.—All patients were GH deficient at initial diagnosis. Sixty-five percent at initial assessment and 60% at reassessment had a peak GH response of less than 9 mU/L. The incidence of severe GH deficiency between assessments increased in patients with radiation-induced GH deficiency and declined in those with idiopathic GH deficiency. Of the 55 patients who had 2 tests at reassessment, 47.3% with a GH peak less than 9 mU/L on 1 test had a GH peak exceeding 9 mU/L on the second test. Additional pituitary hormone deficiencies were found in 15 patients, all of whom had a GH peak of less than 9 mU/L on both tests (Table 3).

Conclusion.—All patients given GH replacement therapy in childhood should be reassessed in young adulthood to determine GH status. Forty percent to 60% may be candidates for GH therapy in adulthood, depending on the definition of severe GH deficiency. Two provocative GH secre-

---

TABLE 3.—The Severity of Growth Hormone Deficiency in 88 Patients Divided According to the Etiology of GH Deficiency

GH Peak (mU/L)	Idiopathic GH deficiency *n* (%)		Radiation-induced GH deficiency *n* (%)		Craniopharyngioma and histiocytosis X *n* (%)	
	Before GH	After GH	Before GH	After GH	Before GH	After GH
< 2	5 (15·6)	10 (31·3)	6 (13·9)	3 (7·0)	6 (23·1)	6 (46·1)
2–4·9	12 (37·5)	2 (6·3)	4 (9·3)	12 (27·9)	3 (23·1)	3 (23·1)
5–8·9	8 (25·0)	5 (15·6)	11 (25·6)	9 (20·9)	2 (15·4)	3 (23·1)
9–20	7 (21·9)	7 (21·9)	19 (44·2)	17 (39·5)	2 (15·4)	1 (7·7)
< 20	—	8 (25·0)	3 (7·0)	2 (4·7)	—	—
Total	32 (100)	32 (100)	43 (100)	43 (100)	13 (100)	13 (100)

Abbreviation: GH, growth hormone.
(Courtesy of Nicolson A, Toogood AA, Rahim A, et al: The prevalence of severe growth hormone deficiency in adults who received growth hormone replacement in childhood. *Clin Endocrinol (Oxf)* 44:311–316, 1996, Blackwell Science Ltd.)

tion tests should be done in patients with isolated GH deficiency. Those with additional anterior pituitary hormone deficiencies need only 1 test.

▶ This editor had never thought too much about what happens to youngsters when they grow up after a period of administration of GH during childhood and adolescence. Pediatricians, in general use GH to achieve adequate stature in those who are GH deficient. We tend to forget that GH deficiency is more than a matter of not having enough inches. Growth hormone is necessary for a wide variety of bodily functions. In adults, GH deficiency is a well-recognized entity characterized by a reduction in lean body mass, an increase in total fat mass, a reduced exercise capacity, a decreased bone mass, and impaired psychological well-being. Worse yet, cardiovascular morbidity and mortality appear to be increased in adults with hypopituitarism who are receiving standard replacement therapy with corticosteroids, thyroxine, and sex steroids, but not GH. Studies of GH replacement therapy in adults have shown beneficial improvements in body composition, an increase in bone mineral density, improved exercise capacity, and improved psychological well-being.

Until recently, the primary indication for GH replacement therapy was GH deficiency causing short stature occurring in childhood. These children were treated until growth stopped. An important issue is whether the world can afford GH replacement therapy beyond this period required for growth. If the data from this article are to be believed, GH replacement might be worthwhile throughout all of one's life right up until doomsday, but the cost implications are monumental. We see from this report that 90% of children with GH deficiency become adults with persistent GH deficiency. You might as well assume that growth hormone deficiency is a permanent disorder in most cases.

The lessons to be learned from this article are pretty straightforward. It is never too late to expect the benefits of GH. If you don't want GH-deficient adults to come up short in their overall well-being, remind the internist or family practitioner who will care for these children as adults to read this report.

Concordance Rates of Insulin Dependent Diabetes Mellitus: A Population Based Study of Young Danish Twins
Kyvik KO, Green A, Beck-Nielsen H (Odense Univ, Denmark)
BMJ 311:913–917, 1995   17–11

Objective.—Twin studies offer an excellent opportunity to gauge the relative influence of genetic and nongenetic factors in the origin of insulin-dependent diabetes. This historical cohort study was based on 20,888 twin pairs born in Denmark between 1953 and 1982. A questionnaire survey was carried out to obtain information on diabetes.

Findings.—The crude probandwise concordance rate was 0.53 for monozygotic twin pairs and 0.11 for dizygotic pairs. After adjusting for age at the onset of diabetes and age at last follow-up of the unaffected twin, the cumulative probandwise risk up to 35 years of age was 0.70 for monozygotic twins and 0.13 for dizygotic twins. Estimated heritability was 0.72.

Conclusion.—Dizygotic twins are at a higher risk of insulin-dependent diabetes than are other first-degree relatives, and monozygotic twins are affected more often than previously realized. In all, this disease is genetically determined to a greater degree than has been appreciated.

▶ Studies of twins can provide powerful insights into the origin of diseases such as diabetes. The problem with most twin studies is that they are biased. Many twin studies are based on obtaining patients by advertising or sampling from diabetic clinics. This has the inherent possibility—in fact, probability—of bias because of a disproportionate sampling of individuals who have health problems.

This report from Denmark was chosen for inclusion in the YEAR BOOK because it has none of the inherent flaws that are seen with most twin studies. In Denmark, all twins are registered at birth. Subsequently, investigators come back to that register to select, in an unbiased manner, populations for surveys or investigations. Between 1953 and 1982, 20,888 twin pairs were registered in Denmark. Thus, it was easy for these investigators to undertake a wholesale survey of this population to determine the likelihood with which a second twin would have diabetes once the initial twin was identified. Amazingly, in studies such as this, which are basically questionnaire analyses, about 95% of the surveyed individuals complete and return the questionnaires!

What we see in this report is amazing in terms of the risks that twins share. The key messages from this Danish investigation are:

The risk for insulin-dependent diabetes mellitus in identical twins is in excess of 50%. For nonidentical twins, it is 11%. These percentages are high enough that patients should be counseled about the probabilities of developing diabetes once one twin is affected.

Although the concordance rate for identical twins is high, it is still less than 100%, implying that there is an environmental component to the cause of diabetes.

The risk to nonidentical twins is higher than to ordinary siblings, indicating a shared environment as a possible contributor to the cause of diabetes.

Lastly, the risk is higher in identical twins than in HLA-identical siblings, indicating that shared environment, genes outside the HLA region, or both, are important in the causation of diabetes.

Data such as these show that twins share a lot more in common than just their parents.

18 The Musculoskeletal System

Effect of Starting Age of Physical Activity on Bone Mass in the Dominant Arm of Tennis and Squash Players
Kannus P, Haapasalo H, Sankelo M, et al (UKK Inst, Tampere, Finland; Tampere Research Ctr, Finland)
Ann Intern Med 123:27–31, 1995   18–1

Background.—The main determinants of peak bone mass in healthy individuals have been suggested to be race, sex, heredity, hormonal status, nutrition, and physical activity. It is important to focus on the environmental factors of nutrition and physical activity, because both can be easily

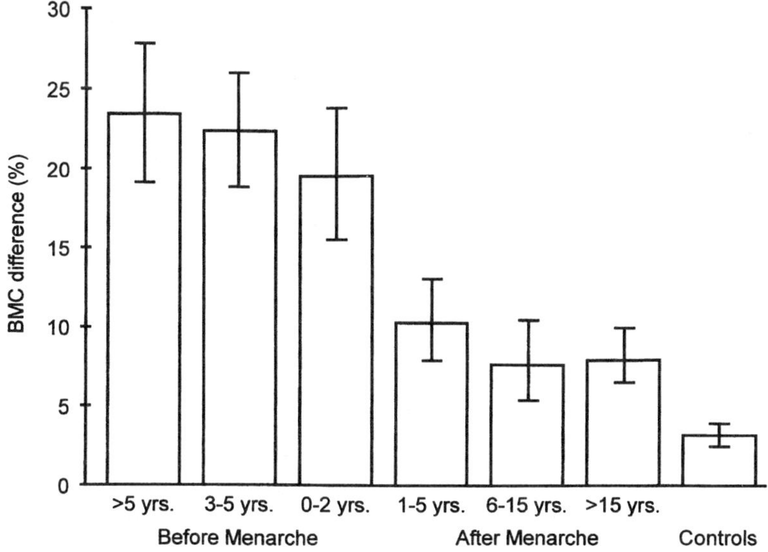

FIGURE 1.—The mean playing-to-nonplaying arm difference in BMC of humeral shaft (percentage difference of BMC) according to biological age at which training was started, i.e., according to starting age of playing relative to age at menarche. *Bars* represent 95% confidence intervals. *Abbreviation:* BMC, bone mineral content (Courtesy of Kannus P, Haapasalo H, Sankelo M, et al: Effect of starting age of physical activity on bone mass in the dominant arm of tennis and squash players. *Ann Intern Med* 123:27–31, 1995.)

controlled. It has not been possible to determine the optimal age or level of exercise needed to achieve maximal peak bone mass precisely. Female tennis and squash players were studied to determine the effect of biological age at which tennis or squash playing was begun on the difference in bone mineral content between players and nonplayers.

Methods.—One hundred five female Finnish national-level players and 50 healthy control subjects were included in the cross-sectional study. Players were divided into 6 groups based on the number of years before or after menarche at which their playing careers began.

Findings.—Compared with control subjects, the players had a significantly greater difference between the dominant and nondominant arms in all sites measured—the proximal humerus, humeral shaft, radial shaft, and distal radius. Group differences in bone mineral content were significant among players. Group means clearly decreased as the biological age of beginning play increased. The difference was 2–4 times greater among players who had begun playing before or at menarche compared with those who started playing more than 15 years after menarche (Fig 1). These trends were unchanged after adjusting for potential confounding factors.

Conclusions.—Active tennis and squash training increases the mineral mass of the bones of the playing extremity. The benefits of playing are about 2 times higher when girls start playing at or before menarche rather than after it.

▶ This report documents why those who exercise vigorously are hard-headed: those who flex their muscles strengthen their bones. If it's hard bones you want, exercise to your heart's desire, but recognize that if you're a woman, you will need to have begun your sporting activity before menarche. To understand this, you need to understand those factors that influence bone mineralization. In healthy individuals, the main determinants of peak bone mass are race, sex, heredity, hormonal status, nutrition, and physical activities. Genetic differences can account for 60% to 80% of the variance between people in the density of their bones. This leaves 20% to 40% of the variation as a result of environmental factors, including nutrition and physical activity. As this report indicates, the more individuals exercise during their period of skeletal growth, the greater the likelihood that their bones will be more dense. The onset of menarche and the completion of longitudinal growth are the first signs that bone mass development is stopping. Approximately 2 years after these developmental milestones are reached, subsequent increases in bone mass are fairly marginal. To say this differently, physical activity during the pubescent years is crucial for maximizing bone mass if the intent is to lessen the risk of osteoporosis later in life.

That's the good news. However, behind every piece of good news, there is some bad news that's not fit to print. In the latter category is the observation of this report that exercise significantly increases bone density only in those bones that have been actively exercised. Thus, if you are a right-handed tennis player, you'll have a good bony mass to your right humerus. Other bones are not likely to be as positively affected. For better symmetry to your body, start using a 2-handed backhand.

This commentary spoke of those who exercise as being hardheaded. Obviously, because exercise only strengthens those bones that are actively exercised, few of us are at risk of becoming hardheaded with the type of physical exercise that most of us engage in.

As an aside, does this report on bone mass qualify as an example of polyauthoritis? The answer to this query is no, but the report is pretty close. The number of journal articles has been increasing with time, as has the number of authors of each article. The latter has assumed morbid proportions—a malady known as polyauthoritis. Sometimes even those who do not contribute to research are listed as co-authors, an additional malady known as giftauthorship.[1] When the 2 maladies coexist, it becomes a syndrome—Polyauthoritis giftosa. Polyauthoritis, however, is defined as more than 10 authors for an original article, and more than 6 for a case report. Thus, the report abstracted does not quite fit the definition. True polyauthoritis has been found to be present in 4% of original articles and 8% of case reports published in the *Journal of Gastroenterology* in 1993. Polyauthoritis does not seem to be confined to any one journal. Five percent of original articles published in the *Annals of Surgery* in that same year suffered from the malady.

Polyauthoritis giftosa is like a disease where 2 organisms (the true author and the honorary author) live as commensals helping each other to survive and grow. It continues to be prevalent because it obliges the honorary authors without harming the interest of the true authors. Remedies for the entity are few and far between. Journals such as *The New England Journal of Medicine* require that if the number of authors exceeds 8 (12 for multicenter articles), each author must sign a statement attesting that he or she fulfills the authorship criteria of uniform requirements. Please note that polyauthoritis giftosa is an infectious entity. Although reactive therapy such as that of *The New England Journal of Medicine* may control the rate of spread of this infectious disease, its cure is in its prevention. The entity is a sign of "publish or perish"; elimination of the infection is only possible with the eradication of academic promotions committee. The sooner, the better.

Reference

1. Shapiro DW, et al: *JAMA* 271:438, 1994.

Usefulness of Magnetic Resonance Imaging for the Diagnosis of Acute Musculoskeletal Infections in Children

Mazur JM, Ross G, Cummings RJ, et al (Nemours Children's Clinic, Jacksonville, Fla; Natl Naval Med Ctr, Bethesda, Md)
J Pediatr Orthop 15:144–147, 1995   18–2

Background.—Early in the illness, acute hematogenous musculoskeletal infection in children is difficult to recognize and localize. The value of MRI in diagnosing acute musculoskeletal infections was studied prospectively during a 2½-year period and compared with the accuracy of bone scans in evaluating children with suspected musculoskeletal infections.

Methods.—Children admitted to the hospital with a clinical diagnosis of musculoskeletal infection underwent radiographs and bone scans (with technetium-99m–labeled diphosphate). Standard spin-echo MR pulse sequences were used in the MRI scan, obtaining T1- and T2-weighted images. The radiologist reading the MRI scan had all the relevant clinical information.

Results.—Forty-three patients (29 boys) with an average age of 6 years (range, 10 days to 15 years) had 31 proven musculoskeletal infections. In osteomyelitis, the involved marrow space showed decreased signal on T1-weighted images and increased signal on T2-weighted images. Magnetic resonance imaging also revealed cortical destruction or thickening and edema or abscess formation in the soft tissues. Septic arthritis showed an increase in joint fluid. An abscess in the soft tissue was associated with an area of low signal on T1-weighted images, a well-demarcated border, and a rim of decreased intensity. Magnetic resonance imaging helped to make the correct diagnosis in 41 of 43 cases. The sensitivity of MRI was 0.97 and the specificity was 0.92, with 1 false positive and 1 false negative result. Bone scans helped make the correct diagnosis in 24 of the 36 cases in which they were done. The sensitivity of bone scans was 0.64 and the specificity was 0.71, with 2 false positive and 10 false negative results. False positive results were caused by errors in patient positioning. False negative results occurred in newborns, and with soft-tissue and joint infection.

Conclusions.—Magnetic resonance imaging is valuable in diagnosing musculoskeletal infection in children and is more sensitive and specific than bone scans. Because of cost and technical limitations, its use should probably be limited to difficult cases. Magnetic resonance imaging is particularly helpful when infection involves the spine or pelvis. Because MRI accurately displays the location of the disease process, it may be essential when débridement and drainage are planned.

▶ One of the great dilemmas for those who provide pediatric care is determining which studies are necessary to appropriately diagnose musculoskeletal infections, particularly osteomyelitis. Is a plain radiograph necessary? Should a bone scan be performed? Does CT or MRI provide better yield? Is there any value at all in an ultrasound study? If the data from this report are true, MRI is the single most useful study for the diagnosis of acute musculoskeletal infections. It has a sensitivity (in this report) of 0.97 and a specificity of 0.92, superior to a bone scan, which has a sensitivity of 0.64 and a specificity of 0.71. A major advantage of MRI is that it defines precisely the spatial extent and localization of an inflammatory process. In the case of osteomyelitis, MRI shows replacement of normal fat in bone marrow with inflammatory exudates. This is particularly valuable information in cases requiring incision and drainage. Bone scans often overestimate the extent of osteomyelitis because of increased blood flow and bone metabolism in adjacent structures. In the case of joint and soft-tissue infection, bone scans are frequently negative because adjacent bone may not be affected.

Please note that MRI is not without some disadvantages. It is expensive (average cost $1,400). Patients must be positioned properly and remain still. Patients who are claustrophobic or who have tattoos should not undergo MRI. Lastly, MRI does not scan the entire body, whereas a bone scan does scan all bones and frequently shows areas of multifocal osteomyelitis.

So what is the best study to perform? As with most things, it depends. It depends on what equipment is available to you, how much money you can expend, what the clinical indications for a particular study are, and lastly, and probably as importantly, how skilled the radiologist is in interpreting the particular study that is to be performed. Some radiologists are terrific at interpreting plain radiographs and MRI but are not so great at interpreting scans (and vice versa). This editor's advice to help you decide what study to perform would be to read the best review available on the role of imaging for musculoskeletal infections, which appeared as an editorial recently by Dr. Ted Harcke, Chief of Radiology at the Alfred I. duPont Institute in Wilmington, Delaware.[1] Dr. Harcke provides the following advice when dealing with a suspected osteomyelitis:

- Always start with good plain films. It is virtually impossible to refute this statement.

- After plain films, do a bone scan. It is most widely accepted as the second step in the diagnosis of osteomyelitis. It is important to note that aspiration of a joint (or bone) can be performed before a scan. There is still a misconception that such a procedure will make a scan falsely positive. Its value in picking up a multifocal infectious process, particularly in a young child without symptoms, cannot be surpassed.

- Although cost must always be considered, prompt identification and treatment prevent sequelae that may cost far more when you delay diagnosis by "going on the cheap."

- There is no substitute for a seasoned orthopedist who is familiar with musculoskeletal inflammatory processes in children.

Reference

1. Harcke HT: *J Pediatr Orthop* 15:141, 1995.

Congenital Dislocation of the Hip in Boys

Borges JLP, Kumar SJ, Guille JT (Alfred I duPont Inst, Wilmington, Del)
J Bone Joint Surg (Am) 77A:975–984, 1995   18–3

Introduction.—Congenital dislocation of the hip occurs 5–8 times more frequently in girls than in boys. There has been no previous study of the specific problems of boys who have congenital dislocation of the hip. The problems associated with treatment of this condition in affected boys were reviewed.

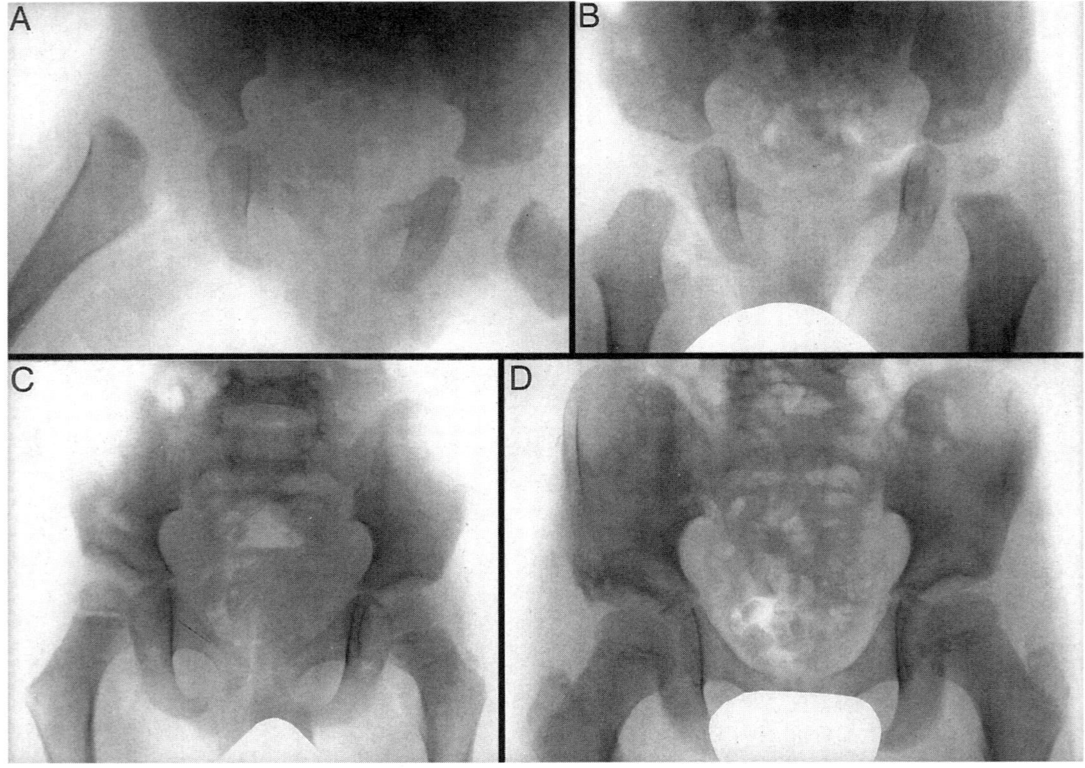

FIGURE 1.—Serial anteroposterior roentgenograms of a boy who had congenital dislocation of the hip. **A**, at the age of 8 months, there was dislocation of the right hip with a delay in the appearance of the ossific nucleus. A closed reduction was performed. **B**, 1 year after the closed reduction, at 20 months of age, there was evidence of avascular necrosis. **C**, when the patient was 5 years old, an innominate osteotomy was performed to treat persistent acetabular dysplasia on the right. **D**, 8 years later, at 13 years of age, the patient had an excellent clinical result, and the hip was rated as Severin class I. (Courtesy of Borges JLP, Kumar SJ, Guille JT: Congenital dislocation of the hip in boys. *J Bone Joint Surg (Am)* 77A:975–984, 1995.)

Methods.—The medical records and roentgenograms of 55 boys with 78 congenitally dislocated hips were reviewed. The patients were classified into 3 groups defined by their initial treatment. Group 1 included 22 children with 30 dislocated hips treated initially with a Pavlik harness. Group 2 included 29 children with 42 hips treated initially with closed reduction and immobilization in a hip-spica cast. Group 3 included 4 children with 6 hips treated initially with open reduction. Treatment outcome, the occurrence and grading of avascular necrosis, and the clinical result at the latest follow-up were reviewed.

Results.—The patients were followed up for an average of 8.5 years (range, 2–21 years). In group 1, the Pavlik harness resulted in a stable reduction of only 2 of the 30 hips in 2 of the 22 children, for a 7% success rate. These 2 patients were 1 week old and 4 months old when treatment began. At the last follow-up, both hips were Severin class I. In group 2, 29 (69%) of the 42 hips were stable after closed reduction. Of these 29, 14 did not need a second operative treatment. In these 14 hips, the clinical results were excellent in 10 and good in 4. The other 15 hips had residual subluxation or persistent acetabular dysplasia requiring a secondary operative procedure. Grade I avascular necrosis developed in 2 hips, requiring further surgery (Fig 1). In group 3, 3 hips were treated with an open reduction alone and 3 were treated with open reduction, a proximal femoral varus-derotation osteotomy, and an innominate osteotomy. Redislocation occurred in 2 of the hips treated with open reduction alone and 1 of the hips in the other subgroup, requiring further surgery. Three of these hips developed avascular necrosis (grade II in 2 hips and grade III in 1 hip). The clinical results were excellent in 2, good in 1, and fair in 3 hips.

Conclusions.—Boys have a significantly higher rate of treatment complications than do girls with congenital dislocation of the hip, with a high prevalence of redislocation. Treatment with a Pavlik harness has a very low success rate, particularly among children older than 7 weeks, with hips that are not initially reducible, and in children with a bilateral dislocation.

▶ When it comes to congenital dislocation of the hip, boys sometimes get "second shuffle," for as every pediatrician knows, girls have a 5–8 times greater risk for congenital dislocation of the hip(s). These investigators at Alfred I. duPont Institute in Wilmington have told us all about what it's like to be a boy with this problem. Only 7% of boys will have a satisfactory reduction of their hips with the use of a Pavlik harness (vs. 50% to 89% success rate in girls). Also, boys will likely have just a 68% success rate after a closed reduction of a dislocated hip joint, again a much lower success rate than would be expected in girls.

This study demonstrates the difficulty associated with the management of boys who have congenital dislocation of the hip. The rate of success for treatment of such hips with a Pavlik harness is sufficiently low that one must balance the use of such harnesses with their risk, the latter being avascular necrosis of the femoral head. These patients should be followed carefully, and other modes of therapy, such as closed or open reduction, should be used when the hip is not reduced after about 4 weeks of full-time use of a

Pavlik harness. Closed and open reductions of the hip are also associated with a higher rate of complications in boys than in girls. The prevalence of redislocation is fairly high as well. This high rate of redislocation may be secondary to an intrinsic deficiency of acetabular development and laxity in boys compared with girls.

All pediatric care providers must be comfortable with the hip examination in the newborn. We must recognize that although there is less risk of congenital dislocation of the hip in boys, the latter are more likely to run a rocky course should they have a bum hip. Pay careful attention to any infant who is born breech or after a pregnancy complicated by oligohydramnios, which are known risk factors for this problem.

Lastly, don't rely too heavily on the use of ultrasound as a substitute for your own examination in the newborn period. The use of ultrasound in the newborn period leads to an unacceptably high rate of false positives (in the range of 70 per 1,000, well beyond the 10 or 12 per 1,000 that is believed to be a reasonable estimate of the rate of discovery of congenital dislocation of the hip in the newborn).[1] Overdiagnosis with ultrasound frequently leads to unnecessary treatment, which translates into considerable expenditure of health care resources, higher risk of problems and complications, and an added emotional burden for the family. Recently, ultrasound when paired with a dynamic clinical examination has been shown to be much more specific.[2] Hopefully the latter will improve the specificity problem related to ultrasound. Something has to help us, because the traditional clinical examination has as its major weakness sensitivity in determining all kids with developmental dysplasia of the hip.

References

1. Hensinger RN: *J Pediatr Orthopaed* 15:723, 1995.
2. Harcke TH, et al: *AJR* 155:837, 1990.

Prospective Study of Recurrent Radial Head Subluxation
Teach SJ, Schutzman SA (State Univ of New York; Harvard Med School, Boston)
Arch Pediatr Adolesc Med 150:164–166, 1996   18–4

Background.—Radial head subluxation (RHS) is an upper extremity injury in children in which the radial head, under forces of forearm pronation and axial traction, slides under the annular ligament and is entrapped. Although several researchers have studied the causes and treatment of acute RHS episodes, no one has prospectively studied a cohort with RHS to determine the recurrence rate or to identify risk factors for recurrence.

Methods.—One hundred seven consecutive children younger than 6 years were included in the study. Ninety-four had definite and 13 had probable RHS. Follow-up lasted at least 12 months.

Findings.—Follow-up information was available for 93 of the patients (86.9%). Mean follow-up was 16.4 months. Twenty-two of these patients (23.7%) had recurrent RHS. Patients with recurrences were significantly younger than those who did not have recurrences. The relative risk for 1 or more recurrences during the study period in children 24 months of age or younger compared with those older than 24 months was 2.6. The groups with and without recurrences did not differ significantly in duration of follow-up, sex, elbow involved in the initial episode, or family history of RHS.

Conclusions.—Radial head subluxation recurs in almost one fourth of children with a diagnosis of RHS. Children aged 24 months or younger are at greatest risk.

▶ This report represents 2 firsts. It is the first study to prospectively evaluate the recurrence rate of radial head subluxation. It is also the first report to identify an age-associated risk of this problem. Younger children are more likely to experience a recurrence than older children. What this report doesn't tell us is why there is such a high recurrence rate (almost 25%) of RHS, although ligamentous laxity remains the likely culprit.

Given the high recurrence rate of this problem, parents of younger children with an acute episode of RHS should be counseled against applying undue traction to either arm of their child. Failure to warn parents about this might allow for another painful episode, one that could easily have been prevented.

Natural History of Untreated Chronic Slipped Capital Femoral Epiphysis
Carney BT, Weinstein SL (Shriners Hosp for Crippled Children, Lexington, KY; Univ of Iowa, Iowa City)
Clin Orthop 322:43–47, 1996   18–5

Background.—A slipped capital femoral epiphysis occurs in adolescents in whom the capital physeal plate has a gradual or acute disruption. Treatment is focused on restoring hip function in the short term and delaying degenerative joint disease in the long term. The long-term development of degenerative joint disease is related to the deformity's severity. To further characterize this relationship, the natural history of untreated chronic slipped capital femoral epiphysis was examined retrospectively.

Methods.—The records of 31 untreated hips with slipped capital femoral epiphysis in 28 patients seen between 1915 and 1952 were reviewed. The slip severity was graded. The Iowa Hip Rating was used to assess hip function at the most recent follow-up. Degenerative joint disease was classified using radiographs.

Results.—The patients were followed for a mean of 41 years after symptom onset, from a mean of 13 years of age at onset to a mean of 54 years of age at the latest assessment. Of the 31 hips, 17 had mild slips, 11 had moderate slips, and 3 had severe slips. During follow-up, there were complications in 4 slips, including severe displacement in 2, chondrolysis in 1, and osteonecrosis in 1. One of these complications occurred in a patient with a mild slip. The mean Iowa Hip Rating scores were 89 points overall, 92 points in the group with mild slips, 87 points in the group with moderate slips, and 75 points in the group with severe slips. There was radiographic evidence of degenerative joint disease in all hips with moderate or severe slips and in 64% of the hips with mild slips.

Conclusions.—When displacement remains mild, a chronic slipped capital femoral epiphysis will often have a favorable natural history. However, even a mild slip can progress to severe complications.

▶ Who would ever have thought that somebody would dig out the records of patients with untreated chronic slipped capital femoral epiphysis that was diagnosed between 1915 and 1952? Well, that's what Drs. Carney and Weinstein did. We see that, although we now know a great deal about the epidemiology, the etiology, and the pathogenesis of this condition, there is no substitute for good and timely treatment. The short-term goal of such treatment of slipped capital femoral epiphysis is to restore the function of the hip; the long-term goal is to delay the development of degenerative joint disease. The latter is directly related to the severity of the initial deformity. Even mild deformity may play a major role in later degenerative disease.

Don't miss slipped capital femoral epiphysis. The long-term term consequences of misdiagnosis are profound. Also recall that the time of the year to keep this disorder in mind is June. Only the Maker knows why slipped capital femoral epiphysis has a seasonal variation, but it does. The mean calendar month of onset is 6.8 ± 2.6 (that is, late June).[1] To say this differently, if slipped capital femoral epiphysis is diagnosed in December, the boat may have been missed by about 6 months.

Reference

1. Loder RT, et al: *Clin Orthop* 322:28, 1996.

Tibial Tuberosity Excision for Symptomatic Osgood-Schlatter Disease
Flowers MJ, Bhadreshwar DR (Barnsley District Gen Hosp, England)
J Pediatr Orthop 15:292–297, 1995   18–6

Introduction.—Osgood-Schlatter disease, a condition involving a traction apophysitis of the tibial insertion of the patellar tendon, typically affects adolescent boys and usually responds to conservative treatment. Various surgical techniques have been used in symptomatic, resistant cases. An excisional procedure was described that may be a useful option when standard conservative treatment fails.

Patients and Methods.—An attempt was made to contact the 47 patients who underwent tibial tubercle excision at the study institution between January 1982 and April 1993. Thirty-five patients responded and were interviewed for long-term outcome (mean, 5 years). All patients were initially treated with immobilization, restriction of activity, analgesics, and physiotherapy. After an average of 13.25 months of conservative treatment, excision was recommended. The mean patient age was 17.4 years, and the male-to-female ratio was 4:1. Both knees were affected in 7 patients. The operative technique starts with exposure of the patellar tendon and tibial tuberosity through a 5-cm vertical, infrapatellar midline incision. The tuberosity is removed using an osteotome, and any remaining osseocartilaginous material is excised. Patients are encouraged to walk the day after surgery.

Results.—Complete pain relief was obtained in 88% of patients and complete reduction of the prominent tuberosity in 52.5%. Two patients reported no change in pain, and 3 had partial relief. Reduction of the prominent tuberosity was incomplete in 14 patients, whereas 2 reported no reduction and 4 believed the prominence was larger postoperatively. All patients, however, were able to participate in sports and leisure activities without restriction. Patients younger than 16 years had a better outcome.

Conclusion.—In approximately 90% of cases, Osgood-Schlatter disease can be treated conservatively until fusion of the apophysis occurs and symptoms usually resolve. The type of excisional surgery described appears to be a successful option for those who fail to respond to conservative therapy or whose symptoms persist into adulthood.

▶ We're soon coming up on the centennial of Osgood and Schlatter's initial description of the disorder that bears their names, for in 2003, it will be exactly 100 years since these individuals separately described a traction apophysitis of the tibial insertion of the patellar tendon.

In the ten decades since its first description, the etiology of Osgood-Schlatter disease remains disputed. Infection, avascularity of the patellar tendon or of the apophysis resulting in osteochondritis, and endocrine abnormalities have all been suggested. The work by Uhry, and Lazerte and Rapp,[1, 2] which suggests that trauma is the cause, generally has the most believers. Certainly a persistent stress resulting from active participation in athletics does play a role in some boys.

Standard treatment of Osgood-Schlatter disease involves conservative approaches including immobilization in plaster or firm splinting for periods of up to 6 weeks, restriction of sporting activities, analgesics, and physiotherapy. For those boys who are liturgically inclined, it may also involve a reprieve from being an altar boy, because kneeling tends to be a most painful experience. The prominence of the tibial tubercle with tenderness on direct pressure and reproduction of symptoms by resisted knee extension are as diagnostic as virtually anything else. Few patients fail to respond to conservative measures, but when a failure does occur, perhaps these authors are correct in their surgical approach (when in doubt, cut it out). Remove the tibial tuberosity all together. No tuberosity, no possibility of continuing Osgood-Schlatter disease.

Such surgery seems a tough price to pay for resolution of this problem. For boys with persistent symptoms, most will opt for this approach because it brings almost immediate relief.

References

1. Uhry E: *Arch Surg* 48:406, 1944.
2. Lazerte GD, Rapp IH: *Am J Pathol* 34:803, 1958.

Limb Length After Fracture of the Femoral Shaft in Children

Corry IS, Nicol RO (Auckland Children's Hosp, New Zealand)
J Pediatr Orthop 15:217–219, 1995   18–7

Background.—In children sustaining femoral shaft fractures, the affected limb may grow faster than the contralateral limb. Reported ranges of overgrowth are 8.1–13.0 mm. Overgrowth in a group of children treated by hip spica immobilization was described.

Patients and Methods.—Fifty children aged 10 years or less were studied. All had sustained isolated fractures of the femoral shaft. Spica casts were applied under general anesthetic within 72 hours of the injury. Scanograms were performed at the time of fracture union and at a mean of 3.9 years later.

Findings.—Forty-four femoral shaft fractures overgrew. Growth was retarded in 5, and 1 showed no growth abnormalities. Fractured femurs showed a mean overgrowth of 6.9 mm, and tibias on the affected side showed a mean overgrowth of −0.6 mm. Overgrowth was greater in

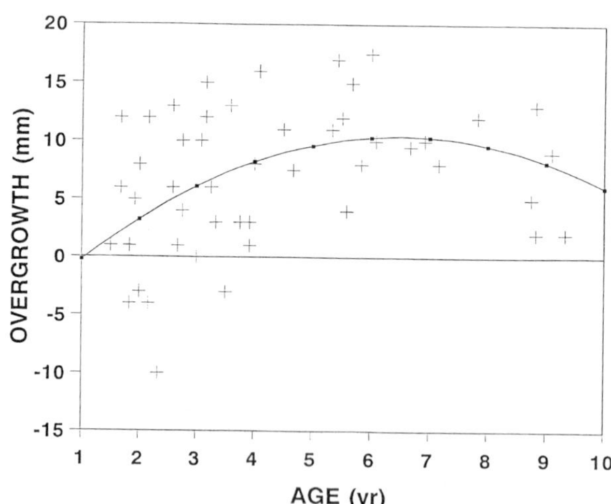

FIGURE 1.—Best-fitting quadratic function of age. (Courtesy of Corry IS, Nicol RO: Limb length after fracture of the femoral shaft in children. *J Pediatr Orthop* 15:217–219, 1995.)

children aged 4–7 years than in children in the 1- to 4-year and 7- to 10-year age groups (Fig 1). Other variables were not associated with overgrowth.

Conclusions.—Clinicians should accept less initial shortening than is commonly recommended in children with femoral shaft fractures, especially in children younger than 4 years and older than 7 years. Ages need to be specified in future reports of femoral shaft overgrowth in children with fractures.

▶ It has been known for a long time that were a child to fracture his or her femur, there was a significant risk that the afflicted extremity would ultimately be longer than the normal leg. Prior estimates gave ranges of mean overgrowth of 8.1–13.0 mm. This report shows an average overgrowth of 6.9 mm (range, 5.2–8.6 mm). As can be seen from Figure 1, a child aged 6–7 years is most likely to sustain the greatest overgrowth.

To my knowledge, this is the first time an orthopedic series has analyzed limb length after fractures of a femur by early and late scans and radiographs, controlling for the same method of fracture treatment. What this report does not tell us is how much overgrowth can be tolerated without producing difficulties for a youngster. The human body can compensate for minor limb length discrepancies, but at a certain point the spine will need to significantly curve to keep the shoulders in balance.

One final comment: although having a broken leg is not good, it is ironic, perhaps, that having 2 broken legs is not all that bad. Imagine growing up to be an adult who is half an inch taller as a perk of having bilateral femoral fractures in mid-childhood...break a leg (or 2).

Humeral Fractures Without Obvious Etiologies in Children Less Than 3 Years of Age: When Is It Abuse?

Strait RT, Siegel RM, Shapiro RA (Med College of Wisconsin, Milwaukee; St Luke Hosp, Fort Thomas, Ky; Univ of Cincinnati, Ohio)
Pediatrics 96:667–671, 1995   18–8

Background.—Four previous studies of humeral fractures in children suggest that from one half to three fourths of children with such injuries are victims of abuse. Abused children most often have spiral/oblique and transverse fractures; supracondylar fractures are comparatively rare. The authors' experience suggested that abuse is in fact much less prevalent than the literature suggests.

Objective.—All 124 children younger than 3 years who were treated for an acute humeral fracture in a 3¼-year period were reviewed to identify those injuries that resulted from abuse. Abuse was identified after independent review by 3 investigators using a wide range of criteria (Table 1), followed by a discussion of each case.

Findings.—Seven injuries were definitely a result of abuse, and 3 others probably represented abuse. Abuse was questionable in 2 instances. In all,

---

TABLE 1.—Criteria Used for Distinguishing Between Abuse and Accidents

---

Abuse
  A. Definite abuse
    Positive skeletal survey—multiple recent fractures and/or fractures of various ages
    Eyewitness
    Multiple internal injuries
    Physical findings—bruises (hand, electrical cord, teeth) or suspicious/unexplained
      burns or scars
    Sibling abused at same time
    A definite intentional act causing physical harm to child
    Parental fight; injury not directed at the child
    Highly* suspicious injury with definite later abuse
  B. Likely abuse
    Original doctors called injury abuse AND history inconsistent:
    History not sufficient for injury, and/or
    Story of accident changes, and/or
    Family members present different versions of history,
      and/or
    Inappropriate delay in seeking care
    Moderately suspicious injury with definite later abuse*
Indeterminate
  C. Questionable abuse
    History inconsistent:
      History not sufficient for injury, and/or
      Story of accident changes, and/or
      Family members present different versions of history,
        and/or
      Inappropriate delay in seeking care
    Low but somewhat suspicious injury with definite later abuse*
  D. Unknown cause
    Insufficient information available in chart
  E. Questionable accident
    Isolated incident, social worker/physician (sw/phy) no suspicion of abuse, story
      somewhat inconsistent with extent of injury, but consistent with type of injury
    Story somewhat inconsistent with extent of injury, sw/phy no suspicion of abuse,
      neglect involved
    Isolated incident, no suspicion of abuse, story not known.
    Injury not necessarily suspicious, but multiple injuries in the past*
    Initial suspicion of abuse, but upon investigation by social service, abuse ruled out*
Not abuse
  F. Likely accident
    Consistent story, sw/phy no suspicion of abuse, isolated injury
    Consistent story, no suspicion of abuse, neglect involved
    Minimal but consistent story, sw/phy no suspicion of abuse, isolated incident
    Consistent story, aggressive or irresponsible behavior involved, but injury not
      directly inflicted
  G. Definite accident
    Motor vehicle accident
    Multiple witnesses (police, ambulance at scene)
    Pedestrian hit by automobile

---

  * Modified from Thomas SA, Rosenfield NS, Leventhal JM, et al: Long-bone fractures in young children: Distinguishing accidental injuries from child abuse: *Pediatrics* 88:471–476, 1991.

  (Courtesy of Strait RT, Siegel RM, Shapiro RA: Humeral fractures without obvious etiologies in children less than 3 years of age: When is it abuse? Reproduced by permission of *Pediatrics*, Vol. 96, pp 667–671, Copyright 1995.)

8% of cases were considered to represent abuse, 73% were not abuse, and 19% were indeterminate. Nine of the 10 abused children were younger than 15 months, much younger than the other children. Three abused children had supracondylar fractures and 7 had spiral/oblique fractures.

Half the abused children had a history of having fallen less than 3 feet. Three of 7 skeletal surveys were positive.

Implications.—Child abuse is a common cause of humeral fractures in children younger than 15 months, but it is uncommon in older children. The presence of a supracondylar fracture in a young child is consistent with abuse.

▶ If you see an infant or a toddler with a fracture of the humerus, bells should go off alerting you to the possibility of child abuse. An adequate number of studies have been performed to substantiate this. In 1991, Thomas et al. published a 5-year review of all long-bone fractures in children younger than 3 years who were treated at Yale–New Haven Hospital.[1] Eleven of the 14 humeral fractures identified were the result of abuse. Kowal-Vern et al. published a similar 5-year review of all children younger than 3 years admitted to Loyola University Medical Center with a fracture.[2] They described 10 humeral fractures, 5 of which were believed to be caused by abuse. Rosenberg et al. published a 1-year review of all children younger than 1 year with fractures seen in their emergency department at the Children's Hospital of Michigan.[3] They reported abuse as the cause in 4 of 6 children with humeral fractures. Most importantly, in 1986, Worlock et al. compared groups of abused and nonabused children.[4] All 10 infants with any type of humeral fracture had been abused, as well as 4 of 5 toddlers with nonsupracondylar fractures. None of the 15 toddlers with supracondylar fractures had been abused. The prevalence of abuse in these 4 studies ranges from 46% to 78% among children with humeral fractures. The most common fracture type seen in the abused children were spiral/oblique and transverse humeral fractures.

The study abstracted above from Milwaukee adds a bit more insight into the problem of fractures of the humerus and the risk of associated child abuse. Although the prevalence of abuse in children seen with humeral fractures was much lower than in other published reports, there still was a good correlation. Furthermore, a high prevalence of supracondylar fractures associated with abuse was seen. Therefore any kind of humeral fracture is potentially associated with child abuse. The relationship between humeral fractures and child abuse holds true for children younger than 15 months and much less so for older children.

References

1. Thomas SA, et al: *Pediatrics* 88:471, 1991.
2. Kowal-Vern A, et al: *Clin Pediatr* 31:653, 1992.
3. Rosenberg N, et al: *Ann Emerg Med* 11:178, 1982.
4. Worlock P, et al: *BMJ* 293:100, 1986.

Athlete Age and Sports Physical Examination Findings

Briner WW Jr, Farr C (Lutheran Gen Sports Medicine Ctr, Park Ridge, Ill)
J Fam Pract 40:370–375, 1995   18–9

Objective.—Up to 7 million high school and 7 million junior high school athletes, along with a much smaller number of collegiate athletes, undergo sports preparticipation examinations (PPEs). Most of these examinations are performed at family physicians' and pediatricians' offices. However, as common as these examinations are, there are few data to help in determining the age range for which they are reasonable. The findings of 937 consecutive PPEs in interscholastic and intercollegiate athletes were analyzed to determine the percentage of athletes with significant findings.

Methods.—Data on the PPEs were reported by the primary care physicians using a standardized form. All the individuals were interscholastic athletes in the junior high, high school, and college age groups. Any finding that resulted in any recommendation for a change in management by the examining physician was considered significant.

Results.—Three percent of the junior high school athletes had significant findings, compared with 15% of the high school athletes and 34% of the college athletes. The most frequent significant findings were, in order, tight hamstring, ankle laxity, patellofemoral pain, shoulder tendinitis, and obesity. Overall, about 2% of athletes were disqualified from any sports participation. This figure did not vary significantly by age group.

Conclusions.—On sports PPEs, significant findings resulting in a recommended change of management are significantly more likely for high school and college athletes than for junior high school athletes. The findings cast uncertainty on the need for annual PPEs for junior high school athletes. Decisions about the age range for which sports PPEs are appropriate should be based on available data rather than on legislative mandate.

▶ It's fascinating to see how legislation has been established to regulate the need for physical examinations upon entry into school-based athletic programs. Individuals can exercise to their heart's content on the sidewalks of New York or in a backyard sandlot, but the second they cross onto school property, they had better have a sports PPE completed. In most of the United States, the periodicity of sports PPEs for high school athletes is determined by state law. Thirty-five states require annual examinations. When state law does not regulate this, school boards may. Most colleges also require their athletes to have annual examinations. The number of such examinations is staggering, estimated to be 7 million at the high school level and a similar number at the junior high school level. Although much smaller in number, there are about 360,000 college PPEs performed each year. Most of these PPEs are performed by family physicians and pediatricians.

This report asks a very interesting question: should requirements determine practice patterns for physicians engaged in this activity? There are virtually no data in the literature that indicate what the yields are on sports PPEs, at least not until this study.

In this report from Illinois, we see that significant findings were found on routine examination in 3.4% of junior high school athletes, 15.4% of high school athletes, and 33.9% of college athletes. Of 130 athletes with findings on examination, 48 had 1 of the following 5 conditions: tight hamstring muscle, ankle ligament laxity, patellofemoral arthralgia, tendinitis, and obesity. Twenty-one athletes who had tight hamstring muscles were advised to begin stretching programs. Eight athletes in whom ankle ligament laxity was noted received basic instructions regarding rehabilitation exercises, or advice about supportive ankle devices, taping, or both. Seven athletes who had patellofemoral arthralgia were advised to do exercises to strengthen the quadriceps, particularly the vastus medialis oblique. Rotator-cuff strengthening exercises were recommended for the 7 athletes with tendinitis of either the biceps or supraspinatus tendons in the shoulder.

Depending on your viewpoint, this report can be interpreted in varying ways. The authors chose to conclude that it may not be worthwhile to do sports PPEs earlier than high school. They may be right. It has been estimated that were you to eliminate these 7 million sports PPEs, there would be significant health care savings nationwide (probably about $140 million per year). Recognize, however, that such examinations may be the hook that brings an adolescent to your practice for the first time in years. Thus, from your vantage point, such examinations could be a surrogate reason for opening discussions of adverse adolescent risk behaviors such as smoking, sexual activity, and drug and substance abuse, including the dangers of anabolic steroids.

Yes, sports PPEs may have low yields, particularly in the youngest of athletes, but common sense dictates that it is wise to continue to endorse doing them. One can use the opportunity afforded by such examinations to cast a wide net of preventive medicine that goes far beyond muscles, joints, and bones.

The Outcome of Children Referred to a Pediatric Rheumatology Clinic With a Positive Antinuclear Antibody Test but Without an Autoimmune Disease
Deane PMG, Liard G, Siegel DM, et al (Univ of Rochester Med Ctr, NY)
Pediatrics 95:892–895, 1995   18–10

Background.—An antinuclear antibody (ANA) test is often performed to look for autoimmune disease in children with musculoskeletal or dermatologic symptoms or signs. The significance of a positive ANA test in children without clinically apparent autoimmune disorder has not been established.

TABLE 1.—Autoimmune Syndromes Diagnosed Among 72 Pediatric Patients With Positive Antinuclear Antibody Test Results at Initial Consultation

Diagnosis	Number of patients (%)
Pauciarticular juvenile arthritis	44 (61)
Systemic lupus erythematosus	16 (22)
Dermatomyositis	3 (4)
UCTD	2 (3)
Uveitis	2 (3)
Other*	5 (7)
	72 (100)

Abbreviation: UCTD, undifferentiated connective tissue disease.

*Comprises 1 case each of Crohn's disease, Hashimoto's thyroiditis, morphea, polyarticular juvenile arthritis, and psoriatic arthritis.

(Courtesy of Deane PMG, Laird G, Siegel DM, et al: The outcome of children referred to a pediatric rheumatogy clinic with a positive antinuclear antibody test but without an autoimmune disease. Reproduced by permission of *Pediatrics*, Vol 95, pp 892–895, Copyright 1995.)

Methods and Findings.—The charts of 500 children undergoing ANA testing between 1978 and 1993 were reviewed retrospectively. One hundred thirteen patients had positive results. Seventy-two patients (64%) had an autoimmune condition diagnosed at their initial clinical visit (Table 1). Another 10 children were lost to follow-up. Thus, 31 children (27%) had no autoimmune condition diagnosed at their initial visit. These children were followed up for a mean of 37 months. Most of these children initially had nonspecific musculoskeletal complaints and hypermobility (Table 2). Routine hematologic testing was normal in most patients. The median ANA titer was 1:160, although the patterns were variable. Symptoms eventually resolved in 81% of the children and improved significantly in 16%. Autoimmune hepatitis ultimately developed in 1 child (Table 3).

Conclusions.—Autoimmune conditions do not subsequently develop in most children with positive ANA test results but no autoimmune condi-

TABLE 2.—Diagnosis on Initial Examination of 31 Patients With Positive Antinuclear Antibody Test Results but Without Autoimmune Syndromes

Diagnosis	Number of Patients (%)
Nonspecific musculoskeletal complaints*	10 (32)
Hypermobility	9 (29)
Dermatologic complaints†	6 (19)
Patellofemoral syndrome	3 (10)
Viral syndrome	2 (7)
Fibromyalgia	1 (3)
	31 (100)

*Musculoskeletal symptoms without evidence of synovitis, myositis, and other defined diagnoses.

†Comprises 2 cases of alopecia and 1 case each of diffuse maculopapular rash, erythema multiforme, facial swelling, and urticaria.

(Courtesy of Deane PMG, Laird G, Siegel DM, et al: The outcome of children referred to a pediatric rheumatogy clinic with a positive antinuclear antibody test but without an autoimmune disease. Reproduced by permission of *Pediatrics*, Vol 95, pp 892–895, Copyright 1995.)

TABLE 3.—Clinical Status at Follow-up of 31 Pediatric Patients With Positive Antinuclear Antibody Test Results but Without Autoimmune Syndromes

Clinical Status At Last Follow-Up	Number	Female:Male Ratio	Mean Age (y) (±SD)	Mean Follow-Up, (mo) (±SD)
No illness	25	21:4	10 (±4)	38 (±28)
Persistent symptoms	5	5:0	11 (±4)	38 (±39)
Autoimmune disease	1	1:0	17	2

(Courtesy of Deane PMG, Liard G, Siegel DM, et al: The outcome of children referred to a pediatric rheumatogy clinic with a positive antinuclear antibody test but without an autoimmune disease. Reproduced by permission of *Pediatrics*, Vol 95, pp 892–895, Copyright 1995.)

tions at initial diagnosis. In children with musculoskeletal or dermatologic problems but no autoimmune conditions, ANA testing does not yield new diagnoses and is therefore an unnecessary use of resources. Children with positive ANA results in the absence of autoimmune conditions have an excellent prognosis.

▶ This report is terrific. There isn't a clinician among us who hasn't faced the problem of what looks like a false positive ANA test. We use the ANA test to screen for autoimmune disease in patients, including children, who have musculoskeletal or dermatologic signs or symptoms. A positive test may indicate that a patient has an autoimmune disease such as oligoarticular juvenile arthritis, juvenile systemic lupus erythematosus, or juvenile dermatomyositis. The rub is that many normal individuals (up to 5%) have a positive ANA test. False positive tests have been seen in various infections, with drug therapies, and in some hematologic disorders. Our internal medicine counterparts have noted that less than 1% of adults with a positive ANA test go on to actually have lupus.

The report abstracted indicates that 64% of children who are referred to a consultant and who have a positive ANA test will have an autoimmune disease. This leaves a large number (36%) of children with what must be called a false positive ANA test. More importantly, these investigators found that the vast majority of children who have a positive ANA test, but who do not have autoimmune conditions at the time of initial diagnosis, will not subsequently have an autoimmune disorder. Antinuclear antibody testing of children who have musculoskeletal or dermatologic problems (in the absence of autoimmune conditions) does not reveal new diagnoses, and in an era of cost consciousness, represents unnecessary laboratory time and expense.

Given the problems of sensitivity and specificity related to the use of the ANA test, one wonders whether it should be used only by those familiar with the ins and outs of this test. Even those in the latter category are often disenchanted with its usefulness.

Before leaving this commentary, which deals with an autoimmune disease that can involve muscles as well as joints, recognize that recently Brown observed that one can use a stethoscope to listen to muscle sounds and that this procedure may have potential diagnostic relevance.[1] In fact, you can hear a quivering muscle better than you can feel it. Actually this is not a new finding, merely a neglected one, having first been reported by the British physician, W. Wolaston, in 1810.[2] Wolaston, who used a primitive stethoscope (a stick and an ear cushion), developed this interest in muscle sound from an initial curiosity about the rumblings he heard when placing a finger in the ear while clenching his hand, a maneuver described a century and a half earlier by Grimaldi.[3] Try this maneuver. On rainy days it will entertain you. This saga about muscle groups would be merely a curiosity were it not for the fact that the distinguished Wellcome Trust is actively investigating the significance of muscle sounds and has traced their history, finding that investigations continued from the 17th century right on until the mid-1970s. Since the 1970s, muscle sound research has focused on two areas: relations between signal-sound characteristics and physiologic conditions of muscle, and the development of techniques for recording and analyzing these signals. To say this differently, muscle groups are a cheap, very cheap version of an electromyelogram. Don't discard these sounds out of hand. Muscle in on the trend. Start listening.

References

1. Brown J: *Lancet* 346:306, 1995.
2. Wolaston WH: *Phil Trans Roy Soc London* 1810:2–5.
3. Grimaldi FM: *Psychomathesis de lumine* Bologna, 1665:383

Amyoplasia, the Most Common Type of Arthrogryposis: The Potential for Good Outcome
Sells JM, Jaffe KM, Hall JG (Univ of Washington, Seattle; Univ of British Columbia, Vancouver, Canada)
Pediatrics 97:225–231, 1996   18–11

Objective.—Arthrogryposis, or multiple congenital joint contractures, occurs in 1 of every 3,000 births. More than one third of all patients with arthrogryposis have amyoplasia, characterized by fatty- and fibrous-tissue replacement of limb muscles, usually in all 4 limbs. The intrauterine and birth histories, therapeutic interventions, and level of functioning of children with amyoplasia were retrospectively reviewed.

Methods.—A total of 38 children (18 boys), from birth to 16 years, were studied.

Results.—Pregnancies and birth histories were unremarkable. There was 4-limb involvement in 84% of the 38 children studied (Figure). Twenty-eight of 35 children with shoulder involvement had internally rotated shoulders. Elbow, wrist, and hand involvement was apparent in 36 patients. In 34 children with lower limb involvement, the hips were affected in 31, with 16 fixed in flexion and 15 fixed in abduction. Thirty children had knee involvement. Other common characteristics were abnormally shaped heads, hemangiomas at birth, micrognathia, genital abnormalities, and congenital spinal problems. There were 17 perinatal fractures, and 15 additional fractures occurred later mainly from falls. Orthopedic surgery was performed in 33 children who had an average of 5.7 procedures each.

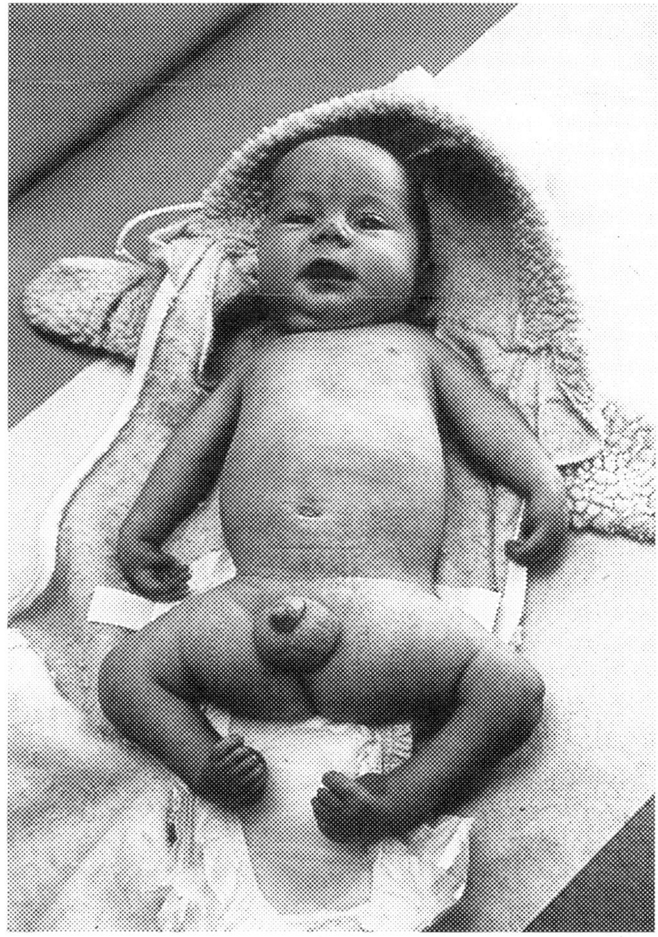

FIGURE.—A young child with typical limb positioning seen in amyoplasia. (From Sells JM, Jaffe KM, Hall JG: Amyoplasia, the most common type of arthrogryposis: The potential for good outcome. Reproduced by permission of *Pediatrics,* Vol 97, pp 225–231, Copyright 1996. Courtesy of Lynn T. Staheli, MD, Children's Hospital and Medical Center, Seattle.)

In addition, 94% had physical therapy, 79% had occupational therapy, 60% had both, and 16% had other therapy. Patients spent an average of 5 years in therapy. Casting was applied to 34 children and splinting to 37. By 5 years of age there were 25 ambulators, 2 partial ambulators, and 11 nonambulators. Most children required some assistance in activities of daily living (Table 9). Thirteen of 15 children 7 years or older were able to read and write. Sixteen of 25 schoolchildren were in regular classes, and 4 were in preschool.

Conclusion.—With surgical and therapeutic interventions, the physical and educational outcomes of children with amyoplasia is much more optimistic than previously thought.

TABLE 9.—Level of Independence in Activities of Daily Living for Children 5 Years of Age and Older

Activity	Independent, %	Intermittent Assist, %	Assist Throughout, %	Not Documented, %
Feeding	75	15	10	0
Grooming	20	55	10	15
Dressing	10	60	20	10
Toileting	35	40	5	20
Bathing	25	55	10	10

(Courtesy of Sells JM, Jaffe KM, Hall JG: Amyoplasia, the most common type of arthrogryposis: The potential for good outcome. Reproduced by permission of *Pediatrics*, Vol 97, pp 225–231, Copyright 1996.)

▶ It has only been in recent years that we have learned that arthrogryposis is not a single diagnosis but rather a descriptive term that encompasses a wide variety of distinct diagnoses. The lumping of all children with contractures as having a single diagnostic entity, arthrogryposis, has confounded reports of therapeutic intervention and functional outcomes. This report is important because it focuses on 1 distinct form of arthrogryposis, known as amyoplasia, the most common diagnostic subgroup. Children with this type of arthrogryposis have fatty and fibrous tissue replacement of their limb muscles. In the initial descriptions, children with amyoplasia typically had 4-limb involvement. The upper limbs tended to have internally rotated shoulders, extended elbows, and flexed wrists. The lower limbs had more variable positioning of the hips and knees, but the feet had severe equinovarus deformities. This form of arthrogryposis has no recognizable pattern of inheritance and is thought to be sporadic. The pregnancies of these infants are largely unremarkable except that about half result in cesarean section because of failure to progress. Some infants are delivered by cesarean section because of fears of fractures. This is a very legitimate concern because inflexibility of the limbs and osteoporosis caused by decreased motion of the limbs result in broken bones during vaginal delivery.

It will not be every day that you see a child with arthrogryposis, because it occurs once in every 3,000 births. The frequency of the disorder is such, however, that most of us will be involved with an affected child at some point in our careers. Accurate diagnosis is imperative because diagnostic subgroups carry very different prognoses. When amyoplasia is the diagnosis, parents can be reassured that it is a sporadic condition for which the cause is unknown and that nothing could have been done during pregnancy to prevent the problem. They should also be told that future pregnancies have no increased risk of this problem. Referral should be made to a tertiary care center accustomed to dealing with the surgical and therapeutic interventions currently available for patients with amyoplasia.

The conclusions of this report include the observation that functional outcome is much more optimistic than has been reported previously. Although a severe birth defect, the clinical course can actually improve with appropriate interventions.

Acute Injuries in Soccer, Ice Hockey, Volleyball, Basketball, Judo, and Karate: Analysis of National Registry Data

Kujala UM, Taimela S, Antti-Poika I, et al (Univ of Helsinki; Helsinki Univ Central Hosp)
BMJ 311:1465–1468, 1995   18–12

Introduction.—Designing strategies and measures to prevent sports injuries requires consistent data collection and recording regarding the varying risks of acute injury associated with particular sports. Information on the types and severity of acute injuries was obtained from insurance registry data on 4 team sports (soccer, ice hockey, volleyball, basketball) plus judo and karate to compare injury risks in these sports.

Methods.—Competitive athletes in Finland were required to obtain a license from the appropriate sports association, which was linked to an insurance policy covering acute sports injuries. Both the injured athlete and the treating physician completed accident reports for each injury. Data from these reports were entered into the insurance computer database, including patient age, sports event, circumstance of injury (training or competition), type of injury, mechanism of injury and the injured body part. The injury rate per 1,000 person years of exposure was calculated by age and sex for each sport.

Results.—During the 5 years of the study, 54,186 acute sports injuries were reported. The highest injury rates were associated with karate and judo, followed by ice hockey, soccer, and basketball (Table 1). The injury rates were highest among athletes aged 20–24 years and were higher among men than women in this age group. However, injury rates were significantly higher in females than in males participating in judo or karate between the ages of 15 and 19 years. Soccer, volleyball, and basketball athletes most commonly had lower limb injuries, whereas upper limb injuries were more common in athletes participating in judo. the most common types of injuries were sprains, strains, and bruises, with nondental fractures comprising 4% to 10.8% of the injuries and occurring most

TABLE 1.—Person-years of Exposure, Numbers of Injuries, and Injury Rate in 6 Sports in Finland (Sports Insurance Data 1987–1991)

Sport	Person years of exposure	No of injuries	Injury rate (95% confidence interval)†
Soccer	296 646	26 330	89 (88 to 90)
Ice hockey	179 798	16 836	94 (92 to 95)
Volleyball	87 668	5 235	60 (58 to 61)
Basketball	39 541	3 472	88 (85 to 91)
Judo	9 936	1 163	117 (111 to 123)
Karate	8 102	1 150	142 (134 to 150)

*Injuries per 1,000 person years of exposure.

(Courtesy of Kujala UM, Taimela S, Antti-Poika I, et al: Acute injuries in soccer, ice hockey, volleyball, basketball, judo, and karate: Analysis of national registry data. *BMJ* 311:1465–1468, 1995.)

frequently among athletes participating in karate, judo, and ice hockey, and least frequently among volleyball athletes. Injury resulting in permanent disability was most common in soccer players, followed by volleyball, judo, karate, ice hockey, and basketball athletes. These injuries most commonly involved the knee.

Conclusions.—Because the injury profiles of the different sports varied greatly, preventive measures should be specifically designed for each sport. However, general preventive measures should include decreasing violent contact between athletes by changing game rules and strict refereeing. Mouth guards should also be used routinely and designed for each sport.

▶ Finland is a remarkable place. What better country to do this type of study than Finland, the land of the fit and hearty, the land where anyone engaging in competitive soccer, ice hockey, volleyball, basketball, judo, or karate must have a license as well as carry sports insurance. Sandlot sporting activities obviously are excluded from this rigorous oversight. Such oversight can produce powerful data that show us how frequently sporting competitors get injured. As importantly, we can tell which sports are likely to be more injurious than others. Karate and judo have the highest injury rates, followed by ice hockey, soccer, and basketball. Volleyball has the lowest injury rate. In team games, 46% to 59% of injuries occur during competitions, whereas in judo and karate around 70% occur during training. Girls have significantly higher injury rates in all sports except for ice hockey, where just about everyone gets hurt given enough time.

Fortunately, most of the injuries described in this report were relatively minor: sprains, strains, and bruises. Insurance carriers awarded no death benefits for an accidental injury during the period of this study, but there was 1 neck fracture in an ice hockey player that led to quadriplegia. There were a fair number (greater than 100) permanent disability awards, most of which resulted from severe knee injuries.

This report also shows us that an ounce of prevention is worth a pound of cure. Given the data from this study, which show who in which sport is most likely to be injured, it would behoove an adolescent girl not to engage in judo. Another preventive measure would be to cut out all training...most injuries occur during training.

Better yet, switch to Formula One race driving. Far fewer Formula One drivers (only 69 in the last 40 years) get killed each year than do skiers.

Yes, Finland is the land of the fit and the hearty, but with injury rates as high as those seen here, it seems fairly clear that those who believe that exercise is good for your health are "mythfits" and "foolhearty".

Snowboarding Trauma

Callé SC, Evans JT (State Univ of New York, Stony Brook; Nassau County Med Ctr, East Meadow, NY)

J Pediatr Surg 30:791–794, 1995   18–13

Background.—Roughly 2 million Americans own a snowboard. The Burton snowboard was introduced in 1978. The original snowboards were narrow, wooden, and shaped like a surfboard. Today, they are either laminated wood or fiberglass. Riders wear snow boots secured by straps or polyurethane hard boots with bindings. Different snowboards are designed for high-speed racing, steep slopes, or aerial acrobatics. Snowboarders can travel faster than 40 mph. When snowboarders do not wear protective gear, severe injuries can result. The incidence and nature of injuries resulting from snowboarding were investigated.

Methods.—Injuries sustained by 487 snowboarders from 6 Vermont ski resorts and 565 cases of snowboarding injuries collected nationally were analyzed and reviewed.

Results.—In the Vermont survey, the mean age of injured snowboarders was 19.1 years; 80% were between 5 and 24 years, and 77.4% were male. More than 42% were novice snowboarders, 31% were intermediate, and the rest were advanced. Of all injuries, 38% were of the upper extremity. In the national survey, the mean age of snowboarders was 17.6 years; more than 80% were between 5 and 24 years, and 83% were male. Of all injuries, 47% were of the upper extremity. In both surveys, fractures, dislocations, and soft-tissue trauma of the upper extremity were the most common injuries. The wrist, ankle, and knee were the most common body parts injured. In the Vermont survey, 19.9% of injuries were of the wrist and 45.2% were of the upper extremity. In the national survey, 20.4% of injuries were of the wrist and 46.2% were of the upper extremity. None of the Vermont snowboarders were wearing protective gear.

Discussion.—More injuries of the upper extremity are sustained by snowboarders today than a few years ago. The nature of injuries was learned by interviewing the snowboarders from Vermont. More than 50% of injuries occur in the afternoon. Ligamentous sprains occur more often when vision is obscured by clouds or snow and riders travel more slowly. Fractures occur more often when vision is good and riders attempt more hazardous maneuvers. Riders can lose balance and fall when an edge of the snowboard gets caught in snow, or when travelling over ice. Going too fast can also result in a loss of control. Colliding with alpine skiers or obstacles can result in severe trauma or death. Beginners sustain more injuries than do advanced riders.

▶ This commentary was written in Chapel Hill, North Carolina, where you are as likely to find a snowboard as you are to find Tonya Harding's image on a box of Wheaties. Read this commentary knowing that this editor has little, actually no, personal experience with snowboards.

Old-timers such as this editor tend to think of snowboarding as a fairly recent innovation, but technically it is not. Snowboarding dates back to the 1920s, when a Frenchman popularized a wooden board for snow riding. The Brunswick Company produced a "snurfer" in the 1960s, but it was hard to control on slopes. A "winterstick" made in 1972 is the forerunner of the modern snowboard, which finally came into existence in 1978, when Jake Burton Carpenter of Vermont produced the first "Burton Snowboard." Since that time, 18 years ago, millions of these have been made and at least 15 additional companies have gotten into the manufacturing act. Unlike alpine skis, snowboards can get by with the use of soft snow boots, although hard shell boots with advanced alpine-type metal bindings are becoming more and more available.

So, what's the problem with snowboards? The problem is that they have been designed to handle virtually any mountain condition, depending on the type you buy. Snowboarders on new equipment can achieve speeds exceeding 40 mph. Their simplicity leads to their use by a lot of novices who sometimes wear a minimum of protective gear. Investigators in this report actually spoke to and interviewed patients with injuries to determine under what circumstances injury occurred. Over half of the injuries happened in the afternoon. Ligamentous sprains occurred more often on cloudy days or when snow obscured vision, when snowboarders were more likely to have traveled slowly. With clear visibility, the snowboarders sustained fractures while attempting more daring and hazardous maneuvers. A common injury occurred when a snowboard edge became caught in snow, causing the rider to lose balance and to fall onto a hyperextended wrist. The left arm or leading extremity was more commonly injured, and wrist fractures predominated. Some lost control by going too fast, resulting in a twist of the lower extremity. Deaths usually occurred when alpine skiers collided with an immovable object. About 1 in 100 injuries resulted in death.

If one adds up all the dollars and cents used to treat the injuries incurred by skiers, it is a fairly substantial sum. It is incumbent upon all of us to try to prevent such injuries. Unfortunately, given the ingenuity of those among us who migrate to the slopes, trying to prevent such downhill mishaps is an uphill battle. As is true of most preventive measures, the correct result is likely to be a 10% improvement in technology and a 90% improvement in the use of common sense.

To learn more about how to save lives on the slopes, see the excellent article by Friermood et al.[1] entitled "Save the trees: A comparative review of skier-tree collisions."

Reference

1. Friermood TG, et al: *J Orthop Trauma* 8:116, 1994.

Don't Twist My Child's Head Off: Iatrogenic Cervical Dislocation
Casey ATH, O'Brien M, Kumar V, et al (Natl Hosp for Neurology and Neurosurgery, London; Hosp for Sick Children, London)
BMJ 311:1212–1213, 1995   18–14

Introduction.—Two otherwise normal children whose necks were excessively rotated while undergoing cervical lymph node biopsy under general anesthesia probably sustained cervical dislocation as a result. Because the injury was not recognized initially, complex spinal surgery proved necessary to correct the deformity.

Case Report.—Girl, 6 years, underwent excisional biopsy of lymph nodes in the right side of the neck because of persistent adenopathy of unknown origin. Torticollis (Fig 1) and neck pain were noted on returning from the operating room. The wry neck

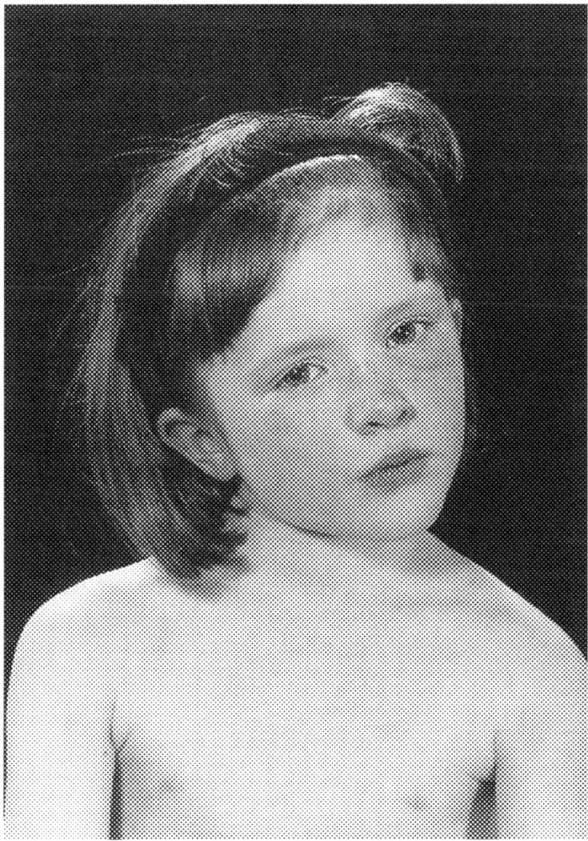

FIGURE 1.—Preoperative picture showing typical cock-robin position. (Reproduced by permission of the patient's parent. Courtesy of Casey ATH, O'Brien M, Kumar V, et al: Don't twist my child's head off: Iatrogenic cervical dislocation. *BMJ* 311:1212–1213, 1995.)

persisted for a few months, at which time electromyography excluded spasmodic torticollis. A CT study 8 months after biopsy demonstrated a rotary atlantoaxial dislocation that could not be reduced by closed methods. Reduction was achieved by an "extreme lateral" approach 1 year after injury. The patient was immobilized in a halo jacket for 10 weeks postoperatively.

Discussion.—This injury presumably occurred when the supine child's head was rotated and held to one side to expose the posterior triangle of the neck. This maneuver also could compromise the vertebral artery or the spinal cord. Torticollis may make it difficult to properly interpret lateral cervical spine radiographs. A CT scan with multiplanar reconstructions will clarify the situation. Any child with a wry neck after surgery should be promptly examined, because delayed treatment may result in asymmetrical facial growth.

▶ This report puts a new twist on an old topic: atlantoaxial dislocation. This editor, and I'm certain the readers of the YEAR BOOK are more than aware of the association between atlantoaxial dislocation and Down syndrome, but I would bet you are not aware that merely turning a normal child's head to a somewhat awkward position under general anesthesia can also dislocate the cervical spine.[1] Similar dislocations have been reported in patients with achondroplasia, particularly in patients treated with growth hormone and in patients with Ehlers-Danlos syndrome.[2, 3]

There are lots of lessons to be learned from the 2 cases described by Casey et al. The first is that extreme care must be taken in positioning the head of an anesthetized and paralyzed child. Second, a child who wakes from surgery with a wry neck should set off all manner of bells in your mind about the potential for that child having had a cervical spine dislocation.

This commentary ends the Musculoskeletal chapter. Because the YEAR BOOK OF PEDIATRICS has rarely given any insights into chiropractic as related to pediatrics, it might be worthwhile to close this chapter by doing so at this time.

Gotlieb et al. searched the world's literature (including use of MEDLINE) to determine how many articles since 1966 onward have dealt with chiropractic and children.[4] There were just 66 discrete documents uncovered that related manipulative therapy to pediatric health conditions. One might say that 66 is 66 too many, particularly when you actually see what chiropractors are doing to kids these days. Samples of these 66 articles are as follows:

- Mierau D, et al: Dysplastic spondylolisthesis: A report of two cases. *J Can Chiropr Assoc* 219:131, 1985. (Two cases of spondylolisthesis in teenage girls, one treated with side posture sacroiliac joint manipulation.)

- Patterson B: Encopresis in a seven-year-old girl: A case study. *Res Forum* Spring:79–82, 1986. (A single case study [7-year-old male treated with full spine manipulation and resolution of encopresis].)

- Banks BD, et al: Sudden infant death syndrome: A literature review with chiropractic implications. *J Manip Physiol Ther* 10:346, 1987.

- Borregard PE: Neurogenic bladder and spina bifida occulta: A case report. *J Manip Physiol Ther* 10:122, 1987. (Single case report, 13-year-old male, of flaccid type neurogenic bladder treated successfully with manipulation.)
- Davies NJ: Chiropractic management of the acute febrile pediatric patient. *J Aust Chiro Assoc* 17:126, 1987. (Reviews the chiropractic protocol of acutely febrile children and how to manage such fever.)
- Klougart N, et al: Infantile colic treated by chiropractors: A prospective study of 316 cases. *J Manip Physiol Ther* 12:281, 1989. (A multicenter study with "strict" inclusion criteria showing the benefits of chiropractic on infantile colic.)
- Goodman RJ, et al: Cessation of a seizure disorder. *J Chiro Res Clin Inv* 6:43, 1990, (A single case report of a 5-year-old white girl with Lennox-Gestalt syndrome with seizures that resolved after manipulation of the spine.)
- Do chiropractors know something that we don't?

References

1. Hardy JB: *Radiology* 183:125, 1992.
2. Okabe T, et al: *Acta Paediatr Jpn* 33:357, 1991.
3. Bhatia SJ, et al: *J Assoc Physicians India* 38:361, 1990.
4. Gotlieb AC, et al: *J Can Chiropr Assoc* 39:154, 1995.

19 Gastroenterology

Prolonged Dysphagia Caused by Congenital Pharyngeal Dysfunction
Mbonda E, Claus D, Bonnier C, et al (Univ of Louvain, Brussels, Belgium)
J Pediatr 126:923–927, 1995   19–1

Background.—Congenital paralysis of the pharyngeal muscles causes a rare but life-threatening swallowing disorder that can last several months or years. Recovery is possible with correct management. Four patients with this disorder were described.

Patients and Outcomes.—The first 2 patients, a boy born at 38 weeks' gestation and a girl born at term, recovered from severe, isolated, congenital dysphagia caused by pharyngeal muscle paralysis at 40 and 20 months of age, respectively. Except for a transient paralysis of the adductors of the vocal cords in 1 child, these children had no other evidence of neurologic or muscular dysfunction. On radiocinematographic assessment, paralysis of the pharyngeal stage of swallowing was observed, with minimal involvement of the oral stage. After apparent radiologic recovery, 1 child refused oral feeding for several months. Another 2 patients, both girls born normally at term, with a similar disorder died of tracheal aspiration at 8 and 4 months of age, respectively. Autopsy findings indicated no CNS abnormalities. The cranial nerves involved in swallowing were normal.

Conclusions.—These patients, along with 5 others previously reported in the literature, had a severe, idiopathic, congenital dysphagia associated with paralysis of the constrictor muscles of the pharynx. Children with this condition can recover after several months or years with proper management. Although the cause of this disorder is unknown, it is probably related to a dysfunction of the CNS. The table lists other disorders that can cause persistent dysphagia in the neonate.

▶ Hopefully, these 4 patients represent a rare phenomenon. Each had a severe, isolated, and persistent congenital inability to swallow related to a paralysis of the constrictor muscles of the pharynx. Most of us have occasionally seen infants who don't seem to swallow or who do not swallow normally. The reason this article was selected for inclusion in the YEAR BOOK OF PEDIATRICS is because of the excellent table, which shows the differential

TABLE.—Causes of Persistent Dysphagia in the Neonate

Nasal-oropharyngeal malformations
   Choanal atresia
   Cleft lip or palate
   Craniofacial syndromes (e.g., Pierre
     Robin syndrome, Crouzon syndrome)
   Hypopharyngeal stenosis
Nasopharyngeal tumors
Foreign bodies
Esophageal and tracheoesophageal
    malformations
   Tracheoesophageal fistula*
   Esophageal stenosis*
   Achalasia of cricopharyngeal muscle*
   Esophageal achalasia
   Esophageal atony
   Gastroesophageal reflux
Vascular malformations
   Aberrant right subclavian artery
   Double aortic arch
   Right aortic arch with left ligament
Neurologic causes
   Supranuclear bulbar palsy:
    Pseudobulbar syndrome*
   Dystonic syndromes
   Chiari malformation with
    myelomeningocele
   Werdnig-Hoffmann spinal muscular
    atrophy
   Möbius syndrome
   Duosyndrome of laryngeal nerve
   Bilateral laryngeal paralysis
   Riley-Day syndrome
   Willi-Prader syndrome*
Muscular causes*
   Familial infantile myasthenia
   Myotonic dystrophy*
   Congenital muscular dystrophy
   Facioscapulohumeral dystrophy
   Nemaline myopathy*
   Myotubular myopathy
   Disproportion, congenital fiber type
Syndrome of congenital persistent
    idiopathic paralysis of the pharynx

*More frequent causes.
(From Mbonda E, Claus D, Bonnier C, et al: *J Pediatr* 126:923–927, 1995. Adapted from Weiss MH: Otolaryngol Clin North Am 21:727–735, 1988; and Volpe JJ: *Neurology of the Newborn,* Philadelphia, WB Saunders, 1987, pp 88–89.)

diagnosis of persistent dysphagia in the newborn. Dig out this table the next time you have occasion to worry about an infant who isn't swallowing properly.

In most patients with prolonged congenital dysphagia, the dysfunction is not limited to just the pharynx or soft palate, but extends upward to include the motility of the tongue. Fortunately, the tendency for the disorder described in this paper is to improve with time, which is in keeping with a progressive adaptation of a central command problem rather than with lesions of the peripheral nerves or of the muscles themselves.

How Valid Are Clinical Signs of Dehydration in Infants?

Duggan C, Refat M, Hashem M, et al (Harvard Med School, Boston; Cairo Univ, Egypt; Johns Hopkins Univ, Baltimore, Md; et al)
J Pediatr Gastroenterol Nutr 22:56–61, 1996   19–2

Background.—Infantile diarrhea causes approximately 4 million deaths each year, primarily in developing countries. The most serious consequence of infantile diarrhea is dehydration. An accurate assessment of dehydration is essential for optimal treatment; however, the lack of laboratory facilities in developing countries makes such assessments difficult. In the current prospective study, the ability of several clinical signs to distinguish among degrees of hydration was determined, and 2 clinical assessment systems were compared (Table 1).

Methods.—One hundred thirty-five boys (age range 3–18 months) were evaluable. All had a history of acute diarrhea, defined as 5 or more watery stools a day for no more than 7 days. The mean duration of illness was 54.5 hours. None had frank protein-energy malnutrition or serious

TABLE 1.—Dehydration Scales

Santosham scale*
  Mild dehydration (6%): one of
    Slightly dry mucous membranes
    Any one sign from the moderate category
  Moderate dehydration (8%): two of
    Loss of skin turgor
    Sunken eyes
    Very dry mucous membranes
    Depressed anterior fontanelle
  Severe dehydration (10%): signs consistent with
      moderate dehydration, plus one or more of
    Thready/absent radial pulse
    Cold extremities
    Coma

Fortin-Parent scale (adapted from reference 8)

	0	1	2
Tongue	Wet	Slightly dry	Dry
Fontanelle	Flat	Slightly sunken	Deeply sunken
Eyes	Normal	Slightly sunken	Deeply sunken
Skinfold	Instant recoil	<2 seconds	2 seconds
Extremities	Warm	Cool	Cold/Blue
Neuro status	Normal	Whimpering	Apathetic
Breathing	Quiet	Fast	Deep
Subtotal			_______
If child is semi comatose or very irritable, add 3			_______
Total			_______
Mild dehydration	= 0–3		
Moderate dehydration	= 4–8		
Severe dehydration	= 9–17		

*Adapted from Santosham M, Brown KH, Sack RB: *Pediatr Rev* 8:273–278, 1987.
(Courtesy of Duggan C, Refat M, Hashem M, et al: How valid are clinical signs of dehydration in infants? *J Pediatr Gastroenterol Nutr* 22:56–61, 1996.)

TABLE 3.—Individual Signs of Dehydration and Their Relationship to Percent Weight Gain

Sign	Score (n)	Mean percent weight gain (SD)	Kruskal-Wallis P
Skinfold	Instant (75)	3.91 (2.2)	< 0.001
	<2 s (50)	4.84 (3.2)	
	>2 s (9)	9.37 (4.6)	
Neuro exam	Normal (107)	4.11 (2.7)	< 0.001
	Whimper (16)	5.69 (3.0)	
	Apathetic (11)	8.06 (4.2)	
Eyes	Normal (35)	3.31 (2.7)	< 0.001
	Slightly sunken (81)	4.78 (2.8)	
	Very sunken (18)	6.49 (3.9)	
Mucosa	Normal (23)	3.26 (2.2)	< 0.001
	Slightly dry (71)	4.35 (2.7)	
	Very dry (40)	5.89 (3.7)	
Pulse	Normal (133)	4.48 (2.9)	0.02
	Weak (2)	13.75 (2.6)	
Breathing	Normal (124)	4.39 (2.9)	0.03
	Fast (7)	7.46 (3.7)	
	Deep (3)	7.57 (4.7)	
Extremities	Warm (121)	4.43 (2.9)	0.11
	Cool (13)	6.45 (4.2)	
Fontanelle	Normal (64)	4.94 (2.7)	0.42
	Slightly sunken (65)	4.24 (3.2)	
	Very sunken (5)	5.54 (6.3)	

(Courtesy of Duggan C, Refat M, Hashem M, et al: How valid are clinical signs of dehydration in infants? *J Pediatr Gastroenterol Nutr* 22:56–61, 1996.)

nongastrointestinal illness or were exclusively breast-fed. On study entry, several clinical signs of dehydration were evaluated. The infants were then rehydrated with oral solution and given a standardized diet until there were no watery or loose stools for 16 hours. The mean length of rehydration was 5.2 hours. Percent body weight gain at rehydration and at resolution of illness was the main outcome measure.

Findings.—In a multiple regression analysis, prolonged skinfold, a change in neurologic status, sunken eyes, and dry oral mucosa were the clinical signs that best correlated with percent dehydration (Table 3). For the 2 assessment systems, average weight gain was 3.6% to 3.9% for mild, 4.9% to 5.3% for moderate, and 9.5% to 9.8% for severe dehydration. Fluid deficits of approximately 3% and 5% occurred in children with clinical signs of mild and moderate dehydration, respectively.

Conclusions.—The best clinical correlates of hydration in infants with diarrhea and prolonged skinfold, altered neurologic status, sunken eyes, and dry oral mucosa. Infants' hydration status, fluid intake, and excess fluid losses must be frequently reassessed during treatment.

▶ Mark this as one of the more useful reports of 1996. Most of us learned that there were three levels of dehydration: mild (5% to 6% and associated with increased thirst and dry mucous membranes), moderate (7% to 8% deficit with decreased skin turgor), and severe (10% or greater deficit, associated with a reduction in blood pressure). These clinical signs and symptoms of dehydration severity have been more or less a sacred cow of pediatrics and are included in virtually every major textbook. However, the scientific basis for these types of correlations is tenuous at best, and recent evidence suggests that early signs of dehydration are clinically evident at just a 3% deficit.

This report goes a long way to make hamburger out of the sacred cow. These investigators determined whether clinical signs of dehydration could distinguish degrees of dehydration in infants with acute diarrhea. They measured the gain in weight of babies when their illnesses were over and after they had been fully rehydrated. It was found that mild dehydration was detected at about three percent dehydration. Signs and symptoms of moderate dehydration occurred at just 5%. At 8% to 9% dehydration there were severe clinical signs and symptoms of dehydration.

Clinical signs of dehydration among infants with acute diarrhea differ in their ability to distinguish among mild, moderate, and severe dehydration. When considered together, skin fold changes, neurologic status, sunken eyes, and dry mucous membranes provide the best combination of physical findings. The presence or absence of a sunken fontanelle is not a helpful indicator of hydration status. The latter observation has also been made by several other authors in recent years.

At the beginning of this decade, the World Health Organization (WHO) also recognized the limitations of using physical findings in the assessment of dehydration. It has revised its guidelines for the assessment of dehydration so that the distinction between mild and moderate dehydration is no longer made. The WHO uses three classes of dehydration: none, some, or severe.[1]

One final comment: you're probably wondering why there has been no mention in any of these discussions about capillary refill time as evidence of dehydration. Saavedra et al., who studied this technique among U.S. children who had been hospitalized for diarrhea, reported an excellent correlation between weight gain (as a measure of dehydration) and capillary refill time ($r = 0.843$).[2] Two problems with capillary refill time, however, limit its usefulness. One problem relates to the impact of environmental temperature. Decreases in ambient temperature within the range found in typical office/emergency room settings may cause a significant prolongation of the capillary refill time in children with a normal circulatory status. The second problem is the high interobserver variability in measuring capillary refill time.[3, 4]

References

1. World Health Organization, Program for Control of Diarrheal Diseases. Geneva, 1990.
2. Saavedra JM, et al: *Am J Dis Child* 145:296, 1991.
3. Schriger DL, et al: *Ann Emerg Med* 17:932, 1988.
4. Gorelick MH, et al: *Pediatrics* 92:699, 1993.

Helicobacter pylori and Recurrent Abdominal Pain in Children

Hardikar W, Feekery C, Smith A, et al (Univ of Melbourne, Australia)
J Pediatr Gastroenterol Nutr 22:148–152, 1996   19–3

Background.—Pediatricians often see patients with recurrent abdominal pain. However, an organic cause can only be found in 10%. *Helicobacter pylori*, which causes gastritis in children and adults, may play a role in unexplained recurrent abdominal pain. This hypothesis was tested in a case-control study.

Methods and Findings.—Ninety-eight children referred to a clinic for recurrent abdominal pain and 98 children without such pain were included in the study. Serum *H. pylori* IgG antibodies were measured by an enzyme immunoabsorbent assay. Adjustments were made in the statistical model for age, sex, ethnicity, and socioeconomic status. Five percent of the case patients and 14.3% of control patients were found to have increased serum IgG antibodies to *H. pylori.* The adjusted odds ratio among the case patients was 0.21.

Conclusions.—This study shows that *H. pylori* is negatively associated with recurrent abdominal pain. Thus this organism is unlikely to be a cause of recurrent abdominal pain.

▶ Caring for children with recurrent abdominal pain is often a source of headache to a care provider. The frequency of this problem is quite high; about 10% of schoolchildren have recurrent abdominal pain. The problem is more prevalent in girls. Recall that the pain is usually periumbilical. It can occur at any time of the day and tends to last several hours. There is no relationship to meals or other activities, and the patient is rarely awakened at night by the pain. Other apparently functional gastrointestinal disorders may also be seen, either in the patient or in his or her immediate family. Children with recurrent abdominal pain tend to be more anxious and internalizing than their peers, but overt psychological problems are fairly uncommon. Physical examination in such children is not helpful, and diagnostic studies are usually within normal limits. In the majority of cases, no organic cause can be found and the disorder runs a benign course, although as many as one third of children will have symptoms right up into adulthood.

What this article is telling us is that *H. pylori* is not the cause of recurrent abdominal pain in children. This is not the first study to examine a potential relationship between *H. pylori* and this symptom in children. Some studies have suggested that there is such a relationship. Nonetheless, the issue of whether *H. pylori* infection and chronic active gastritis cause clinical symptoms in the absence of mucosal ulceration remains contentious. Currently available data, including those abstracted above, on which to base an informed decision are not compelling enough to provide support for the concept that colonization by this organism actually causes a specific symptom complex. Identifying *H. pylori* in a symptomatic patient does not provide evidence that the infection is the cause of symptoms, particularly because there is a comparable rate of infection in asymptomatic, age- and community-matched controls. It must be emphasized that much of the literature in this area is fraught with methodologic limitations. Current recommendations, therefore, do not support the initiation of *H. pylori* eradication therapy in the absence of the endoscopic evidence of peptic ulcer disease.

If you want to read an excellent review of *H. pylori* infection and peptic ulcer disease in children, see the superb article by Bourke et al.[1] You will learn that abdominal pain is clearly in the eye (and tummy) of its beholder, and little, shy of an endoscope, will bring any objectivity to understanding its cause.

Reference

1. Bourke B, et al: *Pediatr Infect Dis J* 15:1, 1996.

Helicobacter pylori Infection in Recurrent Abdominal Pain in Childhood: Comparison of Diagnostic Tests and Therapy

Chong SKF, Lou Q, Asnicar MA, et al (James Whitcomb Riley Hosp for Children, Indianapolis, Ind; Indiana Univ, Indianapolis)
Pediatrics 96:211–215, 1995   19–4

Introduction.—The association of recurrent abdominal pain with *Helicobacter pylori* infection has not been confirmed in many long-term prospective studies with children. Studies have been contradictory; however, methods to detect antibodies against *H. pylori* have helped clinicians to identify infected individuals and follow the response of antimicrobial therapy. The anti–*H. pylori* IgG titers of patients before therapy and 2, 4, and 6 months after completion of therapy were determined. The efficacy of the high–molecular-weight cell-associated protein (HM-CAP) *H. pylori* enzyme immunoassay kit was evaluated as a diagnostic method for *H. pylori* infection.

Methods.—The presence of serum IgG antibody to *H. pylori* was investigated in 456 children during a 3-year period using an HM-CAP *H. pylori* enzyme immunoassay kit. Symptoms of recurrent abdominal pain with or without vomiting were found in 218 children (aged 3–18 years), and no symptoms were found in 238 children. Upper gastrointestinal endoscopy was performed on 111 of the 218 children with recurrent abdominal pain so that mucosal biopsy specimens could be obtained for culture, histologic analysis, *H. pylori* detection by polymerase chain reaction, and CLO test.

Results.—Of 218 children in the recurrent abdominal pain group, 38, or 17.4%, were seropositive for *H. pylori*, as were 25, or 10.5%, of the 238 children in the group without recurrent abdominal pain. In the group of 111 children who had an endoscopy performed, 12 were positive with all 5 assays, and 95 were negative. Two children had negative specimens by culture and the CLO, but had positive specimens with the other 3 assays. Fourteen children had peptic ulcer disease detected by upper gastrointestinal endoscopy, and 12 had antral nodular gastritis detected. All 5 assays showed that only 4 of the 14 children with peptic ulcers were *H. pylori* positive, whereas all 12 children with antral nodular gastritis were found to be positive for *H. pylori*. A combination treatment of bismuth subsalicylate, amoxicillin, and metronidazole for 2 weeks was given to 9 of the 12 *H. pylori*–positive children. A decrease in anti–*H. pylori* serum IgG titer was shown in the sera of the 9 children obtained at 2, 4, and 6 months after treatment. The 3 *H. pylori*–infected children who did not receive any treatment served as the controls, and their IgG levels increased over time or remained elevated.

Conclusion.—The findings suggest that in children, *H. pylori* infection is more frequently associated with gastritis than with peptic ulcer disease, and *H. pylori* gastritis is a cause of recurrent abdominal pain syndrome in children. Screening for the serum IgG antibody to *H. pylori* is a practical method for diagnosing *H. pylori* infection, and serial measurements of the antibody help monitor treatment. Children with recurrent abdominal pain should first be tested for the antibody and retested 1 month later. If the test is positive, the children should be treated and retested 3–6 months later to ensure effectiveness of treatment.

▶ So much has been written about *H. pylori* that it's difficult to tell fact from fiction. One investigator says this organism is a cause of chronic abdominal pain in children. Another says not. This report says "maybe," inasmuch as 17.5% of the children with recurrent abdominal pain vs. 10.5% of those without abdominal pain were *H. pylori* positive. Please note that in reverse, 26.7% of kids with documented *H. pylori* infection have duodenal or gastric ulcer disease; the latter entities certainly being a cause of chronic and recurrent abdominal pain.

What can we conclude about all of this, and what will we do the next time we see a child who has recurrent abdominal pain? Well, lots of children have such pain. Many fewer have *H. pylori* infection as its cause. The trick is to sort out the wheat from the chaff and to do it by some simple means. Diagnostic invasive endoscopy is not entirely simple. Alternatively, one might do serologic testing for *H. pylori*. The problem with serologic testing is that it doesn't help all that much. Antibody titers to *H. pylori* are positive in many patients without symptoms. The titers stay elevated for long periods, even after the organism is eradicated. The latter problem obviates its usefulness in following the effectiveness of therapy. Breath hydrogen analysis is probably the best noninvasive test, but the equipment to do it is not readily available.

Perhaps the test that ultimately will have the greatest attractiveness in making a noninvasive diagnosis of *H. pylori* is the string test, which was described recently. This is the same test used for the diagnosis of *Giardia lamblia*. Swallow the string and leave it down for a while. Pull it back and culture the string for the presence of *H. pylori*. Better yet, because a polymerase chain reaction assay has been developed against *H. pylori*, it's likely that we will soon see a combination of polymerase chain reaction and a string test as a rapid diagnostic procedure.

In the meantime, you're stuck. You could go ahead and simply treat children as if they had *H. pylori* if they're having a difficult time with recurrent pain. As you know, such treatment requires an antibiotic, an antacid, and bismuth. This editor isn't suggesting that you empirically treat every child with recurrent abdominal pain. That would not seem to make sense. However, without the ability to do some of the diagnostic testing alluded to, one might be tempted to use such a therapeutic/diagnostic test. That, as yet, is not standard practice, so if you choose to go that route, carefully document why you are doing what you are doing. Good luck.

High Prevalence of Undiagnosed Coeliac Disease in 5280 Italian Students Screened by Antigliadin Antibodies

Catassi C, Rätsch IM, Fabiani E, et al (Univ Dept of Paediatrics, Ancona, Italy; "G Salesi" Children's Hosp, Ancona, Italy)
Acta Paediatr 84:672–676, 1995   19–5

Background.—The clinical expression of celiac disease is more heterogeneous than has been appreciated. Many cases of this disease go undiagnosed. Screening for celiac disease among children can be done reliably by the combined use of serum IgG and IgA antigliadin antibody (AGA) testing. The prevalence of celiac disease was quantified, and the features of undiagnosed celiac disease were determined.

Methods.—Screening was performed in 3 phases: serum IgG-AGA and IgA-AGA assay, antiendomysium antibody (AEA) and total serum IgA determinations, and jejunal biopsy. A total of 5,280 children, aged 11–15 years, underwent the first screening phase. One hundred thirteen of these children underwent the second tests, and 34 of these had an intestinal biopsy performed.

TABLE 2.—Clinical Findings in the 22 Screening-detected Celiac Patients

Clinical data	n
Iron deficiency	9
Recurrent aphthous stomatitis	8
Transient failure to thrive or diarrhea during infancy	6
Irritability	6
No problems (silent cases)	5
Recurrent abdominal pain	5
Gluten-free diet during infancy	3
Recurrent diarrhea	3
Short stature	1
Pubertal delay	1
Vitiligo	1
Selective IgA deficiency	1

(Courtesy of Catassi C, Rätsch IM, Fabiani E, et al: High prevalence of undiagnosed coeliac disease in 5280 Italian students screened by antigliadin antibodies. *Acta Paediatr* 84:672–676, 1995.)

Findings.—Celiac disease was diagnosed in 22 children. Most of these patients had atypical or silent forms of the disease (Table 2). The prevalence of undiagnosed celiac disease in the screened children was 4.36 per 1,000. In the general population, the prevalence was 5.03 per 1,000. The ratio of known to undiagnosed patients was 1:6.4.

Conclusions.—In Italy, celiac disease is much more common than previously believed. Without serologic screening, most cases will remain undiagnosed. A screening test for celiac disease, such as the AGA or AEA assay, probably should be included in the routine hematologic investigations that are performed at least once during childhood.

▶ What do 1 in 500 Italian children have in common with one another? If you answered celiac disease, you would be right. Also, if you are in the general practice of pediatrics, and if the frequency of celiac disease in an unselected population in the United States is close to that seen in Italy, you would expect to have 3 or 4 patients with this disorder under your care right now. The significance of this report is that if you don't recognize this frequency of celiac disease, chances are that you very well may be missing it. Indeed, the ratio of previously diagnosed to undiagnosed cases, using antigliadin antibodies as the screening test for celiac disease, is approximately 1:6.4. The validity of these estimates, however, hinges on the merits, pro and con, of serologic screening tests for celiac disease.

The serum AGA assay is a simple screening test using an enzyme-linked immunosorbent assay (ELISA), which measures IgG and IgA antibodies. The IgA-AGA assay is more sensitive but less specific for celiac disease than the IgG-AGA assay, which is more specific but less sensitive. Thus, both classes of antibody should be measured if you decide to use these types of antibody tests. Measurement of antireticulin antibody in serum is also used as a screening test and is as sensitive and specific for untreated celiac disease. Antireticulin antibody disappears with mucosal healing and reappears when the disease reappears. The best screening test, however, for celiac disease is measurement of IgA-AEA. It has a high degree of specificity and sensitivity (90% to 100%).

Antibody screening tests aside, a peroral small intestinal biopsy, while on a gluten diet, remains the "gold standard" for the diagnosis of celiac disease. The problem is that it is too rigorous a test to use without a very strong indication.

Whether we should be screening for "asymptomatic" celiac disease is a hotly debated issue. Interestingly, many of the children who have been detected by antibody screening have had recognizable clinical features of this disorder, including recurrent aphthous stomatitis, iron-deficiency anemia, recurrent diarrhea, and short stature.

The data presented indicate that various serum antibody tests for celiac disease are valuable as screening tests in children to detect celiac disease, but jejunal biopsy remains the litmus test. Arguments for population screening will probably increase as these tests become more widely available. The indications for treating asymptomatic patients with celiac disease with a gluten-free diet need to be established. Although symptomatic patients left untreated have a higher risk of long-term problems including malignancy, we really don't know much about those who have this disease but have no clinical problems.

One additional comment about celiac disease. If you run across a child who shows evidence of folic acid deficiency (most often characterized by a macrocytic anemia in the presence of hypersegmented granulocytes), think celiac disease. Folic acid deficiency may very well be the most common feature of malabsorption among patients with symptomatic celiac disease.[1] If you want to learn more about screening tests for this interesting disease, see the excellent review by Challacombe.[2]

Now this commentary closes with a fast fact: What population, other than subjects with celiac disease, is likely to have a 15-fold increased risk of having AGAs? About 2% of individuals in the general population have AGAs, usually without any explanation. One disease in particular, other than celiac disease, has a high frequency of antibodies to gliadin. This disease is rheumatoid arthritis, which in some patients results in intestinal villous atrophy that presumably increases permeability to a variety of antigens. Similarly, raised concentrations of AGAs are found in juvenile chronic arthritis, psoriasis, and IgA nephropathy. However, the entity that has the highest frequency of AGAs is the factor of working in a flour mill. Perfectly normal individuals who work with flour continuously have a 37% chance of having significantly elevated titers of AGAs. Presumably, bakers and cooks would have the same experience. Whether the presence of AGAs and those who cook a lot with flour specifically correlates with the degree of their exposure remains to be seen. Perhaps we'll have to do a double-volume comparison of the Julia Childs of this world vs. the Frugal Gourmets.

References

1. Pittschieler K: *Acta Paediatr* 84:705, 1995.
2. Challacombe DN: *Arch Dis Child* 73:3, 1995.

Longitudinal Evaluation of Serum Trypsinogen Measurement in Pancreatic-insufficient and Pancreatic-sufficient Patients With Cystic Fibrosis
Couper RTL, Corey M, Durie PR, et al (Hosp for Sick Children, Toronto; Univ of Toronto)
J Pediatr 127:408–413, 1995   19–6

Background.—Previous studies suggest that patients with cystic fibrosis (CF) and pancreatic sufficiency (PS) should be monitored for pancreatic disease progression. However, most methods for evaluating exocrine pancreatic function are too invasive or insensitive to be useful. Measuring immunoreactive pancreatic cationic trypsinogen in serum may be useful for monitoring the functional status of the pancreas in patients with CF. Serum trypsinogen levels have been found to strongly predict pancreatic

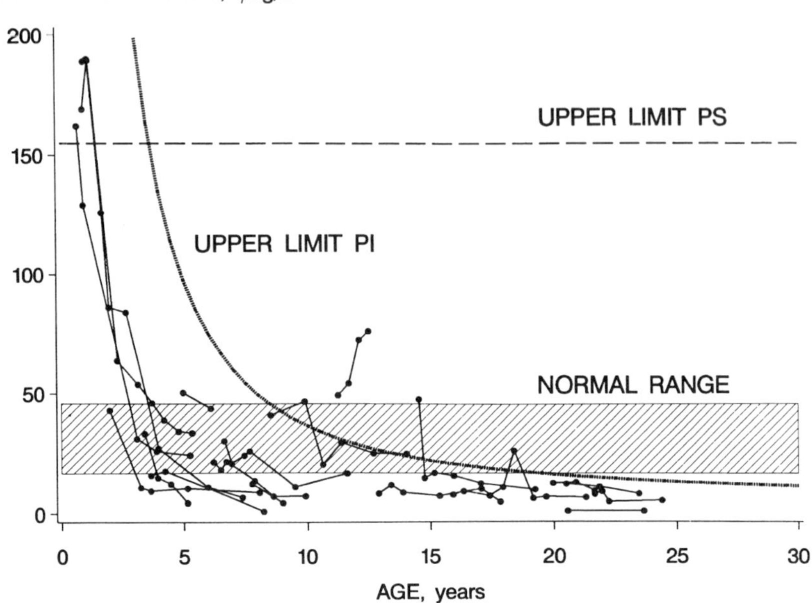

FIGURE.—Serial measurements of serum trypsinogen in 18 patients with cystic fibrosis who were pancreatic sufficient at diagnosis but became pancreatic insufficient during follow-up. *Shaded area* indicates normal range. *Curved line* indicates upper limit for patients with pancreatic insufficiency, based on cross-sectional measurements. *Horizontal dashed line* indicates upper limit for patients with pancreatic sufficiency. *Abbreviations: PI,* pancreatic insufficiency; *PS,* pancreatic sufficiency. (Courtesy of Couper RTL, Corey M, Durie PR, et al: Longitudinal evaluation of serum trypsinogen measurement in pancreatic-insufficient and pancreatic-sufficient patients with cystic fibrosis. *J Pediatr* 127:408–413, 1995.)

status in patients older than 7 years. Serum trypsinogen levels were assessed longitudinally to validate these findings.

Methods.—Trypsinogen serum levels in 329 patients with CF were measured 2–12 times for up to 7 years. The ages of patients ranged from 3 days to 40 years. Based on 72-hour fecal fat studies performed at diagnosis, 233 patients were classified as having pancreatic insufficiency (PI); 78, PS; and 18, PS at diagnosis with PI acquired during follow-up.

Findings.—In infants with PI, serum trypsinogen levels were greatly increased, then decreased sharply in the first years of life. By 7 years of age, more than 95% of these patients had subnormal values. Individual values followed a predictable course, similar to that previously reported. Patients with PS had serum trypsinogen levels that generally stayed within or above the normal range. After 10 years of age, these values in this group were far greater than the upper limit for the patients with PI. Within-patient variance was significantly higher in patients with PS than in those with PI older than 7 years. In the third group of patients, changes generally followed the pattern seen in patients with PI. However, values in older patients tended to be in the higher range (Figure).

Conclusions.—Serial measurement of serum trypsinogen is useful for monitoring the pancreatic status of patients with CF and PS. Pancreatic-insufficient and pancreatic-sufficient patients with CF had distinct differences in serum cationic trypsinogen levels, which were most apparent after 5–7 years of age. Because patients with PS have great variability in serum trypsinogen measures, a single measurement cannot be used to characterize a patient's pancreatic status.

▶ This report is of value because it extends our earlier understanding about the role of serum trypsinogen measurement in patients with CF. Recall that some time ago, serum trypsinogen measurements were validated as a screening tool to detect newborns with CF, at least the 70% to 80% who have evidence of pancreatic insufficiency. Early in life, affected patients with CF and pancreatic insufficiency have elevated serum trypsinogen levels. The precise mechanism by which trypsinogen enters the systemic circulation remains unknown, but the theory is that plugging of small pancreatic ductules so commonly seen in CF, results in a backup of trypsinogen, which leaks into the circulation. Over time, these markedly elevated serum trypsinogen levels eventually decline steeply. This decline probably reflects the loss of pancreatic cells capable of producing trypsinogen.

The value of this report is that it tells us that we can use trypsinogen measurements in blood to do more than detect newborns with CF. We can also use the levels later in life, particularly after 7 years of age, to determine which patients have pancreatic sufficiency and which have pancreatic insufficiency. There are distinct differences in serum trypsinogen levels in such patients. These differences are most apparent after 5–7 years of age, when patients with pancreatic insufficiency invariably have subnormal serum trypsinogen levels progressing to nondetectable levels, whereas patients with pancreatic sufficiency have elevated and extremely variable levels. Longitudinal serum trypsinogen measurements therefore provide a relatively simple and cheap test of pancreatic function in older patients with CF. Multiple longitudinal assays are best used because a single measurement cannot be used to characterize a patient's pancreatic status.

It is important to know how well the pancreas is working in patients with CF. The reason extends far beyond recognizing the need for replacement therapy for nutritional purposes. Pancreatic-sufficient patients have lower sweat chloride values, maintain better pulmonary function with age, are less likely to have pulmonary colonization with *Pseudomonas* infections, and maintain growth into adulthood. Their survival rate is far superior to that of patients with pancreatic insufficiency. Determine the difference.

Improved Steatocrit Results Obtained by Acidification of Fecal Homogenates Are Due to Improved Fat Extraction

Tran M, Forget P, Van den Neucker A, et al (Univ Hosp of Maastricht, The Netherlands)
J Pediatr Gastroenterol Nutr 22:157–160, 1996   19–7

Background.—Studies of the value of steatocrit in the screening of patients for steatorrhea have yielded inconsistent results. The test procedure was recently modified by fecal acidification in an attempt to improve fat extraction and increase test sensitivity.

Methods.—The fat content of fatty and solid layers obtained by centrifugation of 12 acidified and nonacidified steatorrheal stools were compared to determine whether fecal acidification improves fat extraction. The Sudan semiquantitative scoring system was used to assess the fat content of fatty and solid layers.

Findings.—The fatty layers sum of scores was 31 for the acid steatocrit and 16 for the classic steatocrit (Fig 1). The solid layers sum of scores was 13 and 24 for the respective steatocrits. After fecal sample acidification, fat extraction from stool samples was signficantly improved. The results of acid steatocrit were in better agreement with chemically determined fecal fat than were the results of classic steatocrit.

Conclusions.—Fecal acidification improves fat extraction in the centrifugation step of steatocrit and therefore improves the reliability of the test to detect fat malabsorption. The acid steatocrit is a good alternative to the Sudan semiquantitative staining method for measuring chemical fat.

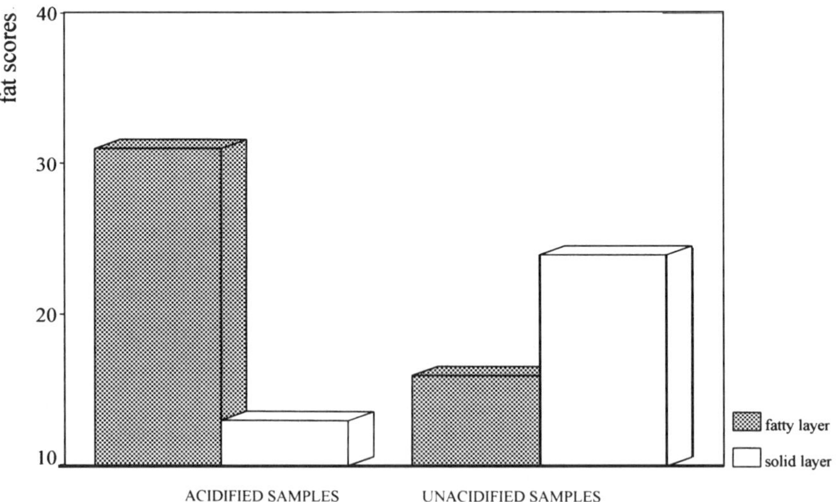

FIGURE 1.—Sum of 12 microscopical Sudan fat globule scores (1, 2, or 3) performed on fatty and solid layers cf acidified and unacidified fecal samples. (Courtesy of Tran M, Forget P, Van den Neucker A, et al: Improved steatocrit results obtained by acidification of fecal homogenates are due to improved fat extraction. *J Pediatr Gastroenterol Nutr* 22:157–160, 1996.)

▶ This is the 15th anniversary of the steatocrit. The steatocrit is the stool fat equivalent test to the hematocrit for percent red cell mass and the cremacrit for the percent fat layer in human milk. In 1981, Phuapradit introduced the steatocrit as a new, simple, and easily repeatable method for measuring fecal fat content.[1] Although several authors have found this method satisfactory for the evaluation of steatorrhea, others have found it unreliable. The authors of the report abstracted had shown previously that acidification would allow a better identification of the fat in a stool when performing a steatocrit.[2] This report takes these observations one step further by taking a large number of steatorrheal stool samples and testing them further. One can conclude that fecal acidification does improve fat extraction and fairly readily distinguishes those who are experiencing malabsorption of fats in their diet.

If you're thinking about setting up the steatocrit procedure in your office, it is fairly simple to do. First, 0.5 g of solid stool should be weighed and diluted with water equal to 2 times the weight of the stool. The stool and water should be mixed well in a Vortex mixer. The mixture then should be homogenized, following which 5-normal perchloric acid is added in a volume equal to one fifth of the homogenate. This acid homogenate then is remixed in a Vortex mixer, following which the homogenate is aspirated into a standard hematocrit capillary tube, which is then centrifuged in a standard hematocrit centrifuge. The upper limit for the hematocrit is 10%.

Although many still consider the steatocrit (acid or not) with skepticism, it sure beats a 72-hour stool collection for a quantitative fecal fat. The latter is pretty unpleasant for a patient and even more so for a parent who has to keep the specimen during the collection period.

One other stool test has emerged recently—stool osmolality—that could be quite useful in certain circumstances. Patients with unexplained chronic diarrhea frequently present diagnostic and therapeutic challenges. One of the causes of such a problem is Munchausen-by-proxy "diarrhea," which usually results from the administration of excessive amounts of laxatives or from intentional dilution of a stool sample to make it look like diarrhea. The diagnosis of either of these two can be made fairly readily by measuring stool osmolality. In a normal child, the osmolality of fresh liquid stool is roughly equivalent to that of serum. After laxative use or after dilution of a stool, the stool osmolality will be quite low. If you're thinking about factitious diarrhea, don't forget to measure stool osmolality. It may be a smelly test to do, but it's a cheap and pretty good test for determining real and nonreal causes of diarrhea.[3]

References

1. Phuapradit P, et al: *Arch Dis Child* 56:725, 1981.
2. Tran M, et al: *Pediatr Gastroenterol Nutr* 19:299, 1994.
3. Topazian M, et al: *N Engl J Med* 330:1418, 1995.

Campylobacter jejuni Infection and Guillain-Barré Syndrome
Rees JH, Soudain SE, Gregson NA, et al (Guy's Hosp, London)
N Engl J Med 333:1374–1379, 1995   19–8

Introduction.—*Campylobacter jejuni* is the organism most frequently associated with Guillain-Barré syndrome. However, the clinical and epidemiologic features of these patients have not been well studied. The characteristics and prognosis of the Guillain-Barré syndrome caused by *C. jejuni* infection were examined in a prospective case-control study.

Methods.—Blood and stool samples were collected from 103 patients with Guillain-Barré syndrome or Miller Fisher syndrome, and from controls identified from patients' households and from age-matched patients hospitalized at the same time who did not have neuropathy or diarrheal illness. The stool samples were cultured for *Campylobacter* organisms, and the serum samples were screened for antibodies against *C. jejuni*. The worst deficits at the peak of illness among the case patients were graded. Electrophysiologic data were obtained from case notes or nerve conduction studies and classified.

Results.—*Campylobacter jejuni* was detected in 26% of the patients, 2% of the household controls, and 1% of the hospital controls. Of the 27 patients positive for *C. jejuni,* 19 (70%) had a diarrheal illness within 12 weeks before the development of Guillain-Barré syndrome, as did 5 of the 76 (7%) patients negative for *C. jejuni. Campylobacter jejuni* infection was more common among men than women. Weakness was the first symptom in 67% of the *C. jejuni*–positive patients and 36% of the *C. jejuni*–negative patients. The 2 groups were similar in the incidence of sensory disturbance, pain, and other symptoms. Compared with the *C. jejuni*–negative patients, the *C. jejuni*–positive patients had a significantly longer convalescence and were more likely to be disabled at 1 year after diagnosis (Table 3), although there were no differences between the 2

TABLE 3.—Outcomes at 1 Year*

Outcome	C. jejuni-Positive (N = 26)	C. jejuni-Negative (N = 75)†	Odds Ratio
	number (percents)		
Not disabled or slightly disabled (disability grades 0 and 1)	9 (35)	51 (68)	1.0
Moderately disabled (disability grade 2)	11 (42)	17 (23)	3.7
Severely disabled (disability grades 3, 4, and 5)	5 (19)	2 (3)	14.2
Death (disability grade 6)	1 (4)	5 (7)	1.1

*Chi-square value for linear trend is 5.1 ($P = 0.02$).
†Percentages do not add up to 100 because of rounding.
(Reprinted by permission of *The New England Journal of Medicine*, from Rees JH, Soudain SE, Gregson NA, et al: *Campylobacter jejuni* infection and Guillain-Barré syndrome. *N Engl J Med* 333:1374–1379, Copyright 1995, Massachusetts Medical Society.)

TABLE 5.—Multivariate Analysis of Factors Contributing to a Poor Outcome After 1 Year

Factor	Good Outcome	Poor Outcome	P Value	Odds Ratio (95% CI)
	number (percent)			
Age	NA	NA	< 0.01	3.0* (1.4–6.1)
C. jejuni positivity				
Yes	20 (23)	6 (46)		
No	68 (77)	7 (54)	0.03	7.3 (1.2–45.1)
Ventilatory support				
Yes	19 (22)	7 (54)		
No	69 (78)	6 (46)	< 0.01	15.9 (2.4–106.7)
Confinement to bed within 2 days				
Yes	20 (23)	9 (69)		
No	68 (77)	4 (31)	0.01	8.6 (1.7–43.7)

*Odds ratio is for age intervals of 10 years.

Abbreviations: NA, not applicable (as a continuous variable); *CI,* confidence interval, *C. jejuni, Canpylobacter jejuni.*

(Reprinted by permission of The New England of Journal of Medicine, from Rees JH, Soudain SE, Gregson NA, et al: *Campylobacter jejuni* infection and Guillain-Barré syndrome. *N Engl J Med* 333:1374–1379, Copyright 1995, Massachusetts Medical Society.)

groups in deficits at the peak of illness. However, sensory symptoms were significantly less severe in *C. jejuni*–positive than in *C. jejuni*–negative patients. The electrophysiologic data indicated more frequent acute motor or motor and sensory axonal neuropathy and axonal degeneration and less frequent acute inflammatory demyelinating polyradiculoneuropathy in the *C. jejuni*–positive patients than in the *C. jejuni*–negative patients. Among patients with acute, inflammatory demyelinating polyradiculoneuropathy, those positive for *C. jejuni* were more likely to have axonal degeneration than were those negative for *C. jejuni.* In multivariate analysis, increasing age, *C. jejuni* positivity, ventilatory support, and confinement to bed within 2 days of neuropathic symptoms were significant predictors of poor outcomes (Table 5).

Conclusions.—Campylobacter jejuni–induced Guillain-Barré syndrome is more likely than other forms of the syndrome to be manifested as a purely motor syndrome, with a longer recovery and a greater likelihood of prolonged disability.

► This report from Great Britain largely involves an adult population of patients with Guillain-Barré syndrome. The reason for including the report in the Year Book of Pediatrics is because with the relative infrequency of this syndrome in children, there is not much written about its potential causes. There is much to be learned from our adult counterparts.

We see that infection with *C. jejuni* precedes Guillain-Barré syndrome 26% of the time. The true frequency of antecedent *C. jejuni* infection is probably higher than 26%, because of the difficulty in confirming a diagnosis of this infection. This frequency makes *C. jejuni* the most common single identifiable pathogen in Guillain-Barré syndrome in adults. The syndrome is more likely to develop in men after *C. jejuni* infection than in women, which suggests a sex-linked predisposition or results from a predominance of males among those with *C. jejuni* infection. The median interval from the onset of diarrhea to the onset of neuropathic symptoms is about 9 days, suggesting that Guillain-Barré syndrome occurs as a consequence of an immune response to *C. jejuni* rather than as a direct effect of the organism or one of its toxins.

The next time you see a child with Guillain-Barré syndrome, obtain appropriate blood and stool specimens to diagnose a preceding *C. jejuni* infection. If children with Guillain Barré syndrome respond in the same way as adults when previously infected with *C. jejuni*, they are more likely to have a purely motor syndrome, defined by an absence of sensory signs and symptoms. They also will be in the subset of children who take longer to recover and are more likely to be severely disabled for a longer period.

Whether *C. jejuni* infection plays a major role in the causation of Guillain-Barré syndrome in children remains to be seen. In the meantime, at least think about the association. We should be hearing more about *C. jejuni* as a predecessor of Guillain-Barré syndrome in children in this country. In rural areas of northern China, a high percentage of children affected with this neurologic disorder have IgG and IgM against *C. jejuni*.[1]

While on the topic of diarrheal illnesses, we recently learned that not only does cooked rice really work to control diarrhea, we know why it works. Investigators at Montreal Children's Hospital have found a substance extracted from rice that inhibits the response of intestinal epithelial crypt cells to adenosine 3'5'-cyclic monophosphate, a major intracellular inhibitor of secretion. Apparently this component of rice reduces cell shrinkage in the gut so fluid isn't squeezed out. The active fraction is a very low molecular weight substance, the nature of which needs to be more fully defined. When it is defined, buy stock in the company that figures out a way to make the substance. Meanwhile, take stock in Uncle Ben's.

Reference

1. McKhann GM, et al: *Ann Neurol* 33:333, 1993.

A Comparison of Symptoms After the Consumption of Milk or Lactose-hydrolyzed Milk by People With Self-reported Severe Lactose Intolerance

Suarez FL, Savaiano DA, Levitt MD (Univ of Minnesota, St Paul; Minneapolis Veterans Affairs Med Ctr)
N Engl J Med 333:1–4, 1995   19–9

Background.—Approximately 75% of adults worldwide have lactose malabsorption. After weaning, a reduction in lactase activity occurs in many individuals. Most individuals with lactose malabsorption have abdominal pain, bloating, flatulence, and diarrhea after consuming large doses of lactose, but their tolerance of smaller doses of lactose is contro-

TABLE 1.—Gastrointestinal Symptoms and Frequency of Flatus in 30 People With Self-reported Severe Lactose Intolerance Who Drank 240 mL of Ordinary Milk or Lactose-hydrolyzed Milk Daily for 1 Week*

Symptom	Ordinary Milk	Lactose-Hydrolyzed Milk	Difference	95% Confidence Interval†
Lactose-malabsorption group (n = 21)				
Bloating‡	0.6 ± 0.1	0.5 ± 0.1	0.1 ± 0.1	−0.2 to 0.4
Abdominal pain‡	0.4 ± 0.1	0.3 ± 0.1	0.1 ± 0.1	−0.1 to 0.3
Diarrhea (episodes/day)	0.1 ± 0.0	0.3 ± 0.1	−0.2 ± 0.1	−0.4 to 0.0
Flatus				
Perceived severity‡	1.1 ± 0.1	0.9 ± 0.1	0.2 + 0.1	0.0 to 0.4
Frequency (episodes/day)	10.1 ± 1.5	7.6 ± 1.2	2.5 ± 1.1	0.2 to 4.8
Lactose-absorption group (n = 9)				
Bloating‡	0.6 ± 0.2	0.5 ± 0.2	0.2 ± 0.2	−0.3 to 0.7
Abdominal pain‡	0.6 ± 0.2	0.4 ± 0.2	0.2 ± 0.1	0.0 to 0.4
Diarrhea (episodes/day)	0.3 ± 0.2	0.2 ± 0.1	0.1 ± 0.2	−0.4 to 0.6
Flatus				
Perceived severity‡	0.9 ± 0.2	1.2 ± 0.2	0.3 ± 0.2	−0.2 to 0.8
Frequency (episodes/day)	11.8 ± 2.3	8.4 ± 1.9	3.4 ± 1.7	−0.53 to 7.3

*Data were analyzed by analysis of variance. Plus-minus values are means ± SEM.

†The 95% confidence intervals for differences between the means for severity or presence of symptoms include zero, indicating nonsignificance.

‡Symptoms were ranked according to severity: 0 indicated no symptoms; 1, trivial symptoms; 2, mild symptoms; 3, moderate symptoms; 4, strong symptoms; and 5, severe symptoms.

(Reprinted by permission of *The New England Journal of Medicine*, from Suarez FL, Savaiano DA, Levitt MD: A comparison of symptoms after the consumption of milk or lactose-hydrolyzed milk by people with self-reported severe lactose intolerance. *N Engl J Med* 333:1–4, Copyright 1995, Massachusetts Medical Society.)

versial. The gastrointestinal symptoms of patients with severe lactose intolerance were investigated in a randomized, double-blind, crossover study.

Methods.—Thirty individuals who reported they had severe lactose intolerance were studied. Their ability to digest lactose was determined by measuring end-alveolar hydrogen concentrations after they drank 15 g of lactose in 250 mL of water. Then, the individuals drank 240 mL of milk each day for two 1-week periods. Milk preparations were either a lactose-hydrolyzed milk with 2% fat, or milk with 2% fat and an artificial sweetener. Individuals rated their gastrointestinal symptoms.

Results.—Of the 30 participants, 21 had lactose malabsorption and 9 were able to absorb lactose according to their breath hydrogen concentrations. The individuals' self-rated symptoms were between trivial and mild for abdominal pain, bloating, flatus, and diarrhea (Table 1). There were no significant differences in severity of symptoms between the 2 study periods.

Discussion.—These findings indicate that some individuals may incorrectly attribute abdominal distress to lactose malabsorption. These individuals were able to tolerate 240 mL of milk per day for 7 days with only mild gastrointestinal symptoms. Lactose-digestive aids may not be necessary when smaller doses of lactose are consumed.

▶ The data and conclusion of this report are believable. The reason they are believable is that were they not, the atmosphere would be permeated by the malodorous flatus of the billions, yes billions, of individuals worldwide who are lactose intolerant. The ability to maintain throughout adult life the levels of lactase characteristic of infancy is inherited through a single, highly penetrant, autosomal dominant gene located on chromosome 2. People of northern European descent have this gene and generally have high lactase levels during adulthood. Most other people become lactase-nonpersistent. About a quarter of adults in the United States and 75% of those worldwide have lactose malabsorption. These figures are not contested. What has been contested is how much milk or milk product you can take before you have symptoms. Many adults swear that the small amount of milk in a coffee creamer is enough to cause abdominal pain, bloating, and flatus.

Well, it just ain't so. What these investigators have done is to show that the average lactase-deficient adult can drink 1 glass (240 mL) of milk without bloating, abdominal pain, or diarrhea. Their flatus index (episodes of flatus per day) is no different than that of the average bloke.

It's not clear how lactase-deficient individuals will receive this report. No longer can they blame lactase deficiency for symptoms such as bloating or the passing of gas. For sure, those who produce lactose-digestive aids will be unhappy with these results. Some 18 cents worth of such products are needed to completely hydrolyze the lactose from 240 mL of milk. The average individual who had been needlessly buying such aids will be able to pocket about $66 a year by avoiding their use.

The real winners in the data from this report are the Baskin Robbins and Ben & Jerry's of this world. Their business is now secure. Furthermore, the owners of these establishments need no longer worry about the danger of hydrogen explosions on their premises.

Pediatric Laparoscopic Splenectomy

Moores DC, McKee MA, Wang H, et al (Loma Linda Univ, Calif; Kaiser Permanente Med Ctr, Fontana, Calif)
J Pediatr Surg 30:1201–1205, 1995   19–10

Background.—Increasing evidence shows that laparoscopic techniques can be successfully applied to children. Laparoscopic methods are associated with less postoperative pain, reduced ileus, fewer pulmonary complications, and shorter hospital stays. Such techniques also appear to be useful for elective splenectomy in patients with hematologic disease or for staging in those with Hodgkin's lymphoma. One series of laparoscopic splenectomies (LS) was described.

Methods and Findings.—Twelve children treated consecutively since 1993 were reviewed retrospectively. The patients ranged in age from 3 to 16 years. Diagnoses were hereditary spherocytosis in 5 patients, idiopathic thrombocytopenia purpura in 4, and autoimmune thrombocytopenia, β-thalassemia, and sickle cell anemia in 1 each. The outcomes of this group were compared with those of 20 children undergoing open splenectomy (OS) for a similar spectrum of diseases. Total operative time and estimated blood loss were greater in the patients undergoing LS, although the amount of IV analgesia needed in the first 48 hours was comparable. Patients undergoing OS had significantly longer times to oral intake followed by regular diet, and longer overall hospital stays. There were no long-term complications in either group.

Conclusions.—Laparoscopic splenectomy can be performed effectively, efficiently, and at a reasonable cost in the hands of experienced laparoscopic surgeons. Compared with OS, LS has a more benign postoperative course and the potential for fewer long-term complications in children requiring splenectomy.

▶ The list of conditions for which minimally invasive surgery can be performed in children grows and grows. If you want your gallbladder out, even as a child, find a surgeon who knows how to do it with a laparoscope. The same applies to those in need of appendectomy, Nissen fundoplication, or those who need to have an undescended testes brought down.

This report by Moores et al. shows us the relative ease with which a spleen can be removed by a skilled operator. It's even possible to do a concomitant cholecystectomy and splenectomy (some patients with hereditary spherocytosis need this done) if you have to. Laparoscopic surgery avoids major incisions, lessens postoperative pain, diminishes postoperative ileus, is associated with fewer respiratory complications, and shortens hospital stays, allowing quicker returns to school or work. Laparoscopic surgery minimizes the risk of subsequent adhesions and therefore postoperative bowel obstructions. Although the actual cost of laparoscopic surgery is higher than that of conventional surgery (mostly because of extra instrumentation and additional operating room time), total costs diminish because of the shorter hospital stay and the fact that most children return to full activity within a week, allowing a parent or parents to return to work in as short a time as possible.

Laparoscopic surgery may seem to you to be better than apple pie and motherhood. In fact, it probably is pretty close. Recognize, however, that there are 3 absolute contraindications to laparoscopic surgery. These include an uncorrectable bleeding diathesis, an inability to tolerate general anesthesia, and an incompetent surgeon. Of the 3, the latter is the greatest risk factor. It was the surgeon, Halsted, who said, "The only recourse for an anesthetized patient against an incompetent surgeon is hemorrhage." Be certain to check out the laparoscopic credentials on someone who is going to be operating on one of your patients.

Early Childhood Appendicitis Is Still a Difficult Diagnosis

Paajanen H, Somppi E (Univ of Tampere, Finland)
Acta Paediatr 85:459–462, 1996　　　　　　　　　　　　　　　19–11

Background.—Acute appendicitis makes up 10% of all surgical emergencies in the pediatric emergency department. The rate of perforated

TABLE 2.—Symptoms and Clinical Signs

	Appendicitis (group A)	Perforated appendix (group B)	Normal appendix (group C)	P
Prehospital symptoms				
Duration (days ± SD)	1.3 ± 0.7	3.1 ± 1.9	1.9 ± 2.2	< 0.05*
Vomiting	15 (60%)	11 (69%)	15 (31%)	< 0.01
Diarrhea	0 (0%)	4 (25%)	5 (10%)	< 0.05†
Fever (> 37°C)	20 (80%)	14 (88%)	35 (71%)	NS
Preoperative clinical signs				
Tenderness in RLQ	22 (88%)	16 (100%)	40 (82%)	NS
Diffuse peritonitis	3 (12%)	7 (44%)	0 (0%)	< 0.001†
Body temperature (°C ± SD)	38.4 ± 0.90	38.4 ± 0.64	37.9 ± 0.80	NS

*Between groups A and B.
†Between groups B and C.
Abbreviations: SD, standard deviation; *RLQ*, right lower quadrant.
(Courtesy of Paajanen H, Somppi E: Early childhood appendicitis is still a difficult diagnosis. *Acta Paediatr* 85:459–462, 1996.)

appendicitis is between 40% and 70% in young children. There are reports of negative pediatric appendectomy rates of 20% to 50%. There is little information on the difficulties of diagnosing appendicitis in very young children. Data from emergency appendectomies in patients younger than 5 years were analyzed in a retrospective review.

Methods.—Emergency appendectomy was performed in 90 consecutive children younger than 5 years of age; 29% of children were younger than 3 years. Patients with acute appendicitis without perforation made up group A, those with perforation made up group B, and patients with a normal appendix at operation made up group C. Medical records were reviewed, and operative and postoperative findings were among the data analyzed.

Results.—In 54% of patients, the outcome of exploration was negative. In 28% of patients, an inflamed nonperforated appendix was removed. In 18% of patients, a perforated appendix was removed. The perforation rate was 60% in children younger than 3 years and 27% in children between 4 and 5 years of age. Tenderness in the iliac fossa, blood leukocytosis, and urinalysis provided little diagnostic information. In children with a perforated appendix, diffuse peritonitis and elevated serum C–reactive protein values were more frequent (Table 2). Postoperative morbidity was between 10% and 20%. There were no deaths.

Conclusion.—It is still difficult to diagnose appendicitis in young children. Prompt diagnosis and treatment can reduce the rate of perforated appendixes in infants with suspected appendicitis; this will result in a high negative exploration rate but a low rate of postoperative complications.

Further research should address the value of noninvasive diagnostic imaging and specific blood tests for bacterial infection.

▶ From time to time, this editor is asked to comment on a case of missed appendicitis, usually by a caring and committed pediatric care provider who had recently failed to establish a correct diagnosis. This report from Finland makes 2 things obvious: First, if someone has done everything right and still appendicitis is missed, there should be little in the way of guilt; second, the diagnosis of appendicitis in early childhood is much more of an art than a science. If medicine, in general, is an art form, pediatrics, in particular, is the ultimate expression of that art.

So what are the rules? A negative abdominal examination does not rule out appendicitis. A normal complete blood cell count, a normal C-reactive protein, a normal urinalysis, a normal ultrasound result, a normal radioactive-tagged leukocyte scan, and a normal cytokine assay, if one is inclined to do such, do not rule out appendicitis.[1] Any young child with ill-defined and nonspecific symptoms that could be consistent with appendicitis should be considered to possibly have appendicitis. Often, only inactivity, lethargy, decreased capillary refill time, and hypothermia mark an appendix that has gone seriously awry.

As long as an accurate diagnosis of early childhood appendicitis remains difficult, we must, and in fact should, expect a relatively high surgical exploration rate in young pediatric patients. Indeed, this may be acceptable because of the low frequency of postoperative complications in these youngsters. At some point, hopefully, the diagnostic value of noninvasive imaging techniques will increase as will specific blood tests for bacterial infection, providing us with the diagnostic acumen that currently comes only from having seen a number of children with appendicitis.

Reference

1. Vinjamuri S, et al: *Lancet* 347:233, 1996.

Open *Versus* Laparoscopic Appendectomy: A Prospective Randomized Comparison
Martin LC, Puente I, Sosa JL, et al (Univ of Miami, Fla)
Ann Surg 222:256–262, 1995   19–12

Introduction.—Although the laparoscopic approach is well accepted for the treatment of cholelithiasis, the efficacy of and indications for laparoscopic appendectomy are still at issue. Previous studies have suggested that laparoscopic appendectomy can significantly shorten hospital stay compared with the conventional open operation. Open and laparoscopic appendectomy were prospectively compared.

Methods.—During a 9-month period, 169 patients aged 15 years or older with a diagnosis of acute appendicitis were studied. The patients were randomly assigned to a laparoscopic (81 patients) or an open surgical

TABLE 2.—Comparison of All Laparoscopic Patients and Open Patients

	Laparoscopic	Open	p Value
No. of patients	81	88	—
OR minutes	102.2	81.7	0.0002
Hospital days	2.2	4.3	0.0007
Days to normal activity	12.2	12.8	0.92
Days to work	23.3	23.6	0.99

Abbreviations: OR, operating room.
(Courtesy of Martin LC, Puente I, Sosa JL, et al: Open versus laparoscopic appendectomy: A prospective randomized comparison. *Ann Surg* 222:256–262, 1995.)

approach (88 patients). Both groups received preoperative antibiotics. Operative time—defined as the time from incision to full wound closure—was compared for the 2 groups, as were hospital stay and the time for return to normal activity. Patients requiring conversion from laparoscopic to open appendectomy were considered separately.

Results.—The demographic characteristics of the 2 groups were similar. Sixteen percent of the laparoscopic group required conversion to open surgery. Acute appendicitis was present in 80% of the open group and 77% of the laparoscopic group; perforative appendicitis was present in 24% of the open group and 12% of the laparoscopic group. Operative time was 82 minutes in the open group vs. 102 minutes in the laparoscopic group (Table 2). Hospital stay was significantly longer in the open group: 4.3 vs. 2.2 days. Although hospital stay was not significantly different for patients who had acute appendicitis vs. those who had a normal appendix but with pelvic inflammatory disease, where was a significant difference for patients with perforative appendicitis: 9.5 days in the open group vs. 1.5 days in the laparoscopic group. The mean hospital cost was $7,227 for open vs. $6,077 for laparoscopic appendectomy (Table 6). The laparoscopic group had no increase in the complication rate. There were no differences in return to normal activity.

Conclusions.—Laparoscopic and open appendectomy are similar in terms of hospital complications, hospital stay, cost, return to activity, and return to work. Operative time is significantly longer with the laparoscopic approach. Diagnostic laparoscopy may be useful for selected patients with vague clinical findings, such as women of childbearing age or obese pa-

TABLE 6.—Cost Analysis of Laparoscopic and Open Patients

	Laparoscopic ($)	Open ($)	P Value
All patients	6,077	7,227	0.164
Acute	6,189	5,277	0.074
Perforated	7,465	13,670	0.05
Normal	5,088	5,515	0.51

(Courtesy of Martin LC, Puente I, Sosa JL, et al: Open versus laparoscopic appendectomy: A prospective randomized comparison. *Ann Surg* 222:256–262, 1995.)

tients, but laparoscopic appendectomy does not offer any significant benefit compared with open appendectomy for the patient with routine appendicitis.

▶ Another report on laparoscopic surgery. Has the pendulum begun to swing away from laparoscopic surgery, particularly when it comes to appendectomy? If the results of this study are to be believed, open appendectomy and laparoscopic appendectomy are equivalent with respect to complications, return to activity, and return to work. The hospital stay was shorter (2.2 days) in the laparoscopic group compared with 4.3 days in the open group, but operative time was significantly longer with the minimally invasive surgery. There appears to be a slight cost advantage to laparoscopic appendectomy ($6,077 vs. $7,227), but overall there is not much that distinguishes between these 2 forms of surgery.

Chances are, with time we will learn that conventional surgery really isn't all that bad in terms of cost and stay in the hospital. There seems to be a mind-set that with the "old" operations, patients need to be hospitalized for as long as they had been in the past. This need not be so, as Professor Alan Johnson of Sheffield, England, has recently pointed out.[1] Dr. Johnson notes that the length of hospital stay is strongly influenced by patients' expectations. He recently finished a clinical trial of open small incision vs. laparoscopic cholecystectomy. To eliminate the psychological influence that was potentially possible, he "blinded" the patients, the surgeons, and the nurses beforehand by randomly assigning patients to one or the other type of surgical approach after they were in the operating room. Afterward, he "blinded" the nurses and patients to which operation had been done by covering the abdomen with identical dressings. He told the patients they could eat, get out of bed, and go home as soon as they felt like it. He found no difference between open incision vs. laparoscopic cholecystectomy. The average stay in the hospital was 2 nights for each, with the same time back to full activity.

The advantages of laparoscopic appendectomy compared with regular surgery are probably more marginal than the advantages of laparoscopic cholecystectomy compared with regular cholecystectomy. In fact, there is some anecdotal experience that the rate of intraabdominal abscess formation may actually be higher after laparoscopic appendectomy. One recent nonrandomized series reported a 45% rate of readmission to the hospital for infectious complications after laparoscopic appendectomy for complicated appendicitis.

After reading all this, were my appendix to be removed, I would ask the surgeon to reach for a regular scalpel blade and to make a 2-inch incision over McBurney's point. Sometimes the classic approach turns out to be the simplest.

Reference

1. Johnson AG: *Ann Surg* 222:261, 1995.

Treatment of Intractable Constipation in Children: Experience With Cisapride

Nurko S, Garcia-Aranda JA, Guerrero VY, et al (Hosp Infantil de Mexico "Federico Gomez," Mexico City)
J Pediatr Gastroenterol Nutr 22:38–44, 1996   19–13

Introduction.—Constipation is a common problem in children, and a substantial portion of these patients will fail to respond to any of the various treatments. Children with intractable constipation can be very difficult to treat; they may become dependent on laxatives, undergo surgery, and experience social problems. The prokinetic agent cisapride has proven useful in the treatment of constipation in adults. Cisapride was evaluated for the treatment of children with chronic constipation.

Methods.—The prospective open trial included 27 children with chronic constipation that had not improved with at least 12 weeks of medical treatment. There were 14 boys and 13 girls, mean age about 8 years. Those with pelvic floor dyssynergia were excluded. All patients received cisapride, 0.2 mg/kg 3 times a day for 12 weeks, and were followed up for at least 1 year.

TABLE 1.—Main Characteristics Before and After 12 Weeks of Cisapride Administration According to the Clinical Outcome

	Asymptomatic	Partial improvement	No improvement
# Patients	18	7	2
Sex (M/F)	8/10	6/1	0/2
Age at time of study (months)	85 ± 43‖	93 ± 39	150 ± 76
Onset of constipation (months)	24 ± 29	41 ± 37	0.2 ± 0.2
Duration of constipation (months)	59 ± 39	53 ± 28	150 ± 76
Fecal mass (%)			
Before	12 (67)	4 (57)	2 (100)
After	0 (0)*	1 (14)	2 (100)§
Encopresis (%)			
Before	15 (83)	6 (86)	2 (100)
After	0 (0)*	6 (86)	2 (100)§
BM/week			
Before	1.5 ± 0.5	1.3 ± 0.5	0.9 ± 0.2
After	7.4 ± 4.0*	5.8 ± 4.0‡	0.9 ± 0.2§
Accidents/day			
Before	2.2 ± 1.8	4.4 ± 4.0	3.8 ± 3.2
After	0 ± 0*	0.9 ± 0.7	3.8 ± 3.2
Laxative doses/week			
Before	13.8 ± 5.2	14.9 ± 7.9	17.5 ± 4.9
After	1.5 ± 3.8†	6.0 ± 10.2	10.5 ± 14.9

*$P < 0.001$.
†$P < 0.01$.
‡$P < 0.05$ comparing before vs. after cisapride administration.
§$P < 0.05$ comparing between groups.
‖ Mean ± standard deviation.
Abbreviation: BM, bowel movements.
(Courtesy of Nurko S, Garcia-Aranda JA, Guerrero VY, et al: Treatment of intractable constipation in children: Experience with cisapride. *J Pediatr Gastroenterol Nutr* 22:38–44, 1996.)

Results.—Cisapride treatment increased the number of bowel movements per week significantly, from about 1.5 to 6.5. Significant declines in accidents and laxative use were observed as well (Table 1). Encopresis resolved for 65% of children and improved for another 26%. Sixty-nine percent of children were able to cease laxative use. At the end of the 12-week treatment period, 67% of patients were symptom-free, 26% had some improvement, and 7% had no improvement. Cisapride had only a few minor side effects

At a mean follow-up of 20 months, 37% were asymptomatic and no longer taking laxatives or cisapride. Another 30% still had symptoms but were still taking drug treatment. None of the initial patient characteristics distinguished between children who did and did not respond fully to cisapride.

Conclusions.—The prokinetic drug cisapride appears to be a useful treatment alternative for some children with intractable constipation, as long as they do not have pelvic floor dyssynergia. Further studies of the use of cisapride in children with intractable constipation are warranted. Children who cannot stop taking cisapride without the need for other medications probably have an underlying gastrointestinal functional problem that has not been addressed.

▶ It has been estimated that constipation accounts for up to 25% of outpatient visits to the average pediatric gastrointestinal clinic. Such children with chronic constipation and encopresis are referred to univerity medical centers because of poor response to the types of conventional treatments that we use. Treatment options, including disimpaction, prevention of reaccumulation of feces by added dietary fiber, laxatives, and alteration of toilet behavior sometimes do not work. There are many refractory patients, including those who comply with all aspects of such conventional treatment programs. For these children, cisapride may be the treatment of choice.

Cisapride, a prokinetic drug like metoclopramide and domperidone, acts on the myenteric plexus, enhancing the motility of the gut. The action of cisapride involves the facilitation of acetylcholine release in the intramural plexuses. This enhances gastrointestinal peristalsis. Cisapride can be used for a variety of gastrointestinal disturbances. It promotes esophageal clearance of acid in patients with reflux. It accelerates gastric emptying in patients with gastroparesis. It accelerates small-bowel transit in patients with chronic intestinal pseudo-obstruction. In addition to colonic pseudo-obstruction, it has been widely used for irritable bowel syndrome and post-operative ileus. It relieves constipation by making the colon contract.

Please consider this report from Boston to be a preliminary one. Nurko et al. are the first to tell us that cisapride may be an effective treatment for intractable constipation in some children. Any new therapeutic advance requires clear proof of effectiveness from well-designed, well-conducted trials. All too often, initial reports of new therapies are overly optimistic, and confirmation must be obtained through additional studies. While waiting for this to happen, however, cisapride may very well be light at the end of the alimentary tunnel for some kids who have great difficulty in pooping.

This is one of the rare editions of the YEAR BOOK OF PEDIATRICS in which the Gastroenterology chapter does not include any abstracts of articles dealing with inflammatory bowel disease. This is not to say that the literature doesn't teach us some interesting facts, which are now shared with you:

* Smoking might help those with ulcerative colitis.[1] Smokers are less likely to have ulcerative colitis, and smoking may ameliorate the clinical manifestations of this disease. Flare-ups of colitis are common in those who stop smoking.

* Those who grow up in dirty households have a lower risk of inflammatory bowel disease. Investigators in England did a properly controlled study in which they asked individuals whether each of first 3 homes that they had lived in after birth had tap water, central plumbing, flushing toilets, hot water, or separate bathrooms.[2] Having hot water increases the risk of regional enteritis fivefold. Having a separate bathroom increases the risk 3.4-fold. It appears that those raised in homes with "amenities" may grow up to be adults who have had limited exposure to certain kinds of enteric organisms, thereby rendering the bowel more susceptible to bowel disease later in life. Whether this is fact or fiction is obviously speculative. Nonetheless, there are good data to show that infants who get down and dirty are at lesser risk of inflammatory bowel disease later in life.

* If you ever have occasion to do an MR scan of the brain of an individual with Crohn's disease and find hyperdense white matter lesions, go no further. Such findings, which appear to be fairly benign and unassociated with any neurologic symptoms, are noted now in some patients with Crohn's disease.[3] These lesions appear to be virtually identical to those seen in patients with multiple sclerosis. Similar lesions have also been found in those with systemic lupus erythematosus. They presumably result from episodes of brain vasculitis.

* Measles vaccination may place you at a higher risk of having inflammatory bowel disease. In a study that compared more than 10,000 individuals who had received measles vaccine in 1964 with a similar number who had not, the relative risk of having Crohn's disease in the vaccinated group was 3 time greater than that in the unvaccinated group. The risk of ulcerative colitis was 2.5 times greater.[4] If all this seems far-fetched, realize that measles virus may persist in intestinal lymphatic tissue. Certainly this viral infection can cause prolonged disruption of immune function, particularly of helper T-cell responses. It just goes to show you that if the natural disease doesn't get you, what is used to prevent it might very well do so.

* Lastly, if you ever care for a child with short bowel syndrome as a result of extensive bowel resection, a consequence of surgery for regional enteritis or as a consequence of surgery for other reasons, look to growth hormone to help you. Recently, a combination of a modified diet, glutamine, and growth hormone was described to be an adjunctive therapy, allowing a number patients with short bowel syndrome who were total parenteral nutrition dependent to discontinue hyperalimentation altogether. Apparently, glutamine is a major nutrient for this bowel. Supplying it permits the bowel

mucosa to hypertrophy after small bowel resection. Growth hormone will stimulate intestinal growth and enhance its transport of nutrients across the small bowel. When all else fails, use growth factors and nutrients together to enhance the small bowel and its function. Growth hormone works not only for short kids, but for kids with short bowels. Growth hormone clearly can stretch a bowel beyond its limits.

References

1. Hanauer SB: *N Engl J Med* 330:856, 1994.
2. Gent AE, et al: *Lancet* 343:766, 1994.
3. Geissler A, et al: *Lancet 345:897, 1995.*
4. Thompson MP, et al: *Lancet* 345:1071, 1995.

Subject Index*

A

Abdomen
    air gun injuries, penetrating, pitfalls in
        recognition and management,
        97: 208
    intraabdominal (*see* Intraabdominal)
    pain (*see* Pain, abdominal)
Abortion
    during adolescence in U.S., 1980, 1985
        and 1990, 97: 308
    in toxoplasmosis, maternal, 96: 118
Abscess
    peritonsillar, incidence, management,
        and treatment guidelines proposal,
        97: 556
Abuse
    alcohol, during adolescence,
        self-reported health problems and
        physical symptomatology in,
        96: 365
    child (*see* Child abuse)
    dextromethorphan, over-the-counter, by
        teenagers, 95: 269
    sexual (*see* Sexual abuse)
    substance (*see* Substance abuse)
Academic
    correlates of sports participation in
        urban high school, 97: 323
    medicine, promotion of women
        physicians in, 96: 219
Acanthamoeba
    keratitis, risk factors in contact lens
        users, 97: 519
Acanthosis
    nigricans, 97: 157
Accident
    department, experience with asthma
        major outbreak in thunderstorm,
        97: 169
Acetaminophen
    analgesia for newborn circumcision,
        95: 301
    for febrile children, body temperature
        and infectious outcome in, 95: 178
    for febrile seizure recurrence prevention,
        97: 261
Achondroplasia
    growth hormone therapy in, 95: 488
Acid
    reflux disease and dental erosion,
        96: 555
    steatocrit, much improved method for,
        96: 660

    suppression, in treatment efficacy for
        Helicobacter pylori infection,
        96: 655
Acidification
    of fecal homogenates, in steatocrit
        improved results, due to fat
        extraction improvement, 97: 646
Acidosis
    with methemoglobinemia,
        life-threatening, in infant, 96: 665
Acquired immunodeficiency syndrome (*see*
    AIDS)
ACTH
    vs. prednisone for infantile spasms,
        97: 259
ACTOBAT
    prenatal, for newborn respiratory
        disease prevention, 96: 22
Acyclovir
    oral, for postexposure prophylaxis of
        varicella in family contact, 95: 52
Adenoidectomy
    ambulatory, 97: 554
ADHD (*see* Attention deficit hyperactivity
    disorder)
Adhesive
    tissue, cost in facial laceration repair,
        97: 228
Adolescence, 95: 245
    affective disorder, seasonal, rates for,
        97: 286
    alcohol abuse during, self-reported
        health problems and physical
        symptomatology in, 96: 365
    alcoholic beverages obtained during,
        95: 260
    anabolic steroid use, strength training
        and multiple drug use during, in
        U.S., 97: 321
    anorexia nervosa during
        medical complications, in males,
            97: 310
        psychological characteristics and
            DSM-III-R diagnoses, 6 year
            follow-up , 95: 185
    of Asian Americans, ethnic differences
        in psychiatric diagnosis during,
        95: 181
    attention deficit hyperactivity disorder
        driving related risks and outcomes of,
            follow-up, 95: 215
        persistence into, predictors of,
            97: 271

** All entries refer to the year and page number(s) for data appearing in this and previous
editions of the* YEAR BOOK.

Author Index

A

B

C

D